Foot and Ankle
SPORTS MEDICINE

Foot and Ankle SPORTS MEDICINE

EDITORS

David W. Altchek, MD

Co-Chief, Sport Medicine and Shoulder Surgery
Attending Orthopaedic Surgeon, The Hospital for Special Surgery
Professor of Clinical Orthopaedic Surgery, Weill Cornell Medical College
Medical Director for the New York Mets
New York, New York

Christopher W. DiGiovanni, MD

Professor of Orthopaedic Surgery, The Warren Alpert School of Medicine at Brown University
Director, Brown University Orthopaedic Residency Program
Chief, Foot and Ankle Service, Department of Orthopaedic Surgery, The Rhode Island Hospital
Director, Foot and Ankle Fellowship, Department of Orthopaedic Surgery, The Rhode Island Hospital
Providence, Rhode Island

Joshua S. Dines, MD

Orthopedic Surgeon, Sports Medicine and Shoulder Service, The Hospital for Special Surgery
Orthopedic Surgery Director
Joe DiMaggio Sports Medicine Foot and Ankle Center, Hospital for Special Surgery
Assistant Professor of Orthopedic Surgery, Weill Cornell Medical College
Team Orthopedist, LI (NY) Ducks Baseball Team
Consultant Orthopedic Surgeon, LA Dodgers Baseball Team
New York, New York

Rock G. Positano, DPM, MSc, MPH

Director of the Non-Surgical Foot and Ankle Service, Hospital for Special Surgery, New York, New York
Joe DiMaggio Sports Medicine Foot and Ankle Center, Hospital for Special Surgery
Director of the Non-Surgical Foot and Ankle Service, Department of Orthopaedics
The Warren Alpert School of Medicine at Brown University
Providence, Rhode Island
Professor and Chairman, Department of Academic Orthopedic Science
New York College of Podiatric Medicine, New York, New York

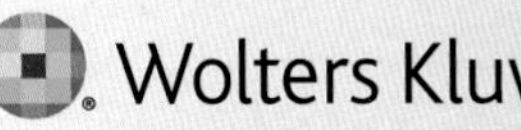

Lippincott Williams & Wilkins

Philadelphia • Baltimore • New York • London
Buenos Aires • Hong Kong • Sydney • Tokyo

Acquisitions Editor: Brian Brown
Product Manager: Dave Murphy
Marketing Manager: Lisa Lawrence
Vendor Manager: Alicia Jackson
Manufacturing Manager: Benjamin Rivera
Design Manager: Steve Druding
Production Services: Aptara, Inc.

Two Commerce Square
2001 Market Street
Philadelphia, PA 19103 USA
LWW.com

Printed in China

Library of Congress Cataloging-in-Publication Data
Foot & ankle sports medicine / [edited by] David W. Altchek, Christopher DiGiovanni, Joshua Dines.
p. ; cm.
Foot and ankle sports medicine
Includes bibliographical references and index.
ISBN 978-0-7817-9752-8 (alk. paper)
I. Altchek, David. II. DiGiovanni, Christopher W. III. Dines, Joshua S.
IV. Title: Foot and ankle sports medicine.
[DNLM: 1. Ankle Injuries. 2. Foot Injuries. 3. Athletic Injuries. WE 880]
617.1′027–dc23

2012036582

DISCLAIMER
Care has been taken to confirm the accuracy of the information presented and to describe generally accepted practices. However, the authors, editors, and publisher are not responsible for errors or omissions or for any consequences from application of the information in this book and make no warranty, expressed or implied, with respect to the currency, completeness, or accuracy of the contents of the publication. Application of the information in a particular situation remains the professional responsibility of the practitioner.

The authors, editors, and publisher have exerted every effort to ensure that drug selection and dosage set forth in this text are in accordance with current recommendations and practice at the time of publication. However, in view of ongoing research, changes in government regulations, and the constant flow of information relating to drug therapy and drug reactions, the reader is urged to check the package insert for each drug for any change in indications and dosage and for added warnings and precautions. This is particularly important when the recommended agent is a new or infrequently employed drug.

Some drugs and medical devices presented in the publication have Food and Drug Administration (FDA) clearance for limited use in restricted research settings. It is the responsibility of the health care provider to ascertain the FDA status of each drug or device planned for use in their clinical practice.

To purchase additional copies of this book, call our customer service department at (800) 638-3030 or fax orders to (301) 223-2320. International customers should call (301) 223-2300.

Visit Lippincott Williams & Wilkins on the Internet: at LWW.com. Lippincott Williams & Wilkins customer service representatives are available from 8:30 am to 6 pm, EST.

10 9 8 7 6 5 4 3 2 1

To the person I most look up to in so many ways, my wife Sudie, and to my four wonderful boys Nicholas, Cameron, Peter-Luca, and William. I am incredibly fortunate to have each of you in my life every day, and I love you all.
—C.W.D.

To the residents, fellows, and medical students who constantly inspire me to be a better clinician, surgeon, and educator. And, to Kathryn, my parents, Allison and Humphrey . . . thank you for being the most loving, supporting family one could ask for.
—J.D.

To the iconic New York Yankee legend, Joe DiMaggio, whose famous heel spur injury inspired the development of the specialty of foot and ankle sports medicine and to the brilliant Neil Young for his numerous contributions to children's health, music, art, and mankind.
—R.G.P.

Carmen Alcala, BA
Medical Student, Stony Brook University School of Medicine
Stony Brook University Hospital
Stony Brook, New York

Answorth A. Allen, MD
Associate Professor, Department of Orthopaedic Surgery
Weill Cornell College of Cornell University
Associate Attending, Department of Orthopaedic Surgery
The Hospital for Special Surgery
Head Team Orthopedist, NY Knicks
New York, New York

Basil J. Alwattar, MD
Oakland Bone and Joint Specialist
Attending Surgeon
Oakland California

Robert Anderson, MD
Founder, Foot and Ankle Institute, OrthoCarolina
Head Team Physician, Carolina Panthers
Ortho Carolina Medical Center
Charlotte, North Carolina

Sherry I. Backus, PT, DPT, MA
Leon Root, MD Motion Analysis Laboratory
Rehabilitation Department
The Hospital for Special Surgery
New York, New York

John S. Blanco, MD
Associate Attending Orthopaedic Surgeon
The Hospital for Special Surgery
Associate Professor of Orthopaedic Surgery
Weill Cornell Medical College
New York, New York

Michael Brage, MD
Associate Professor, Department of Orthopaedic Surgery
University of Washington School of Medicine
Seattle, Washington

Sepp Braun, MD
Department of Orthopaedic Sports Medicine
Hospital Rechts der Isar
Technical University of Munich
Munich, Germany

Robert H. Brophy, MD
Assistant Professor, Department of Orthopedic Surgery
Washington University Orthopedics
Chesterfield, Missouri

Mark A. Caselli, DPM
VA Hudson Valley Health Care System
Montrose, New York
Adjunct Professor of Orthopedic Sciences
New York College of Podiatric Medicine
New York, New York

Gilbert Chan, MD
Pediatric Orthopaedic Surgeon
Children's Orthopaedics of Louisville
Louisville, Kentucky

Edward S. Chang, MD
Department of Sports Medicine
The Hospital for Special Surgery
New York, New York

Timothy P. Charlton, MD
Assistant Professor of Clinical Orthopaedics
Keck School of Medicine
University of Southern California
Los Angeles California

Meaghan M. Colletti, BS
Non-surgical Foot and Ankle Service
Joe DiMaggio Sports Medicine Foot and Ankle Center
The Hospital for Special Surgery
New York, New York

Stephen L. Comite, MD, FAAD
Assistant Clinical Professor
The Mount Sinai Department of Dermatology
Mount Sinai School of Medicine
New York, New York

Christopher Cook, DO
Regional Anesthesia Fellow, Department of Anesthesiology
The Hospital for Special Surgery
New York, New York

Thomas M. DeLauro, DPM
Chairman, Department of Medical Sciences
New York College of Podiatric Medicine
New York, New York

Joshua S. Dines, MD
Orthopedic Surgeon, Sports Medicine and Shoulder Service, The Hospital for Special Surgery
Orthopedic Surgery Director
Joe DiMaggio Sports Medicine Foot and Ankle Center, Hospital for Special Surgery
Assistant Professor of Orthopedic Surgery, Weill Cornell Medical College
Team Orthopedist, LI (NY) Ducks Baseball Team
Consultant Orthopedic Surgeon, LA Dodgers Baseball Team
New York, New York

Christopher C. Dodson, MD
Assistant Professor
Thomas Jefferson University Hospital
Assistant Team Physician, Philadelphia Eagles, Philadelphia Flyers
Philadelphia, Pennsylvania

Shevaun M. Doyle, MD
Resident, Department of Orthopaedics
The Hospital for Special Surgery
New York, New York

Mark Drakos, MD
Assistant Attending Orthopedic Surgeon
The Hospital for Special Surgery
Instructor of Orthopaedic Surgery
Weill Cornell Medical College
New York, New York

Pete Draovitch, MS, ATC, PT
Clinical Supervisor, Hip Disorders
Sports Rehabilitation and Performance Center
Department of Rehabilitation
The Hospital for Special Surgery
New York, New York

Randall Farac, MD
Resident
UC Davis, Department of Orthopaedics
University of California, Davis
Sacramento, California

Brian Fullem, DPM
Fellow, American Academy Podiatric Sports Medicine
Fellow, ACFAS
Private Practice
Bayshore Podiatry Center
Tampa, Florida

Bethany Gallagher, MD
Resident, Department of Orthopaedic Surgery
Washington University School of Medicine
St. Louis, Missouri

Michael J. Gardner, MD
Assistant Professor, Department of Orthopaedic Surgery
Washington University Orthopaedics
St. Louis, Missouri

David N. Garras, MD
Foot and Ankle Fellow
OrthoCarolina
Charlotte, North Carolina

Eric Giza, MD
Assistant Professor, Department of Orthopaedics
Chief, Foot and Ankle Service, Department of Orthopaedics
University of California, Davis, Medical Center
Sacramento, California

Daniel W. Green, MD, MS, FAAP, FACS
Associate Attending Orthopedic Surgeon
The Hospital for Special Surgery
Associate Professor of Orthopaedic Surgery
Weill Cornell Medical College
New York, New York

Matthew H. Griffith, MD
Clinical and Research Fellow, Department of Orthopaedics and Sports Medicine
Harvard University
Massachusetts General Hospital
Boston, Massachusetts

Brian Halpern, MD
Medical Director
Joe DiMaggio Sports Medicine Foot and Ankle Center
The Hospital for Special Surgery
New York, New York

David L. Helfet, MD
Attending Orthopaedic Surgeon
Chief of Combined Orthopaedic Trauma
Department of Orthopaedic Surgery
The Hospital for Special Surgery
Professor of Surgery (Orthopaedics)
Weill Cornell Medical College
New York, New York

Iftach Hetsroni, MD
Department of Orthopaedic Surgery
Meir General Hospital,
Sapir Medical Centre
Sackler Faculty of Medicine
Tel Aviv University
Tel Aviv, Israel

Howard J. Hillstrom, PhD
Director, Leon Root, MD Motion Analysis Laboratory
Rehabilitation Department
The Hospital for Special Surgery
New York, New York

Greg Horton, MD
Associate Professor
Department of Orthopaedic Surgery
University of Kansas Medical Center
Kansas City, Kansas

Clifford Jeng, MD
Attending Orthopedic Surgeon
The Institute for Foot and Ankle Reconstruction at Mercy
Mercy Medical Center
Baltimore, Maryland

Anne H. Johnson, MD
Department of Orthopaedic Surgery
Foot and Ankle Service
Massachusetts General Hospital
Harvard Medical School
Boston, Massachusetts

Rupali Joshi, PT, PhD
Clinician
Rehabilitation Department
The Hospital for Special Surgery
New York, New York

Kenneth S. Jung, MD
Orthopaedic Surgeon
Kerlan-Jobe Orthopaedic Clinic
Los Angeles, California

Justin M. Kane, MD
Resident
Thomas Jefferson Medical College
Philadelphia, Pennsylvania

Jonathan Kaplan, MD
Keck School of Medicine
University of Southern California
Los Angeles, California

Bryan Kelly, MD
Associate Attending Orthopedic Surgeon
Co-Director, Center for Hip Preservation
The Hospital for Special Surgery
Associate Professor of Orthopedic Surgery
Weill Cornell Medical College

Tamar Kessel, MD
Department of Physiatry
The Hospital for Special Surgery
New York, New York

Andrew P. Kraszewski, MS
Leon Root, MD Motion Analysis Laboratory
Rehabilitation Department
The Hospital for Special Surgery
New York, New York

Hannah N. Ladenhauf, MD
Fellow, Department of Orthopaedics
The Hospital for Special Surgery
New York, New York

Kaj TA. Lambers, MD
Department of Orthopaedic Surgery
Foot and Ankle Service
Massachusetts General Hospital
Harvard Medical School
Boston, Massachusetts

Jian-Ren Liu, MD
Associate Professor of Neurology
Zhejiang University School of Medicine
Second Affiliated Hospital
Hangzhou, PR China

Dean G. Lorich, MD
Assistant Professor, Department of Orthopaedic Surgery
Weill Cornell College of Medicine
Cornell University
Associate Director Trauma Service, Department of Orthopaedic Surgery
The Hospital for Special Surgery
New York, New York

Gregory Lutz, MD
Physiatrist-in-Chief Emeritus
Associate Attending Physiatrist
The Hospital for Special Surgery
Associate Professor of Clinical Rehabilitation Medicine
New York-Presbyterian Hospital
New York, New York

Nicola Maffulli, MD, MS, PhD, FRCS(Orth)
Professor of Trauma and Orthopaedic Surgery
Department of Trauma and Orthopaedic Surgery
Keele University School of Medicine
University Hospital of North Staffordshire
Staffordshire, United Kingdom

Elizabeth Manejias, MD
Assistant Attending Physiatrist
Department of Physiatry
The Hospital for Special Surgery
Clinical Instructor
Weill Cornell Medical College
New York, New York

Moira McCarthy, MD
Resident
The Hospital for Special Surgery
New York, New York

Ashley Mehl, MS
Tufts University School of Medicine
Boston, Massachusetts

Peter J. Millett, MD, MSc
The Steadman Clinic
Vail, Colorado

Douglas N. Mintz, MD
Associate Attending Radiologist
The Hospital for Special Surgery
Associate Attending Radiologist
New York Presbyterian Hospital
Associate Professor of Clinical Radiology
Weill Medical College of Cornell University
New York, New York

Rajshree Mootanah, PhD
Postgraduate Medical Institute
Faculty of Science and Technology
Rivermead Campus
Anglia Ruskin University
Chelmsford, United Kingdom

Natalia Mozol, BS
Brooklyn, New York

Melanie, Ng, BA
Brooklyn, New York

Kirstina Olson, MD
Department of Orthopaedic Surgery
University of California—San Francisco
San Francisco, California

Daryl C. Osbahr
Clinical Associate, Department of Orthopaedic Surgery
Weill Medical College of Cornell University
Resident, Department of Orthopaedic Surgery
The Hospital for Special Surgery
New York, New York

Amar Patel, MD
Private Practice
Rockhill Orthopaedics
Lee's Summit, Missouri

Helene Pavlov, MD, FACR
Radiologist-In-Chief
Radiology and Imaging
Attending Radiologist
The Hospital for Special Surgery
Attending Radiologist
New York Presbyterian Hospital
Professor of Radiology
Professor of Radiology in Orthopedic Surgery
Weill Medical College of Cornell University

David I. Pedowitz, MD
Rothman Institute Lankenau Medical Center
Foot and Ankle Surgeon
Wynnewood, Pennsylvania

Elynor Giannin Perez, DPM, MS
Podiatric Medicine and Surgery Resident
New York College of Podiatric Medicine
New York, New York

Rock C.J. Positano, BA
Joe DiMaggio Sports Medicine Foot and Ankle Center
Hospital for Special Surgery
New York College of Podiatric Medicine
New York, New York

Rock G. Positano, DPM, MSc, MPH
Director of the Non-Surgical Foot and Ankle Service, Hospital for Special Surgery, New York, New York
Joe DiMaggio Sports Medicine Foot and Ankle Center, Hospital for Special Surgery
Director of the Non-Surgical Foot and Ankle Service, Department of Orthopaedics
The Warren Alpert School of Medicine at Brown University
Providence, Rhode Island
Professor and Chairman, Department of Academic Orthopedic Science
New York College of Podiatric Medicine, New York, New York

Mark L. Prasarn, MD
Department of Orthopaedic Surgery
University of Texas
Houston, Texas

Smita Rao, PT, PhD
Department of Physical Therapy
Steinhardt School of Culture, Education and Human Development
New York University
New York, New York

Keri Reese, MD
South County Orthopedic Specialists
Laguna Woods, California

Jordan Reichman, MD
Resident
New York Presbyterian Hospital Weill Cornell Medical Center
Department of Neurology
New York, New York

Keith R. Reinhardt, MD
Department of Orthopedic Surgery
The Hospital for Special Surgery
Weill Cornell Medical College
New York, New York

Robin J. Reiter, DPT, ATC, CFT
Owner and Chief Physical Therapist
Reiter Rehabilitation P.T. D.C

Andrew J. Rosenbaum, MD
Resident
Department of Orthopedic Surgery
Albany Medical Center
Albany New York

Michael K. Ryan, MD
NYU Hospital for Joint Diseases
Department of Orthopaedic Surgery
New York, New York

Gregory R. Saboeiro, MD
Chief
Division of Interventional Radiology and CT
Assistant Attending Radiologist
The Hospital for Special Surgery
Assistant Professor of Radiology
Weill Cornell Medical College
New York, New York

Amol Saxena, DPM, FACFAS, FAAPSM
Department of Sports Medicine, Palo Alto Division
Palo Alto Medical Foundation
Palo Alto, California

Pankaj Sharma, MBBS, FRCS (Tr and Orth)
Specialist Registrar in Trauma and Orthopaedic Surgery
University Hospital of Southampton
Southampton, Hampshire, United Kingdom

Jessica Siegelheim, BA, MD Candidate 2013
Temple University School of Medicine
Philadelphia, Pennsylvania

Carolyn M. Sofka, MD
Director of Education, Radiology and Imaging,
Associate Attending Radiologist
The Hospital for Special Surgery
Associate Attending Radiologist
New York Presbyterian Hospital
Associate Professor of Radiology
Weill Cornell Medical College

Jinsup Song, DPM, PhD
Director
Gait Study Center
Temple University School of Podiatric Medicine
Philadelphia, Pennsylvania

Dexter Sun, MD
Assistant Professor of Neurology
New York Presbyterian Hospital
Weill Cornell Medical Center
The Hospital for Special Surgery
New York, New York
Adjunct Professor of Neurology
Zhejiang University School of Medicine
Hangzhou, Xhejiang Province, PR China

George Theodore, MD
Department of Sports Medicine
Massachusetts General Hospital
Harvard University Medical School
Boston, Massachusetts

David B. Thordarson, MD
Professor
Department of Surgery
Division of Orthopaedics
Cedar Sinai Medical Center
Beverly Hills, California

Michael J. Trepal, DPM
Vice-President for Academic Affairs and Dean
New York College of Podiatric Medicine
New York, New York

Lauren Turteltaub, MD
Clinical Assistant Professor of Anesthesiology
Weill Medical College of Cornell University
Attending Anesthesiologist, Department of Anesthesiology
The Hospital for Special Surgery
New York, New York

Russell F. Warren, MD
Professor of Orthopaedics
Weill Medical College of Cornell University
Professor of Orthopaedics
Surgeon in Chief Emeritus, Department of Orthopaedics
The Hospital for Special Surgery
Team Physician, NY Giants
New York, New York

Clément ML. Werner, MD
Department of Orthopaedics
University of Zurich, Balgrist
Zurich, Switzerland

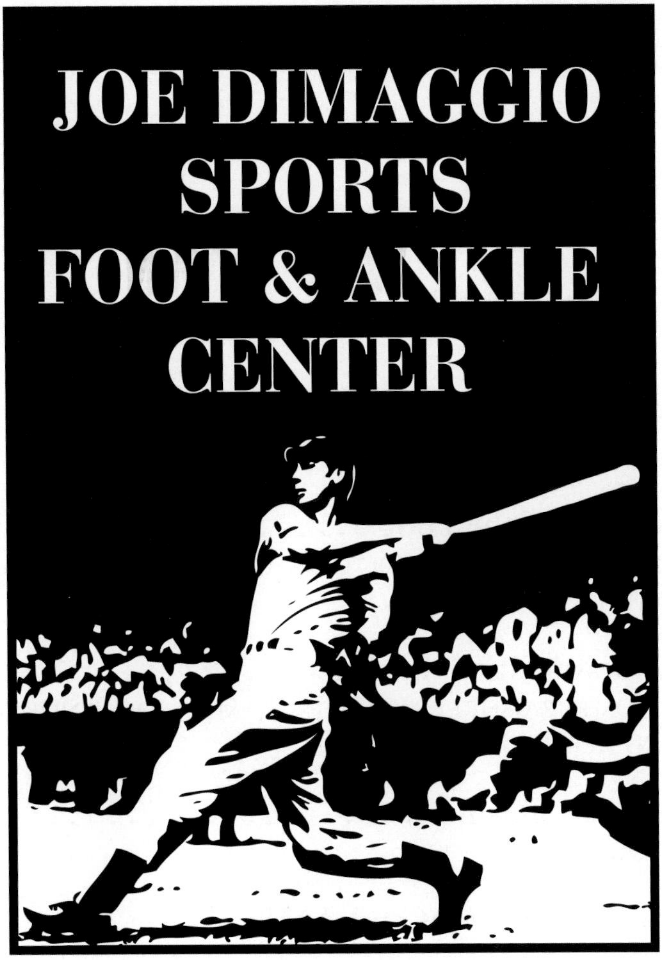

"I must have confidence and I must be worthy of the great DiMaggio who does all things perfectly even with the pain of the bone spur in his heel . . . Do you believe the great DiMaggio would stay with a fish as long as I will stay with this one? . . . I am sure he would and more since he is young and strong. Also, his father was a fisherman. But would the bone spur hurt him too much?"

The Old Man and The Sea

Ernest Hemingway-1952

Contents

Introduction

As all sports medicine professionals know, foot and ankle is the foundation of every athlete's performance.

Foot and ankle injuries in athletes are often difficult to diagnose and complex to treat.

This book, championed by Dr. Rock Positano, goes a long way to solve these difficult problems we all face in treating our athletic patients.

This book provides the coverage and details and the insights into the diagnoses and treatment of these issues.

David W. Altchek, MD
Co-Chief Sports Medicine & Shoulder Service
Hospital for Special Surgery

CHAPTER

1

Amar Patel
Greg Horton

Anatomy of the Foot and Ankle

INTRODUCTION

This chapter will focus on aspects of anatomy that are relevant regarding common pathology often encountered by those treating sports-related foot and ankle conditions.

ANKLE AND HINDFOOT

BONY ANATOMY

The distal ends of the tibia and fibula form the scaffolding upon which the ankle is built. The lateral malleolus forms a pyramid, whose apex is most prominent posteriorly. It extends 1 to 1.5 cm more distal than the medial malleolus (1). The medial portion of the lateral malleolus is covered with articular cartilage distally and just above the joint line, this structure fits into the incisural notch of the distal tibia. The posterior border of the fibula serves as a conduit for the peroneal tendons as they make their way from the lower leg to their attachments in the foot. The contour of the distal fibula is variable with 82% of samples in one anatomic study having a sulcus for these tendons, while the remainder had either a flat or convex surface (2). This anatomic configuration may have implications regarding the surgical repair of dislocated or subluxated peroneal tendons.

The distal portion of the tibia is wider laterally than medially with the anterior border longer than the posterior. The lateral distal tibial angle, or the angle between the distal articular surface and the tibial shaft is normally 89 degrees (3) (Fig. 1.1). The lateral portion of the distal tibia forms the incisural notch.

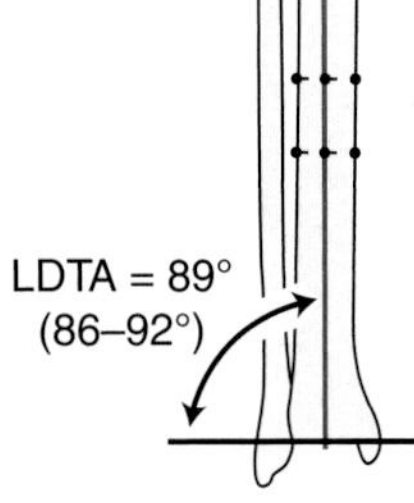

Figure 1.1. The lateral distal tibial angle. Adapted from Paley D. Principles of deformity correction. In: Browner B, Jupiter J, Levine A, Trafton P, eds. *Skeletal Trauma*. 4th ed. Philadelphia, PA: Saunders; 2009:2781.

The anterior portion of the tubercle of this notch is larger than the posterior, and tends to overlap the fibula, which is evident on anterior–posterior radiographs of the ankle. The medial malleolus is formed by the anterior and the posterior colliculus, of which the anterior colliculus descends lower. The superficial deltoid takes its attachment from the medial border of the anterior colliculus of the medial malleolus.

The talus is a complex bone that is tethered between the fibula and distal tibia. The body of the talus is wider anteriorly than posteriorly by an average of 4.2 mm in one series (1). This point should be considered when performing stabilization of the syndesmosis. The lateral portion of the body gives rise to the lateral process of the talus, which forms an articular facet with the distal fibula as well as a facet with the underlying calcaneus. This portion of the talus is often difficult to visualize on plain film and can cause persistent pain when injured. The posterior portion of the talar body is defined by the posterolateral and posteromedial processes that form a groove for the flexor hallucis longus (FHL) tendon. The posterolateral process is the larger of the two processes and may have an accessory bone, the os trigonum, associated with it. A large posterior talar process or a separate os trigonum can be a source of posterior ankle impingement and occult pain following injury. Injuries to the ankle may result in destabilization of a previously asymptomatic os trigonum or a fracture of the posterior talar process. A stenosing tenosynovitis of the traversing FHL tendon may cause pain and a triggering phenomenon referred to as hallux saltans. The talar neck slopes plantarly and medially away from the talar body and gives rise to the talar head that articulates with the navicular.

The calcaneus is the largest bone in the foot. Its axis is directed laterally. The lateral wall is relatively flat, however, and has a raised peroneal tubercle that divides the peroneus brevis tendon which runs superior to it from the peroneus longus tendon. The medial portion of the calcaneus contains the sustentaculum tali. Under this projection runs the FHL, which may be endangered with overly long screws used in lateral wall calcaneal fracture fixation (Fig. 1.2).

LIGAMENTOUS ANATOMY

The distal tibiofibular joint is stabilized by the anterior inferior tibiofibular (AITF) ligament, the posterior inferior tibiofibular (PITF) ligament, and the interosseous ligament. The AITF ligament runs from the anterior tubercle of the incisural notch to

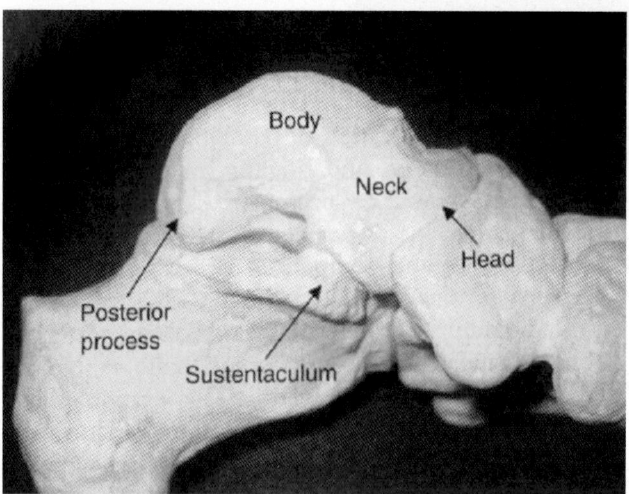

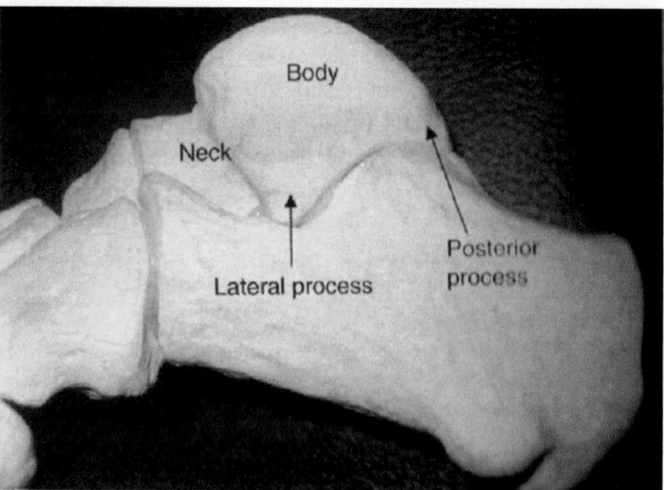

Figure 1.2. Medial and lateral views of the talus and calcaneus. Adapted from Banerjee R, Nickisch F, Easley ME, et al. Foot injuries. In: Browner B, et al., eds. *Skeletal Trauma.* 4th ed. Philadelphia, PA: Saunders; 2009:2588.

the anterior portion of the fibula. The PITF ligament is much broader in its tibial origin and is divided into a superior and deep portion. The stoutest and shortest of these three ligaments is the interosseous ligament, which is continuous with the interosseous membrane (Fig. 1.3). These injuries can occur in isolation or in conjunction with ankle fractures or injuries to the deltoid ligament complex.

The talus and calcaneus are anchored to the distal tibia and fibula laterally by the anterior talofibular ligament (ATFL), the calcaneofibular ligament (CFL) and the posterior talofibular ligament (PTFL). The ATFL is a flat ligament that is formed by an upper and a lower portion. This ligament courses at a 75-degree angle from the distal anterior portion of the fibula to the lateral body of the talus (4). The CFL is only one of these three that crosses the subtalar joint and courses slightly posteriorly from the inferior portion of the lateral malleolus to a tubercle of the calcaneus just superior to the peroneal tubercle. The CFL courses deep to the peroneal tendons. Procedures that attempt an anatomic repair of the CFL require mobilization and protection of the peroneal tendons. The PTFL extends from the posterior aspect of the distal fibula to the posterior talus, just anterior to the posterolateral process (Fig. 1.4).

The deltoid ligament complex is covered by the anterior tibial tendon, the posterior tibial tendon as well as by the flexor digitorum longus tendon. The superficial component, of which there are three components, originates from the anterior colliculus of the medial malleolus and extends to

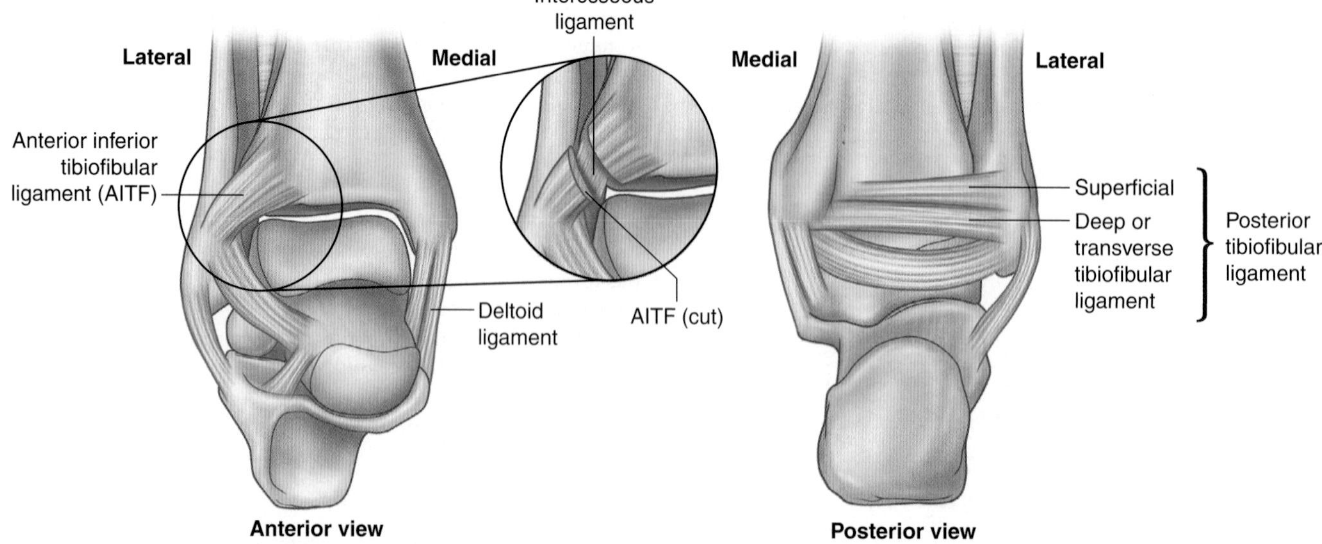

Figure 1.3. Syndesmotic ligament complex. Adapted from Clanton T, McGarvey W. Athletic injuries to the soft tissues of the foot and ankle. In: Coughlin M, Mann R, Saltzman C, eds. *Surgery of the Foot and Ankle.* 8th ed. Philadelphia, PA: Mosby; 2007:1472.

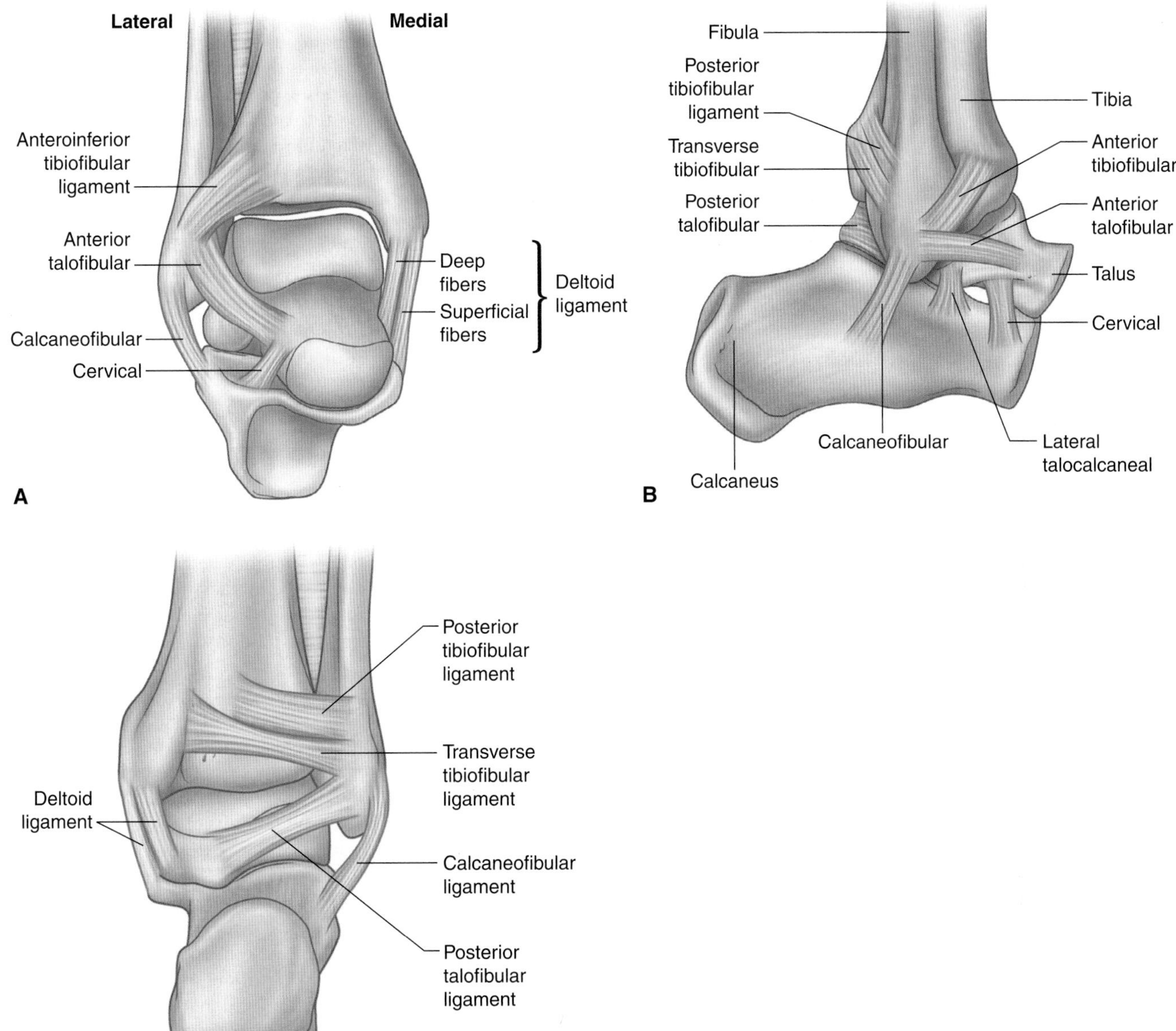

Figure 1.4. Lateral ankle ligament complex. Adapted from Clanton T, McGarvey W. Athletic injuries to the soft tissues of the foot and ankle. In: Coughlin M, Mann R, Saltzman C, eds. Surgery of the Foot and Ankle. 8th ed. Philadelphia, PA: Mosby; 2007:1452.

the talar neck and body of the navicular. Portions of this ligament contribute to the calcaneonavicular or spring ligament (5). The deep deltoid, which originates more posterior to the superficial portion, is divided into an anterior portion and a posterior portion which is the sternest portion of this medial ligament complex. This ligament originates on the posterior surface of the anterior colliculus and inserts both onto the medial aspect of the talus just distal to the articular cartilage and on the posteromedial tubercle (Fig. 1.5). Deltoid instability may occur in conjunction with lateral ligament injuries, fractures, or surgical approaches to the medial malleolus. Chronic deltoid instability should be suspected in those with longstanding hindfoot valgus or in those with chronic lateral ankle instability.

MUSCULAR ANATOMY

The anterior ankle is spanned by the tibialis anterior medially, the extensor hallucis longus, the extensor digitorum longus and the peroneus tertius. The tibialis anterior courses under the extensor retinaculum and inserts onto the medial cuneiform and the first metatarsal base. The extensor hallucis longus is just lateral and deep to the tibialis anterior tendon and extends to the distal hallucal phalanx. The extensor digitorum longus tendon divides just proximal to the superior extensor retinaculum and then again under the inferior retinaculum to form the individual tendons to the lesser toes (6). The peroneus tertius, present in about 90% of the population, is the most lateral anterior tendon and inserts onto the fifth metatarsal base (6).

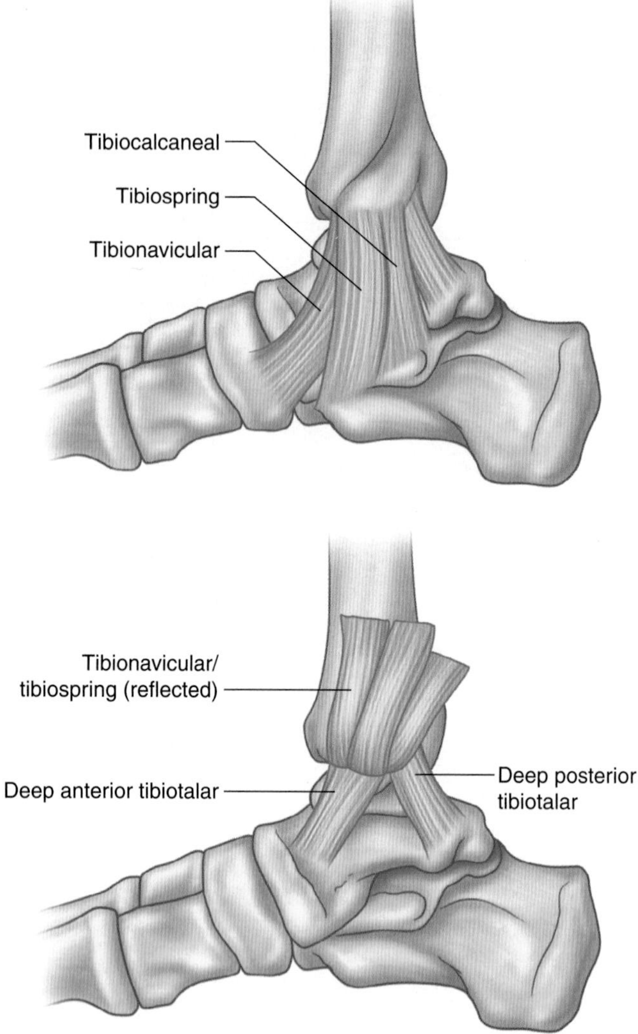

Figure 1.5. Superficial and deep medial ankle ligament complex. Adapted from Clanton T, McGarvey W. Athletic injuries to the soft tissues of the foot and ankle. In: Coughlin M, Mann R, Saltzman C, eds. Surgery of the Foot and Ankle. 8th ed. Philadelphia, PA: Mosby; 2007:1486.

The lateral portion of the foot and ankle contains the peroneal tendons and the muscle belly of the extensor digitorum brevis. The peroneus brevis is just posterior to the lateral malleolus, is superficial to the CFL and passes above the peroneal tubercle to the base of the fifth metatarsal. The peroneus longus runs along the posterior aspect of the brevis tendon at the level of the distal fibula, courses distally under the peroneal tubercle and abuts the cuboid where it then turns medially toward the base of the first metatarsal. The superior peroneal retinaculum is a retromalleolar structure that maintains the relationship of the fibula to these tendons. Injury to this structure may result in subluxation of these tendons and must be suspected in those with chronic lateral ankle pain and in those with calcaneal fractures in which the peroneal tendons are displaced (Fig. 1.6).

The medial aspect of the ankle is the conduit for the flexors. The tibialis posterior, the flexor digitorum longus and the FHL cross over the medial portion of the talus in their own fibro-osseous sheaths. The posterior tibial tendon lies directly against the medial malleolus in its own sheath. This intimate location puts the tendon at risk when performing procedures about the medial malleolus. The position of the tendon should be considered when percutaneous fixation of the medial malleolus is used. The FHL tendon is the most posterior of the three and runs through the posterior groove in the talus formed by the posteromedial and posterolateral processes, and then continues under the sustentaculum tali. This fibro-osseous tunnel also contains the tibial nerve and accompanying posterior tibial artery. One anatomic variant is the finding of an accessory soleus muscle which is a potential space occupying mass that may cause intrinsic compression upon the tibial nerve.

The Achilles tendon is the largest tendon unit of the hindfoot and has a broad insertion onto the calcaneus. It is covered posteriorly by a relatively thick sheath of paratenon. This sheath becomes contiguous with that of the underlying FHL muscle belly found directly anterior to the tendon. The paratenon is very important allowing for smooth excursion of the tendon during activity. Repair of the paratenon following procedures about the Achilles can be facilitated by the release of the posterior encasement of the FHL muscle, which allows for greater mobilization of the paratenon when performing the repair. The Achilles insertion is crescent shaped with the medial side exhibiting more extensive tendon substance, which may be due to the contribution of the plantaris tendon to the medial-sided insertion (7). A bursa is typically formed in the retrocalcaneal area posterior to the calcaneus and anterior to the tendon above its insertion.

NERVOUS AND VASCULAR ANATOMY

The posterior tibial, anterior tibial, and the peroneal arteries provide the vascular supply to the foot. The anterior tibial artery lies roughly halfway between each malleoli. Above the ankle joint, the artery lies between the tendons of the extensor hallucis longus and the tibialis anterior. The extensor hallucis longus crosses over the artery at the level of the ankle joint when the artery lies between the extensor hallucis longus and the extensor digitorum longus. At this level, the artery becomes the dorsalis pedis artery. The posterior tibial artery lies between the FHL and the flexor digitorum longus. When it enters the plantar aspect of the foot, it divides into the lateral and medial plantar arteries.

There are five major nerves that cross the ankle. The tibial and deep peroneal nerves are found deep to the investing fascia. The superficial peroneal (with various branches), the sural, and the saphenous nerve are located in the subcutaneous layer. The saphenous nerve, which is the terminal branch of the femoral nerve, runs with the long saphenous vein anterior to the medial malleolus. The superficial peroneal nerve supplies the dorsal skin of the foot and runs along the anterolateral aspect of the ankle joint. It divides into the medial dorsal and intermediate dorsal cutaneous nerves which can be easily damaged during portal placement during ankle arthroscopy (Fig. 1.7). Most commonly, the superficial peroneal nerve branches exit the crural fascia 4 to 5 mc above the ankle joint. There are, however, a number of significant variations which may have surgical implications. In 25% to 30% of patients, the medial and intermediate dorsal cutaneous nerves arise independently with unique fascial exit sites. While usually exiting the lateral compartment, one or more of the nerve branches may also be found exiting the anterior compartment. The intermediate branch may be found within the intermuscular septum or even crossing the fibula. Knowledge of these variations may help to avoid iatrogenic

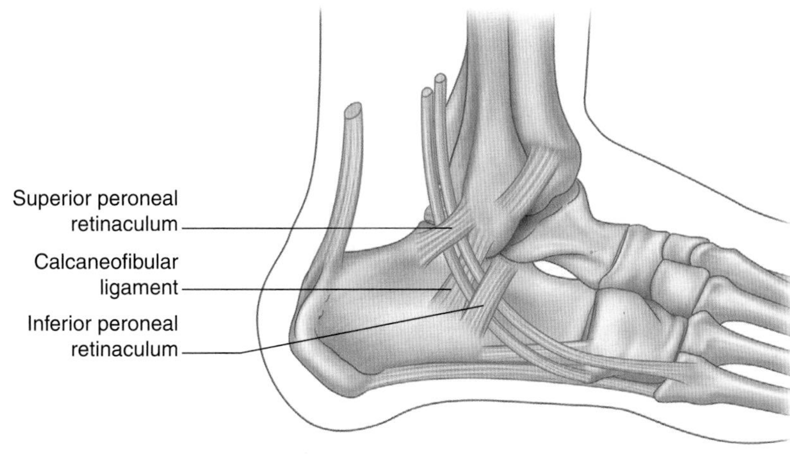

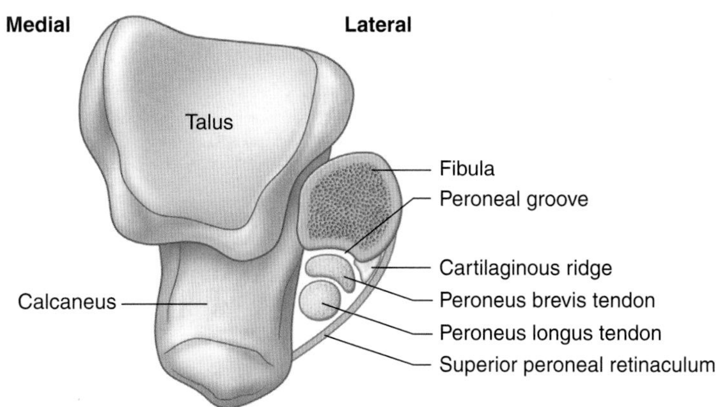

Figure 1.6. Lateral and coronal views of peroneal tendons. Adapted from Clanton T, McGarvey W. Athletic injuries to the soft tissues of the foot and ankle. In: Coughlin M, Mann R, Saltzman C, eds. *Surgery of the Foot and Ankle.* 8th ed. Philadelphia, PA: Mosby; 2007:1501.

injury during a lateral approach to the fibula. The sural nerve accompanies the lesser saphenous vein posterior to the lateral malleolus. It is consistently located adjacent to the lateral aspect of the Achilles tendon at a distance of 7 to 10 cm above the tip of the lateral malleolus and as it travels distally, it runs inferior to the sheath of the peroneal tendons. Branches of the nerve consistently cross superficial to the peroneal tendons more distally. The deep peroneal nerve lies adjacent to the dorsalis pedis artery while the tibial nerve lies just posterior to the posterior tibial artery. This nerve then divides into the medial and lateral plantar nerves as well as into a calcaneal branch. This branching occurs just proximal to the medial malleolus; however, it can occasionally occur up to 14 cm above the medial malleolus. In addition, multiple calcaneal branches may originate from both the medial and lateral plantar nerve branches.

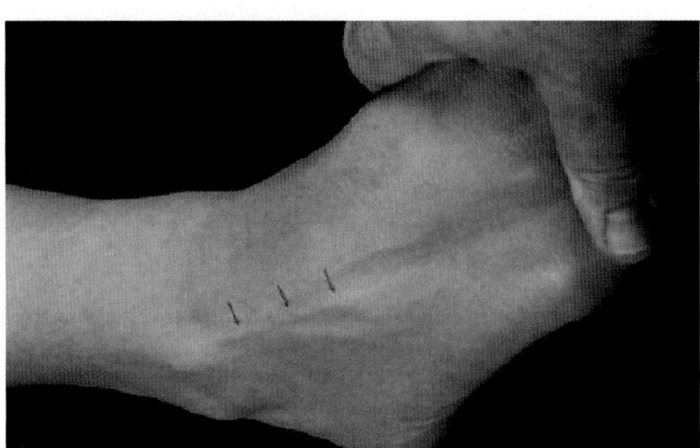

Figure 1.7. The intermediate branch of the superficial peroneal nerve may be visualized along the anterior aspect of the ankle. Adapted from de Leeuw PA, Golanó P, Sierevelt IN, et al. The course of the superficial peroneal nerve (*arrows*) in relation to the ankle position: anatomical study with ankle arthroscopic implications. *Knee Surg Sports Traumatol Arthrosc* May 2010;18(5):612–617.

MIDFOOT

BONY ANATOMY

The cuboid and navicular bones begin the transition into the midfoot. The cuboid extends from the calcaneus to the bases of the fourth and fifth metatarsals. It forms the basis for the lateral column of the foot and can articulate with the navicular in some cases. The tendon of the peroneus longus curves along the cuboid's lateral surface as it courses toward the base of the first metatarsal. Injury to this bone should be considered in those with Lisfranc injuries.

The navicular articulates with the head of the talus as well as with the three cuneiform bones. The medial portion of this bone is the anchor point for the tibialis posterior tendon. Variations in the size and morphology of the navicular tuberosity often arise and in one such variation, there is complete separation of a portion of the tuberosity which gives rise to an accessory navicular bone which when injured may cause persistent

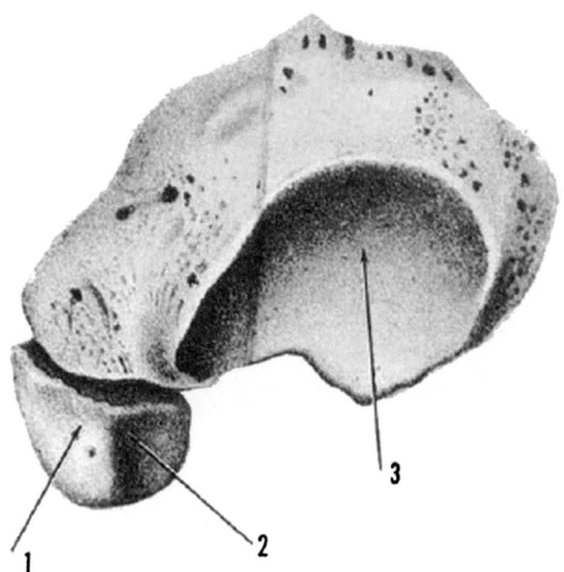

Figure 1.8. Accessory navicular. *1, 2* point to the facets of the accessory navicular while *3* points to the navicular body. Adapted from Sarrafian S, Kelikian A. Osteology. In: A. Kelikian, ed. *Anatomy of the Foot and Ankle: Descriptive, Topographic, Functional.* 3rd ed. Philadelphia, PA: Lippincott Williams and Wilkins; 2011:102. From Pfitzner W. Beiträge zur Kenntnis des Menschlichen Extremitätenskelets: VI. Die Variationen in Aufbau des Fussskelets. In: Schwalbe, ed. Morphologische Arbeiten. Jena: Gustav Fischer; 1896:245–527.

medial foot pain and swelling (Fig. 1.8). The three cuneiforms contribute to the transverse arch of the foot. The middle cuneiform is the smallest of the three and extends the least distal, allowing for the second metatarsal base to be partially recessed between the surrounding cuneiform bones (Fig. 1.9). The anatomic alignment of the metatarsal bases to the cuneiforms and cuboid should be critically assessed on weight-bearing radiographs in those with suspected midfoot ligamentous instability.

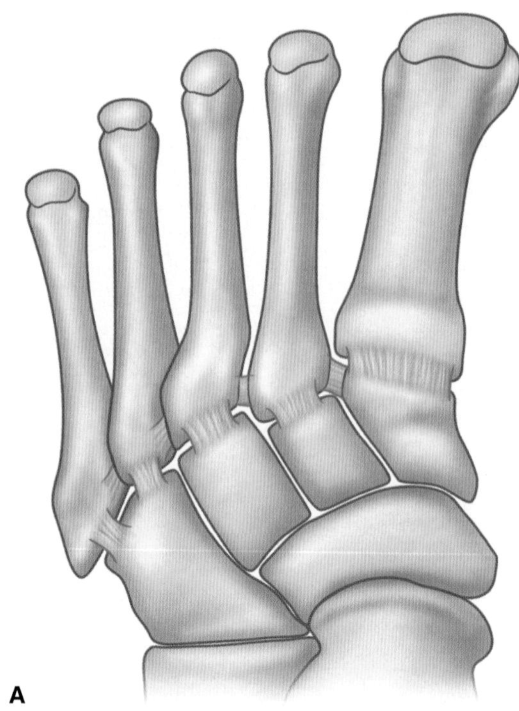

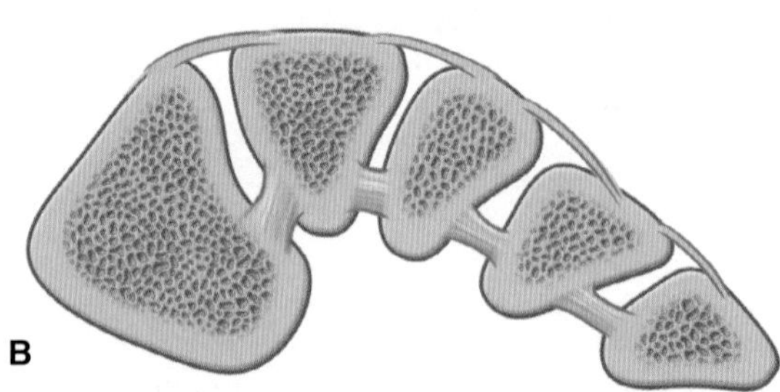

Figure 1.9. Configuration of the tarsometatarsal articulation in the AP (**A**) and coronal (**B**) planes. Adapted from Sayeed SA, Khan FA, Turner NS 3rd, et al. Midfoot arthritis. *Am J Orthop* 2008;37(5): 251–256.

LIGAMENTOUS ANATOMY

A major ligamentous structure of the midfoot is the calcaneonavicular ligament, or the spring ligament. This ligament contains a stronger superior medial ligament as well as an inferior portion (8). A second large ligamentous complex of the midfoot is the calcaneocuboid ligament which arises from the anterior process of the calcaneus and inserts onto the dorsal aspect of the cuboid.

The third large ligamentous complex of the midfoot and the most notorious is the Lisfranc complex which encompasses the five metatarsal bases and their respective cuboid or cuneiform articulations. The stability of these articulations is provided by both the stout ligamentous attachments as well as the bony configuration of the joints themselves. The ligamentous anatomy can be divided into plantar, interosseous, and dorsal components (9). The interosseous intermetatarsal ligaments are the strongest stabilizers of this construct with the dorsal ligaments regarded as the weakest (10). In the coronal plane, the bones of the Lisfranc joints have a Roman arch configuration with the apex at the second metatarsal. This particular metatarsal has a recessed base in relationship to the surrounding cuneiforms, adding to its overall stability. Furthermore, there is an absence of 1 to 2 intermetatarsal base ligaments. There is, instead, a second metatarsal base–medial cuneiform oblique ligament. This area is vulnerable to injury from torsion of the forefoot and axial load due to this biomechanical construct.

MUSCULAR ANATOMY

On the lateral aspect of the dorsum of the foot is the origin and muscle belly of the extensor digitorum brevis. The tendons of this muscle course laterally to the long extensors and insert onto the proximal phalanges of the toes. The remainder of the dorsal tendons course under the inferior extensor retinaculum toward their insertions in the midfoot and forefoot. The anterior tibialis tendon has a broad insertion onto the navicular, medial cuneiform, and base of the first metatarsal. The extensor hallucis longus courses toward the distal phalanx of the great toe.

The peroneus longus tendon bends around the lateral border of the cuboid as it courses toward the base of the first metatarsal. Within this tendon at this location is an os peroneum that can be fully ossified in up to 20% of feet (1) (Fig. 1.10). This articulation of the os peroneum and cuboid can itself be a cause of lateral foot pain.

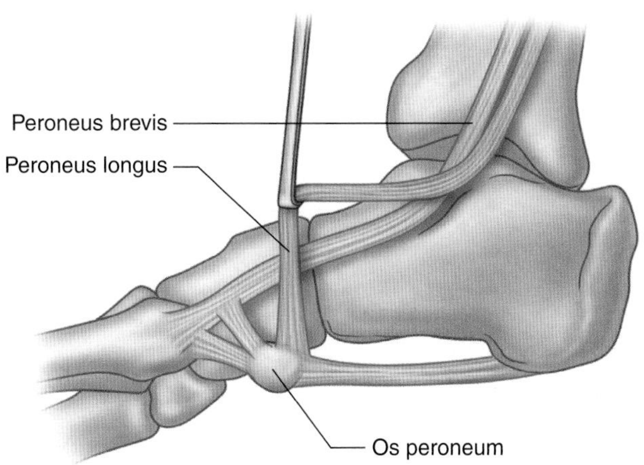

Figure 1.10. Anatomic diagram of os peroneum. Adapted from Coughlin M. Sesamoids and accessory bones of the foot. In: Coughlin M, Mann R, Saltzman C, eds. *Surgery of the Foot and Ankle.* 8th ed. Philadelphia, PA: Mosby; 2007:572.

In the midfoot, the flexors enter the transverse arch of the foot. The tibialis posterior tendon inserts into the tuberosity of the navicular but can have insertional slips distal to this bone as well. Just inferior to the sheath of the posterior tibial tendon, the flexor digitorum longus tendon lies in a separate sheath. The flexor digitorum longus can be followed distally to find the FHL. The medial plantar nerve is located in the dissection directly inferior to these tendons. Dissection in a plane superior to the flexor digitorum longus helps to avoid injury to the medial plantar nerve and the venous plexus found more inferiorly. The flexor digitorum longus and the FHL intersect at the Master Knot of Henry with varying degrees of connection between the two. With consistency, a slip of the FHL connects to the flexor digitorum longus of the second toe. This typically obviates the need to perform any type of tenodesis when harvesting the flexor digitorum longus for regional tendon transfer. In the midfoot, various muscles originate on the plantar aspect of the calcaneus and interact with the extrinsic flexors in the midfoot. The most superficial of these muscles is the flexor digitorum brevis. Just deep to this muscle are the abductor hallucis medially, the abductor digiti minimi muscle laterally, and the quadratus plantae in the deep layer. The oblique head of the adductor hallucis originates in the longitudinal arch with attachments on the cuneiforms and inserts distally on the fibular sesamoid (Figs. 1.11, 1.12).

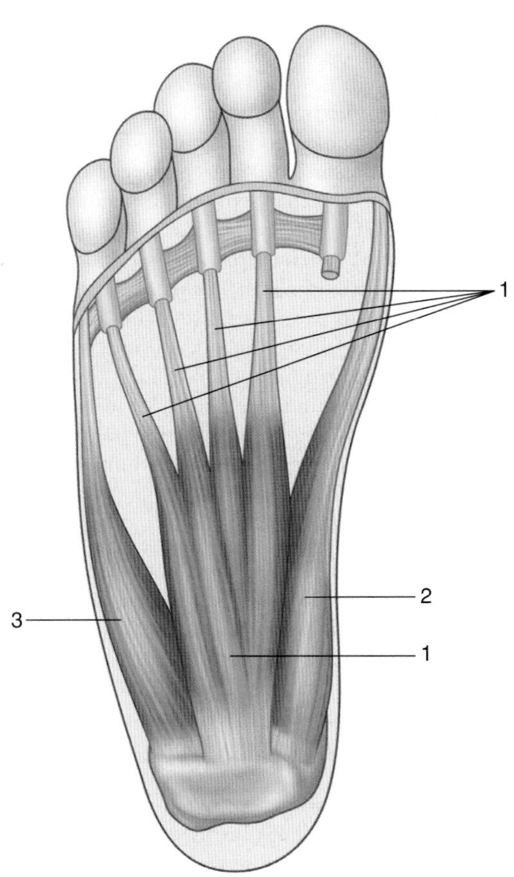

Figure 1.11. Flexor digitorum brevis. *1,* flexor digitorum brevis muscle, *2* abductor hallucis muscle, *3* abductor of the fifth toe. Adapted from Sarrafian S, Kelikian A. Myology. In: A. Kelikian, ed. *Anatomy of the Foot and Ankle: Descriptive, Topographic, Functional.* 3rd ed. Philadelphia, PA: Lippincott Williams and Wilkins; 2011:257.

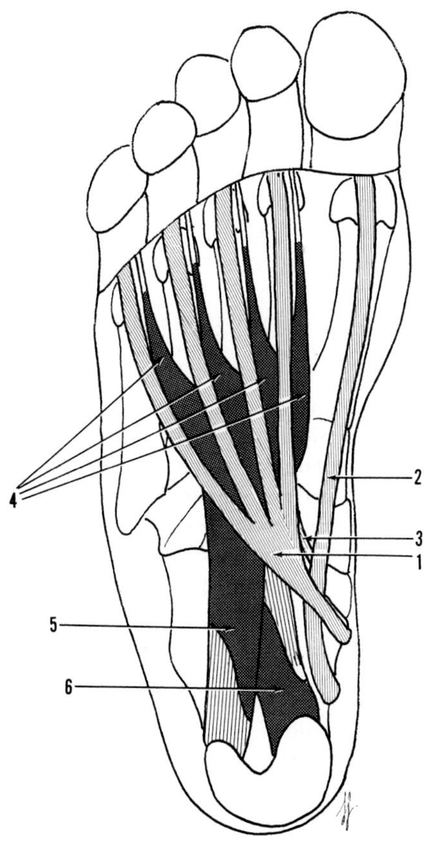

Figure 1.12. Flexor digitorum longus and FHL tendons. *1* Flexor digitorum longus tendon, *2* FHL tendon, *3* connection between *1* and *2* at the Knot of Henry, *4* lumbrical muscles, *5* lateral head of quadratus plantae muscle, *6* medial head of quadratus plantae muscle. Adapted from Sarrafian S, Kelikian A. Myology. In: A. Kelikian, ed. *Anatomy of the Foot and Ankle: Descriptive, topographic, functional.* 3rd ed. Philadelphia, PA: Lippincott Williams and Wilkins; 2011:249.

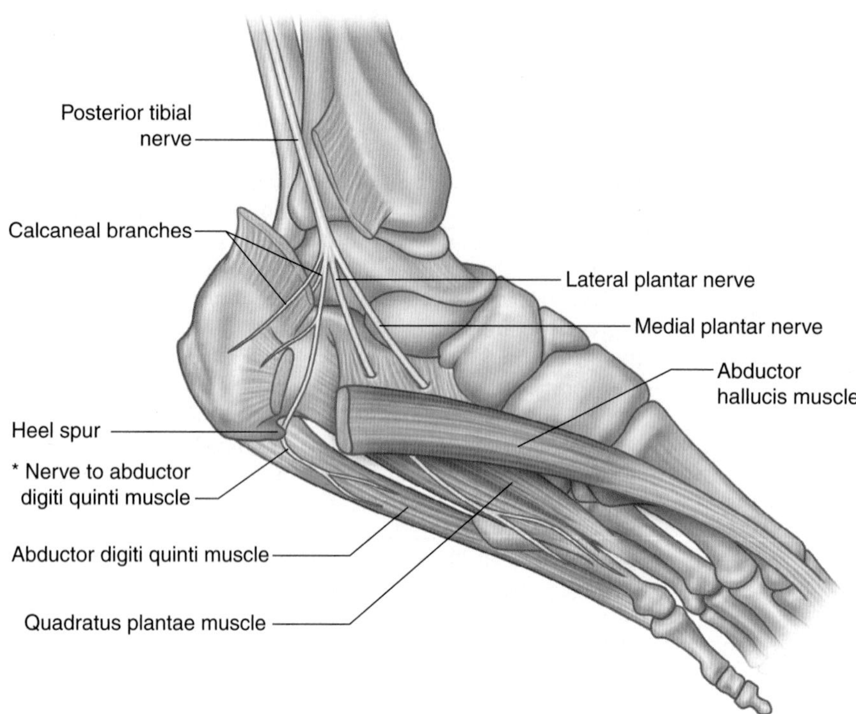

Figure 1.13. Posterior tibial nerve. Adapted from Baxter DE, Thigpen CM. Heel pain–operative results. Foot Ankle. 1984;5(1):16–25.

NEUROLOGIC AND VASCULAR ANATOMY

The dorsalis pedis artery continues toward the first interspace where it dives into the plantar aspect of the foot as the first intermetatarsal artery. The posterior tibial artery bifurcates in the region adjacent to the sustentaculum tali into the larger lateral plantar artery and the smaller medial plantar branch. These two plantar branches continue to form the deep plantar arterial arch that then gives rise to each of the digital arteries.

The tibial nerve gives rise to the medial and lateral plantar nerves as well as a medial calcaneal branch within the tarsal tunnel. This area is located behind the medial malleolus where the flexor retinaculum encloses both the neurovascular structures as well as the tendons of the foot flexors. The medial plantar nerve is the largest branch and is located adjacent to the medial plantar artery. Near the base of the first metatarsal, the medial plantar nerve gives rise to the first three digital nerves. The lateral plantar nerve gives rise to the innervating branch of the abductor digiti quinti which lies just distal to the origin of the plantar fascia on the lateral plantar portion of the calcaneus (Fig. 1.13). Compression of this nerve may cause pain located just distal to the origin of the plantar fascia and should be evaluated in those with chronic heel pain. This branch also provides the common digital nerves to the two most lateral digits with varying degrees of contribution to the third digital nerve, which may explain the propensity of symptomatic neuromas in the 3 to 4 interspace.

FOREFOOT

BONY ANATOMY

The bases of the metatarsals at their tarsometatarsal articulations form an arch with the apex at the second metatarsal base, which is also slightly recessed between the medial and lateral cuneiforms. The second metatarsal is also usually the longest in length, with either the first or third following in length. The base of the fifth metatarsal contains a styloid of varying size which allows for the insertion of the peroneus brevis tendon. The head of the first metatarsal contains a plantar groove that serves as the articulation for the plantar sesamoids. The heads of the lesser metatarsals also have plantar extensions with the lateral extension often extending further plantar than the medial, a factor that can lead to painful calluses. The first ray contains two phalanges with the distal phalanx serving as the terminal attachment for the FHL and extensor hallucis longus tendons. The lesser toes each contain three phalanges with the proximal and middle phalanges acting as the insertion point for the short flexors, the interossei muscles as well as the lumbrical muscles.

LIGAMENTOUS ANATOMY

The ligaments that stabilize the metatarsophalangeal (MTP) joints are divided into the collateral ligaments and the suspensory ligaments with those on the lateral side stronger than those on the medial side.

The plantar plate of the first MTP joint is a thick confluence of multiple ligaments that contain the two hallucal sesamoids (Fig. 1.14). The attachment of this complex on the proximal phalanx is stronger than that on the head of the metatarsal. The plantar plate contains a groove for the FHL tendon to pass distally while the flexor hallucis brevis tendon blends into the proximal phalanx insertion. Those with unstable injuries to the plantar plate should be carefully evaluated for FHL tendon tears.

MUSCULAR ANATOMY

The tibialis anterior tendon inserts onto the first metatarsal base as well as on the medial cuneiform. Occasionally, this

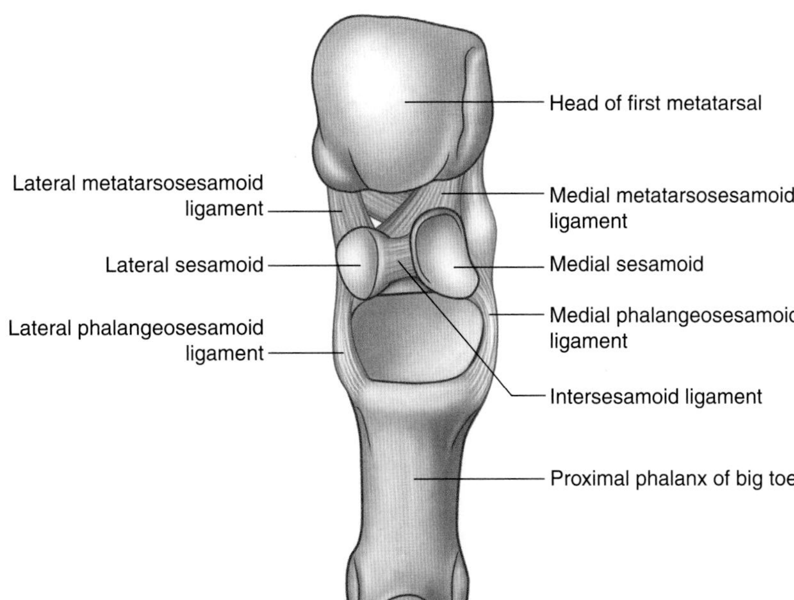

Figure 1.14. Plantar plate complex of first MTP joint. Adapted from Clanton T, McGarvey W. Athletic injuries to the soft tissues of the foot and ankle. In: Coughlin M, Mann R, Saltzman C, eds. *Surgery of the Foot and Ankle.* 8th ed. Philadelphia, PA: Mosby; 2007:1531.

insertion may be bifid. The base of the first metatarsal also serves as the insertion of peroneus longus tendon plantarly. Dorsally, the extensor hallucis longus tendon enlarges as it courses distally from the ankle to insert onto the base of the distal phalanx of the great toe. At the level of the first MTP joint, an extensor aponeurosis anchors this tendon along its course. This band of tissue blends in with the thick joint capsule that encircles this joint.

The extensor digitorum longus tendons course toward the distal phalanx of each toe. The extensor brevis tendons run parallel and lateral to the longus tendons at the level of the MTP joints. At the middle phalanx, these tendons form a trifurcation of tendons that insert into the distal phalanx centrally with lateral slips that act as insertion points for the lumbrical muscles (Fig. 1.15).

The flexor digitorum longus tendon divides into four individual tendons after intersecting the FHL at the Master Knot of Henry. These four tendons then act as the origin of the lumbrical muscles as well as the insertion of the quadratus plantae muscle. The flexor digitorum brevis muscle, which arises from the plantar medial aspect of the calcaneus, also gives rise to four tendons that are situated superficial to the deeper longus tendons. The superficialis tendon bifurcates in the area of the proximal phalanx to allow for the deeper longus tendon to pass between the two heads before inserting onto the base of the distal phalanx. The brevis tendons then fan out onto the middle phalanx. The four dorsal interossei and three plantar interossei as well as the four lumbrical tendons make up the intrinsic muscles of the toes. The dorsal and plantar interossei muscles occupy the interspaces between each of the metatarsals and attach to the extensor retinacular complex at the proximal phalanges. These muscles course dorsal to the deep intermetatarsal ligament. The lumbrical tendons are located plantar to the deep intermetatarsal ligament and insert onto the extensor hood as well as contribute to the lateral extensor slip (Fig. 1.15).

Like the flexor digitorum brevis tendons, the flexor hallucis brevis tendon gives rise to two heads with the medial head larger than the lateral head (6). Each head contains a sesamoid bone just proximal to the MTP joint. These heads then terminate within the plantar plate complex on the base of the proximal phalanx. The adductor hallucis is formed via two muscular heads as well. The oblique head inserts into the lateral sesamoid while the transverse head inserts both onto the lateral sesamoid as well as on the lateral base of the proximal phalanx. The abductor hallucis originates on the planatarmedial aspect of the calcaneus and inserts onto the medial sesamoid as well as onto the medial aspect of the proximal phalanx (Fig. 1.16). Knowledge of this anatomy is important when performing hallux valgus procedures that employ the release of the lateral structures. Mobilization of the sesamoid complex may require both release of the adductor insertion onto the lateral sesamoid as well as release of the transverse intermetatarsal ligament.

NEUROLOGIC AND VASCULAR ANATOMY

The four plantar metatarsal arteries branch from the deep plantar arch at the mid-metatarsal level. Further branching then gives rise to the plantar digital arteries which supply the majority of the vasculature to the lesser toes. The arcuate artery, a branch of the dorsalis pedis artery, gives rise to the corresponding dorsal digital arteries. The first dorsal metatarsal artery is the termination of the dorsalis pedis artery and provides contributions to the great and second toes.

The medial plantar nerve at the level of the first metatarsal divides into a medial and lateral branch. The medial branch terminates as the medial cutaneous nerve of the great toe. The lateral division gives rise to the common digital nerves of the first three toes, with branches to the lesser toes traveling under the deep transverse metatarsal ligaments. The lateral plantar nerve provides the common digital branches to the fourth and fifth toes with varying contributions to the third toe.

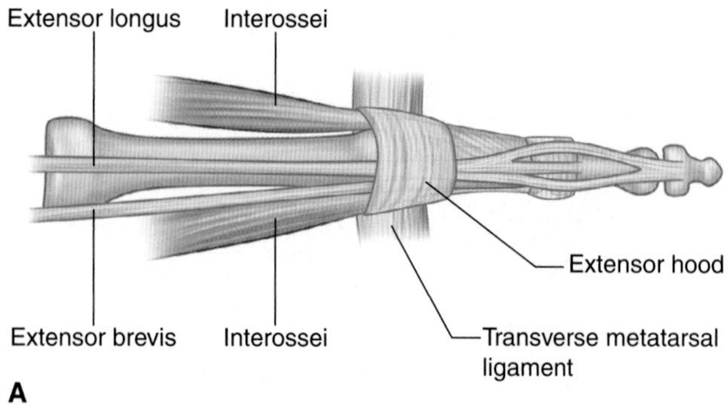

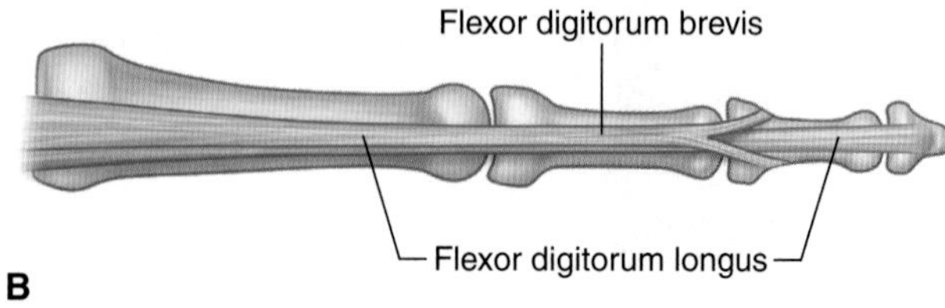

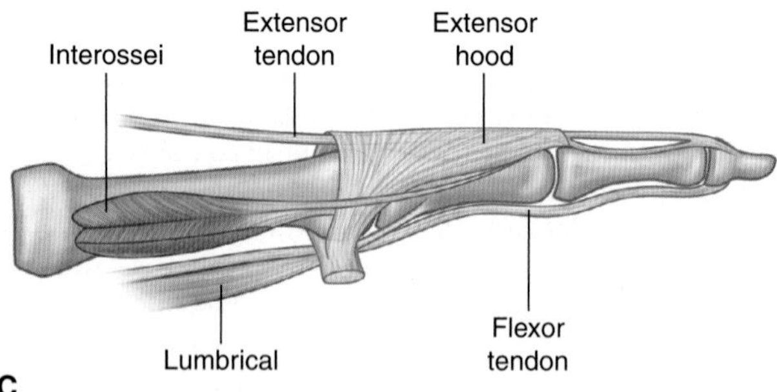

Figure 1.15. Anatomy of distal flexor and extensor insertions. **A:** Dorsal view. **B:** Plantar view. **C:** Lateral view. Adapted from Coughlin M. Lesser toe deformities. In: Coughlin M, Mann R, Saltzman C, eds. *Surgery of the Foot and Ankle.* 8th ed. Philadelphia, PA: Mosby; 2007:370–371.

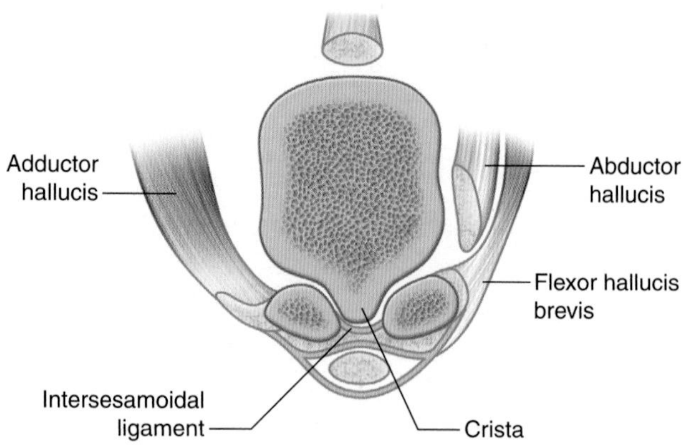

Figure 1.16. Cross-section of sesamoid complex at the first metatarsal head. Adapted from Coughlin M. Sesamoids and accessory bones of the foot. In: Coughlin M, Mann R, Saltzman C, eds. *Surgery of the Foot and Ankle.* 8th ed. Philadelphia, PA: Mosby; 2007:533.

REFERENCES

1. Sarrafian S, Kelikian A. Osteology. In: Kelikian A, ed. *Anatomy of the Foot and Ankle: Descriptive, Topographic, Functional.* 3rd ed. Philadelphia, PA: Lippincott Williams and Wilkins; 2011:14–119.
2. Edwards M. The relation of the peroneal tendons to the fibula, calcaneus, and cuboideum. *Am J Anat* 1927;42:213–252.
3. Paley D. Principles of deformity correction. In: Browner B, Jupiter J, Levine A, Trafton P, eds. *Skeletal Trauma.* 4th ed. Philadelphia, PA: Saunders; 2009:2779–2842.
4. Lassiter TE Jr, Malone TR, Garrett WE Jr. Injury to the lateral ligaments of the ankle. *Ortho Clin North Am* 1989;20:629–640.
5. Clanton T, McGarvey W. Athletic injuries to the soft tissues of the foot and ankle. In: Coughlin M, Mann R, Satzman C, eds. *Surgery of the Foot and Ankle.* 8th ed. Philadelphia, PA: Mosby; 2007:1425–1563.
6. Sarrafian S, Kelikian A. Myology. In: Kelikian A, ed. *Anatomy of the Foot and Ankle: Descriptive, Topographic, Functional.* 3rd ed. Philadelphia, PA: Lippincott Williams and Wilkins; 2011:223–291.
7. Lohrer H, Arentz S, Nauck T, et al. The Achilles tendon insertion is crescent shaped: An in vitro anatomic investigation. *Clin Orthop relat Res* 2008;466:2230–2237.
8. Taniguchi A, Tanaka Y, Takakura Y, et al. Anatomy of the spring ligament. *J Bone Joint Surg Am* 2003;85-A(11):2174–2178.
9. Sarrafian S. Syndesmology. In: Sarrafian S, ed. *Anatomy of the Foot and Ankle: Descriptive, Topographic, Functional.* Philadelphia, PA: Lippincott Company; 1993:159–217.
10. Desmond EA, Chou LB. Current concepts review: Lisfranc injuries. *Foot Ankle Int* 2006; 27:653–660.

Rupali Joshi
Jinsup Song
Rajshree Mootanah
Smita Rao
Sherry I. Backus
Howard J. Hillstrom

CHAPTER 2

Structure and Function of the Foot

INTRODUCTION

The human foot is one of the most anatomically complex structures in the body. The foot is comprised of 28 bones, 33 joints and 112 ligaments, which are controlled by 13 extrinsic and 21 intrinsic muscles. The forefoot is formed by the metatarsals as well as proximal, intermediate, and distal phalanges. The midfoot is comprised of medial, intermediate, and lateral cuneiforms as well as navicular and cuboid. The hindfoot includes the calcaneus, talus, tibia, and fibula. These bones and the adjoining soft tissues together comprise the medial, lateral, and transverse arches. The structural alignment of the bones and tissues of the foot are thought to be related to foot function (1–4). The primary functions of the human foot include weight bearing, shock absorption, propelling the body away from the ground and serving as a mobile adaptor to unsure surfaces (5–7). The foot is a triplanar mechanism which exhibits different functions based on its structure (e.g., alignment). Given the anatomical complexity, no one objective measure can completely describe the intricacies of how a foot functions. The purpose of this chapter is to describe in more detail how one may assess foot structure and function as well as the relationship between these measurements.

The primary reason for assessing foot structure and function is that specific foot alignments have been clinically associated with overuse injuries and pathologies. For example, in a study of Navy Seals undergoing training, Kauffman et al. (8) reported that the incidence of stress fractures was nearly twice as high in subjects with either planus or cavus foot types compared to those with normal arches. Another commonly occurring clinical problem is diabetic foot ulcers (9–12). Occurrence and location of diabetic neuropathic foot ulcers, which precipitate 85% of lower limb amputations, have also been shown to be linked to altered foot structure and function (13–16). In fact, foot ulcers tend to occur in areas of excessive plantar pressure in the presence of peripheral neuropathy that results in loss of feeling. The location of diabetic neuropathic foot ulcers is correlated with hindfoot alignment (17). Specifically, an everted standing alignment was associated with ulcer formation under the medial metatarsal areas and an inverted hindfoot alignment was associated with lateral metatarsal ulcers (18). Sub-hallucial neuropathic foot ulceration has been associated with limited joint mobility of the first metatarsophalangeal joint (18).

In addition to the association of specific foot alignments with overuse injuries and pathologies, correction of biomechanical foot malalignment with the use of foot orthoses appears to delay or prevent specific foot deformities (19). For example, in individuals recently diagnosed with rheumatoid arthritis (RA), the incidence of hallux valgus deformity decreased 73% with use of orthoses that maintained the foot in neutral position (20). In a study by Rao et al. (21) full length carbon graphite orthoses which stiffened the foot significantly improved pain and function in a cohort of patients with midfoot arthritis compared with an age-, sex-, and BMI-matched control group (21).

These studies suggest (1) the potential link between biomechanical foot structure and function to pedal pathologies and (2) the potential benefit of early diagnosis and intervention of altered foot biomechanics in prevention and/or delay of foot complications.

MEASUREMENT OF FOOT STRUCTURE

Whether evaluating foot pathology or trauma, one of the first assessments that a clinician will perform on the patient is a determination of foot structure. The fundamental tools include the clinical biomechanical examination and plain radiographic measures. Advanced tools for assessing foot structure (ultrasound, computed tomography, and magnetic resonance imaging) can also be quite informative but are beyond the scope of this chapter.

Clinical Biomechanical Examination

In general, and unless noted otherwise, the following measures should be quantified with a 1 degree resolution goniometer and a 1 mm resolution tape measure. The increments on goniometers with 5 degrees of resolution are too large to capture measures that may well be only several degrees.

1) Resting calcaneal stance position (RCSP):

RCSP is the angle between a line bisecting the calcaneus and the horizontal (ground) in degrees (Fig. 2.1) during quiet standing. The intra-tester (0.85) and intertester (0.68) reliabilities have been previously reported (22). One of the largest sources of error for this measurement is drawing the calcaneal bisection but this error may be reduced using digital calipers (23). RCSP values are used to classify low- (planus), normal-, and high-arched (cavus) feet (6). Planus feet are typically in a valgus hindfoot alignment (RCSP ≥4 degree valgus). Rectus feet are closer to neutral in hindfoot alignment (0 degree ≤RCSP ≤2 degree valgus). Cavus feet may be neutral or varus in hindfoot alignment (RCSP ≥0 degree varus) (24).

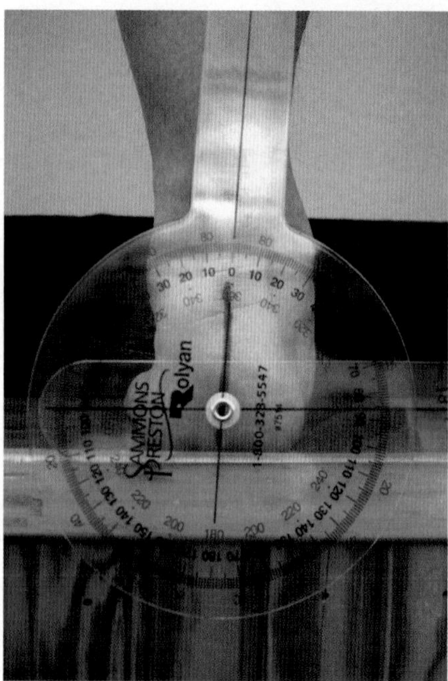

Figure 2.1. RCSP is measured by a goniometer in an individual's natural angle and base of support.

2) Forefoot to Rearfoot position (FF–RF):

FF–RF position is the angle between the forefoot and the rearfoot in the transverse plane. The FF–RF position is measured while the subject is prone and their subtalar joint is held in neutral position (Fig. 2.2). The hinge of the goniometer is aligned with the fifth metatarsal head for varus forefeet or the first metatarsal head for valgus forefeet. The lower arm of the goniometer is placed perpendicular to the calcaneal bisection and parallel to the plantar heel while the upper arm of the goniometer is placed parallel to the first through fifth metatarsal heads. The resulting angle, the FF–RF position, is considered one of the most difficult measures of foot structure to perform. The intra-tester reliability has been reported as 0.89 (left) and 0.90 (right) (25). FF–RF values are used to classify low- (planus), normal-, and high-arched (cavus) feet (6). Planus feet are typical in a varus forefoot alignment (FF–RF ≥5 degree varus). Rectus feet are closer to neutral in forefoot alignment (0 degree ≤RCSP ≤4 degree varus). Cavus feet are in a valgus forefoot alignment (FF–RF ≥1 degree valgus) (24).

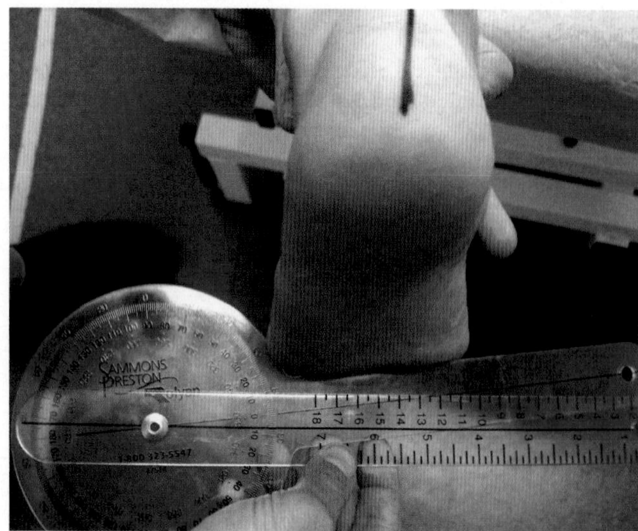

Figure 2.2. FF–RF is measured by a goniometer with the subject prone and the subtalar joint in neutral position.

3) Range of motion (ROM):

Assessing passive ankle dorsiflexion is important to discriminate contracture from spasticity in the individual with cerebral palsy, evaluating the idiopathic toe-walker, and understanding potential sources of plantar fasciitis and Achilles tendonitis. The measurement is typically done with the individual supine and the subtalar joint in neutral position. One arm of the goniometer is aligned with the lateral plantar border of the foot while the other passes through the lateral malleolus. Based on dorsiflexion ROM, the Silfverskiöld examination is a clinical test to distinguish between gastrocnemius and soleus tightness. Examination is carried out with knee in full extension and also in 90 degrees of knee flexion. Lack of passive dorsiflexion (<10 degrees) with the subtalar joint in neutral and the knee in full extension and the knee at 90 degrees of flexion indicates that the individual has soleus equinus. Lack of passive dorsiflexion with the knee in full extension, but not with the knee in 90 degrees of flexion, indicates that the individual has gastrocnemius equinus. Normal dorsiflexion with the knee extended should be ≥10 degrees and ≥20 degrees with knee flexed (26). Plantarflexion is measured in the same position as dorsiflexion. Normal range for plantarflexion is 30 to 50 degrees. Assessment of plantarflexion is important to determine if there is contracture of the anterior capsule or posterior boney impingement. Inversion and eversion are the terms often used to describe motion at the subtalar joint. A common misconception is that all plantar–dorsiflexion occurs at the ankle joint and all inversion–eversion occurs at the subtalar joint. In fact both motions occur in both joints (27).

For this reason, it is more appropriate to test for inversion–eversion, as well as dorsiflexion–plantarflexion, at the hindfoot (i.e., the ankle–subtalar joint complex). Hindfoot inversion–eversion is measured with the individual prone and the goniometer measuring the arc between the posterior tibial bisection and the calcaneal bisection. Normal hindfoot inversion should approach 20 degrees while eversion approaches 10 degrees (28).

Since the foot and ankle is a triplanar mechanism its combined motion is often described as supination and pronation. Supination describes plantarflexion, inversion and adduction motions in the open-kinetic chain to provide rigidity. As a result of this positional rigidity, supination allows the foot and ankle to be in a closed packed position for an efficient gait pattern (29). Pronation describes the dorsiflexion, eversion, and abduction motions in the open-kinetic chain which provide flexibility to absorb shock and adapt to flat and uneven surfaces (29,30).

First metatarsophalangeal (MTP) joint dorsiflexion ROM is measured by a goniometer. Healthy individuals with a normal ROM should have ≥65 degrees of dorsiflexion with the subtalar joint in neutral position in both weight bearing and non–weight-bearing (31–35). If the first MTP ROM is normal in non–weight-bearing but decreases in weight bearing then the condition is diagnosed as functional hallux limitus (36). Dorsiflexion range of <45 degrees in non–weight-bearing will be categorized as hallux limitus (37,38). Dorsiflexion range of

≤20 degrees in non–weight-bearing is categorized as hallux rigidus (seen frequently in individuals with first metatarsophalangeal joint (MTPJ) osteoarthritis (37,38).

4) Limb-length discrepancy (LLD)
LLD is hypothesized to be one of the primary reasons for asymmetry in foot structure and function. Clinically, actual limb length is measured with a tape measure from the anterior superior iliac spine (ASIS) to the lowest point on the medial malleolus with the subject in supine position (39). As an alternative, apparent limb length may be measured with a tape measure from the umbilicus to the medial malleoli.

The comparison between tape measurements and radiographic techniques has shown poor to moderate correlation (40,41). Tape measures, although easy, safe, non-invasive and handy, are less reliable and therefore clinicians are advised to use the average value of repeated measurements to ensure reliability when using a tape measure to assess LLD (42).

A weight-bearing measure of limb length may also be performed from the ASIS to the lateral first MTPJ while the individual stands at their comfortable angle of foot progression and base of support.

Limb-length asymmetry is not considered pathologic. Discrepancies of 1 to 1.5 cm are common, typically do not lead to any symptoms, and may not need management (43). A limb-length inequality >2.0 cm results in asymmetrical gait patterns; nonetheless, the extent of asymmetry varies for each individual (44).

5) Manual muscle function testing (MMT):
MMT is recommended to evaluate the prime movers of the foot and ankle. Gastrocnemius–soleus (plantarflexion and inversion) and tibialis anterior (dorsiflexion), extensor hallucis longus (first MTPJ dorsiflexion), and flexor hallucis longus and brevis (first MTPJ plantarflexion), peroneus longus and brevis (eversion) and posterior tibialis (plantarflexion and inversion) strength are typically evaluated. The distal limb segment motion is resisted while the individual performs a maximal contraction. The strength is graded by the examiner according to the following scale: (5) Normal—*subject completes ROM against gravity with maximal resistance,* (4) Good—*completes ROM against gravity with moderate resistance,* (3) Fair—*completes ROM against gravity without manual resistance,* (2) Poor—*completes ROM with gravity eliminated,* (1) Trace—*muscle contraction can be palpated but there is no joint movement,* (0) Zero—*no palpable muscle* contraction (45).

Malleolar Valgus Index (MVI)

Biomechanical alignment of the hindfoot and forefoot are important determinants of foot function. MVI is a measure of static hindfoot alignment in weight-bearing position.

MVI is measured while the test subject is standing in his/her comfortable angle and base of support on a 7/8″ thick Plexiglas® table over a flatbed scanner (Fig. 2.3A). An adjustable aluminum jig is placed about the hindfoot, which registers the lateral and medial malleoli to the plantar surface to be scanned. MVI is the deviation from the midpoint of the transmalleolar axis to the midpoint of the hindfoot normalized to the ankle width in this region. MVI is calculated from the scanned image (Fig. 2.3B), which depicts the transverse plane plantar foot and the registration points for the medial and lateral malleoli. The fourth level of an 8-bit grey scale image is used to define the contact area from which the medial, lateral, inferior and superior borders of the foot are established to define the foot coordinate system. MVI is calculated according to the following formula:

$$MVI\ (\%) = \frac{(LA - LF)}{LM} \times 100$$

where LA is the distance from the lateral malleolus to the midpoint of the transmalleolar axis, LF is the distance from the lateral malleolus to the foot coordinate system midpoint along the transmalleolar axis, and LM is the length of the transmalleolar axis. MVI is a reliable measure (ICC = 0.97) (2,3) of static

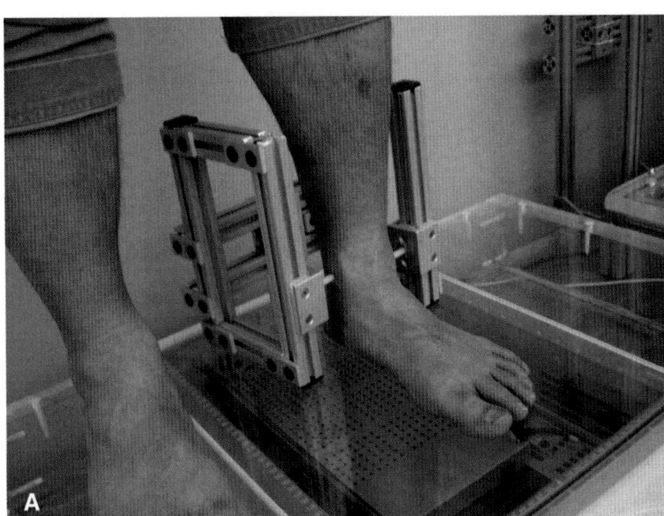

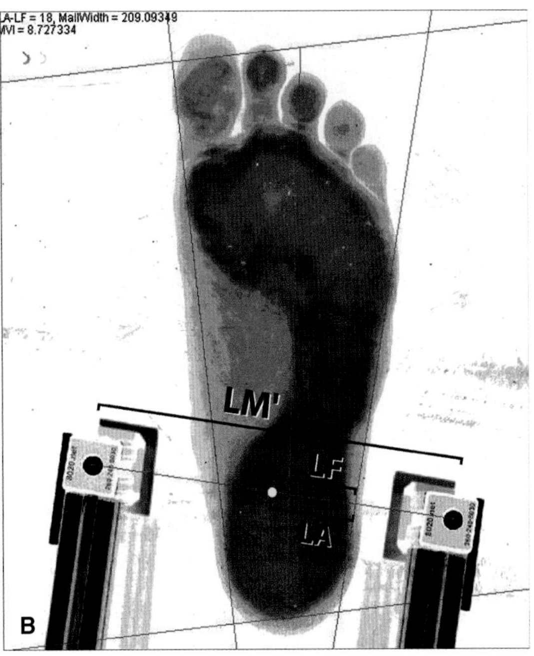

Figure 2.3. **A:** MVI is a measure of hindfoot alignment in weight bearing while the test subject is standing in their comfortable angle and base of support. **B:** MVI is calculated from a flatbed scanner image of the plantar foot.

TABLE 2.1 Malleolar Valgus Indices (MVI)

	Pes Planus		Rectus		Pes Cavus	
	Mean	**SD**	**Mean**	**SD**	**Mean**	**SD**
MVI (%)	13.34*#	5.37	7.40*	3.88	6.73#	3.52

Note: Significant differences ($p < 0.05$) illustrated by *#.

foot alignment and also correlates with RCSP (46). In a recent study it has been shown that MVI (Table 2.1) could significantly distinguish between planus and rectus as well as planus and cavus foot types in asymptomatic healthy individuals (47). The center of pressure excursion index (CPEI) is a measure of dynamic foot function during gait and does not correlate with MVI (46). This suggests that diagnosis and/or treatment based on static parameters alone may not always reflect dynamic foot biomechanical function (47). Thus it is important for clinicians to perform static as well as dynamic foot function tests as a part of assessment.

Radiographic Parameters

Radiographic techniques are considered the "clinical gold standard" for evaluating potential fractures and bony alignment of the foot in static weight bearing (48). Angular foot measurements obtained from x-rays are frequently used to confirm clinical measures of foot posture (49–51). The lateral view (Fig. 2.4A) provides a measure of sagittal plane alignment of the hindfoot, midfoot, and forefoot while the anteroposterior view reveals a transverse plane alignment of the midfoot and forefoot (Fig. 2.4B) (52).

The well-aligned foot on a lateral view, has a calcaneal inclination of 18 to 20 degrees, talar declination angle of 21 degrees, and a linear appearance of the medial column with a continuous lazy s-shaped Cyma line (2,53). On anterior–posterior view, the well-aligned foot demonstrates a talocalcaneal angle of 17 to 21 degrees, metatarsus adductus angle of 10 to 20 degrees, an intermetatarsal angle of 8 degrees adducted, a hallux valgus angle of ≤15 degrees abducted, normal sesamoid position, and an elliptical metatarsal length pattern (2,53).

Pedal x-ray parameters are sensitive to foot type (e.g., calcaneal inclination, talar declination) but their use is reserved for individuals where a pathology is expected due to the, albeit low levels of, ionizing radiation.

About 35% of the variance in peak plantar pressure under the heel and first metatarsal head during walking can be explained by just a few structural (e.g., radiographic) measurements (54). These structural measurements include: Decreased soft-tissue thickness (calcaneal or sesamoid height), medial longitudinal arch height (first metatarsal inclination) and placement of the first metatarsal head in relation to the second (intermetatarsal angle). These findings suggest that dynamic foot function can be predicted by static structural variables (54).

Arch Height Index (AHI)

AHI can be measured by placing the subject's feet within a pair of custom-made anodized aluminum jigs with their heels seated within each heel cup (Fig. 2.5A). The most anterior adjustable bar is set to maximum foot length (FL). A small adjustable cup is positioned at the first MTPJ to denote truncated foot length (TFL). Finally, a vertical bar, which is positioned at one half of FL, is lowered upon the dorsal aspect of the foot to measure

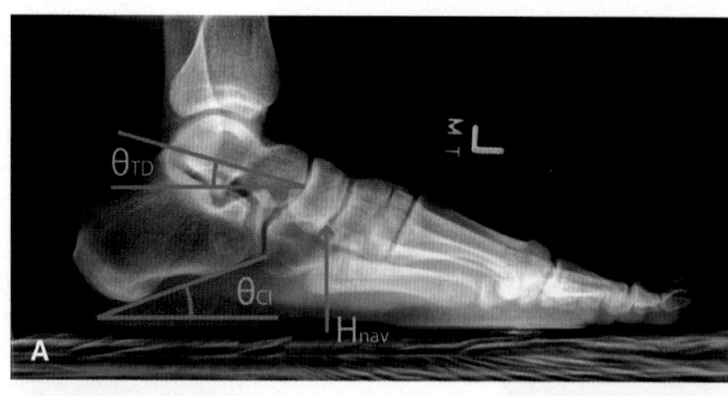

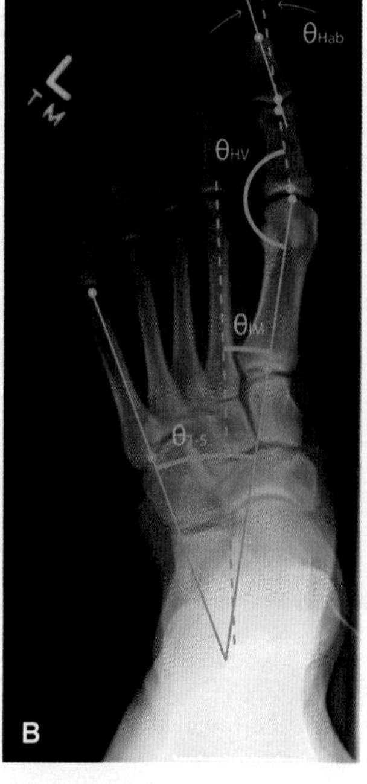

Figure 2.4. **A:** Medial–lateral x-ray view provides several measures of foot structure including talar declination (θ_{TD}), calcaneal inclination (θ_{CI}), and navicular height (H_{nav}). **B:** Anterior–posterior x-ray view provides several measures of forefoot and midfoot structures including hallux abductus angle (θ_{Hab}), hallux valgus angle (θ_{HV}), intermetatarsal angle (θ_{IM}), and the first through fifth metatarsal angle (θ_{1-5}).

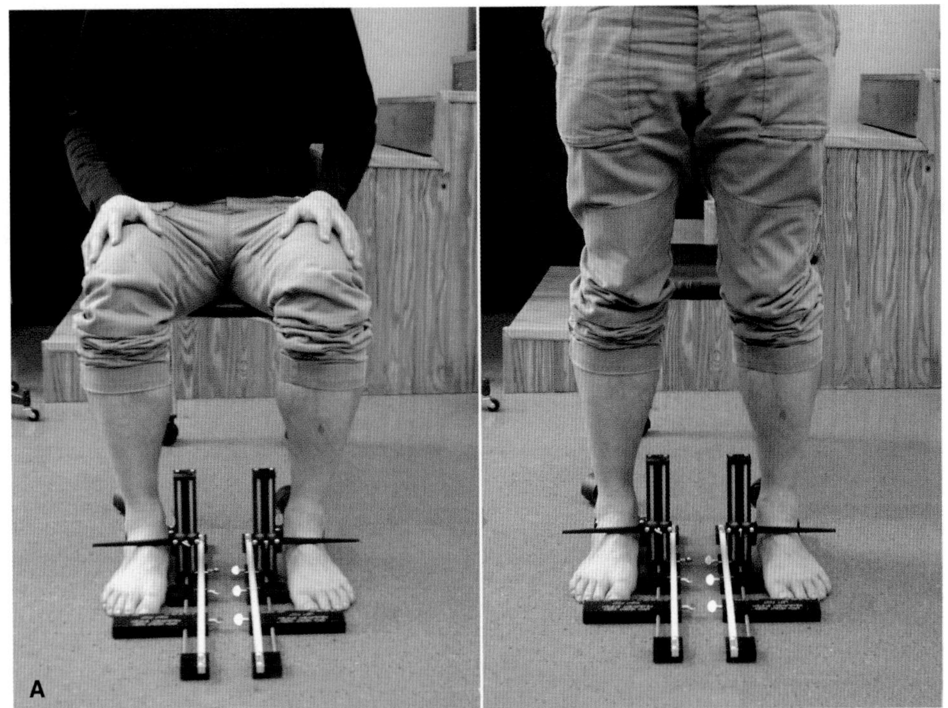

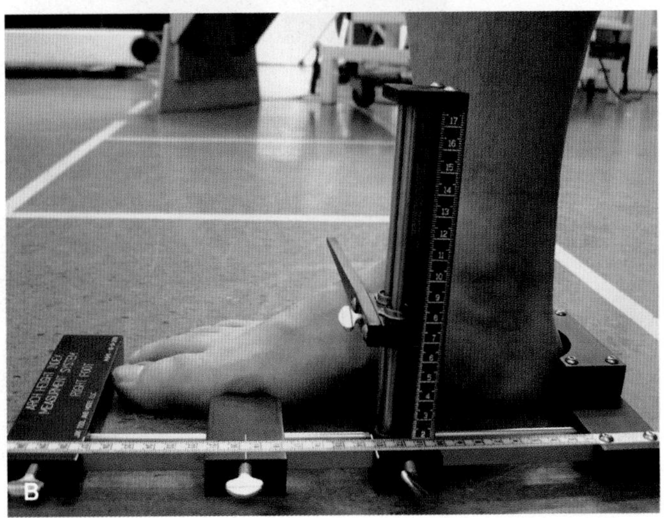

Figure 2.5. **A:** AHI measured while sitting and standing. **B:** Close-up view of graticule scaled in centimeters for measuring dorsal arch height at one half of foot length.

arch height (AH). Linear graticules scaled in centimeter are laminated to the jig for visual measurement of each parameter. AHI is defined as the dorsal arch height (AH) at one-half of FL normalized by the TFL (55) while sitting ($AH_{sitting}$) and standing ($AH_{standing}$). AHI sitting and standing (Fig. 2.5B) are calculated according to the following formulae:

$$AHI_{sitting} = \frac{(AH_{sitting})}{TFL} \times 100$$

$$AHI_{standing} = \frac{(AH_{standing})}{TFL} \times 100$$

AHI (Table 2.2) can objectively distinguish planus, rectus, and cavus foot types in asymptomatic healthy individuals (47).

AHI values that are 1.5 standard deviations larger than the mean correlate with lower extremity overuse injuries in runners (56). Studies have shown that running injuries are multi-factorial but differences in injury pattern have occurred as a function of arch height. Individuals with high-arched feet had an increased tendency for bony injuries such as tibial and femoral fractures (57), anterior knee pain, and injury to the lateral structures of the lower extremity (56) whereas low-arched feet were more susceptible to metatarsal fractures (57), medial tibial stress syndrome, knee pain, and other injuries involving the medial and soft-tissue structures of the lower extremity (56).

Arch Height Flexibility (AHF)

AHF (mm/kN) is the change in arch height between sitting and standing normalized to the change in load, which has been estimated to be 40% of body weight (55). AHF is calculated

TABLE 2.2 Arch Height Indices (AHI)

	Pes Planus		Rectus		Pes Cavus	
	Mean	SD	Mean	SD	Mean	SD
$AHI_{sitting}$	0.35*#	0.03	0.38*^	0.03	0.40#^	0.03
$AHI_{standing}$	0.33*#	0.03	0.36*^	0.03	0.38#^	0.03

*: significant differences between pes planus and rectus; #: significant differences between pes planus and pes cavus ; ^: significant differences between rectus and pes cavus.

according to the following formula:

$$AHF\ (mm/kN) = \frac{(AH_{standing} - AH_{standing})}{0.4 \times BW} \times 100$$

where BW is the body weight. Although this parameter was not significantly different across foot type amongst asymptomatic individuals in the previous research (47), this parameter is anticipated to be very useful for distinguishing pathologic feet (e.g., osteoarthritis) from healthy.

Zifchock et al. showed that women have less arch stiffness compared to men (55). Increased arch flexibility is related to soft-tissue injuries of the foot and ankle (58). Posterior tibial syndrome, a condition linked with flexible flat feet, is more common in women (59).

First MTPJ Flexibility

In addition to first MTPJ ROM, flexibility may enhance our understanding of joint function. First MTPJ flexibility is assessed by a custom test jig that simultaneously permits application of joint moment and measurement of the resulting angular excursion about the axis of plantarflexion–dorsiflexion (Fig. 2.6A). A variable resistor (potentiometer) measures the angular excursion whereas a strain gauge–based extension socket torque transducer measures the applied moment (60). First MTPJ flexibility is the slope of the angular displacement versus applied moment curve (Fig. 2.6B). The slope of the angle versus moment curves in the initial 25% of the joint's ROM was termed "early flexibility (°/N·cm)", and during the final 25%, "late flexibility (°/N·cm)". First MTPJ flexibility is associated with improved hallucal loading during walking (35). Low-arched feet result in increased hallucal loading (61) and shift of the first metatarsal axis (62), thus predisposing the first MTPJ to osteoarthritis (63). First MTPJ flexibility differs across foot types (60). In standing, individuals with low arch have higher first MTPJ late flexibility compared to normal arch structure (60).

MEASURE OF FOOT FUNCTION

Foot function may be measured in several different but complimentary ways. The global effect of the foot upon gait pattern may be evaluated by measuring the temporal-distance parameters of locomotion. The kinematics local to the foot are typically measured with a motion capture system and may focus upon the hindfoot or assess multiple segments within the foot to reveal its intricate function. With ground reaction forces measured by a force plate, the kinetics (moments and powers) may be computed at the hindfoot, and with some underlying assumptions, at multiple segments within the foot. One of the most revealing measures of foot function is the plantar pressure distribution, which may be assessed either barefoot or within a shoe and is capable of providing both differential diagnostic and treatment efficacy data. Each of these measures contributes to our overall understanding of how the foot functions in healthy, athletic, and individuals with pathology.

Temporal-distance Footfall Parameters

A healthy foot and ankle, within the context of an asymptomatic lower extremity, will promote symmetrical gait patterns. The gait pattern is comprised of stance phase, when the foot makes contact with the ground from heel strike to toe-off and swing phase, when the foot is swinging in a pendulum-like manner to advance the body and prepare for the next stance phase. A gait cycle, or stride, encompasses one stance

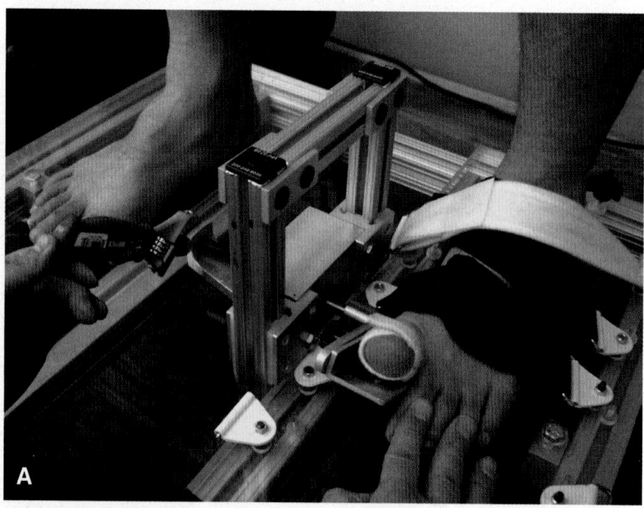

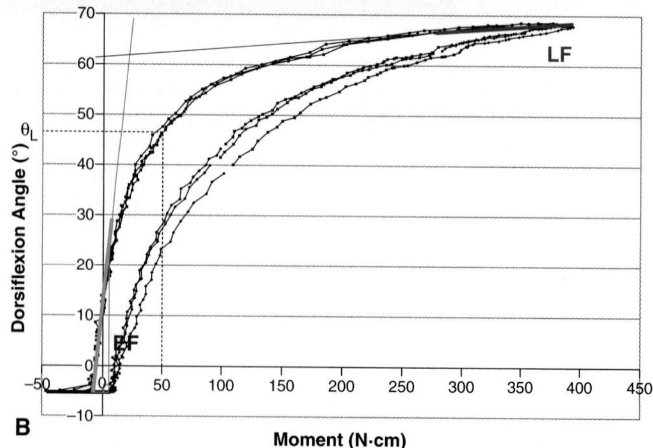

Figure 2.6. **A:** First MTPJ flexibility is assessed by mechanically grounding the foot with Velcro straps and applying a moment about the joint axis of rotation using a wrench to the limits of passive ROM. **B:** the slope of the resulting angle versus moment curve serves as a measure of early (EF) and late (LF) first MTPJ flexibility.

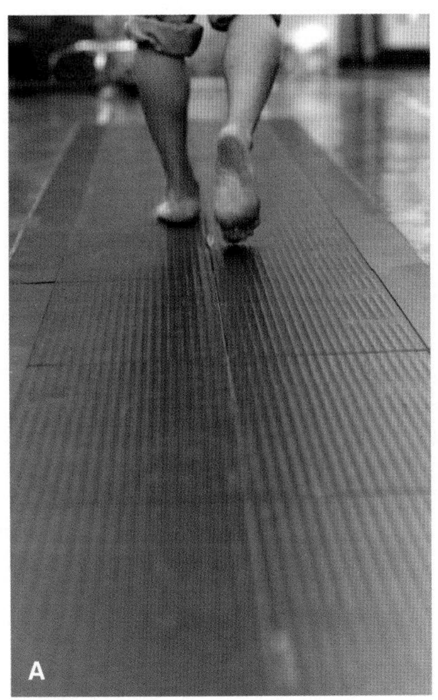

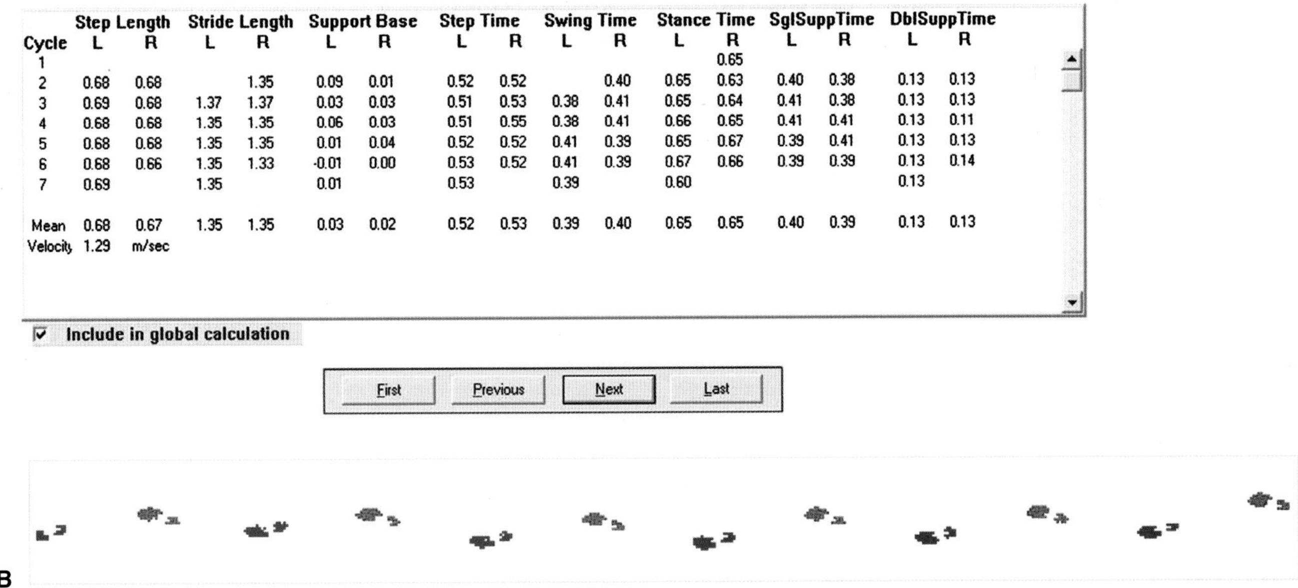

Cycle	Step Length L	Step Length R	Stride Length L	Stride Length R	Support Base L	Support Base R	Step Time L	Step Time R	Swing Time L	Swing Time R	Stance Time L	Stance Time R	SglSuppTime L	SglSuppTime R	DblSuppTime L	DblSuppTime R
1												0.65				
2	0.68	0.68		1.35	0.09	0.01	0.52	0.52		0.40	0.65	0.63	0.40	0.38	0.13	0.13
3	0.69	0.68	1.37	1.37	0.03	0.03	0.51	0.53	0.38	0.41	0.65	0.64	0.41	0.38	0.13	0.13
4	0.68	0.68	1.35	1.35	0.06	0.03	0.51	0.55	0.38	0.41	0.66	0.65	0.41	0.41	0.13	0.11
5	0.68	0.68	1.35	1.35	0.01	0.04	0.52	0.52	0.41	0.39	0.65	0.67	0.39	0.41	0.13	0.13
6	0.68	0.66	1.35	1.33	-0.01	0.00	0.53	0.52	0.41	0.39	0.67	0.66	0.39	0.39	0.13	0.14
7	0.69		1.35		0.01		0.53		0.39		0.60				0.13	
Mean	0.68	0.67	1.35	1.35	0.03	0.02	0.52	0.53	0.39	0.40	0.65	0.65	0.40	0.39	0.13	0.13
Velocity	1.29	m/sec														

Figure 2.7. **A:** An individual walking across an instrumented walkway such as the GaitMat II (EQ Inc, Chalfont, PA, USA). **B:** Resulting temporal-distance parameters of an individual's gait pattern.

and one swing phase, which in healthy individuals typically accounts for 60% and 40% of stride, respectively. Although an individual's temporal-distance parameters of walking may be measured with the use of a stopwatch and a tape measure from the footprints left in the sand from walking along the beach, more modern computerized approaches are available to the clinician and researcher.

As shown in Fig. 2.7A, an individual may walk across an instrumented walkway such as the GaitMat II (EQ Inc, Chalfont, PA, USA) which is comprised of a matrix of normally open switches that close upon foot contact. Spatial (position of initial contact) and temporal (time of initial contact) events are recorded within a microcomputer. The system displays the footprints on a computer monitor in real time while the temporal-distance parameters are computed immediately after collection of the trial (Fig. 2.7B). The following parameters are provided for each walking trial:

Stride Length (m) is calculated as the length from the initial contact on the ipsilateral limb to the next initial contact on that same limb.

Step Length (m) is calculated as the length from the initial contact on the ipsilateral limb to the next initial contact on the contralateral limb.

Double Support Time (s) is calculated as the time when both feet are in contact with the ground. Double support time values are also normalized by gait cycle (stride) time and expressed as a percentage of stride.

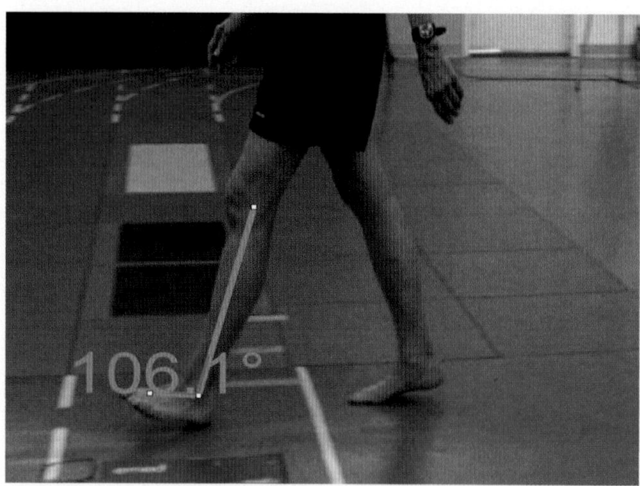

Figure 2.8. Video-based 2D analysis of kinematics using stick figure like representations may be done with a camcorder and software such as DARTFISH (Alpharetta, GA, USA).

Stance Time (s) is calculated as the time from initial (e.g., heel strike) to the final (e.g., toe off) time that the foot is in contact with the ground. Stance time values are also normalized by gait cycle (stride) time and expressed as a percentage of stride.

Swing Time (s) is calculated as the time when both feet are in contact with the ground. Swing time values are also normalized by gait cycle (stride) time and expressed as a percentage of stride.

Velocity (m/s), or more specifically the magnitude of velocity (walking speed), is calculated as the distance traveled per unit time.

As shown in Fig. 2.7B, healthy asymptomatic individuals have symmetrical gait patterns, which exhibit characteristic behavior such as a 1–1.4 m/sec walking speed. Parameters such as stride and step length are a function of stature (i.e., limb length) so they are expected to vary with height unless normalized. In a recent study assessing foot structure and function there were no significant differences in gait pattern parameters across planus, rectus, and cavus foot types in asymptomatic healthy individuals (47).

Pedal pathology, especially when associated with pain (e.g., lateral ligament injury, posterior tendon rupture, plantar fasciitis, etc.), can result in asymmetrical temporal-distance parameters. Temporal-distance parameters elucidate the effect that a given pedal pathology has upon one's gait pattern (64). Thus individuals with foot pain use pain-avoidance strategies such as reduced walking speed or a limp to avoid exacerbating foot pain (65,66).

Kinematics

Kinematics is the study of joint motion without reference to the forces that are responsible for that motion. Kinematics of the hindfoot, usually referred to as the ankle, may be assessed in a variety of ways. If one is interested in a two-dimensional (2D) representation of either the sagittal or frontal plane motion, then very simplified "stick–figure-like" representations may be obtained from a camcorder (Fig. 2.8). A software system that assists with the qualitative analysis of such 2D stick figures is DARTFISH (Alpharetta, GA, USA). Although this information is limited given the anatomical complexity of the foot and ankle, it is cost-effective and can be done in a clinician's office or outside on the athletic field through the use of a laptop computer.

Quantification of the kinematics of the foot and ankle requires a larger investment in both the cost of equipment as well as time and expertise required to use the equipment. The study of the hindfoot in three dimensions (3D) requires a minimum of a two-camera motion capture system although a larger number of cameras is preferred to minimize data drop out and allow for observation of complex motions from any perspective. An example of such technology at the Leon Root, MD Motion Analysis Laboratory is a 12-camera Motion Analysis Corporation (Santa Rosa, CA, USA) system (Fig. 2.9). Six of these cameras have 1.3 megapixel resolution and 6 have 4 megapixel resolution. The cameras may be configured in a wide variety of data capture volumes referred to as fields of view depending on the subject of interest. A foot and ankle focused analysis requires a $1 \times 1 \times 0.5\ m^3$ field of view while a whole body analysis during running requires a $2 \times 2 \times 6.4\ m^3$ field of view.

Before performing 3D motion capture the field of view is calibrated which typically results in 3D residual errors of <0.5 mm. A typical lower extremity kinematic analysis may have >30 passive retro-reflective markers, some of which are used to track the limb segment movements while others are used to define the joint coordinate systems (Fig. 2.10A).

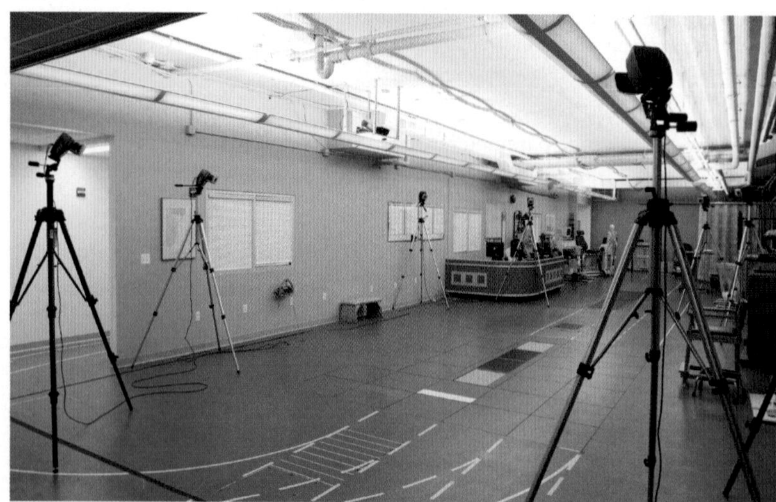

Figure 2.9. A 12-camera Motion Analysis Corporation (Santa Rosa, CA, USA) system at the Leon Root, MD Motion Analysis Laboratory.

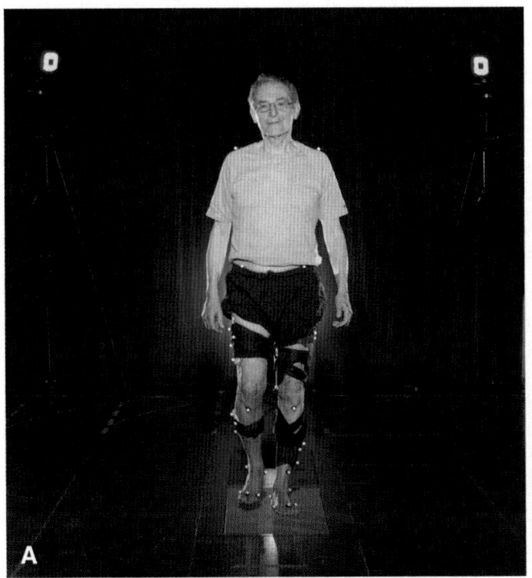

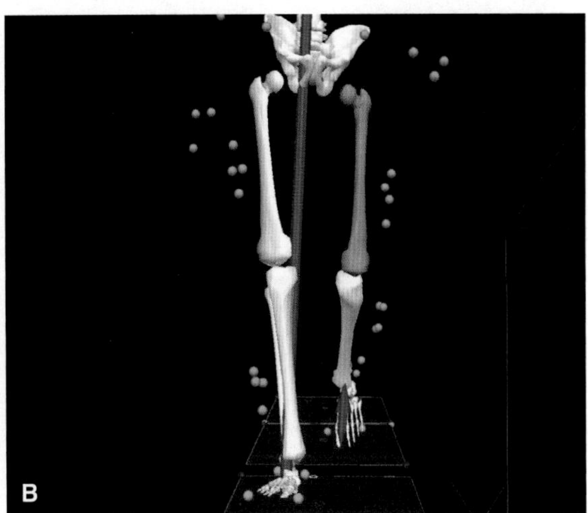

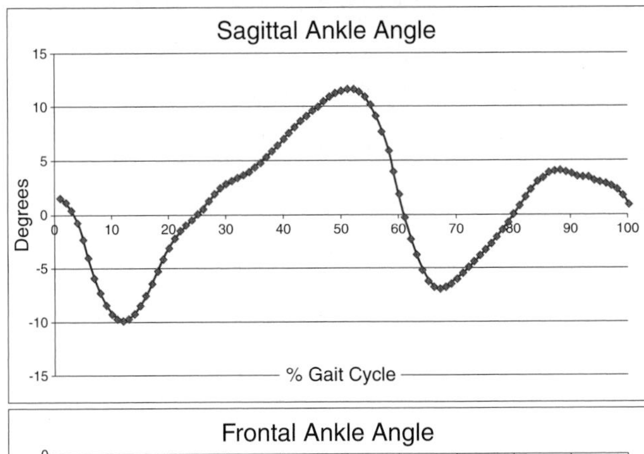

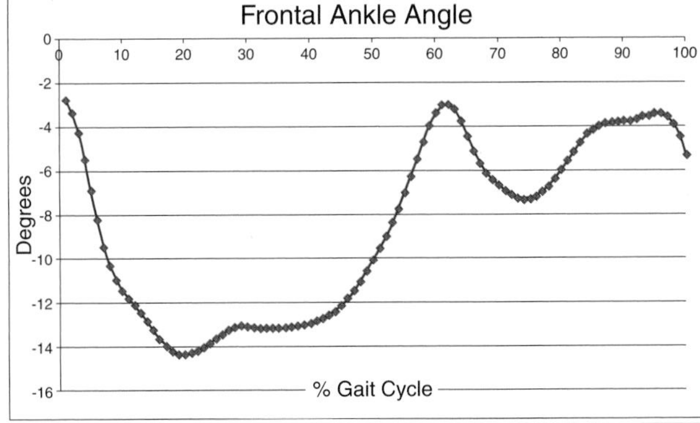

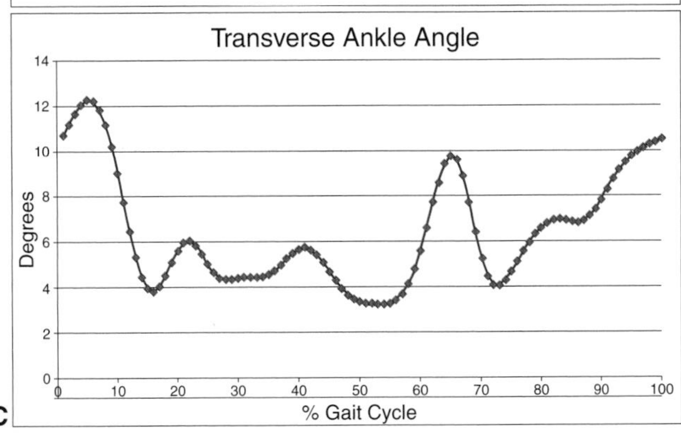

Figure 2.10. **A:** Passive retro-reflective markers on anatomical landmarks of a patient to permit tracking and calculation of 3D kinematics after motion capture. **B:** Frontal plane perspective of motion capture data using kinematic and kinetic analysis software known as Visual 3D (C-Motion, Germantown, MD, USA), (**C**) Typical curves of sagittal (plantar–dorsiflexion), frontal (varus–valgus), and transverse (internal–external) plane rotations are shown.

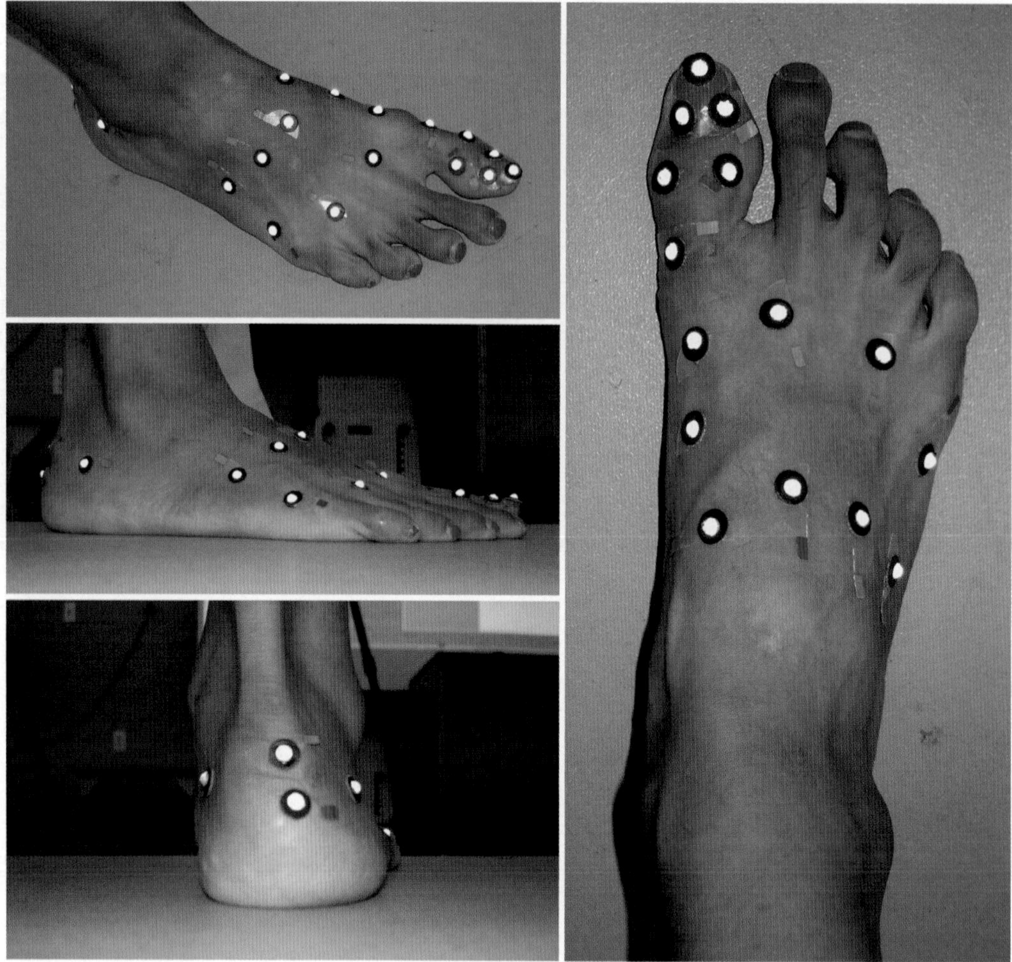

Figure 2.11. Multisegment foot kinematic marker set that permits measurement of motions between the tibia and calcaneus, calcaneus and first metatarsal, calcaneus and second to fourth metatarsals, calcaneus and fifth metatarsal, and the first metatarsal and hallux to measure more detailed motions within the foot.

Hindfoot Kinematics

The minimum number of markers required to study 3D hindfoot kinematics is three on the calcaneus and three on the tibia for tracking plus those required to define the joint coordinate system (lateral and medial malleolus, and dorsal fifth metatarsal head). A frontal plane perspective display for a lower extremity 3D motion analysis is shown here (Fig. 2.10B). Typical curves of sagittal (plantar–dorsiflexion), frontal (varus–valgus), and transverse (internal–external) plane rotations are shown (Fig. 2.10C).

Multisegment Kinematics

The inherent assumption when studying hindfoot kinematics is that the foot is a rigid body (from calcaneus to hallux). Since the anatomical structures within the foot are obviously not a rigid body and are very complex, this has led to the development of multisegment kinematic measurement systems.

In recent years, *in vivo* multisegment foot kinematics (Fig. 2.11) have been studied using 3D motion analysis. Two recent reviews have examined the evidence for the use of multisegment foot models (67,68). Consequently only salient features are highlighted in the following paragraphs.

The foot has been modeled using two (forefoot and hindfoot, (69)), three (hallux, forefoot and hindfoot, e.g., Oxford foot model (70)) and the Milwaukee foot model (71), four (hallux, forefoot, midfoot and hindfoot, (72)), and five (hallux, medial forefoot, lateral forefoot, midfoot and hindfoot segments (73)).

This wide variation in the number of segments and description of motion between segments led to several concerns regarding the repeatability and validity of early applications of multisegment foot models. However, recent studies indicate good intra- and inter-reliability (74,75), particularly with the Oxford foot model in children (76,77) and adults (78). Some researchers have proposed the use of standardized marker placement using plaster casts (79) or custom devices (80) to improve reliability. In addition, recent studies have also established the reliability of multisegment foot models in specific clinical populations (81,82). Taken together, the findings of these studies suggest that trial-to-trial and intertester variability should be no more than 3 to 4 degrees (83).

Most models address kinematic validity in terms of face validity (i.e., by comparing their results to previously published reports) (84,85); however, a few models have been validated in both static and dynamic conditions against a robotic or *in vitro* (cadaveric) "gold standard" (86,87).

At this juncture, it should be noted that there is no consensus when it comes to a gold standard to establish kinematic validity. *In vitro* cadaver robotic simulations (88,89), fluoroscopy (90), invasive *in vivo* methods (91,92) and most recently, 3D magnetic resonance imaging (93) have all been used to assess motion between individual foot bones. These invasive and imaging *in vivo* and robotic *in vitro* studies question the validity of modeling the forefoot as a single rigid segment (88,89,92). Overall, the calcaneus, first metatarsal and hallux have (relatively) low soft-tissue tracking errors. Relatively large soft-tissue artifacts may be seen at toe off at the navicular, highlighting the need for judicious interpretation when using midfoot segments (90).

Overall, the Oxford foot model has several strengths and is increasingly used in clinical and research studies (70,76–78). Its main strengths are its well-established repeatability and a clear reference position. Its main weaknesses are that it models the forefoot as a single rigid body, and does not model the hallux as a rigid body. Consequently, based on the specific research question and area of interest, a modified version of the Oxford foot model may need to be used to allow for 3D tracking of the segments of interest while minimizing violations of the rigid body assumption and/or soft-tissue artifacts (73).

Kinetics

To determine the forces that cause motion, kinetics, an individual must walk across a 3D force plate to measure the ground reaction force vector. Vertical, anterior–posterior, and medial–lateral forces are obtained to solve the equations of motion and permit the calculation of joint moments and powers.

Hindfoot Kinetics

Fig. 2.12A illustrates the basic calculation ($M_a = F \times d$) for ankle moment. Fig. 2.12B depicts typical curves for sagittal, frontal, and transverse plane hindfoot moments. Sagittal hindfoot

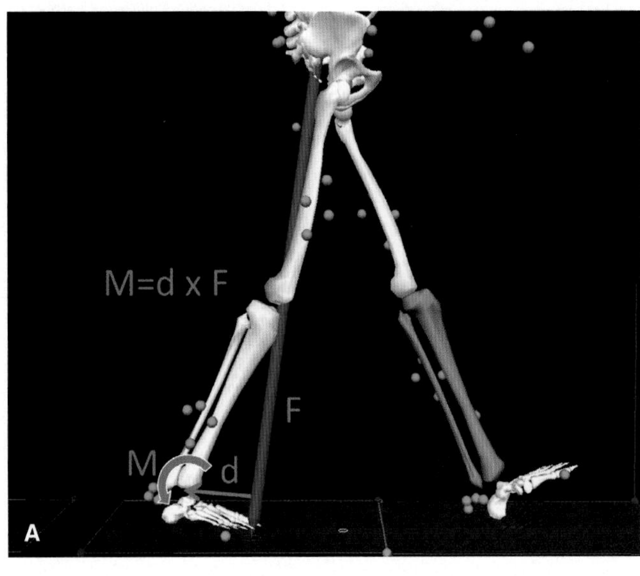

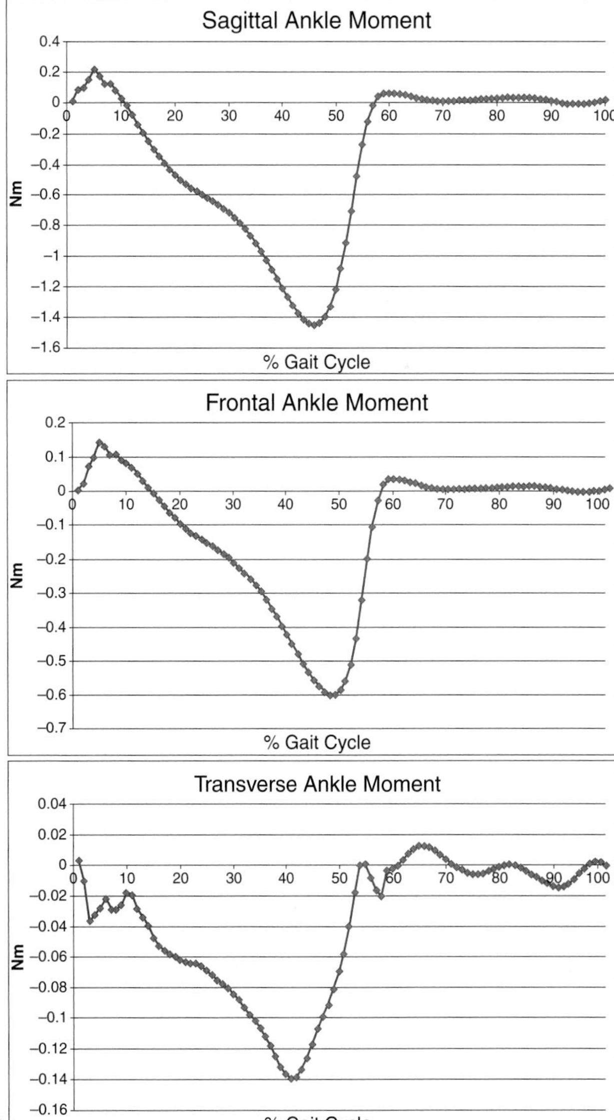

Figure 2.12. **A:** Ankle moment calculation is illustrated using Visual 3D (C-Motion, Germantown, MD, USA). $M_a = F \times d$, where M_a is the ankle moment, F is the ground reaction force vector as measured by a force plate, and d is the moment arm. **B:** Typical ankle moment curves are depicted for the sagittal, frontal, and transverse planes.

moment is very sensitive to spasticity and contracture in individuals with cerebral palsy, hemiparetic stroke, or significant tendo-Achilles tightness. (94) For example, the initial dorsiflexion (positive) peak of hindfoot moment will be absent in a "toe walker" because the ground reaction force vector will never be behind the ankle joint.

Multisegment Kinetics

The issue of defining segments outlined above is central to the decision of how net ground reaction forces are partitioned (95). Three main approaches have been used: First, ground reaction forces have been partitioned proportional to the vertical force obtained from a pedobarograph (96). In this method, kinematic segments of interest should correspond to the "masks" (regions of interest) defined to analyze plantar pressure. Second, a split force platform method with precise targeting has been used to define midfoot and metatarsophalangeal kinetics (85,97). Lastly, specific intervals of the gait cycle have been studied (98,99). Taken together, these studies suggest that single-segment models of the foot may overestimate hindfoot power generation. Multisegment kinetic models suggest that the midfoot and hindfoot both play a significant role in power generation, while the first metatarsophalangeal joint absorbs power at push off.

Plantar Pressures

Pressure is defined as force per unit area (e.g., N/cm^2).

Plantar Loading Parameters: Plantar pressure data can be acquired when an individual walks across a plantar pressure measuring device (Fig. 2.13A). Trials where the individual appears to be targeting the measuring device should be discarded. The following plantar loading parameters maybe calculated from this data.

CPEI (%), is a measure of dynamic foot function calculated in custom software that generates a plot of the maximum pressure throughout stance phase (46). The center of pressure (COP) at each instant of time (shown in red) is superimposed with this maximum pressure plot (Fig. 2.13B). CPEI (%) is calculated as follows;

$$CPEI\ (\%) = (CPE/FW) \times 100$$

where CPE is the displacement between the COP curve and construction line (between the initial and final centers of pressure points) at the anterior third of foot length and FW is the foot width at the CPE. Overpronation is demonstrated by a COP curve with diminished concavity. Oversupination is demonstrated by excessive concavity of the COP curve (100).

Peak Plantar Pressure, PP (N/cm^2) is calculated in each masked region of the maximum pressure throughout stance phase plot. A 12-segment mask (a scalable geometrically based template) has been developed, using Novel software, to permit automated calculations of PP for each anatomical segment of each subject (Fig. 2.13C). The PP values may also be normalized by the total PP (i.e., peak pressure beneath the entire foot) in each anatomical segment.

In a recent study it has also been demonstrated that PP can objectively distinguish planus, rectus, and cavus foot types in asymptomatic healthy individuals (47,60).

Foot Functional Indices and Self-assessments

Foot self-assessments/indices are subjective reports of function completed by patients. Self-assessments are becoming an important outcome measure for health care practitioners (101–103) particularly due to third party payer needs for objective measures of an individual's health-related quality of life. These self-assessment tools quantify dysfunction at the individual's level and allow clinicians to evaluate changes in functional limitations following clinical interventions (104). There are several region-specific scales and the reader is referred to a recent review (105). Briefly, self-reported outcome scales quantify foot health across the dimensions of pain, stiffness, psychosocial issues, and participation restrictions. While a number of outcome scales are available, psychometric properties such as reliability, validity and sensitivity are poorly established.

- The Foot and Ankle Disability Index (FADI) evaluates functional limitations associated with foot and ankle conditions by assessing activities of daily living, and the more specific FADI sport assesses more complex tasks that are critical to sports (106).
- The foot function index (FFI) is a validated, reliable tool of self-assessment for foot disorders in individuals with ankle rheumatoid arthritis (RA) (107,108). The FFI consists of 23 items that evaluate pain, disability, and activity limitation, with items scored on a visual analog scale (107,109).
- The revised version of the foot function index (FFI-R) includes the original domains but is modified to use a Likert scale with 34 questions. The FFI-R modified version of FFI has been used for individuals with ankle osteoarthritis (OA) (110).
- Foot posture index is a measure of foot structure, not self-reported function. The foot posture index evaluates standing foot posture by six criterion-based observations of the rearfoot and forefoot in a relaxed standing position (3).

RELATIONSHIP BETWEEN FOOT STRUCTURE AND FUNCTION

Several studies have shown that biomechanical measures of foot structure and function are related in asymptomatic healthy individuals. Song et al. (46) utilized MVI and CPEI values to successfully discriminate planus from rectus feet in a cohort of 21 young and healthy subjects.

Cavanagh et al. (54), showed that 31% and 38% of the variance of peak plantar pressure at the heel and first metatarsal head, respectively, during walking could be explained by radiographic measures of foot structure, especially arch-related measurements and soft-tissue thickness. This study confirmed that dynamic foot function can be predicted by static structural variables to some extent (54). By combining measures of foot structure from radiographic measurements and function on asymptomatic subjects between 20 and 70 years, these investigators predicted approximately 50% of the variance in peak plantar pressure under the heel, first metatarsal head and hallux (4).

In a recent study of healthy asymptomatic subjects assessing the relationship between foot structure and function, a number of measures of foot structure (arch height indices during sitting and standing, RCSP, FF–RF, total contact area)

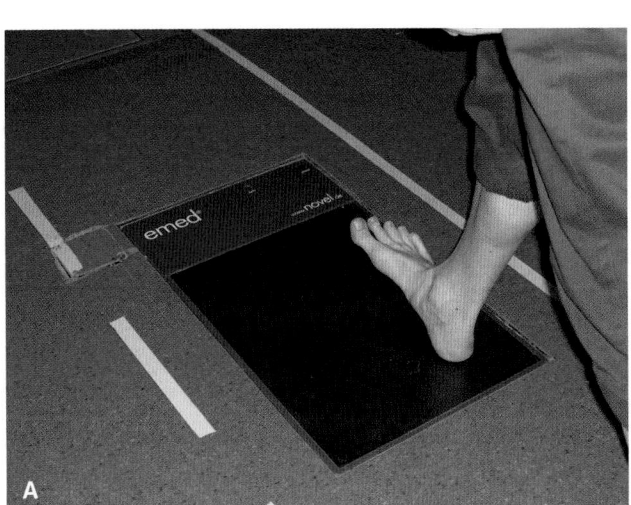

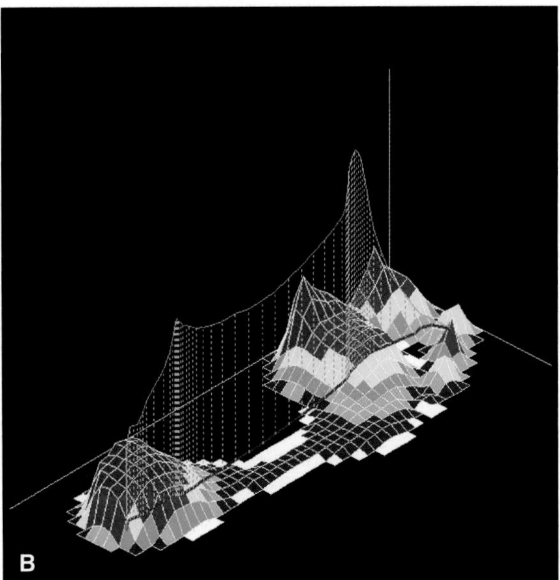

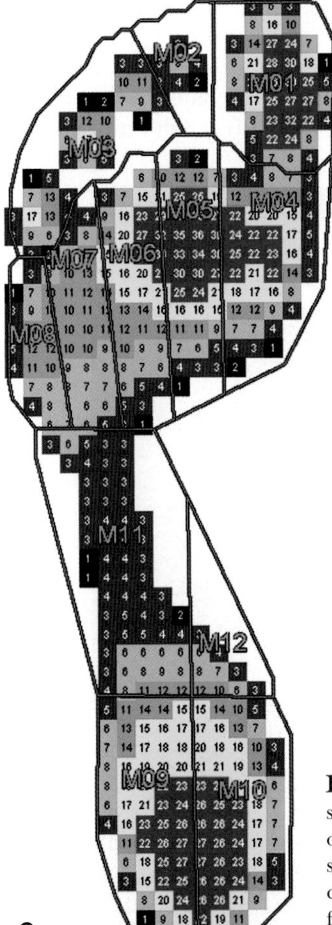

Figure 2.13. **A:** Individual walking over a plantar pressure measuring device such as the emed-X manufactured by Novel (Munich, Germany). **B:** The center of pressure curve is shown superimposed with the maximum pressure throughout stance phase plot. The CPEI is a measure of the concavity of the center of pressure curve **C:** The masking algorithm depicts the regions of interest within the plantar foot that comprise the toes, forefoot, arch, and hindfoot. Pressure, force and area calculations maybe made for any and all of those regions.

and anthropometrics (height, age, and weight) explained 45% to 77% of the model variance (adjusted R^2) for gait pattern parameters (95). Similarly, 7% to 47% of the model variance for plantar pressure parameters and 16% to 64% of the model variance for maximum force parameters can also be explained by measures of foot structure and anthropometrics (111). These results confirm that biomechanical measures of foot structure and function are related in asymptomatic healthy individuals. The structural parameters used in this study were measurements that do not require ionizing radiation and can be employed in a clinical office setting (112).

Measures of foot structure are clinically practical and often less costly than those of foot function. The ability to relate foot structure to foot function would assist the clinician who can practically measure foot structure but not function with differential diagnosis of foot pathologies, treatment planning, and determination of treatment efficacy.

STRUCTURE AND FUNCTION OF PATHOLOGY

Many pathologies that afflict the foot and ankle have a biomechanical origin. By understanding the association between foot structure and function one may begin to understand the pathomechanics underlying many of the maladies involving this anatomy. The following section will discuss some common foot pathologies and usefulness of biomechanical tools to quantify the structural alterations to improve our understanding of foot function.

Posterior Tibial Dysfunction

Posterior tibial tendon dysfunction (PTTD) is a progressive deformity that can result in the development of adult acquired flatfoot (113). PTTD is a result of weakening of the posterior tibial tendon and the adjacent structures that maintain the medial longitudinal arch (114). This condition has a triplanar effect on the structure and function of the foot. Structurally, these individuals present with a valgus hindfoot (RCSP typically >10 degrees), varus FF–RF position (typically >10 degrees), and a decreased AH (Fig. 2.14A). Radiographically, these individuals have a declinated talus and first metatarsal with an abducted forefoot believed in part to result from the tendon rupture and associated ligamentous damage (56,61). Functionally, these individuals have medially directed ground reaction forces during the stance phase of gait which significantly reduces CPEI (Fig. 2.14B). In extreme cases, CPEI can actually be negative implying a convex (as opposed to the typical concave) center of pressure excursion throughout stance.

Anomalous stress on the midfoot eventually results in stretching of the passive support structures and if left undiagnosed or untreated, results in acquired flatfoot deformity (112).

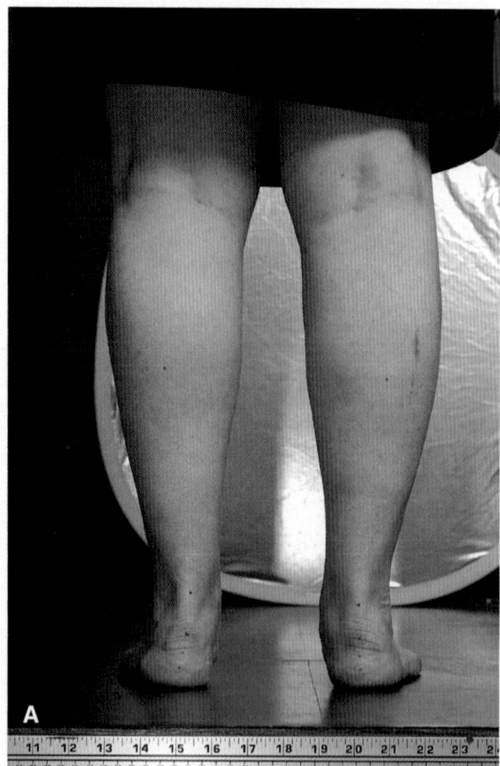

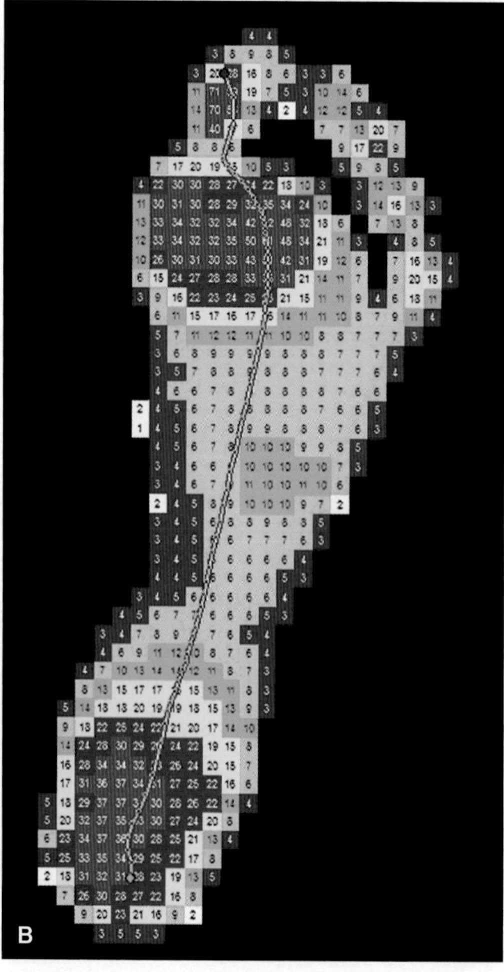

Figure 2.14. **A:** Patient with PTTD illustrating the valgus hindfoot orientation. **B:** The maximum pressure throughout stance phase plot illustrating a reduced concavity of the CPEI and larger peak pressures beneath the medial structures (heel, first and second metatarsal heads, and hallux) for this PTTD patient.

Static foot measures like AHI (115), radiographic angles like talar declination angle, or Meary's angle (116) are not useful measures as changes in these angles become evident only in later stages (stage 2 and 3) (116). On clinical examination, assessing ankle inverter strength is useful in adults; however, (117,118) it may be insensitive in young and active individuals (115).

The maximum pressure throughout stance phase will demonstrate higher peak pressures in the medial structures as well as a medial shift in center of pressure (reduced CPEI) secondary to the abnormal loading present in flat foot (119). If detected early, the development of PTTD can be prevented. The medial to lateral forefoot loading ratio is increased in individuals with PTTD suggesting reduced support of the arch. Increased loads within the arch that occur after the posterior tibial tendon is compromised, may be the underlying mechanical factors that stretch the foot ligaments leading to acquired flatfoot deformity. Hindfoot kinematics are excessively everted during the stance phase of gait (115). Peak rearfoot eversion increases with PTTD progression. There is a 3.1 degrees increase in rearfoot eversion for stage-I PTTD (115) and a 6.2 degrees increase for stage-II PTTD (120) compared to healthy controls.

Hallux Valgus

Hallux valgus (HV), commonly referred to as a bunion, refers to an increase in the intermetatarsal (IM) angle greater than 15 to 20 degrees and a hallux abductus (HA) angle exceeding 8 to 9 degrees (121). HV may be genetic in origin or caused by extrinsic factors (e.g., poor-fitting foot wear) or intrinsic factors (e.g., hypermobility of the first ray, ligamentous laxity, bony alignment, or osteoarthritis of the first MTPJ) (122). While the precise etiology of HV remains unproven, there are several theories including the presence of hypermobility (i.e., excessive superior and inferior displacement of the first metatarsal) that are thought to lead to the medial drifting of the first MTPJ. Feet with hypermobility often have diminished peak pressures beneath the first MTPJ and excessive peak pressures beneath the second MTPJ which is left to do the brunt of load bearing for the medial forefoot (Fig. 2.15). Fig. 2.15A depicts the increased IM an HA angles radiographically while Figs. 2.15B and 2.15C demonstrate the reduced CPEI and larger peak pressure at the second metatarsal head compared with the first metatarsal head suggesting over-pronation and first ray hypermobility to some extent.

This transverse plane deformity not only represents aberrant structure but also causes irritation of skin, joint redness and pain around the bunion and always results in pain during walking. It is also coupled with changes in the soft-tissue arch, sesamoid mechanism and metatarso-cuneiform joint. Conservative management includes rest and ice along with changes in shoe gear, corrective separators and inserts (over the counter or custom molded) (121).

Motion at the first metatarso-cuneiform joint occurs in the sagittal and transverse planes. A motion greater than 4 degrees in the sagittal plane and greater than 8 degrees in the transverse plane indicates excessive motion (123). Clinically, hypermobility is evaluated by determining sagittal motion (the grasping test) and transverse motion (the clinical squeeze test) and by identifying signs such as the presence of a dorsal bunion, intractable plantar keratosis beneath the second metatarsal head, and arthritis of the first and second metatarso-cuneiform joints.

Radiographically, hypermobility is evaluated by measurements from the modified Coleman block test (for sagittal motion) and the radiographic squeeze test (for transverse motion). It can also be identified by signs, such as cortical hypertrophy along the medial border of the second metatarsal shaft, a cuneiform split, the presence of intermetatarseum, and the round shape and increased medial slope of the first metatarso-cuneiform joint (123). Radiographically, first ray elevation is considered a sign of progressive worsening of the first MTPJ function (124).

Sagittal plane kinematics has shown how first ray deformity can affect gait patterns during weight bearing in individuals with hallux valgus (125). Multisegment foot kinematics reveal that individuals with hallux valgus have prolonged stance phase along with decreased velocity and stride length (126). Pain and clinical results are known to be associated with dynamic plantar pressures where mean pressure under the hallux is significantly higher in individuals with hallux valgus (73,76,127,128). Thus quantitative measures like clinical tests, radiographic measures, plantar pressures and having an understanding of joint kinematics can be a critical part of evaluating hallux valgus and can help prevent progression by early intervention.

Diabetes

Foot structure and function also play a critical role in the development of neuropathic foot ulcer(s) and lower limb amputation (LEA) in subjects with diabetes. Diabetic foot complications are a common, complex, and costly problem. Diabetes is the leading cause of non-traumatic LEA in the United States. In 2006 alone, approximately 65,700 cases of LEA occurred in subjects with diabetes (129). It is known that 85% of LEAs are precipitated by diabetic foot ulcers—skin breakdown, characterized by the absence of pain (130). Diabetic peripheral polyneuropathy and loss of feeling in feet is a key risk factor since it permits injuries to occur without the subject's awareness. Because foot ulcers commonly occur at load-bearing sites (e.g., areas beneath metatarsal heads and the big toe) and are typically surrounded by thick hyperkeratotic lesions, it was long suspected that diabetic neuropathic foot ulceration might be related to abnormal foot biomechanics (131,132). Studies have shown that high plantar pressures were common in diabetic patients, especially those with a history of foot ulceration. A 30-month prospective investigation has shown that diabetic neuropathic patients with high plantar pressures (>12.3 kg/cm^2) were much more likely to develop a foot ulcer (4). Obesity, very common in type 2 diabetes, has been suspected to be associated with increased peak plantar pressure and diabetic foot ulceration. Although heavier body weights were noted in diabetic neuropathic patients with a history of ulceration, Cavanagh and colleagues demonstrated that body weight was a poor predictor of high peak plantar pressure (133). Rather, excessive plantar pressures were commonly associated with the presence of foot deformities or restriction joint mobility. Furthermore, Bevans noted that the location of ulcers was associated with abnormal foot structure, as indicated by RCSP values (134). Specifically, an everted RCSP was associated with ulcers under the medial metatarsal areas and an inverted RCSP was associated with ulcers under metatarsal heads 4 and 5 ($r = 0.87$: $P < 0.001$).

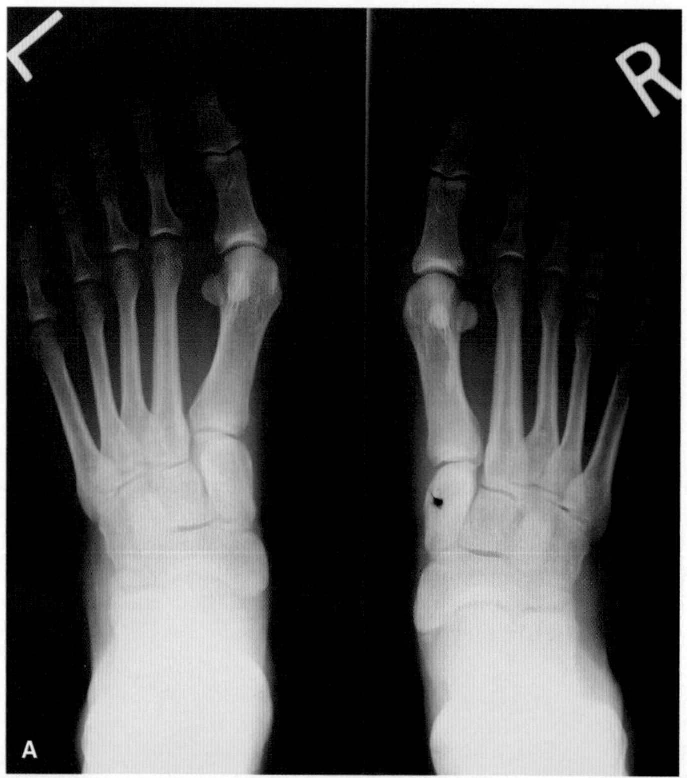

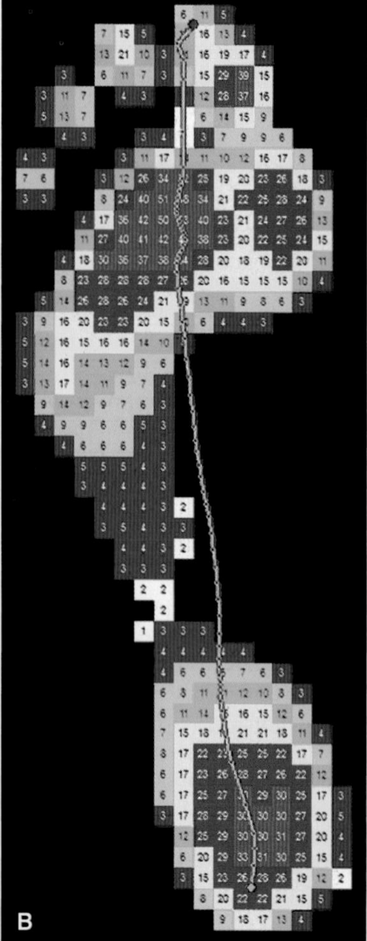

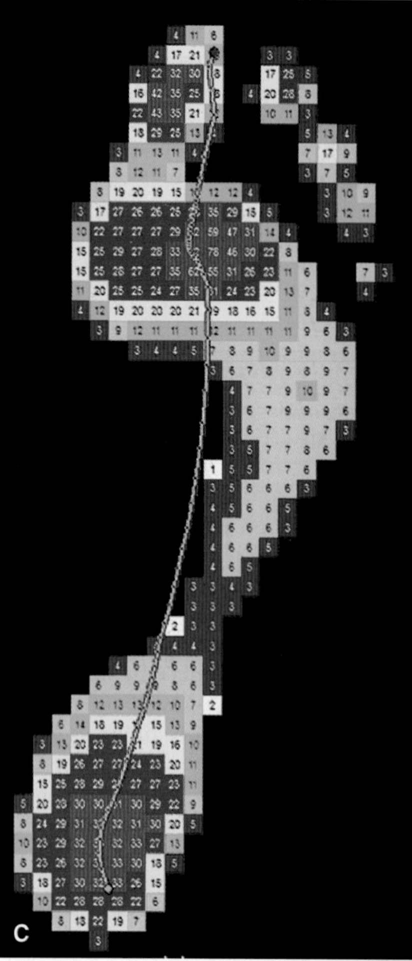

Figure 2.15. (**A**) AP radiograph of a patient with increased intermetatarsal(IM) and hallux abductus (HA) angles consistent with hallux valgus, (**B**) maximum pressure throughout stance phase with reduced CPEI and increased second metatarsal head pressures on the left, and (**C**) right feet.

There is a consensus among investigators that the majority of pedal ulcers result from a combination of factors. Lavery et al. reported significantly greater incidences of ulcerations, infections, amputations and hospitalization in those subjects with foot deformities and neuropathy versus those subjects with diabetic neuropathy alone during a mean follow-up period of 27.2 months (135). In a separate study of causal pathways among three multi-disciplinary foot care centers, Reiber et al. found that neuropathy, deformity, and trauma were the most frequent component causes for diabetic foot ulcerations (136). Assessment and management of aberrant foot structure and function, along with a comprehensive diabetes and multidisciplinary foot care team approach, are critical in reducing serious diabetic foot complications and improving the quality of life.

SUMMARY

There are several measures of foot structure and function that have been applied to distinguish asymptomatic healthy individuals with different foot types, differentiate pathology from healthy, and identify injury in the athlete. Coupled with self-assessments, these tools are anticipated to refine our knowledge of the origin and progression of disease within the foot and ankle as well as document which conservative and surgical treatments are most effective for the management of a specific pedal pathology.

ACKNOWLEDGMENTS

Funding from the National Institutes of Health (1R03HD053135-01, R01AR047853-06, 2U01AG018820-08, 1R01AR060492-01).

The years of experience and expertise from the staff of both the Gait Study Center at the Temple University School of Podiatric Medicine and the Leon Root, MD Motion Analysis Laboratory at the Hospital for Special Surgery.

REFERENCES

1. Dananberg HJ. Gait style as an etiology to chronic postural pain. part I. functional hallux limitus. *J Am Podiatr Med Assoc* 1993;8:433–441.
2. Christman RA. Principles of biomechanical radiographic analysis of the foot. In: *Foot and Ankle Radiology.* 1st ed. St. Louis, MO: Churchill Livingstone; 2003:261–270.
3. Redmond AC, Crosbie J, Ouvrier RA. Development and validation of a novel rating system for scoring standing foot posture: The foot posture index. *Clin Biomech (Bristol, Avon)* 2006;1:89–98.
4. Veves A, Murray HJ, Young MJ, et al. The risk of foot ulceration in diabetic patients with high foot pressure: A prospective study. *Diabetologia* 1992;7:660–663.
5. Morris JM. Biomechanics of the foot and ankle. *Clin Orthop Relat Res* 1977;122:10–17.
6. Root ML. *Normal and Abnormal Function of the Foot.* 1st ed. Los Angeles, LA: Clinical Biomechanics Corp; 1977.
7. McPoil TG, Knecht HG. Biomechanics of the foot in walking: A function approach. *J Orthop Sports Phys Ther* 1985;2:69–72.
8. Kaufman KR, Brodine SK, Shaffer RA, et al. The effect of foot structure and range of motion on musculoskeletal overuse injuries. *Am J Sports Med* 1999;5:585–593.
9. Pecoraro RE, Reiber GE, Burgess EM. Pathways to diabetic limb amputation. Basis for prevention. *Diabetes Care.* 1990;5:513–521.
10. American Diabetes Association. Consensus development conference on diabetic foot wound care: 7-8 April 1999, Boston, MA. *Adv Skin Wound Care* 1999;7:353–361.
11. Larsson J, Agardh CD, Apelqvist J, et al. Long-term prognosis after healed amputation in patients with diabetes. *Clin Orthop Relat Res* 1998;350:149–158.
12. Margolis DJ, Allen-Taylor L, Hoffstad O, et al. Diabetic neuropathic foot ulcers and amputation. *Wound Repair Regen* 2005;3:230–236.
13. Cavanagh PR, Simoneau GG, Ulbrecht JS. Ulceration, unsteadiness, and uncertainty: The biomechanical consequences of diabetes mellitus. *J Biomech* 1993;26 Suppl 1: 23–40.
14. Salsich GB, Brown M, Mueller MJ. Relationships between plantar flexor muscle stiffness, strength, and range of motion in subjects with diabetes-peripheral neuropathy compared to age-matched controls. *J Orthop Sports Phys Ther* 2000;8:473–83.
15. Vlassara H, Brownlee M, Cerami A. Nonenzymatic glycosylation: Role in the pathogenesis of diabetic complications. *Clin Chem* 1986;32 (10 Suppl):B37–B41.
16. Nube VL, Molyneaux L, Yue DK. Biomechanical risk factors associated with neuropathic ulceration of the hallux in people with diabetes mellitus. *J Am Podiatr Med Assoc* 2006;3:189–197.
17. Bevans JS, Bowker P. Foot structure and function: Etiological risk factors for callus formation in diabetic and non-diabetic subjects. *Foot* 1999;3:120–127.
18. Mueller MJ, Diamond JE, Delitto A, et al. Insensitivity, limited joint mobility, and plantar ulcers in patients with diabetes mellitus. *Phys Ther* 1989;69(6):453–459; discussion 459–462.
19. Vicenzino B. Foot orthotics in the treatment of lower limb conditions: A musculoskeletal physiotherapy perspective. *Man Ther* 2004;4:185–196.
20. Budiman-Mak E, Conrad KJ, Roach KE, et al. Can foot orthoses prevent hallux valgus deformity in rheumatoid arthritis? A randomized clinical trial. *J Clin Rheumatol* 1995;6:313–322.
21. Rao S, Baumhauer JF, Tome J, et al. Orthoses alter in vivo segmental foot kinematics during walking in patients with midfoot arthritis. *Arch Phys Med Rehabil* 2010;4:608–614.
22. Sell KE, Verity TM, Worrell TW, et al. Two measurement techniques for assessing subtalar joint position: A reliability study. *J Orthop Sports Phys Ther* 1994;3:162–167.
23. LaPointe SJ, Peebles C, Nakra A, et al. The reliability of clinical and caliper-based calcaneal bisection measurements. *J Am Podiatr Med Assoc* 2001;3:121–126.
24. Kraszewski AP, Chow SB, Lenhoff MW, et al. The effect of foot type on plantar loading. 2010. Available at: http://www.asbweb.org/conferences/2010/abstracts/491.pdf. Accessed 07/20, 2012.
25. Mueller MJ, Host JV, Norton BJ. Navicular drop as a composite measure of excessive pronation. *J Am Podiatr Med Assoc* 1993;4:198–202.
26. Baggett BD, Young G. Ankle joint dorsiflexion. establishment of a normal range. *J Am Podiatr Med Assoc* 1993;5:251–254.
27. Udupa JK, Hirsch BE, Hillstrom HJ, et al. Analysis of in vivo 3-D internal kinematics of the joints of the foot. *IEEE Trans Biomed Eng* 1998;11:1387–1396.
28. Schwarz NA, Kovaleski JE, Heitman RJ, et al. Arthrometric measurement of ankle-complex motion: Normative values. *J Athl Train* 2011;2:126–132.
29. Bluman EM, Title CI, Myerson MS. Posterior tibial tendon rupture: A refined classification system. *Foot Ankle Clin* 2007;2:233–249.
30. Arangio GA, Chen C, Salathe EP. Effect of varying arch height with and without the plantar fascia on the mechanical properties of the foot. *Foot Ankle Int* 1998;10:705–709.
31. Buell T, Green DR, Risser J. Measurement of the first metatarsophalangeal joint range of motion. *J Am Podiatr Med Assoc* 1988;9:439–448.
32. Hopson MM, McPoil TG, Cornwall MW. Motion of the first metatarsophalangeal joint. reliability and validity of four measurement techniques. *J Am Podiatr Med Assoc* 1995;4: 198–204.
33. Joseph J, Nightingale A. Electromyography of muscles of posture: Leg and thigh muscles in women, including the effects of high heels. *J Physiol* 1956;3:465–468.
34. Mann RA, Hagy JL. The function of the toes in walking, jogging and running. *Clin Orthop Relat Res* 1979;142:24–29.
35. Shereff MJ, Bejjani FJ, Kummer FJ. Kinematics of the first metatarsophalangeal joint. *J Bone Joint Surg Am* 1986;3:392–398.
36. Van Gheluwe B, Dananberg HJ, Hagman F, et al. Effects of hallux limitus on plantar foot pressure and foot kinematics during walking. *J Am Podiatr Med Assoc* 2006;5:428–436.
37. Muscarella V, Hetherington VJ. Hallux limitus and hallux rigidus. In: Hetherington VJ, ed. *Hallux Valgus and Forefoot Surgery.* 1st ed. London: Churchill Livingstone; 1994:313–325.
38. Saxena A. The valenti procedure for hallux limitus/rigidus. *J Foot Ankle Surg* 1995;5: 485–488; discussion 511
39. Gogia PP, Braatz JH. Validity and reliability of leg length measurements. *J Orthop Sports Phys Ther* 1986;4:185–188.
40. Rondon CA, Gonzalez N, Agreda L, et al. Observer agreement in the measurement of leg length. *Rev Invest Clin* 1992;1:85–89.
41. Cleveland RH, Kushner DC, Ogden MC, et al. Determination of leg length discrepancy. A comparison of weight-bearing and supine imaging. *Invest Radiol* 1988;4:301–304.
42. Beattie P, Isaacson K, Riddle DL, et al. Validity of derived measurements of leg-length differences obtained by use of a tape measure. *Phys Ther* 1990;3:150–157.
43. Dahl MT. Limb length discrepancy. *Pediatr Clin North Am* 1996;4:849–865.
44. Kaufman KR, Miller LS, Sutherland DH. Gait asymmetry in patients with limb-length inequality. *J Pediatr Orthop* 1996;2:144–150.
45. Kendall FP. McCreary EK, Provance PG and Rodgers MM. *Muscles: Testing and Function with Posture and Pain.* 5th ed. Baltimore, MD: Lippincott Williams & Wilkins; 2005.
46. Song J, Hillstrom HJ, Secord D, et al. Foot type biomechanics. comparison of planus and rectus foot types. *J Am Podiatr Med Assoc* 1996;1:16–23.
47. Hillstrom HJ, Song J, Kraszewski AP, et al. Foot type biomechanics part 1: Structure and function of the asymptomatic foot. *Gait Posture In Review.*
48. Menz HB. Alternative techniques for the clinical assessment of foot pronation. *J Am Podiatr Med Assoc* 1998;3:119–129.
49. McPoil TG, Cornwall MW, Vicenzino B, et al. Effect of using truncated versus total foot length to calculate the arch height ratio. *Foot (Edinb)* 2008;4:220–227.
50. Menz HB, Munteanu SE. Validity of 3 clinical techniques for the measurement of static foot posture in older people. *J Orthop Sports Phys Ther* 2005;8:479–486.
51. Scharfbillig R, Evans AM, Copper AW, et al. Criterion validation of four criteria of the foot posture index. *J Am Podiatr Med Assoc* 2004;1:31–38.
52. Murley GS, Menz HB, Landorf KB. A protocol for classifying normal- and flat-arched foot posture for research studies using clinical and radiographic measurements. *J Foot Ankle Res* 2009;4:22–34.

53. Christman RA. Foot segmental relationships and bone morphology. In: *Foot and Ankle Radiology*. 1st ed. St. Louis, MO: Churchill Livingstone; 2003:272–299.
54. Cavanagh PR, Morag E, Boulton AJ, et al. The relationship of static foot structure to dynamic foot function. *J Biomech* 1997;3:243–250.
55. Zifchock RA, Davis IS, Hillstrom HJ, et al. The effect of gender, age, and lateral dominance on arch height and arch stiffness. *Foot Ankle Int* 2006;5:367–372.
56. Williams DS,3rd, McClay IS, Hamill J. Arch structure and injury patterns in runners. *Clin Biomech (Bristol, Avon)* 2001;4:341–347.
57. Simkin A, Leichter I, Giladi M, et al. Combined effect of foot arch structure and an orthotic device on stress fractures. *Foot Ankle* 1989;1:25–29
58. Franco AH. Pes cavus and pes planus: Analyses and treatment. *Phys Ther* 1987;5:688–694.
59. Funk DA, Cass JR, Johnson KA. Acquired adult flat foot secondary to posterior tibial-tendon pathology. *J Bone Joint Surg Am* 1986;1:95–102.
60. Rao S, Song J, Kraszewski AP, et al. The effect of foot structure on 1st metatarsophalangeal joint flexibility and hallucal loading. *Gait Posture* 2011;1:131–137.
61. Ledoux WR, Hillstrom HJ. The distributed plantar vertical force of neutrally aligned and pes planus feet. *Gait Posture* 2002;1:1–9.
62. Glasoe WM, Nuckley DJ, Ludewig PM. Hallux valgus and the first metatarsal arch segment: A theoretical biomechanical perspective. *Phys Ther* 2010;1:110–120.
63. Mahiquez MY, Wilder FV, Stephens HM. Positive hindfoot valgus and osteoarthritis of the first metatarsophalangeal joint. *Foot Ankle Int* 2006;12:1055–1059.
64. Katoh Y, Chao EY, Laughman RK, et al. Biomechanical analysis of foot function during gait and clinical applications. *Clin Orthop Relat Res* 1983;177:23–33.
65. Canseco K, Long J, Marks R, et al. Quantitative characterization of gait kinematics in patients with hallux rigidus using the Milwaukee foot model. *J Orthop Res* 2008;4: 419–427.
66. Brodsky JW, Baum BS, Pollo FE, et al. Prospective gait analysis in patients with first metatarsophalangeal joint arthrodesis for hallux rigidus. *Foot Ankle Int* 2007;2:162–165.
67. Rankine L, Long J, Canseco K, et al. Multisegmental foot modeling: A review. *Crit Rev Biomed Eng* 2008;2:127–181.
68. Deschamps K, Staes F, Roosen P, et al. Body of evidence supporting the clinical use of 3D multisegment foot models: A systematic review. *Gait Posture* 2011;3:338–349.
69. Kitaoka HB, Crevoisier XM, Hansen D, et al. Foot and ankle kinematics and ground reaction forces during ambulation. *Foot Ankle Int* 2006;10:808–813.
70. Carson MC, Harrington ME, Thompson N, et al. Kinematic analysis of a multi-segment foot model for research and clinical applications: A repeatability analysis. *J Biomech* 2001;10: 1299–1307.
71. Kidder SM, Abuzzahab FS Jr, Harris GF, et al. A system for the analysis of foot and ankle kinematics during gait. *IEEE Trans Rehabil Eng* 1996;1:25–32.
72. Leardini A, Benedetti MG, Berti L, et al. Rear-foot, mid-foot and fore-foot motion during the stance phase of gait. *Gait Posture* 2007;3:453–462.
73. De Mits S, Segers V, Woodburn J, et al. A clinically applicable six-segmented foot model. *J Orthop Res* 2012;4:655–661.
74. Caravaggi P, Benedetti MG, Berti L, et al. Repeatability of a multi-segment foot protocol in adult subjects. *Gait Posture* 2011;1:133–135.
75. Deschamps K, Staes F, Bruyninckx H, et al. Repeatability in the assessment of multi-segment foot kinematics. *Gait Posture* 2012;2:255–260.
76. Stebbins J, Harrington M, Thompson N, et al. Repeatability of a model for measuring multi-segment foot kinematics in children. *Gait Posture* 2006;4:401–410.
77. Curtis DJ, Bencke J, Stebbins JA, et al. Intra-rater repeatability of the oxford foot model in healthy children in different stages of the foot roll over process during gait. *Gait Posture* 2009;1:118–121.
78. Wright CJ, Arnold BL, Coffey TG, et al. Repeatability of the modified oxford foot model during gait in healthy adults. *Gait Posture* 2011;1:108–112.
79. Saraswat P, Macwilliams BA, Davis RB. A multi-segment foot model based on anatomically registered technical coordinate systems: Method repeatability in pediatric feet. *Gait Posture* 2012;4:547–555.
80. Telfer S, Morlan G, Hyslop E, et al. A novel device for improving marker placement accuracy. *Gait Posture* 2010;4:536–539.
81. Sawacha Z, Cristoferi G, Guarneri G, et al. Characterizing multisegment foot kinematics during gait in diabetic foot patients. *J Neuroeng Rehabil* 2009;6:37.
82. Hyslop E, Woodburn J, McInnes IB, et al. A reliability study of biomechanical foot function in psoriatic arthritis based on a novel multi-segmented foot model. *Gait Posture* 2010;4:619–626.
83. Long JT, Eastwood DC, Graf AR, et al. Repeatability and sources of variability in multicenter assessment of segmental foot kinematics in normal adults. *Gait Posture* 2010;1:32–36.
84. Woodburn J, Nelson KM, Siegel KL, et al. Multisegment foot motion during gait: Proof of concept in rheumatoid arthritis. *J Rheumatol* 2004;10:1918–1927.
85. Bruening DA, Cooney KM, Buczek FL. Analysis of a kinetic multi-segment foot model. part I: Model repeatability and kinematic validity. *Gait Posture* 2012;4:529–534.
86. Umberger BR, Nawoczenski DA, Baumhauer JF. Reliability and validity of first metatarsophalangeal joint orientation measured with an electromagnetic tracking device. *Clin Biomech (Bristol, Avon)* 1999;1:74–76.
87. Myers KA, Wang M, Marks RM, et al. Validation of a multisegment foot and ankle kinematic model for pediatric gait. *IEEE Trans Neural Syst Rehabil Eng* 2004;1:122–130.
88. Nester CJ. Lessons from dynamic cadaver and invasive bone pin studies: Do we know how the foot really moves during gait?. *J Foot Ankle Res* 2009;2:18
89. Okita N, Meyers SA, Challis JH, et al. An objective evaluation of a segmented foot model. *Gait Posture* 2009;1:27–34.
90. Shultz R, Kedgley AE, Jenkyn TR. Quantifying skin motion artifact error of the hindfoot and forefoot marker clusters with the optical tracking of a multi-segment foot model using single-plane fluoroscopy. *Gait Posture* 2011;1:44–48.
91. Nester C, Jones RK, Liu A, et al. Foot kinematics during walking measured using bone and surface mounted markers. *J Biomech* 2007;15:3412–3423.
92. Wolf P, Stacoff A, Liu A, et al. Functional units of the human foot. *Gait Posture* 2008;3:434–441.
93. Hu Y, Ledoux WR, Fassbind M, et al. Multi-rigid image segmentation and registration for the analysis of joint motion from three-dimensional magnetic resonance imaging. *J Biomech Eng* 2011;10:101005.
94. Hillstrom HJ, Perlberg G, Siegler S, et al. Objective identification of ankle equinus deformity and resulting contracture. *J Am Podiatr Med Assoc* 1991;10:519–524.
95. Buczek FL, Walker MR, Rainbow MJ, et al. Impact of mediolateral segmentation on a multi-segment foot model. *Gait Posture* 2006;4:519–522.
96. MacWilliams BA, Cowley M, Nicholson DE. Foot kinematics and kinetics during adolescent gait. *Gait Posture* 2003;3:214–224.
97. Bruening DA, Cooney KM, Buczek FL. Analysis of a kinetic multi-segment foot model part II: Kinetics and clinical implications. *Gait Posture* 2012;4:535–540.
98. Stokes IA, Hutton WC, Stott JR. Forces acting on the metatarsals during normal walking. *J Anat* 1979;3:579–590.
99. Bohm I, Landsiedl F. Revision surgery after failed unicompartmental knee arthroplasty: A study of 35 cases. *J Arthroplasty* 2000;8:982–989.
100. Wong L, Hunt A, Burns J, et al. Effect of foot morphology on center-of-pressure excursion during barefoot walking. *J Am Podiatr Med Assoc* 2008;2:112–117.
101. Marx RC, Mizel MS. What's new in foot and ankle surgery. *J Bone Joint Surg Am* 2008;4: 928–942.
102. SooHoo NF, Shuler M, Fleming LL, et al. Evaluation of the validity of the AOFAS clinical rating systems by correlation to the SF-36. *Foot Ankle Int* 2003;1:50–55.
103. Saltzman CL, Domsic RT, Baumhauer JF, et al. Foot and ankle research priority: Report from the research council of the American orthopaedic foot and ankle society. *Foot Ankle Int* 1997;7:447–448.
104. Hale SA, Hertel J. Reliability and sensitivity of the foot and ankle disability index in subjects with chronic ankle instability. *J Athl Train* 2005;1:35–40.
105. Riskowski JL, Hagedorn TJ, Hannan MT. Measures of foot function, foot health, and foot pain: American academy of orthopedic surgeons lower limb outcomes assessment: Foot and ankle module (AAOS-FAM), Bristol foot score (BFS), revised foot function index (FFI-R), foot health status questionnaire (FHSQ), Manchester foot pain and disability index (MFPDI), podiatric health questionnaire (PHQ), and rowan foot pain assessment (ROFPAQ). *Arthritis Care Res* 2011;11:S229–S239.
106. Martin RL, Burdett RG, Irrgang JJ. Development of the foot and ankle disability index (FADI). *J Orthop Sports Phys Ther* 1999;A32–A33.
107. Budiman-Mak E, Conrad KJ, Roach KE. The foot function index: A measure of foot pain and disability. *J Clin Epidemiol* 1991;6:561–570.
108. Agel J, Beskin JL, Brage M, et al. Reliability of the foot function index: A report of the AOFAS outcomes committee. *Foot Ankle Int* 2005;11:962–967.
109. Saag KG, Saltzman CL, Brown CK, et al. The foot function index for measuring rheumatoid arthritis pain: Evaluating side-to-side reliability. *Foot Ankle Int* 1996;8:506–510.
110. Domsic RT, Saltzman CL. Ankle osteoarthritis scale. *Foot Ankle Int* 1998;7:466–471.
111. Mootanah R, Song J, Kraszewski AP, et al. Foot type biomechanics part 2: Is structure and anthropometrics related to function?. *Gait Posture In review.*
112. Baumhauer J. Adult flatfoot: Posterior tendon dysfunction-pathologic anatomy. *Foot Ankle Clin* 1997;2:217–225.
113. Kohls-Gatzoulis J, Angel JC, Singh D, et al. Tibialis posterior dysfunction: A common and treatable cause of adult acquired flatfoot. *BMJ* 2004;7478:1328–1333.
114. Lapidus PW. Misconceptions about the "springiness" of the longitudinal arch of the foot: Mechanics of the arch of the foot. *Arch Surg* 1943;3:410–421.
115. Rabbito M, Pohl MB, Humble N, et al. Biomechanical and clinical factors related to stage I posterior tibial tendon dysfunction. *J Orthop Sports Phys Ther* 2011;10:776–784.
116. Shibuya N, Ramanujam CL, Garcia GM. Association of tibialis posterior tendon pathology with other radiographic findings in the foot: A case-control study. *J Foot Ankle Surg* 2008;6: 546–553.
117. Alvarez RG, Marini A, Schmitt C, et al. Stage I and II posterior tibial tendon dysfunction treated by a structured nonoperative management protocol: An orthosis and exercise program. *Foot Ankle Int* 2006;1:2–8.
118. Houck JR, Nomides C, Neville CG, et al. The effect of stage II posterior tibial tendon dysfunction on deep compartment muscle strength: A new strength test. *Foot Ankle Int* 2008;9:895–902.
119. Imhauser CW, Siegler S, Abidi NA, et al. The effect of posterior tibialis tendon dysfunction on the plantar pressure characteristics and the kinematics of the arch and the hindfoot. *Clin Biomech (Bristol, Avon)* 2004;2:161–169.
120. Tome J, Nawoczenski DA, Flemister A, et al. Comparison of foot kinematics between subjects with posterior tibialis tendon dysfunction and healthy controls. *J Orthop Sports Phys Ther* 2006;9:635–644.
121. Bascarevic ZL, Vukasinovic ZS, Bascarevic VD, et al. Hallux valgus. *Acta Chir Iugosl* 2011;3: 107–111.
122. Perera AM, Mason L, Stephens MM. The pathogenesis of hallux valgus. *J Bone Joint Surg Am* 2011;17:1650–1661.
123. Myerson MS, Badekas A, Schon LC. Treatment of stage II posterior tibial tendon deficiency with flexor digitorum longus tendon transfer and calcaneal osteotomy. *Foot Ankle Int* 2004;7:445–450.
124. Shurnas PS. Hallux rigidus: Etiology, biomechanics, and nonoperative treatment. *Foot Ankle Clin* 2009;1:1–8.
125. Deschamps K, Birch I, Desloovere K, et al. The impact of hallux valgus on foot kinematics: A cross-sectional, comparative study. *Gait Posture* 2010;1:102–106
126. Canseco K, Rankine L, Long J, et al. Motion of the multisegmental foot in hallux valgus. *Foot Ankle Int* 2010;2:146–152.
127. Martinez-Nova A, Sanchez-Rodriguez R, Perez-Soriano P, et al. Plantar pressures determinants in mild hallux valgus. *Gait Posture* 2010;3:425–427.
128. Mickle KJ, Munro BJ, Lord SR, et al. Gait, balance and plantar pressures in older people with toe deformities. *Gait Posture* 2011;3:347–351.

129. CDC - 2011 National Estimates - 2011 National diabetes fact sheet - publications - diabetes DDT. Available at: http://www.cdc.gov/diabetes/pubs/estimates11.htm. Accessed 06/05/2012.
130. Reiber GE, Boyko EJ, Smith DG. Lower extremity foot ulcers and amputations in diabetes. In: National Diabetes Data Group, National Institute of Diabetes and Digestive and Kidney Diseases, National Institutes of Health, eds. Diabetes in America. 2nd ed. Bethesda, MD.: National Institutes of Health, National Institute of Diabetes and Digestive and Kidney Diseases; 1995:409–428.
131. Kelly PJ, Coventry MB. Neurotrophic ulcers of the feet; review of forty-seven cases. *J Am Med Assoc* 1958;4:388–393.
132. Ctercteko GC, Dhanendran M, Hutton WC, et al. Vertical forces acting on the feet of diabetic patients with neuropathic ulceration. *Br J Surg* 1981;9:608–614.
133. Cavanagh PR, Sims DS, Jr, Sanders LJ. Body mass is a poor predictor of peak plantar pressure in diabetic men. *Diabetes Care* 1991;8:750–755.
134. Bevans JS. Biomechanics and plantar ulcers in diabetes. *Foot* 1992;3:166–172.
135. Lavery LA, Peters EJ, Williams JR, et al. Reevaluating the way we classify the diabetic foot: Restructuring the diabetic foot risk classification system of the international working group on the diabetic foot. *Diabetes Care* 2008;1:154–156.
136. Reiber GE, Vileikyte L, Boyko EJ, et al. Causal pathways for incident lower-extremity ulcers in patients with diabetes from two settings. *Diabetes Care* 1999;1:157–162.

CHAPTER

3

Jinsup Song
Rupali Joshi
Rajshree Mootanah
Smita Rao
Andrew P. Kraszewski
Sherry I. Backus
Howard J. Hillstrom

Plantar Pressure Assessment of the Athlete

INTRODUCTION

Our feet serve as the interface between our bodies and the ground. The athlete challenges this interface with squatting, jumping, absorbing shock when landing from a jump, running, and pivoting during rapid changes in direction. Plantar pressures, in conjunction with a comprehensive clinical examination to assess foot structure and function, can assist with differential diagnosis, provide understanding of pathology onset and progression, assist with treatment planning, and document the efficacy of surgical and conservative treatment for the management of pedal pathologies of an athletic nature. The purpose of this chapter is to review basic plantar pressure measurement principles, describe how this information can bring clarity to sports-related pedal pathologies, examine clinical indications for pressure measurements, and discuss cases of athletic injuries of the foot and ankle.

PLANTAR PRESSURE MEASUREMENT DEFINITIONS

PRESSURE

Pressure is force per unit area (Fig. 3.1, left). Plantar forces range from about 50% of body weight (BW) for quiet, bipedal standing up to 500% BW for running. Almost all plantar pressure measurement devices measure only vertical force. *Area* is the size of the region of the plantar foot that makes contact with the ground. The area of each sensor defines the *resolution* of the measurement system, which can affect the magnitude of pressure that the system can detect. For example, if 50 newtons (N) of force are applied to a transducer with a 1×1 cm^2 area, then 50 N/cm^2 of pressure will result. If 50 N of force is distributed in different amounts ranging from 5 N to 30 N over four transducers with a 0.5×0.5 cm^2 area then the resulting pressures will range from 20 N/cm^2 to 120 N/cm^2 (Fig. 3.1, right). The SI unit of force is the newton (the force required to give a mass of 1 kg an acceleration of 1 m/s^2) and the corresponding pressure unit is the pascal (1 N/m^2). Since plantar pressures result from hundreds of newtons distributed over a fraction of a square meter, the results are most often expressed in kilopascals (1 kPa = 1,000 Pa) and megapascals (1 MPa = 1,000,000 Pa). Several other units of pressure have been employed including kilograms per square centimeter (1 kg/cm^2 = 98.1 kPa) and pounds per square inch (1 psi = 6.9 kPa).

From a clinical perspective, excessive pressure, or stress, may be one of the more destructive antagonists to both external (plantar foot) and internal (cartilage within a joint) soft tissues. To illustrate the relationship between force and area for the development of pressure, consider a 600 N woman standing barefoot upon a plantar pressure measurement device (Fig. 3.2, top left). The peak pressure from her BW is <20 N/cm^2 and located beneath her rearfoot (Fig. 3.2, bottom left). If this same woman is wearing high heels (Fig. 3.2, top right), the pressure measured beneath the high heel on the ground is 127 N/cm^2 (Fig. 3.2, bottom right), effectively the maximum value recordable by this plantar pressure measurement device. The force did not change (50% BW) but the area beneath her rearfoot went from ~30 cm^2 when barefoot to ~1.5 cm^2 beneath the high heel. Fortunately, this excessive pressure beneath the high heel is not directly transferred to the plantar surface of the foot. The increased area of contact between the inside of the shoe and the foot effectively distributes the load and thus reduces the stress to plantar tissues. In addition, wearing high heels increases forefoot loading and stress to tissues in the toe-box region of the shoe (1,2). As a consequence, epidemiologists have found increased pain associated with the use of poor shoes (e.g., high heels) and a decreased use of such shoes with each decade of life (1).

CENTER OF PRESSURE

The *center of pressure* (COP) is the centroid or spatial average at any one instant in time of all the pressures measured beneath the foot. The COP is a function of the magnitude and area of loaded force sensors. At heel strike (or initial contact), the COP of an asymptomatic individual is typically located just lateral to the center of the heel (Fig. 3.3). As the gait cycle continues through loading response, for the first 50 msec of stance phase, initial pronation occurs and the COP travels medially. The individual with a rectus, or well-aligned foot, will then begin to resupinate as midfoot and/or forefoot loading occur and midstance begins. The COP moves anterior and lateral throughout

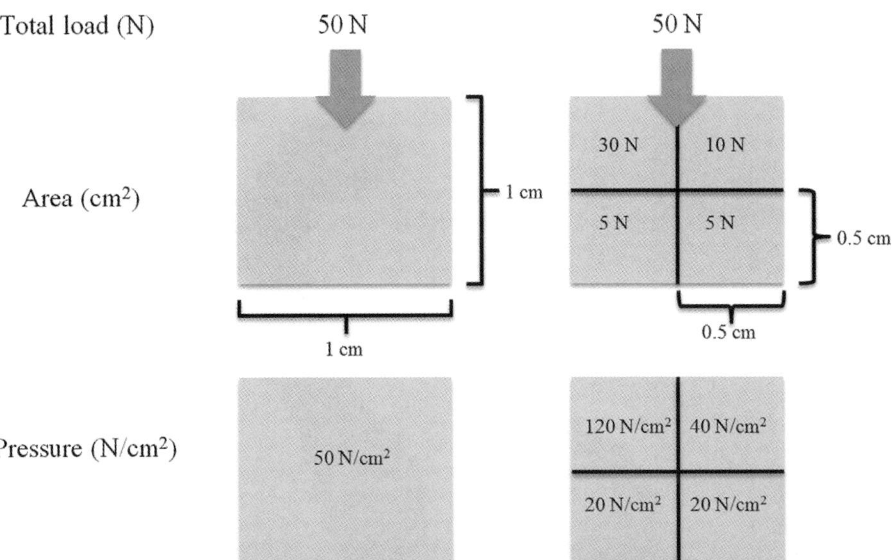

Figure 3.1. Plantar Pressure and Resolution. Pressure is force per unit area. The measurement of pressure may be quite different for transducers of different areas (resolution).

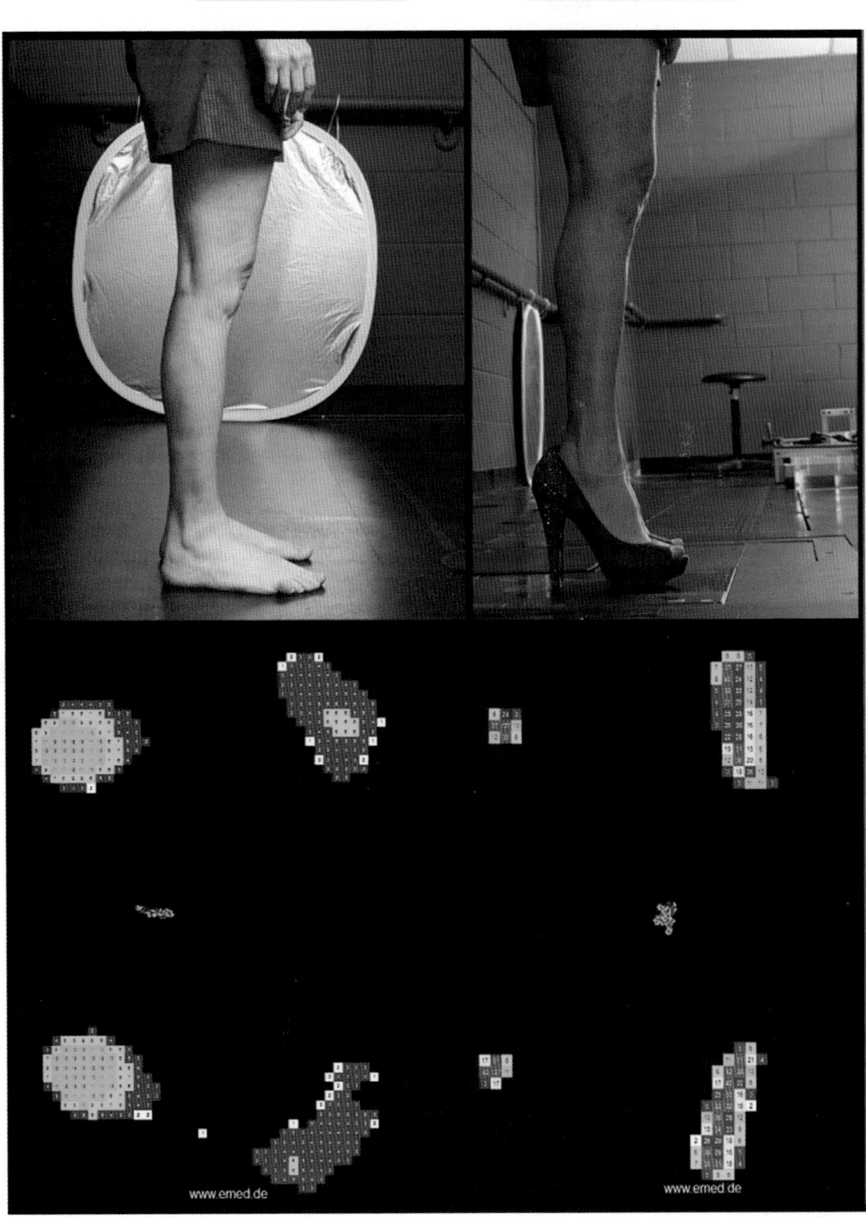

Figure 3.2. Pressure Beneath the Bare Foot vs a High Heel. The spike high heel results in concentrated loads on the ground that exceed the maximum measurement capability (saturation) of the plantar pressure measuring device (127N/cm^2).

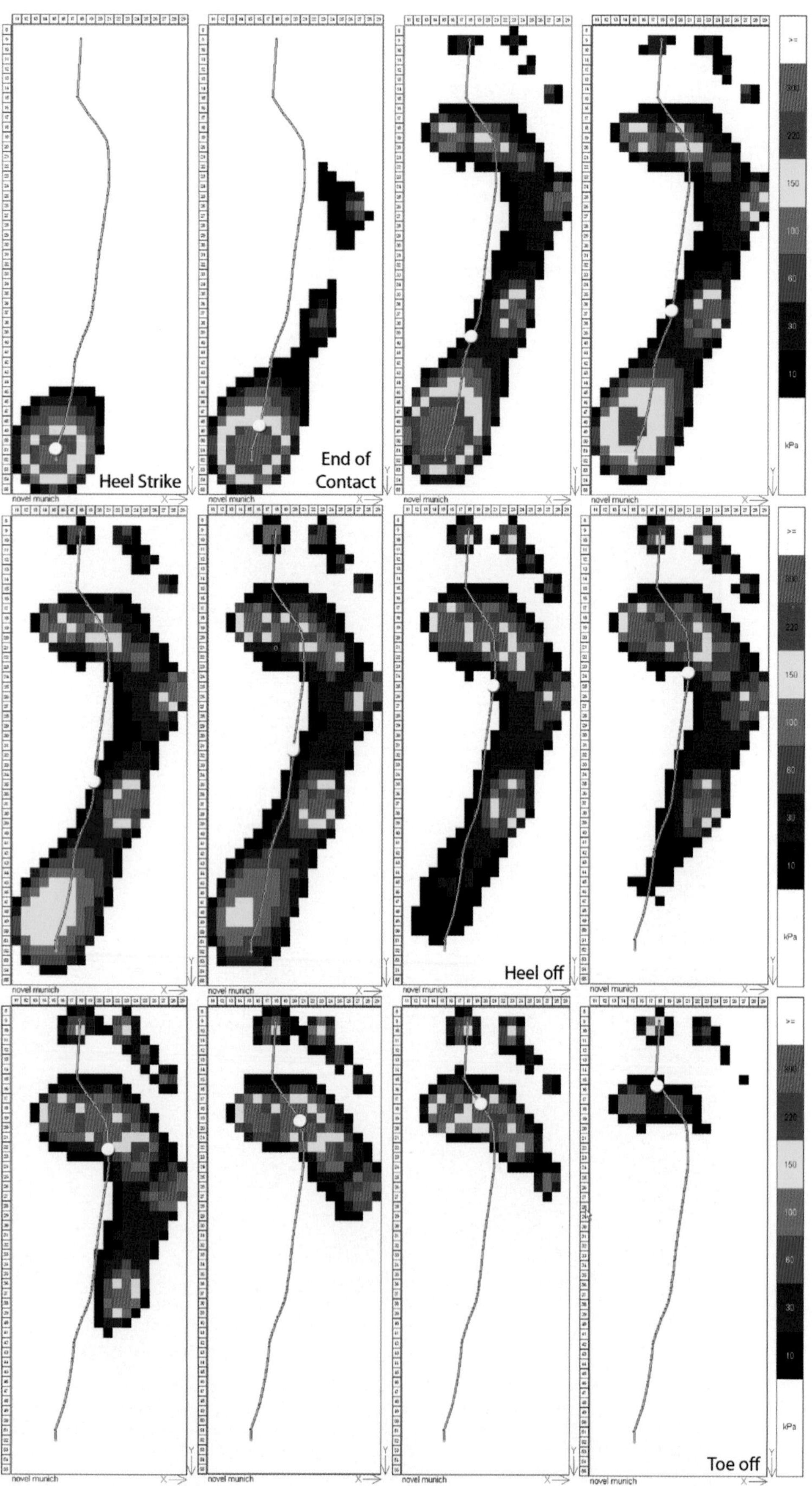

Figure 3.3. Plantar Pressures and the Center of Pressure throughout Stance Phase. Plantar pressures and the center of pressure (white dot) are depicted for an entire stance phase beginning with heel strike and ending with toe off.

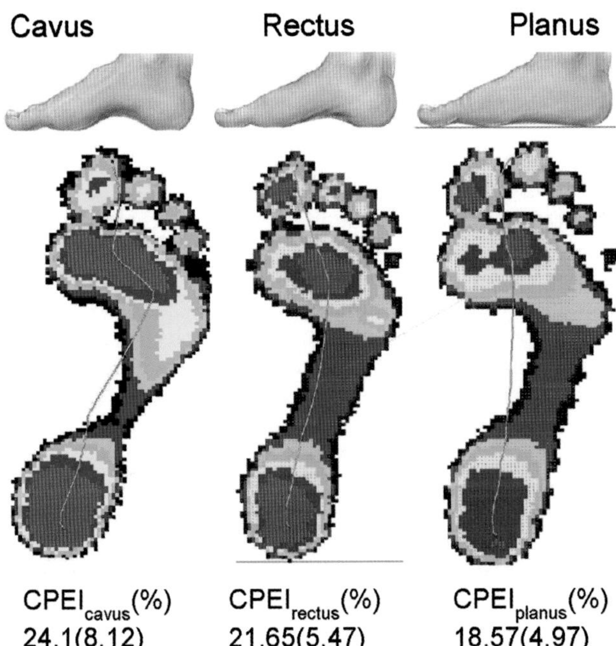

Figure 3.4. Center of Pressure Excursion Index (CPEI) Across Foot Types. Mean CPEI values are displayed for individuals with cavus, rectus, and planus foot types (61 subjects, 122 feet).

midstance. At heel off, the beginning of propulsion, the forefoot loads increase and the COP moves anteriorly and medially. At toe off, the end of stance phase, the COP moves between the first and second digits.

As illustrated in Figure 3.3, the COP moves in a concave pattern throughout stance phase from heel strike (or initial contact) to toe off. The center of pressure excursion index (CPEI), (see Chapter 2) is a measure of the degree of COP concavity. As a dynamic measure of foot function, CPEI has demonstrated sensitivity to foot type (Fig. 3.4) (3). Individuals with cavus feet (high-arched feet) typically oversupinate, have a large CPEI value, and the origin of the ground reaction force vector moves towards the lateral border of the foot (4). Such a loading profile may predispose an individual to lateral ligament injuries (5). Individuals with planus feet (flat feet) typically overpronate, have smaller CPEI values, and have a ground reaction force that is closer to the medial border of the foot (4). Pathologies involving the medial structures of the foot (e.g., hallux valgus, first metatarsal–phalangeal joint osteoarthritis [OA]) may be more prevalent under these loading conditions (6,7).

Since many pedal pathologies in athletes are related to overuse, a systematic method to study how plantar loads are distributed is important. A 12-segment mask (a scalable geometrically based template) has been developed to permit standardized calculations of plantar loading for specifically defined anatomical structures or "masked region" of the plantar foot (Fig. 3.5). A radiographic-based validation study confirmed that each region appropriately represents its corresponding anatomical region (8). Loading parameters are calculated for each masked region. These parameters include peak plantar pressure (PP [N/cm^2]), maximum force (MF [N]), pressure–time integral (PTI [Ns/cm^2]), force–time integral (FTI [Ns]), and area (A

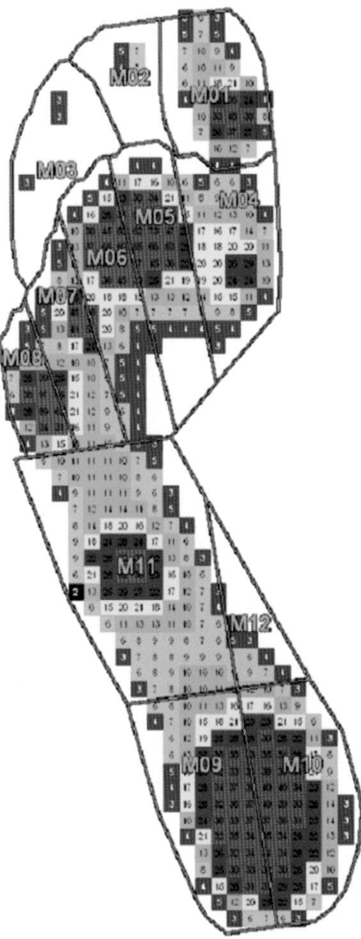

Figure 3.5. Masking Algorithm. A masking algorithm is used to geometrically separate regions of the plantar loading data that correspond to anatomical structures for automated analysis of physical quantities (pressure, force, area, etc.) in each masked region.

[cm^2]). Each parameter may be normalized by the maximum value throughout the entire foot as well. The choice of parameter used depends on the clinical question. For example, is it more of a risk to have a higher peak pressure acting over a short time or a lower one acting for a longer time?

PRESSURE TRANSDUCER PRINCIPLES

The most simplistic plantar pressure measurement technique is based upon the Harris–Beath mat (9). A rubber mat is stretched across a support frame covering an ink pad. The underside of the mat has ridges of three different heights. The largest ridges are visible when loaded with light pressures while the smaller ridges become visible only with increased pressure. The primary advantage of this approach is its low cost. The disadvantage is that only qualitative impressions of the highest plantar pressure locations were possible. A modern version of this concept (PressureStat®, Visual Footcare Technologies, New York, NY) uses a carbon paper–based system. Although not considered a transducer-based measurement of pressure, the clinician then has an archival record of the location of the highest plantar loads.

The majority of pressure transducers capable of measuring plantar forces per unit area are essentially force transducers that cover a defined area. In general applications, force is often detected as a displacement. As an example, an old-fashioned bathroom scale uses internal springs and the principle of Hooke's law:

$$F = kx,$$

where F is the force, k is the spring stiffness, and x is the displacement of the spring.

Plantar pressure transducers are typically much thinner than a physical spring-based system so that the sensors fit within a mat, a plate-based instrument, or a shoe. The most common transducers for measuring plantar pressures are force sensitive resistors (FSRs), strain gauges, piezoelectric transducers, optical transducers, and capacitive transducers.

FORCE SENSITIVE RESISTORS

An FSR is made of a conductive polymer whose resistance changes when a force is applied. Electrically conductive and non-conductive submicron-sized particles are homogenously dispersed as a polymer sheet or screen-printed ink. As the surface of the sensing film is loaded, these particles touch the conducting electrodes, which change the resistance of the film in proportion to the applied load. The advantages of FSRs in plantar pressure measurement devices are that the FSRs require a relatively simple electronic interface, are less expensive to produce compared with other transducers, can operate in hostile environments (e.g., increased temperature and humidity within a shoe), have good shock resistance, and are extremely thin (e.g., 0.5 mm). FSRs have several disadvantages when used in plantar pressure measurement devices. Shear loads (e.g., those experienced during gait) can disrupt the homogeneity of the conductive and non-conductive particles, which at best, alters the transducer's calibration and, at worst, damages the measuring devices. FSRs can also become damaged if pressure is applied for extended time periods (e.g., hours). In comparison to other force transducers (e.g., strain gauges, load cells, etc.), FSRs have relatively low precision so that repeated measurements can differ by 10% or more. FSRs exhibit a power law relationship between conductance (1/resistance) and applied load, which results in saturation at higher loading levels and necessitates more complex calibration strategies to be incorporated within plantar pressure measuring devices. Several companies have developed plantar pressure measuring plate and insole systems based upon the FSR including TekScan® (TekScan, Inc., South Boston, MA), Medilogic (T&T medilogic, Medizintechnik, Germany), and footscan® (RSscan INTERNATIONAL, Olen, Belgium).

STRAIN GAUGES

A strain gauge is an insulated flexible-backed device which supports a metallic foil in a "serpentine" pattern used to measure the strain (displacement under load) of an object. The gauge is typically affixed to the object by glue like cyanoacrylate. Under a compressive load, the object becomes thinner, the foil thickens, and the electrical resistance decreases. This resistance change is often measured using a Wheatstone-bridge circuit. Most strain gauge–based force technology can be very accurate and is used in several commercially available force plate systems (AMTI, Watertown, MA and Bertec Corporation, Columbus, OH). However, for the purpose of plantar pressure measurement, the expense associated with the development of a strain gauge matrix and the corresponding signal-processing circuits is prohibitive. Thus no systems using this approach are commercially available.

PIEZOELECTRIC TRANSDUCERS

Piezoelectric transducers translate small mechanical movements (vibrations) based on distortion of a crystal into an electrical charge. They are typically produced as semiconductor strain gauges for measurements using piezoresistors, which are often preferred over foil gauges. The piezoresistor transduces mechanical loads into varying resistances instead of voltages. Piezoresistive transducers are more sensitive to strain, but more expensive in cost, more sensitive to temperature changes, and more fragile than foil gauges. Semiconductor technology employs such crystals (germanium and silicon) in digital and analog circuits. Piezoresistive commercial devices such as pressure and acceleration transducers have been developed based upon these principles. The paroTec® (The London Orthotic Consultancy Ltd, Kinston upon Thames, Surrey, England) insole system, based upon piezoresistive transducers, measures plantar pressures within a shoe.

OPTICAL TRANSDUCERS

Optical transducers may also be employed for pressure measurement. One such device has a plastic interface with a dimpled undersurface placed upon an obliquely illuminated plate of glass (10). Beneath the glass is a mirror at 45 degrees, with the image on the mirror recorded by a video camera. As load is placed upon the plastic interface, more dimples are in contact with the glass so that the refracted light is proportional to the load. The advantage of this technology is that it has high resolution. The disadvantages are its bulky size and complex alignment calibration process. Although once commercially available, this technology is no longer manufactured.

CAPACITIVE TRANSDUCERS

Capacitive transducers are formed by two parallel conductive plates which are separated by a dielectric layer. When used as a pressure transducer, the force applied to the top plate compresses the dielectric material, brings the two plates closer together, and changes the capacitance. Hand-held digital multi-meters measure capacitances in the range 100 pF to 1 F with an accuracy of about 1% using a 2-lead approach. The current in a capacitor (I_c) is

$$I_c = C\, dV/dt,$$

where C is the unknown capacitance and dV/dt is the change in voltage with respect to time. The capacitance is calculated from the charging time required for the transducer to reach a threshold voltage in response to a constant current. The largest source of error is stray capacitance, typically in the range 10 pF to 10 nF. Stray capacitance can be minimized with cable- and chassis-shielding techniques. Capacitive sensors are the most precise of all electrical sensors and measure a wide range of loads for a moderate cost. A capacitor can be designed to be non-dissipative and therefore free of thermal noise, free from self-heating, linear with applied voltage, and temperature independent. Several manufacturers utilize capacitive transducers to measure plantar pressures in both plate and insole systems including Novel (Munich, Germany) and AM Cube (AM^3, Berkshire, UK).

There are many different transducer technologies that have been incorporated in plantar pressure measurement systems. The choice of system depends upon the application, performance requirements, and budget. In addition to current literature searches, manufacturers should be able to provide published accuracy (measurement error with respect to a gold standard) and reliability (repeatability) studies.

RATIONALE FOR ASSESSMENT OF PEDAL PATHOLOGIES

Plantar pressure assessment may be indicated to examine the effect of foot type, activity and shoes on plantar load distribution. In a large sample of asymptomatic, physically active individuals (n = 1,000), a multivariate regression model was developed to describe the association between dynamic plantar pressures and static foot posture ($R^2 = 0.32$) (11). Recent studies assessing loads at the foot–floor interface during a number of athletic tasks such as running, jumping, and cutting showed that sports-related movements load the plantar surface of the foot more than straight-ahead running (12). Footwear design, orthoses and taping have been shown to affect plantar load distribution. Queen et al. (13) reported increased maximum force, particularly at the lateral forefoot in racing flats. Similarly, augmented low-dye taping increased lateral midfoot loading (14). Lacing patterns can also influence plantar loading patterns (15–17). In a recent clinical trial, orthoses were effective in the prevention of lower-limb overuse injury in a military trainee population with an absolute risk reduction of 0.49 (16).

In addition to foot type, previous activity and injury may also affect load distribution. In a study evaluating 200 marathon runners, Nagel et al. (17) found that post-race peak pressure was higher in the forefoot regions and reduced under the toes. Individuals with chronic ankle instability demonstrated a more lateral loading pattern during barefoot running gait compared to individuals with a previous ankle sprain or asymptomatic controls (18). Increased lateral loading has also been hypothesized to predispose one to the risk of fifth metatarsal fractures (Jones fractures) (19). Conversely, lower middle forefoot loading has been reported in women with a previous fracture of the second metatarsal (20). While increased loading has been postulated to be related to increased injury risk and decreased loading may be indicative of pain avoidance or inadequate rehabilitation, no prospective studies have established the predictive value of plantar pressure.

PATHOLOGIES OF THE FOOT AND ANKLE DURING ATHLETICS AND SPORTS

TURF TOE

Turf toe is a sprain to the first metatarsal–phalangeal joint (MTPJ) (21) and is commonly seen in American football. Turf toe has also been reported in basketball, dancing, soccer, tennis, volleyball, and wrestling (22). The neck of the great toe is the weakest physiologic portion of the joint capsule (21). The common mechanism of injury is hyperextension (23) or increased flexion of the first toe beyond its biomechanical limits leading to capsular tears (24). Hyperextension of the forefoot may also result in injury to articular cartilage, subchondral bone, and fractures of the sesamoid bones (25). Turf toe results in decreased passive MTPJ dorsiflexion on goniometric measures and increased hallucial plantar pressure (26). Such measurements may help detect subtle and early alterations in first toe mechanics that may help clinicians to provide treatment aimed at preventing degradation to hallux rigidus or first MTPJ osteoarthritis (27–30). In a study of 44 professional football players, first MTPJ dorsiflexion was reduced and peak hallucial pressure increased (Fig. 3.6, bottom) in those athletes with turf toe compared to those without turf toe (Fig. 3.6, top) (26).

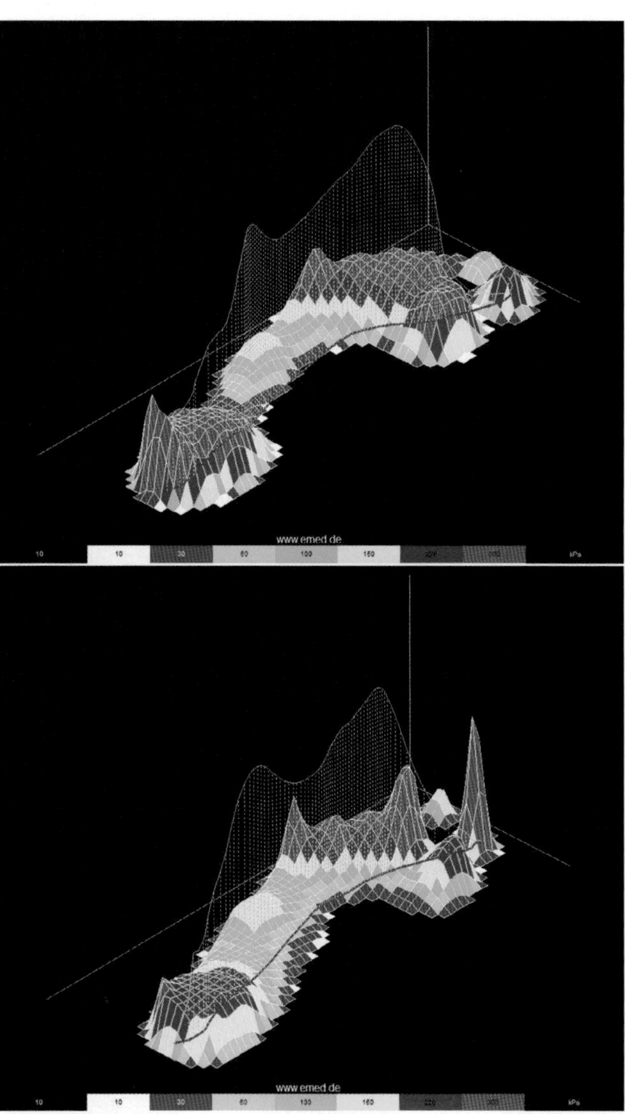

Figure 3.6. Plantar Loading in Football Players with and without Turf Toe. The top segment is the maximum pressure throughout stance phase for a professional football player without a history of turf toe. The bottom segment is the maximum pressure throughout stance phase for a professional football player with a history of turf toe. The change in 1st MTPJ function due to a turf toe injury typically reduces range of motion and increases hallucial loading.

PLANTAR FASCIITIS

Plantar fasciitis is a relatively common injury seen in running athletes with repetitive microtrauma or with limited dorsiflexion (31) and is also seen in obese individuals or those prone to prolonged standing (32). Cumulative overload stress in the form of excessive tensile loading (33,34) results in acute or chronic injury to the origin of the plantar fascia resulting in inferior heel pain on weight bearing and tenderness around the medial calcaneal tuberosity (35). Osteophytes ("heel spurs") may be present in individuals with plantar fasciitis (36) and are detected in plain radiographs. Radiographic osteophytes alone cannot be used as a diagnostic test for plantar fasciitis osteophytes as they are present in 15% to 25% of asymptomatic individuals and absent in many symptomatic individuals (37). Ultrasonography of the heel is particularly useful in confirming diagnosis (38), objectively measuring changes in the plantar-fascia structure (39), determining the response to treatment, and serving as a guide for placement of steroid injections (40,41). Goniometric measurement to determine ankle motion are important to prevent greater fascia stretching secondary to range of motion deficits of the plantar flexors (42). Plantar pressure measurement can detect high pressures under the arches and can influence orthotic recommendations to control loading in plantar fascia (32). Foot kinematics and kinetics may also be useful to monitor disease progression. Higher vertical peak forces and loading rates have been shown in female runners with a history of plantar fasciitis (43). Figure 3.7 depicts a typical pes planus individual with plantar fasciitis. The CPEI value is reduced and the medial arch bears load consistent with overpronation. One plausible mechanism for plantar fasciitis is excessive initial pronation (seen as a lateral COP at heel strike that moves medially in the first 50 ms of stance), reduction of arch height during midstance commensurate with a flexible flatfoot, and torsion about the long axis of the foot, all of which contribute to stretching the plantar fascia. This stretching causes an enthesopathy at the calcaneal insertion which is believed to be responsible for the symptom of pain (44). In-shoe orthoses can prevent the initial pronation, reduction in arch height, and excessive torsional loading at toe off, which may explain the 86.3% success rate in pain relief in individuals with plantar fasciitis (45).

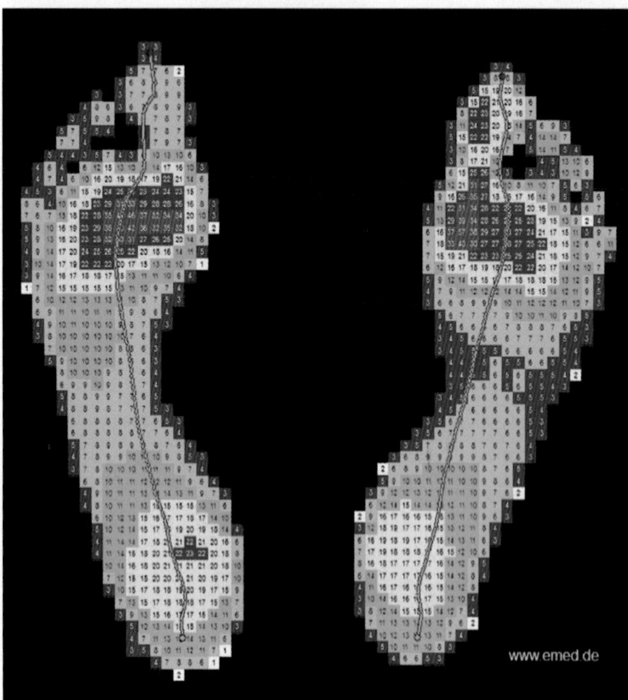

Figure 3.7. Plantar Loading in an Individual with Plantar Fasciitis. The maximum pressure throughout stance phase illustrates overpronation by the reduced CPEI and medial column loading which is consistent with an individual that overpronates.

POSTERIOR TIBIAL TENDON RUPTURE

Partial or complete tibialis posterior tendon rupture is rare in the younger athletic population (46,47), but when rupture occurs, it has a large functional impact. The posterior tibial tendon is a dynamic stabilizer of the hindfoot against eversion forces. Loss of tibialis posterior function puts increased stress on the static stabilizers of the hindfoot, i.e., the interosseous ligaments, thus impeding athletic activities demanding strong push-off action. An inability to perform a symmetric single-heel raise indicates functional loss of tibialis posterior (48). Progression of a partial rupture results in severe pes planus and forefoot pronation (49). Early diagnosis and intervention can help prevent further structural progression into a collapsing pes valgus. Quantitative measures, such as arch height index (AHI), CPEI, malleolar valgus index (MVI) (50) and peak pressure can document the state and progression of the foot with a partially or completely ruptured posterior tibial tendon (Fig. 3.8A). Typically in these individuals, resting calcaneal stance position (RCSP) is greater than 10-degree valgus, CPEI is less than 16% (which in extreme circumstances may be negative when the COP is convex [Fig. 3.8B]), and medial arch undergoes substantial loading. Potentially, these data may be used to customize orthosis, surgical, or rehabilitation therapy to prevent further deterioration of foot structure.

ACHILLES TENDINOSIS

While historically called Achilles tendinitis, this condition is more appropriately termed Achilles tendinosis after the histologic changes seen in the tendon (51). Achilles tendinosis is characterized by degenerative changes in the tendon (52) secondary to microtrauma or failure of this tissue leading to partial tears and subsequent symptoms (53). Apart from injuries, certain pedal pathologies such as hyperpronation (54,55) and limited subtalar joint mobility (56) predispose an athlete to increased risk of Achilles-tendon injuries. Post-injury changes include decreased dorsiflexion and altered dynamic plantar pressures (57) during gait.

Achilles tendinosis results in pain, usually localized to the middle third of the tendon, which is aggravated by dorsiflexion and results in limited ankle motion (58). It is important to note that a paradoxical increase in passive dorsiflexion can occur as a result of a severe degenerative process that results in repetitive partial ruptures (59). Goniometric measures, patient history and appropriate radiographic studies along with goniometric measures of ankle motion, subtalar joint neutral position on static examination with foot kinematics, CPEI, and plantar pressure distribution during gait provides objective

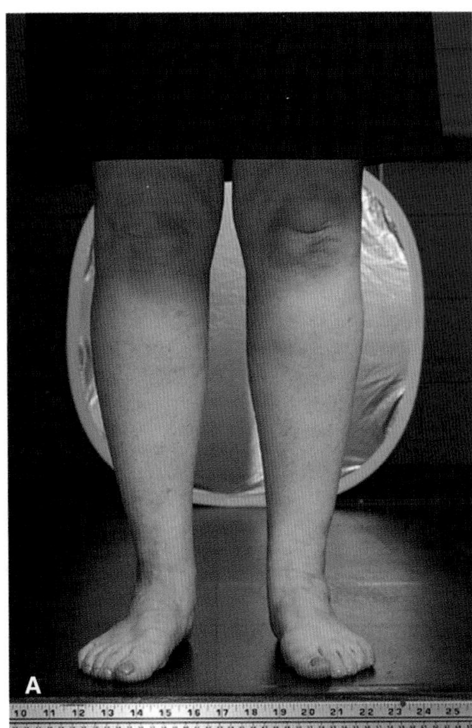

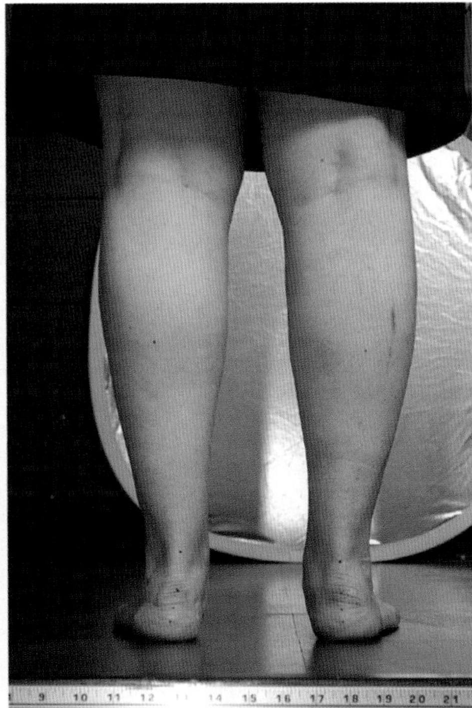

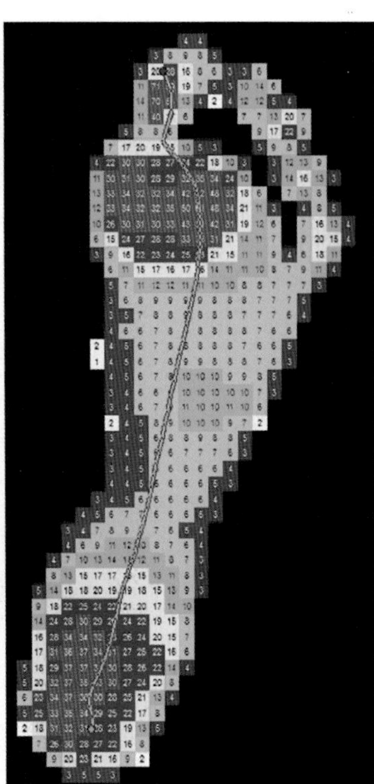

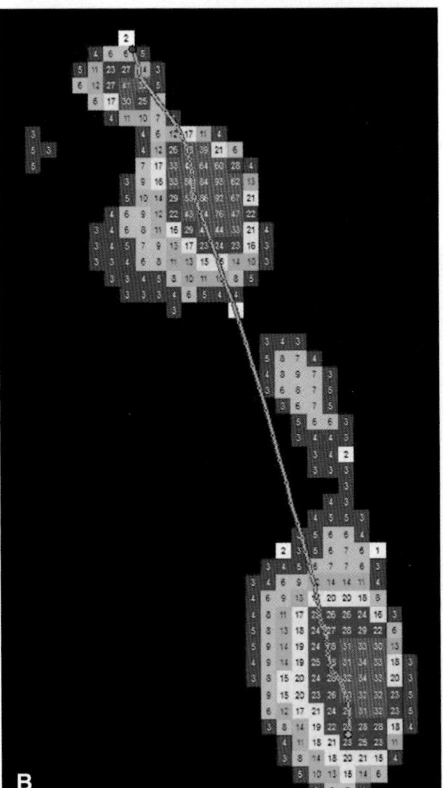

Figure 3.8. **A:** Individual with Posterior Tibial Tendon Insufficiency and Corresponding Plantar Pressures. The photographs illustrate the collapsing pes valgus posture (RCSP>10°) while the plantar pressure distribution demonstrates the significantly reduced CPEI consistent with moderately overpronating feet. **B:** Plantar Pressure Distribution for a Patient with Severe Posterior Tibial Dysfunction. This data is of the individual's left foot. CPEI is negative (convex instead of concave), the forefoot is markedly abducted, and the navicluar region of the medial midfoot is bearing load, which is consistent with severe overpronation.

assessment of the dysfunction to fully document the severity of the tendinosis.

In Figure 3.9 (left only), the COP pattern has oscillations throughout stance phase which are likely due to an antalgic gait. Note the increased loading at heel strike.

In the case of a complete Achilles-tendon rupture, a propulsive gait pattern is not possible. A 28-year-old male had a non-contact left Achilles-tendon rupture while playing basketball. Seven weeks' status post Achilles-tendon repair (Fig. 3.10), the patient still exhibits negligible forefoot loading.

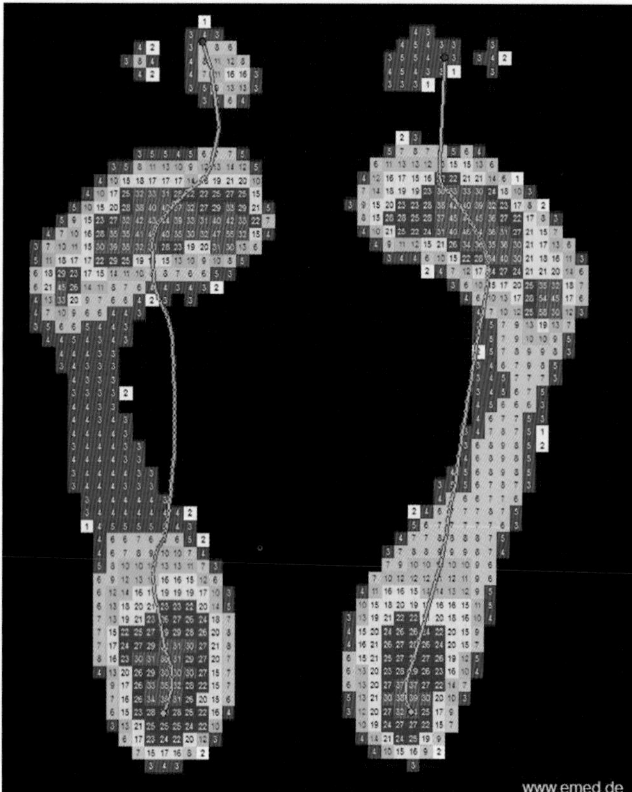

Figure 3.9. Plantar Pressure Distribution in a Patient with Achilles Tendonitis. The center of pressure pattern is oscillatory on the left foot probably due to an antalgic gait. Large pressures are present at heelstrike.

Return to symmetry may be considered a functional measure of recovery.

STRESS FRACTURES

Stress fractures are commonly seen in runners and often occur in the tibia, fibula, femur, metatarsals, tarsals, and sesamoid bones (35). Stress fractures could be a result of overuse or recent alterations in the training regimen. Individuals with stress fractures present with insidious onset of focal-bone tenderness (60). Since stress fractures take time (~13 weeks) to diagnose (35), an understanding of the foot structure, function, and training regimen that may make an athlete susceptible to developing this pathology is helpful. Individuals with high arches (cavus) are more likely to develop stress fractures than low-arched (planus) individuals (61). Tibial, femoral and fifth metatarsal fractures are more common with cavus, and second and third metatarsal injuries occur more frequently with a planus foot type (62). MVI, CPEI, and AHI can be useful tools to predict which individuals may be at risk for stress fractures. Radiographs, magnetic resonance imaging (MRI) and bone scans are commonly used diagnostic tools (35,60). Conservative management, along with shoe modifications and orthotics, is a common method of treatment (35,60).

LATERAL ANKLE SPRAINS

Lateral ankle sprains are one of the most common injuries among athletes and other young, active adults (63–68). Studies report that 10% to 30% of individuals with ankle sprains progress to chronic ankle instability (69,70). Lapointe et al. (71)

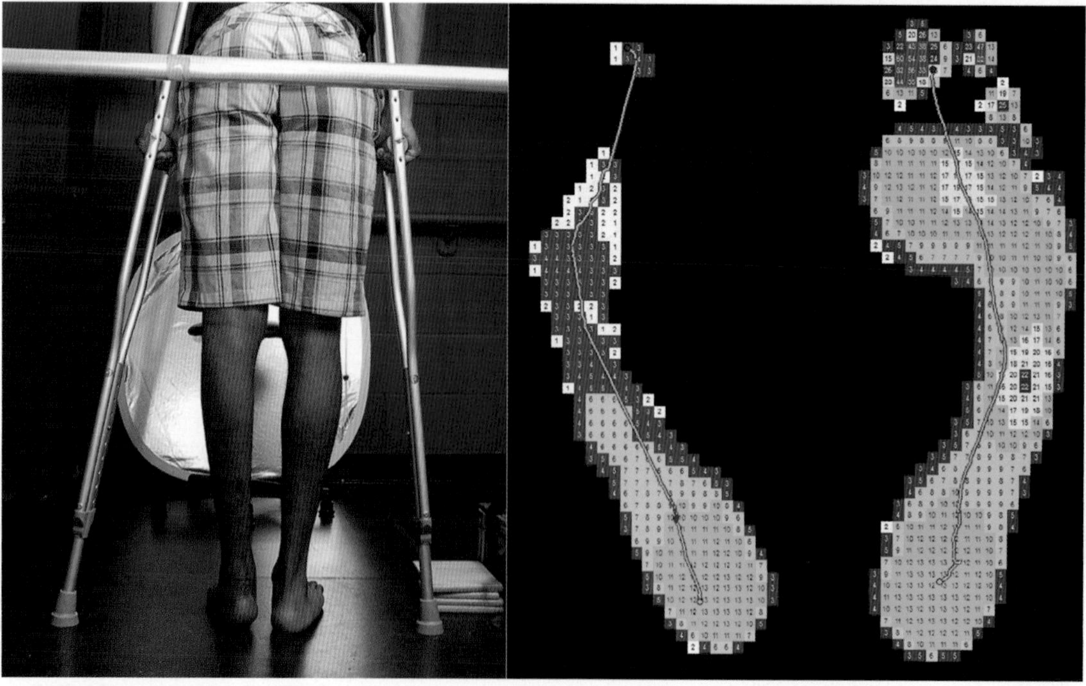

Figure 3.10. Achilles Tendon Rupture Repair. This patient is seven weeks status post Achilles tendon rupture repair.

used a six-degree-of-freedom instrumented linkage capable of measuring the flexibility characteristics of the ankle complex in vivo. In vivo flexibility testing was conducted on five patients with unilateral ankle ligament injuries and reported significant changes in patients with lateral ankle injuries. Functionally, individuals with chronic ankle instability may either have a cavus foot type or exhibit excessive supination as indicated by calcaneal varus and/or forefoot valgus with a larger CPEI value during gait (Fig. 3.4).

SPORTS-SPECIFIC CONSIDERATIONS

SPORTS-SPECIFIC SHOE DESIGNS

The rise in fitness and running activities in the early 1970s and resulting association with bone fractures (72) and soft tissue injuries (73,74) have triggered an increasing demand in research activities including footwear biomechanics to improve sports shoe design (75). Jogging has been associated with a number of lower-limb injuries including overuse or repetitive loading stress and stress fractures of the metatarsals (76,77). Two-thirds of chronic injuries have been attributed to high mileage, workout intensity and running on inclined and hard surfaces (78). Until the mid-1990s, research attempting to address sports injury through footwear design was purely mechanical and focused on lower-extremity kinematics (79), kinetics (80–83), energy dissipation (84,85), rearfoot stability (86), and the relationship between biomechanical parameters and injuries (87,88). Impact forces (83,89) and pressure (90) on the lower limbs associated with repetitive loading were found to be responsible for overuse injuries in the musculoskeletal system. Results of these studies led to shoe designs that reduced movement-related injuries by improving cushioning and rearfoot stability, minimizing impact loading and foot eversion, and guiding take-off inversion. As a result, sports shoes in the mid-1990s were built with stiff heel stabilizers and several "pronatory control" technologies, some of which may have actually increased eversion (91).

More recent footwear research has focused on additional sports activities, including soccer. Many newer studies have examined the interaction between the foot and the shoe for specific functional tasks (92,93) and included muscle activity instead of minimizing foot eversion (94), introduced comfort as an important functional variable (95), related impact loading to soft tissue vibrations and muscle tuning (96), and included the effects of speed and inclination on plantar pressure distribution (97,98). Butler et al. (99) studied kinematics and kinetics of 14 male and 14 female competitive soccer players while performing a jump head task when wearing three different footwear (running shoe, bladed cleat, and turf shoe). Their results suggest that landing mechanics are influenced by gender, footwear and type of landing and that sport-specific footwear should be taken into consideration to reduce lower-extremity injury (99). A similar study by Sims et al. (19) on 17 men and 17 women wearing the Nike Victoria® hard cleat during a side cut showed significantly higher force and FTI in men beneath the lateral midfoot and forefoot during the cross-over cut task, as well as in the middle forefoot during the side cut task. Results of this study could explain the higher incidence of fifth metatarsal stress fractures in men and suggest that gender differences in loading should be taken into consideration in footwear research (19).

Plantar pressure measurement has been used, sometimes in conjunction with other kinematics and kinetics measurements, in the assessment of sports shoe design. For example, plantar pressure and force plate measurements on different golf shoe outer sole design features during the golf swing on natural grass showed significant differences in torque generation at the back foot and back and front insole pressures (100). These studies suggest that gender differences, age, level of training and the types of sports activities should be considered during sports shoe design.

Ho et al. (97) reported that an increase in jogging speed resulted in an increase in maximum force and pressure under all foot regions as well as foot inversion during stance phase (97). In a barefoot walking investigation of 200 marathon runners, Nagel et al. (17) reported increased plantar pressures beneath the metatarsal heads (17). Fourchet and co-investigators (98) studied plantar pressure distribution in 11 highly trained adolescent runners at jogging [11.2 ± 0.9 km/hr] and running [17.8 ± 1.4 km/hr] pace on a treadmill. They reported an increase in relative load under the medial and central forefoot regions while jogging, suggesting that adolescent runners should avoid excessive mileage at jogging speed (98). One of the contemporary topics in running research today is whether shoe gear should be used at all.

BALLET: EN POINTE

Ballet is a highly challenging activity involving a unique balance of athleticism and artistry. In the classical ballet technique, *en pointe,* the dancer rises to the tips of other toes. Other ballet movements include full pointe (maximum plantarflexion of the forefoot, midfoot, and ankle joints with weight bearing on the tips of the great toes) and grande plie (foot flat with maximum dorsiflexion of the ankle and full knee flexion). The pressure beneath the hallux and shoe is increased when in en pointe or full pointe (Fig. 3.11). The ballerina is in the first position in her ballet slippers (Fig. 3.11, left) while her heels are on the ground as well as on the ball of her feet. The pressures between the slippers and the ground (Fig. 3.11, left middle) were measured with an emed-x (Novel, Munich, Germany) while the pressures between the foot and the slipper (Fig. 3.11, left bottom) were measured with the pedar-x (Novel, Munich, Germany). The same postures were performed while wearing pointe shoes (Fig. 3.11, right). The excessive pressures beneath the toes are clearly illustrated (Fig. 3.11, right bottom).

PLANTAR PRESSURES DURING BIKING

In order for a cyclist to be effective at producing crank power, the end effector—the foot—must allow effective power transmission from the hip, knee, and ankle. Given the task of cycling, the cyclist has the ability to produce load in multiple directions over the crank cycle which loads both plantar and dorsal surfaces (e.g., down-stroke push vs. up-stroke pull). The plantar foot experiences the bulk of loading, particularly in the forefoot region underneath the hallux and first metatarsal, most likely because the pedal spindle axis is usually beneath the ball of the foot (Fig. 3.12) (101).

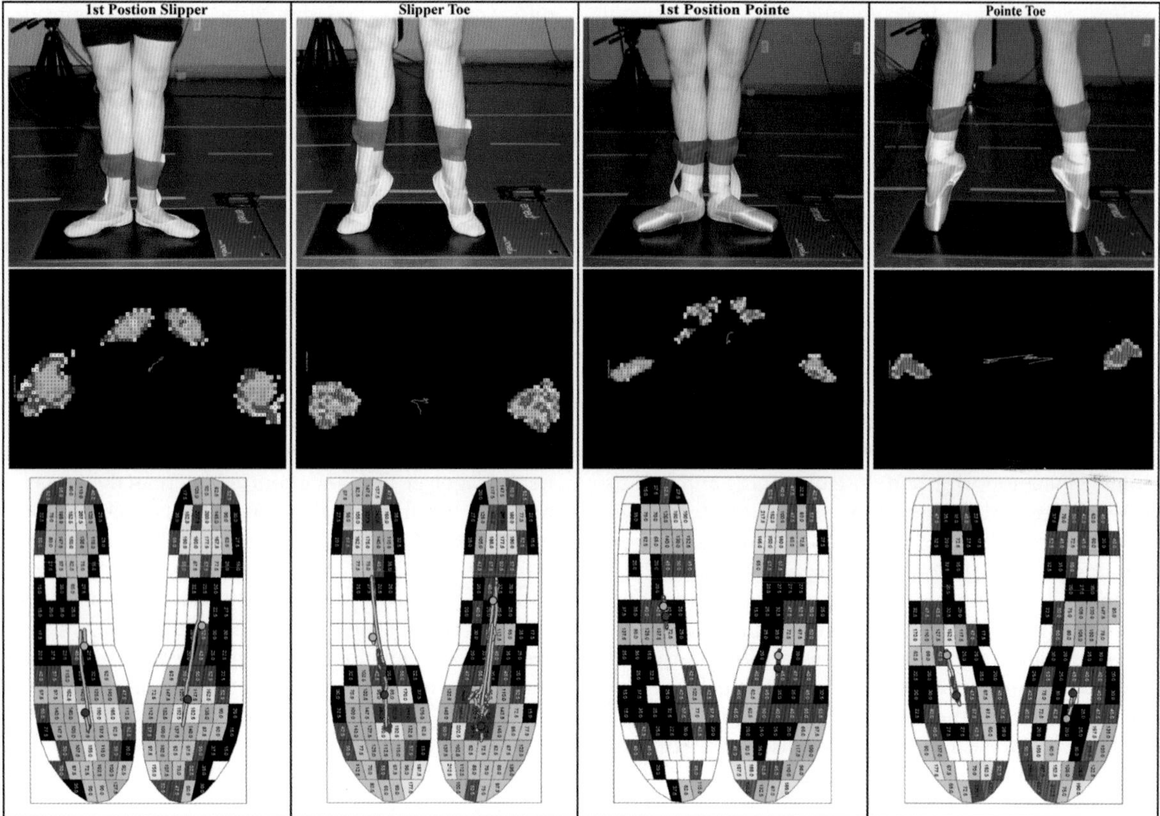

Figure 3.11. Plantar Loading of a Ballerina in First Position while Wearing Traditional Slippers and en Pointe Shoes. The ballerina is demonstrating first position in her ballet slippers (left) while her heels are on the ground and she is standing on the balls of her feet. The pressures between the slipper and the ground are depicted in the middle and the pressures between each foot and the slipper are shown on the bottom. The ballerina is in the same poses while wearing her en pointe shoes (right). As expected, the in-shoe pressures are extremely high in the toe region.

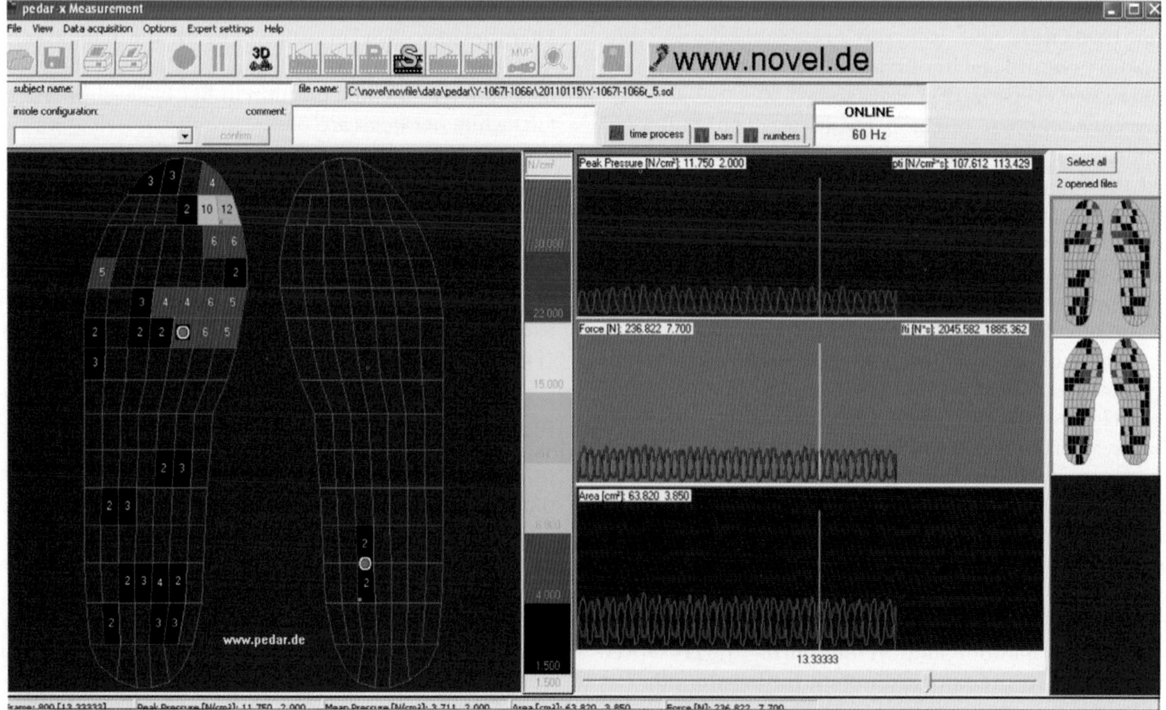

Figure 3.12. A cyclist wearing clipless-pedal type shoes demonstrates the in-shoe cyclic loading that occurs while maintain a 90 revolution per minute pace.

The predominant design used by competitive cyclists and that studied in the literature is the "no-clip" road shoe design where the foot is fixed tightly to the sole with straps, buckles, or other mechanisms. Once the shoe is clipped to the pedal, it is mechanically constrained to two motions, rotation about the spindle and slight toe in/out excursion. Foot loading magnitude and distribution depend on not only power output but also the rider configuration on the bike (seated vs. standing) and the material properties and geometry of the insole. Insole material and geometry will vary depending on the cycling application (indoor, mountain biking, road) and the performance level of the cyclist. Elite-level shoes are constructed of lightweight carbon fiber with deformation-reducing geometries meant to allow for optimal efficient power transmission to the crank. In contrast, recreational-type shoes are heavier and made from plastic, aluminum or a combination with more simple geometry and are consequently less stiff, and therefore less efficient. Sanderson and colleagues (101) quantified differences in plantar loading between recreational and competitive cyclists revealing that "the absence of group differences indicated that pressure distribution was not the result of training, but reflected the intrinsic relationship between the foot, the shoe, and the pedal" (101). To maximize power transfer, bike shoe insoles naturally have minimal padding, leaving much of the pressure distribution dependent on the physiologic whole foot compliance which, alone, does little to address morphologic differences. The effect of cycling shoe stiffness on plantar pressure was investigated by Jarboe and Quesada (102), who reported that a carbon-fiber shoe increased peak plantar pressure by 18% when compared to an identical plastic model. This suggests that a less-compliant shoe will concentrate load under the foot and users with pedal pathology such as metatarsalgia or ischemia must be aware so as not to aggravate these types of foot conditions. Shoe manufacturers have responded with advertised "ergonomic" insole designs that conform to the foot's plantar shape and, ideally, redistribute plantar load to prevent stress concentrations. The implementation is usually in the form of increased arch support, and while in principle, this should attenuate peak loads the human foot has a range of morphologic variability where custom insole technology may be more appropriate. In general, little information is available in the scientific literature on basic epidemiology to characterize cyclist foot type and pedal-injury prevalence across the spectrum of abilities; functional plantar loading changes associated with rider posture and/or bike geometry; relationships between clinical foot structure and function to performance; in-shoe whole and multi-segment foot motion during steady-state cycling and possible compensatory changes during fatigue; and loading of other pedal surfaces.

OTHER SPORT SHOE CONSIDERATIONS

Soccer, or "football" as commonly referred to in Europe, presents an excellent example of the shoe-fitting issue. Many soccer players prefer to wear shoes that are ½ to 1 size smaller than their feet because this gives them a "better feel of the ball". Unfortunately this distorts pedal alignment while wearing the cleated soccer shoe (Fig. 3.13). On the left is an individual's AP radiograph while standing barefoot. On the right is that same individual while wearing their soccer shoes. Note the crowding of the digits, metatarsal heads two to five, and the more valgus position of the hallux. The potential for creating digital deformities (hallux valgus, tailor's bunion, and hammertoes) is obvious. Once hallux valgus (commonly referred to as a

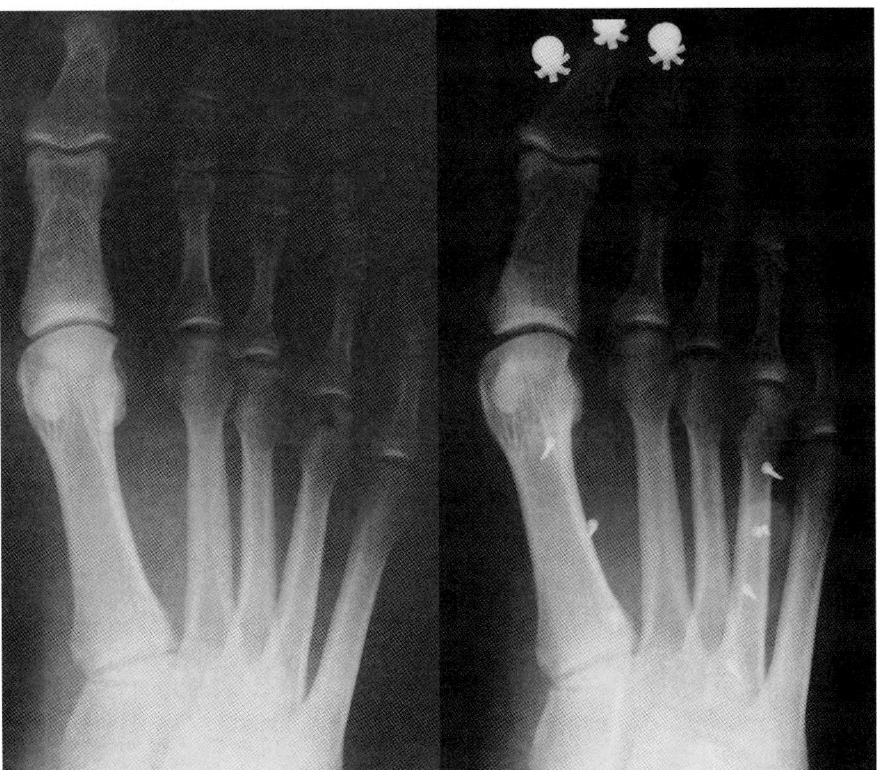

Figure 3.13. AP radiographs of an individual standing barefoot (left) and in his soccer shoes (right). This image underscores the common practice of wearing a soccer shoe that's ½ to 1 size smaller and how that can affect foot structure.

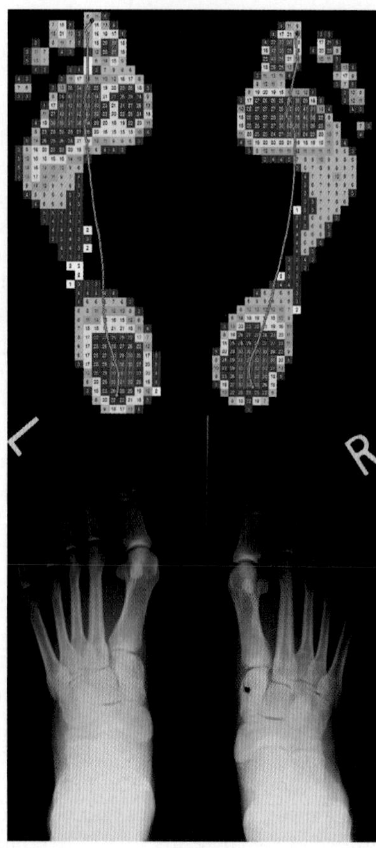

Figure 3.14. AP radiographs of an Individual with Hallux Valgus and His Corresponding Plantar Pressures. Overpronation is considered the most likely mechanism for developing hallux valgus which is clearly shown by the reduced CPEI values and increased medial forefoot loading in the plantar pressure data.

bunion) has developed (Fig. 3.14), management of overpronation (reduced CPEI) will be required. Custom foot orthoses can reduce the overpronation by improving hindfoot alignment and supporting the arch. Surgical procedures at the metatarsal head or if severe enough base may be required.

SUMMARY

Plantar pressure assessments, both barefoot and in-shoe, can provide differential diagnostic, prognostic, and treatment planning insight to help manage the athlete. Pressure is not a quantity that can be seen; it must be measured. Knowledge of a foot type (structure) and associated biomechanics (function) are powerful tools for providing the proper care of patient athletes with pedal pathologies. Exercise and sports are not only a source of joy and stress relief but vital to our health. As the United States population ages it becomes even more important to maintain the ability to achieve aerobic health through even basic exercises such as walking. The structure and function of the foot and ankle, as well as the foot–shoe–ground interface, are important considerations towards maintaining the ability to perform sports, maintain health, return to sport after injury, and perform sports competitively. Plantar pressure assessment should be a primary tool in the clinician's tool bag to achieve these goals.

REFERENCES

1. Dufour AB, Broe KE, Nguyen US, et al. Foot pain: Is current or past shoewear a factor? *Arthritis Rheum* 2009;61:1352–1358.
2. Ko PH, Hsiao TY, Kang JH, et al. Relationship between plantar pressure and soft tissue strain under metatarsal heads with different heel heights. *Foot Ankle Int* 2009;30:1111–1116.
3. Song J, Hillstrom HJ, Secord D, et al. Foot type biomechanics. Comparison of planus and rectus foot types. *J Am Podiatr Med Assoc* 1996;86:16–23.
4. Mootanah R, Frey J, Ziffchock R, et al. The effects of foot type of normal subjects on foot contact dynamics. 2010 34th Annual Meeting of American Society of Biomechanics, Providence, RI.
5. Nawata K, Nishihara S, Hayashi I, et al. Plantar pressure distribution during gait in athletes with functional instability of the ankle joint: Preliminary report. *J Orthop Sci* 2005;10:298–301.
6. Golightly YM, Hannan MT, Dufour AB, et al. Foot disorders associated with over-pronated and over-supinated foot types: The Johnston County Osteoarthritis Project. *Arthritis Rheum.* 2012;64; (in press).
7. Cacace L. The association of pes planus with hallux valgus, hallux rigidus, and plantar fasciitis. The Framingham foot study. *Hunter College*, New York, NY, MS Essay 2012:1–21.
8. Ellis SJ, Stoecklein H, Yu JC, et al. The accuracy of an automasking algorithm in plantar pressure measurements. *HSS J* 2011;7:57–63.
9. Silvino N, Evanski PM, Waugh TR. The Harris and Beath footprinting mat: Diagnostic validity and clinical use. *Clin Orthop Relat Res* 1980;151:265–269.
10. Veves A, Boulton AJ. The optical pedobarograph. *Clin Podiatr Med Surg* 1993;10:463–470.
11. Teyhen DS, Stoltenberg BE, Eckard TG, et al. Static foot posture associated with dynamic plantar pressure parameters. *J Orthop Sports Phys Ther* 2011;41:100–107.
12. Orendurff MS, Rohr ES, Segal AD, et al. Regional foot pressure during running, cutting, jumping, and landing. *Am J Sports Med* 2008;36:566–571.
13. Queen RM, Abbey AN, Wiegerinck JI, et al. Effect of shoe type on plantar pressure: A gender comparison. *Gait Posture* 2010;31:18–22.
14. Kelly LA, Racinais S, Tanner CM, et al. Augmented low dye taping changes muscle activation patterns and plantar pressure during treadmill running. *J Orthop Sports Phys Ther* 2010;40:648–655.
15. Hagen M, Hennig EM. Effects of different shoe-lacing patterns on the biomechanics of running shoes. *J Sports Sci* 2009;27:267–275.
16. Franklyn-Miller A, Wilson C, Bilzon J, et al. Foot orthoses in the prevention of injury in initial military training: A randomized controlled trial. *Am J Sports Med* 2011;39:30–37.
17. Nagel A, Fernholz F, Kibele C, et al. Long distance running increases plantar pressures beneath the metatarsal heads: A barefoot walking investigation of 200 marathon runners. *Gait Posture* 2008;27:152–155.
18. Morrison KE, Hudson DJ, Davis IS, et al. Plantar pressure during running in subjects with chronic ankle instability. *Foot Ankle Int* 2010;31:994–1000.
19. Sims EL, Hardaker WM, Queen RM. Gender differences in plantar loading during three soccer-specific tasks. *Br J Sports Med* 2008;42:272–277.
20. Queen RM, Abbey AN, Chuckpaiwong B, et al. Plantar loading comparisons between women with a history of second metatarsal stress fractures and normal controls. *Am J Sports Med* 2009;37:390–395.
21. Clanton TO, Ford JJ. Turf toe injury. *Clin Sports Med* 1994;13:731–741.
22. Wilson L, Dimeff R, Miniaci A, et al. Radiologic case study: First metatarsophalangeal plantar plate injury (turf toe). *Orthopedics* 2005;28:344,417–419.
23. Rodeo SA, O'Brien S, Warren RF, et al. Turf-toe: An analysis of metatarsophalangeal joint sprains in professional football players. *Am J Sports Med* 1990;18:280–285.
24. Frey C, Andersen GD, Feder KS. Plantarflexion injury to the metatarsophalangeal joint ("sand toe"). *Foot Ankle Int* 1996;17:576–581.
25. Childs SG. The pathogenesis and biomechanics of turf toe. *Orthop Nurs* 2006;25:276–282.
26. Brophy RH, Gamradt SC, Ellis SJ, et al. Effect of turf toe on foot contact pressures in professional American football players. *Foot Ankle Int* 2009;30:405–409.
27. Dananberg HJ. Gait style as an etiology to chronic postural pain. Part I. Functional hallux limitus. *J Am Podiatr Med Assoc* 1993;83:433–441.
28. Dananberg HJ. Gait style as an etiology to chronic postural pain. Part II. Postural compensatory process. *J Am Podiatr Med Assoc* 1993;83:615–624.
29. Dananberg HJ. Functional hallux limitus and its relationship to gait efficiency. *J Am Podiatr Med Assoc* 1986;76:648–652.
30. Van Gheluwe B, Dananberg HJ, Hagman F, et al. Effects of hallux limitus on plantar foot pressure and foot kinematics during walking. *J Am Podiatr Med Assoc* 2006;96:428–436.
31. Glazer JL, Brukner P. Plantar fasciitis: Current concepts to expedite healing. *Phys Sportsmed* 2004;32:24–28.
32. Riddle DL, Pulisic M, Pidcoe P, et al. Risk factors for plantar fasciitis: A matched case-control study. *J Bone Joint Surg Am* 2003;85:872–877.
33. Wearing SC, Smeathers JE, Urry SR, et al. The pathomechanics of plantar fasciitis. *Sports Med* 2006;36:585–611.
34. Young CC, Rutherford DS, Niedfeldt MW. Treatment of plantar fasciitis. *Am Fam Physician* 2001;63:467–474, 477–478.
35. Thomas JL, Christensen JC, Kravitz SR, et al. The diagnosis and treatment of heel pain: A clinical practice guideline-revision 2010. *J Foot Ankle Surg* 2010;49(Suppl):S1–S19.
36. Johal KS, Milner SA. Plantar fasciitis and the calcaneal spur: Fact or fiction?. *Foot Ankle Surg* 2012;18:39–41.
37. Rutherford DJ, Hubley-Kozey C. Explaining the hip adduction moment variability during gait: Implications for hip abductor strengthening. *Clin Biomech (Bristol, Avon)* 2009;24:267–273.
38. Cardinal E, Chhem RK, Beauregard CG, et al. Plantar fasciitis: Sonographic evaluation. *Radiology* 1996;201:257–259.
39. Buchbinder R, Ptasznik R, Gordon J, et al. Ultrasound-guided extracorporeal shock wave therapy for plantar fasciitis: A randomized controlled trial. *JAMA* 2002;288:1364–1372.
40. Kane D, Greaney T, Bresnihan B, et al. Ultrasound guided injection of recalcitrant plantar fasciitis. *Ann Rheum Dis* 1998;57:383–384.

41. Hammer DS, Adam F, Kreutz A, et al. Ultrasonographic evaluation at 6-month follow-up of plantar fasciitis after extracorporeal shock wave therapy. *Arch Orthop Trauma Surg* 2005;125:6–9.
42. Kibler WB, Goldberg C, Chandler TJ. Functional biomechanical deficits in running athletes with plantar fasciitis. *Am J Sports Med* 1991;19:66–71.
43. Pohl MB, Hamill J, Davis IS. Biomechanical and anatomic factors associated with a history of plantar fasciitis in female runners. *Clin J Sport Med* 2009;19:372–376.
44. Scherer PR, Sanders J, Eldredge DE, et al. Effect of functional foot orthoses on first metatarsophalangeal joint dorsiflexion in stance and gait. *J Am Podiatr Med Assoc* 2006;96:474–481.
45. Al-Bluwi MT, Sadat-Ali M, Al-Habdan IM, et al. Efficacy of EZStep in the management of plantar fasciitis: A prospective, randomized study. *Foot Ankle Spec* 2011;4:218–221.
46. Lysholm J, Wiklander J. Injuries in runners. *Am J Sports Med* 1987;15:168–171.
47. Simpson RR, Gudas CJ. Posterior tibial tendon rupture in a world class runner. *J Foot Surg* 1983;22:74–77.
48. Johnson KA. Tibialis posterior tendon rupture. *Clin Orthop Relat Res* 1983;177:140–147.
49. Marcus RE, Pfister ME. The enigmatic diagnosis of posterior tibialis tendon rupture. *Iowa Orthop J* 1993;13:171–177.
50. Ledoux WR, Hillstrom HJ. The distributed plantar vertical force of neutrally aligned and pes planus feet. *Gait Posture* 2002;15:1–9.
51. Clancy WG Jr., Tendon trauma and overuse injuries. In: Leadbetter WB, Buckwalter JA, Gordon SL, Foundation for Sports Medicine Education and Research, American Orthopaedic Society for Sports Medicine, National Institute of Arthritis and Musculoskeletal and Skin Diseases, eds. *Sports-Induced Inflammation: Clinical and Basic Science Concepts*. Park Ridge, IL: American Academy of Orthopaedic Surgeons; 1990:609–618.
52. Strocchi R, De Pasquale V, Guizzardi S, et al. Human Achilles tendon: Morphological and morphometric variations as a function of age. *Foot Ankle* 1991;12:100–104.
53. Kannus P, Jozsa L. Histopathological changes preceding spontaneous rupture of a tendon. A controlled study of 891 patients. *J Bone Joint Surg Am* 1991;73:1507–1525.
54. Nigg BM, Segesser B. The influence of playing surfaces on the load on the locomotor system and on football and tennis injuries. *Sports Med* 1988;5:375–385.
55. Van Ginckel A, Thijs Y, Hesar NG, et al. Intrinsic gait-related risk factors for Achilles tendinopathy in novice runners: A prospective study. *Gait Posture* 2009;29:387–391.
56. Kvist M. Achilles tendon injuries in athletes. *Ann Chir Gynaecol* 1991;80:188–201.
57. Munteanu SE, Barton CJ. Lower limb biomechanics during running in individuals with Achilles tendinopathy: A systematic review. *J Foot Ankle Res* 2011;4:15.
58. Schepsis AA, Leach RE. Surgical management of Achilles tendinitis. *Am J Sports Med* 1987;15:308–315.
59. Myerson MS, McGarvey W. Disorders of the Achilles tendon insertion and Achilles tendinitis. *Instr Course Lect* 1999;48:211–218.
60. Matheson GO, Clement DB, McKenzie DC, et al. Stress fractures in athletes. A study of 320 cases. *Am J Sports Med* 1987;15:46–58.
61. Giladi M, Milgrom C, Stein M. The low arch, a protective factor in stress fractures- a prospective study of 295 military recruits. *Orthop Rev* 1985;14:709–712.
62. Simkin A, Leichter I, Giladi M, et al. Combined effect of foot arch structure and an orthotic device on stress fractures. *Foot Ankle* 1989;10:25–29.
63. Balduini FC, Tetzlaff J. Historical perspectives on injuries of the ligaments of the ankle. *Clin Sports Med* 1982;1:3–12.
64. Garrick JG. The frequency of injury, mechanism of injury, and epidemiology of ankle sprains. *Am J Sports Med* 1977;5:241–242.
65. Fong DT, Hong Y, Chan LK, et al. A systematic review on ankle injury and ankle sprain in sports. *Sports Med* 2007;37:73–94.
66. Holmer P, Sondergaard L, Konradsen L, et al. Epidemiology of sprains in the lateral ankle and foot. *Foot Ankle Int* 1994;15:72–74.
67. Jackson DW, Ashley RL, Powell JW. Ankle sprains in young athletes. relation of severity and disability. *Clin Orthop Relat Res* 1974;101:201–215.
68. Weiker GG. Ankle injuries in the athlete. *Prim Care* 1984;11:101–108.
69. Marder RA. Current methods for the evaluation of ankle ligament injuries. *Instr Course Lect* 1995;44:349–357.
70. Peters JW, Trevino SG, Renstrom PA. Chronic lateral ankle instability. *Foot Ankle* 1991;12: 182–191.
71. Lapointe SJ, Siegler S, Hillstrom HJ, et al. Changes in the flexibility characteristics of the ankle complex due to damage to the lateral collateral ligaments: An in vitro and in vivo study. *J Orthop Res* 1997;15:331–341.
72. Burgess I, Ryan MD. Bilateral fatigue fractures of the distal fibulae caused by a change of running shoes. *Med J Aust* 1985;143:304–305.
73. Wilk BR, Fisher KL, Gutierrez W. Defective running shoes as a contributing factor in plantar fasciitis in a triathlete. *J Orthop Sports Phys Ther* 2000;30:21–28; discussion 29–31.
74. Yeung EW, Yeung SS. A systematic review of interventions to prevent lower limb soft tissue running injuries. *Br J Sports Med* 2001;35:383–389.
75. Rome K, Handoll HH, Ashford R. Interventions for preventing and treating stress fractures and stress reactions of bone of the lower limbs in young adults. *Cochrane Database Syst Rev* 2005;2:CD000450.
76. van Mechelen W, Hlobil H, Kemper HC. Incidence, severity, aetiology and prevention of sports injuries. A review of concepts. *Sports Med* 1992;14:82–99.
77. Marti B, Vader JP, Minder CE, et al. On the epidemiology of running injuries. the 1984 Bern Grand-Prix study. *Am J Sports Med* 1988;16:285–294.
78. James SL, Bates BT, Osternig LR. Injuries to runners. *Am J Sports Med* 1978;6:40–50.
79. Clarke TE, Frederick EC, Hamill CL. The effects of shoe design parameters on rearfoot control in running. *Med Sci Sports Exerc* 1983;15:376–381.
80. Bobbert MF, Schamhardt HC, Nigg BM. Calculation of vertical ground reaction force estimates during running from positional data. *J Biomech* 1991;24:1095–1105.
81. Bobbert MF, Yeadon MR, Nigg BM. Mechanical analysis of the landing phase in heel-toe running. *J Biomech* 1992;25:223–234.
82. Paul JP. Forces predicted at the ankle during running. *Med Sci Sports Exerc* 1983;15:vii.
83. Cavanagh PR, Lafortune MA. Ground reaction forces in distance running. *J Biomech* 1980;13:397–406.
84. Williams KR. The relationship between mechanical and physiological energy estimates. *Med Sci Sports Exerc* 1985;17:317–325.
85. Williams KR, Cavanagh PR. Relationship between distance running mechanics, running economy, and performance. *J Appl Physiol* 1987;85:1236–1245.
86. Hamill J, Freedson PS, Boda W, et al. Effects of shoe type on cardiorespiratory responses and rearfoot motion during treadmill running. *Med Sci Sports Exerc* 1988;20:515–521.
87. Robbins SE, Gouw GJ. Athletic footwear and chronic overloading. A brief review. *Sports Med* 1990;9:76–85.
88. Schwellnus MP, Jordaan G, Noakes TD. Prevention of common overuse injuries by the use of shock absorbing insoles. A prospective study. *Am J Sports Med* 1990;18:636–641.
89. Nigg BM, Bahlsen HA, Luethi SM, et al. The influence of running velocity and midsole hardness on external impact forces in heel-toe running. *J Biomech* 1987;20:951–959.
90. Messier SP, Pittala KA. Etiologic factors associated with selected running injuries. *Med Sci Sports Exerc* 1988;20:501–505.
91. Nigg BM, Morlock M. The influence of lateral heel flare of running shoes on pronation and impact forces. *Med Sci Sports Exerc* 1987;19:294–302.
92. Stacoff A, Nigg BM, Reinschmidt C, et al. Tibiocalcaneal kinematics of barefoot versus shod running. *J Biomech* 2000;33:1387–1395.
93. Bergmann G, Kniggendorf H, Graichen F, et al. Influence of shoes and heel strike on the loading of the hip joint. *J Biomech* 1995;28:817–827.
94. Nigg BM. The role of impact forces and foot pronation: A new paradigm. *Clin J Sport Med* 2001;11:2–9.
95. Mundermann A, Nigg BM, Humble RN, et al. Orthotic comfort is related to kinematics, kinetics, and EMG in recreational runners. *Med Sci Sports Exerc* 2003;35:1710–1719.
96. Wakeling JM, Nigg BM. Soft-tissue vibrations in the quadriceps measured with skin mounted transducers. *J Biomech* 2001;34:539–543.
97. Ho IJ, Hou YY, Yang CH, et al. Comparison of plantar pressure distribution between different speed and incline during treadmill jogging. *J Sports Sci Med* 2010;9:154–160.
98. Fourchet F, Kelly L, Horobeanu C, et al. Comparison of plantar pressure distribution in adolescent runners at low vs. high running velocity. *Gait Posture* 2012;35:685–687.
99. Butler RJ, Russell ME, Queen RM. Effect of soccer footwear on landing mechanics. *Scand J Med Sci Sports* 2012 doi: 10.1111/j.1600-0838.2012.01468.x.
100. Worsfold PR, Smith N, Dyson R. Kinetic assessment of golf shoe outer sole design features. *J Sports Sci Med* 2009;8:607–615.
101. Sanderson DJ, Hennig EM, Black AH. The influence of cadence and power output on force application and in-shoe pressure distribution during cycling by competitive and recreational cyclists. *J Sports Sci* 2000;18:173–181.
102. Jarboe NE, Quesada PM. The effects of cycling shoe stiffness on forefoot pressure. *Foot Ankle Int* 2003;24:784–788.

CHAPTER

4

Pankaj Sharma
Nicola Maffulli

Basic Science of Tendon Healing

Tendon injuries account for considerable morbidity, and often prove disabling for several months. Significant advances have been made in our understanding of tendon healing, in recent times. Improved knowledge of the basic science underlying tendon healing should allow the development of management modalities that can enhance the process of tendon healing (1,2). This chapter presents a synopsis of current knowledge of the complex interplay involved in tendon healing.

TENDON HEALING

Tendon healing occurs in three overlapping phases. In the initial inflammatory phase, erythrocytes and inflammatory cells, particularly neutrophils, enter the site of injury. In the first 24 hours, monocytes and macrophages predominate, and phagocytosis of necrotic materials occurs. Vasoactive and chemotactic factors are released with increased vascular permeability, initiation of angiogenesis, stimulation of tenocyte proliferation, and recruitment of more inflammatory cells (3). Tenocytes gradually migrate to the wound, and type III collagen synthesis is initiated (4).

After a few days, the regenerative stage begins. Synthesis of type III collagen peaks during this stage, which lasts for a few weeks. Water content and glycosaminoglycan concentrations remain high during this stage (4). After approximately 6 weeks, the remodeling stage commences. During this stage, the healing tissue changes in size and shape. A corresponding decrease in cellularity, collagen, and glycosaminoglycan synthesis occurs. The remodeling phase can be divided into a consolidation and maturation stage (5). The consolidation stage commences at about 6 weeks and continues up to 10 weeks. In this period, repair tissue changes from cellular to fibrous, tenocyte metabolism remains high, and tenocytes and collagen fibers become aligned in the direction of stress (6). A higher proportion of type I collagen is synthesized during this stage (7). After 10 weeks, the maturation stage occurs, with gradual change of fibrous tissue to scar-like tendon tissue over the course of 1 year (6). During the latter half of this stage, tenocyte metabolism and tendon vascularity decline (8).

Tendon healing can occur intrinsically, via proliferation of epitenon and endotenon tenocytes, or extrinsically, by invasion of cells from the surrounding sheath and synovium (9). Epitenon tenoblasts initiate the repair process through proliferation and migration (10). Healing in severed tendons can be performed by cells from the epitenon alone, without relying on adhesions for vascularity or cellular support (11). Internal tenocytes contribute to the intrinsic repair process and secrete larger and more mature collagen than epitenon cells (12). Although both fibroblasts in the epitenon and internal tenocytes synthesize collagen during repair, it is possible that different cells produce different collagen types at different time points. Initially, collagen is produced by epitenon cells, with endotenon cells synthesizing collagen later (13). The relative contribution of each cell type may be influenced by the type of trauma sustained, anatomical position, presence of a synovial sheath, and the amount of stress induced by motion after repair has taken place (14).

Intrinsic healing results in improved biomechanics and fewer complications. In particular, a normal gliding mechanism within the tendon sheath is preserved (15). In extrinsic healing, the scar tissue results in adhesion formation, which disrupts tendon gliding (16). Different healing patterns may predominate in particular locations. For example, extrinsic healing tends to prevail in torn rotator cuffs (17).

MODULATORS OF HEALING

Matrix metalloproteinases (MMPs) are important regulators of extracellular matrix remodeling, and their levels are altered during tendon healing (18). Fluctuation in the levels of various different MMPs suggests that these proteolytic enzymes play a key role in the sequence of events that occurs during tendon healing (19). Wounding and inflammation provokes release of growth factors and cytokines from platelets, neutrophils, macrophages and other inflammatory cells (20). These growth factors induce neovascularization and chemotaxis of fibroblasts and tenocytes and stimulate fibroblast and tenocytes proliferation and synthesis of collagen (21).

Nitric oxide is a short-lived free radical, with many biologic functions: It increases collagen synthesis by human tenocytes in vitro, and also affects tenocyte adhesion (22,23). Inhibition of nitric oxide synthase–reduced healing, resulting in decreased cross-sectional area and a reduced failure load after tenotomy of rat Achilles tendons (24). Delivery of nitric oxide using glyceryl trinitrate patches produces beneficial effects in patients with Achilles tendinopathy at 6 months (25).

In a rat Achilles tendon rupture model, peak nerve fiber formation occurred between weeks 2 and 6, in concert with peak levels of the neuronal isoform of nitric oxide synthase (26). These nerve fibers presumably deliver neuropeptides which act as chemical messengers and regulators, and may play an important role in tendon healing. Substance P and calcitonin gene–related peptide (CGRP) are pro-inflammatory and cause vasodilation and protein extravasation (27,28). In addition, substance P enhances cellular release of prostaglandins, histamines, and cytokines (29). Peak levels of substance P and CGRP occur during the regenerative phase, suggesting a possible role during this phase.

LIMITATIONS OF HEALING

Synovial sheath disruption at the time of injury or surgery allows granulation tissue and tenocytes from surrounding tissue to invade the repair site, leading to adhesion formation (30). Exogenous cells predominate over endogenous tenocytes, allowing the surrounding tissues to attach to the repair site resulting in adhesion formation. Despite remodeling, the biochemical and mechanical properties of healed tendon tissue never match those of intact tendon. In spontaneously healed transected sheep Achilles tendons, rupture force was only 56.7% of normal at 12 months (31). One possible reason for this may be the absence of mechanical loading during the period of immobilization.

REFERENCES

1. Sharma P, Maffulli N. The future: rehabilitation, gene therapy, optimization of healing. *Foot Ankle Clin* 2005;10(2):383–397.
2. Sharma P, Maffulli N. Tendinopathy and tendon injury: The future. *Disabil Rehabil* 2008;9: 1–13.
3. Murphy PG, Loitz BJ, Frank CB, et al. Influence of exogenous growth factors on the synthesis and secretion of collagen types I and III by explants of normal and healing rabbit ligaments. *Biochem Cell Biol* 1994;72(9–10):403–409.
4. Oakes BW. Tissue healing and repair: tendons and ligaments. In: Frontera WR, ed. *Rehabilitation of Sports Injuries: Scientific Basis.* Oxford, UK: Blackwell Science; 2003:56–98.
5. Tillman LJ, Chasan NP. Properties of dense connective tissue and wound healing. In: Hertling D, Kessler RM, eds. *Management of Common Musculoskeletal Disorders.* Philadelphia, PA: Lippincott; 1996:8–21.
6. Hooley CJ, Cohen RE. A model for the creep behaviour of tendon. *Int J Biol Macromol* 1979;1:123–132.
7. Abrahamsson SO. Matrix metabolism and healing in the flexor tendon. Experimental studies on rabbit tendon. *Scand J Plast Reconstr Surg Hand Surg* 1991;Suppl 23:1–51.
8. Amiel D, Akeson W, Harwood FL, et al. Stress deprivation effect on metabolic turnover of medial collateral ligament collagen. *Clin Orthop* 1987;172:25–27.
9. Gelberman RH, Manske PR, Vande Berg JS, et al. Flexor tendon repair in vitro: a comparative histologic study of the rabbit, chicken, dog, and monkey. *J Orthop Res* 1984;2(1):39–48.
10. Manske PR, Gelberman RH, Lesker PA. Flexor tendon healing. *Hand Clin* 1985;1(1):25–34.
11. Gelberman RH, Manske PR, Akeson WH, et al. Flexor tendon repair. *J Orthop Res* 1986; 4(1):119–128.
12. Fujita M, Hukuda S, Doida Y. Experimental study of intrinsic healing of the flexor tendon: collagen synthesis of the cultured flexor tendon cells of the canine. *Nippon Seikeigeka Gakkai Zasshi* 1992;66(4):326–333.
13. Ingraham JM, Hauck RM, Ehrlich HP. Is the tendon embryogenesis process resurrected during tendon healing? *Plast Reconstr Surg* 2003;112(3):844–854.
14. Koob TJ. Biomimetic approaches to tendon repair. *Comp Biochem Physiol A Mol Integr Physiol* 2002;133(4):1171–1192.
15. Koob TJ, Summers AP. Tendon-bridging the gap. *Comp Biochem Physiol A Mol Integr Physiol* 2002;133(4):905–909.
16. Strickland JW. Flexor tendons: Acute injuries. In: Green D, Hotchkiss R, Pedersen W, eds. *Green's Operative Hand Surgery.* New York, NY: Churchill Livingstone; 1999:1851–1897.
17. Uhthoff HK, Sarkar K. Surgical repair of rotator cuff ruptures. The importance of the subacromial bursa. *J Bone Joint Surg Br* 1991;73(3):399–401.
18. Riley GP, Curry V, DeGroot J, et al. Matrix metalloproteinase activities and their relationship with collagen remodelling in tendon pathology. *Matrix Biol* 2002;21(2):185–195.
19. Oshiro W, Lou J, Xing X, et al. Flexor tendon healing in the rat: a histologic and gene expression study. *J Hand Surg Am* 2003;28(5):814–823.
20. Evans CH. Cytokines and the role they play in the healing of ligaments and tendons. *Sports Med* 1999;28(2):71–76.
21. Molloy T, Wang Y, Murrell G. The roles of growth factors in tendon and ligament healing. *Sports Med* 2003;33(5):381–394.
22. Xia W, Szomor Z, Wang Y, et al. Nitric oxide enhances collagen synthesis in cultured human tendon cells. *J Orthop Res* 2006;24(2):159–172.
23. Molloy TJ, de Bock CE, Wang Y, et al. Gene expression changes in SNAP-stimulated and iNOS-transfected tenocytes-expression of extracellular matrix genes and its implications for tendon healing. *J Orthop Res* 2006;24(9):1869–1882.
24. Murrell GA, Szabo C, Hannafin JA, et al. Modulation of tendon healing by nitric oxide. *Inflamm Res* 1997;46(1):19–27.
25. Murrell GA. Using nitric oxide to treat tendinopathy. *Br J Sports Med* 2007;41:227–231.
26. Ackermann PW, Li J, Lundeberg T, et al. Neuronal plasticity in relation to nociception and healing of rat achilles tendon. *J Orthop Res* 2003;21(3):432–441.
27. Nakamura-Craig M, Smith TW. Substance P and peripheral inflammatory hyperalgesia. *Pain* 1989;38(1):91–98.
28. Brain SD, Williams TJ, Tippins JR, et al. Calcitonin gene-related peptide is a potent vasodilator. *Nature* 1985;313(5997):54–56.
29. Vasko MR, Campbell WB, Waite KJ. Prostaglandin E2 enhances bradykinin-stimulated release of neuropeptides from rat sensory neurons in culture. *J Neurosci* 1994;14(8):4987–4997.
30. Manske PR. Flexor tendon healing. *J Hand Surg Br* 1988;13(3):237–245.
31. Bruns J, Kampen J, Kahrs J, et al. Achilles tendon rupture: experimental results on spontaneous repair in a sheep-model. *Knee Surg Sports Traumatol Arthrosc* 2000;8(6):364–369.

CHAPTER

5

Tamar Kessel
Elizabeth Manejias
Gregory Lutz

Physical Examination of the Foot and Ankle

INTRODUCTION

A thorough and methodical history and physical examination is crucial to making the correct diagnosis of foot and ankle conditions. This chapter focuses on the physical examination of the foot and ankle, and reveals a systematic approach that will enable physicians to minimize incorrect diagnoses and maximize efficiency.

PATIENT HISTORY

Like any other physical examination in medicine, a thorough examination of the foot and ankle begins with a detailed medical history. Although a comprehensive history is always helpful, there are certain key elements specific to the foot and ankle that should be ascertained. Patient age, gender, occupation, recreational activities, occupational requirements, and shoe-wear preference should be elicited. Of course, the chief complaint should also be discussed. Usually pain is the primary complaint that leads people to seek medical advice; however, other complaints including numbness, deformity, swelling, instability, and stiffness may be of concern. Aggravating and alleviating factors, timing of episodes, and prior therapies should be revealed. Relevant medical history should also be obtained, specifically including a history of diabetes, vascular disease, inflammatory arthritis, and neurologic conditions. Any prior surgery to the foot and ankle should be asked directly. Pain drawing can also be helpful, especially when assessing for possible referred pain from the spine (1).

INSPECTION

The foot and ankle examination should always be performed in both standing and seated positions. The examination begins with observing the patient's stance, mobility, and gait. The foot and ankle should always be inspected with the shoes and socks removed, and the leg should be exposed from knee down. The patient's gait should be observed from the front, side, and back with and without shoes. The observing physician should be watching for any asymmetry, limitation, or avoidance of weight bearing. General body alignment should also be noted. The position of the trunk and hips should be observed. In addition to evaluation of hip and knee alignment, any leg length discrepancies should be noted. Any misalignment or anatomic variation should be noted, as they can give clue to risk factors for certain overuse injuries, or may represent a compensatory change in response to an injury (2).

SEATED INSPECTION

Inspection can begin with the patient seated on an elevated table, with the leg at eye level for the examining physician. Swelling, deformity, erythema, or bruising should be noted. Color differences may represent chronic venous stasis or cyanotic changes. Swelling may be diffuse from peripheral edema, or localized as seen in tendinitis or arthritis. Previous wounds or surgical scars should be noted, as they give clue to prior injury and risk factors for current pathology. Skin and nail health should also be noted. Shiny and hairless skin can be a sign of vascular disease. Fungal infection of the toenails can be a sign of diabetes. The examining physician should pay very close attention to callus formation, as their presence is a clue to preferential weight bearing. It is considered normal to have mild callusing under the first metatarsal head or heel. Callus formation under the second metatarsal head may be a sign of first-ray hypermobility or instability. Heavy callusing under the first metatarsal head may be a sign of a high arched foot, whereas heavy callusing under the heel may be a sign of a weak Achilles. Callusing under the navicular may be seen with a collapsed arch or pathologic flatfoot.

Foot strength can also be determined by visual inspection. An intrinsic plus foot is strong and has narrowing of the metatarsals and straightening of the toes. The opposite is true of an intrinsic minus foot which is weak and has splaying of the metatarsals and clawing of the toes. In addition to observing the patient's feet, you should also inspect their shoes. Often patients with forefoot deformities wear shoes that are too small for their feet. Simply switching to a proper size shoe may alleviate their pain. Wear patterns on shoes also give invaluable information. Wear under the lateral side of the shoe suggests a cavus or varus alignment, whereas medial side wear suggests valgus or flatfoot deformity (3).

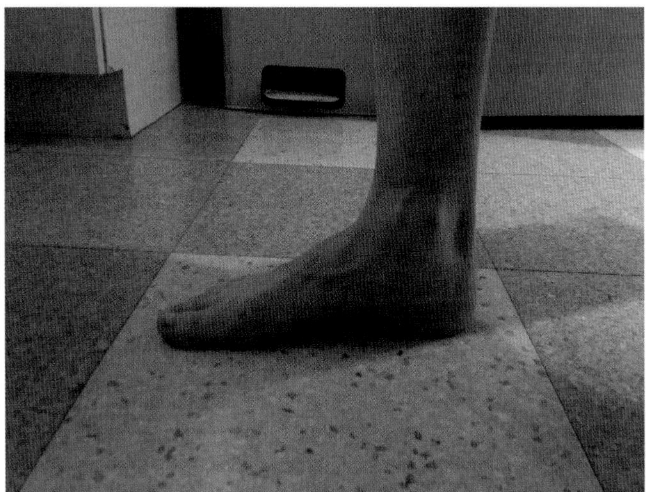

Figure 5.1. Normal arch; note that the height of the apex of the medial longitudinal arch is approximately 1 cm when the patient is weight bearing.

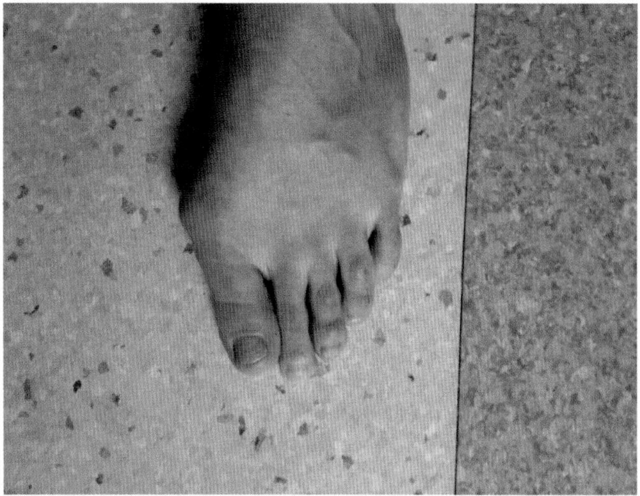

Figure 5.3. Foot shape demonstrating bunion, hallux valgus, and metatarsus primus varus.

ARCHES

For the next part of the examination, attention should be paid to the arches of the feet. The medial arch is examined in both weight-bearing and non–weight-bearing positions. The height of the apex of a normal medial longitudinal arch is approximately 1 cm when the patient is weight bearing (Fig. 5.1). A low arch (pes planus) may be congenital, or may be associated with trauma, posterior tibial tendon dysfunction, rheumatoid arthritis, or contraction of the Achilles tendon. Pes planus (flatfeet) should be characterized into one of the two groups, flexible or rigid. A patient who has a flexible flatfoot will appear to have a normal or near-normal arch when non–weight bearing, but will have a substantial loss of arch height when weight bearing (Fig. 5.2). A high arch (pes cavus) may be idiopathic or associated with congenital or neurologic diseases. A convex, or rocker bottom foot, can be seen in diabetic patients who have Charcot neuropathic arthropathy. Both pes planus and pes cavus do not require any treatment if asymptomatic. However, both conditions place people at a slightly increased risk for overuse injuries such as plantar fasciitis and shin splints, because they are thought to decrease the dissipation of the forces of impact loading on the foot (4).

FOOT SHAPE

Next, the examiner should pay attention to foot shape. There are five predominate shapes. An Egyptian foot is one in which the great toe is the longest. A Greek foot, or Morton's foot, is when the second toe is the longest. A squared foot, or peasant's foot, is when the great toe and second toe are the same length. A simian foot with metatarsus primus varus is the bunion-prone foot (Fig. 5.3). And a model's foot is a narrow foot with an exaggerated taper in metatarsal length from the first to the fifth rays. Foot shapes give information about load

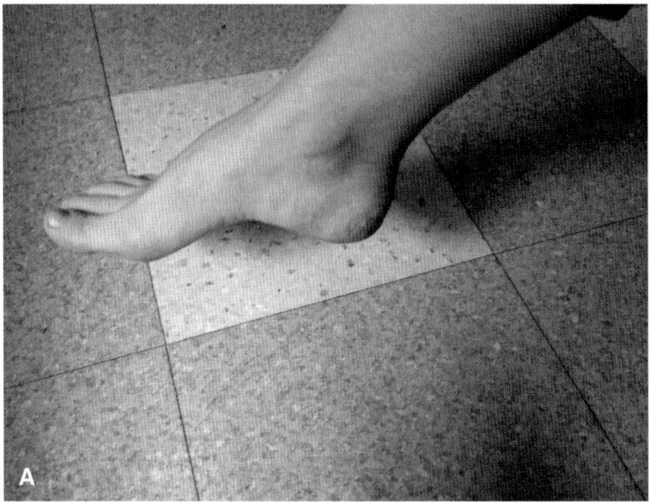

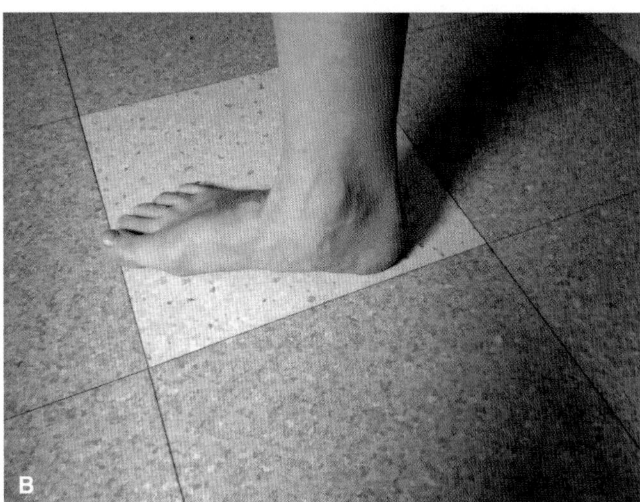

Figure 5.2. Flexible flatfoot appears to have a normal or near-normal arch when non–weight bearing, but has a substantial loss of arch height when weight bearing. **A:** Flexible flatfoot appears to have a normal or near-normal arch when non–weight bearing, **B:** but has a substantial loss of arch height when weight bearing.

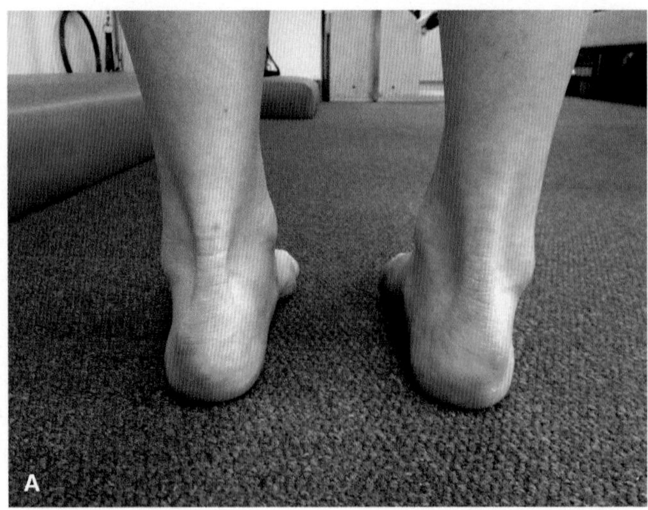

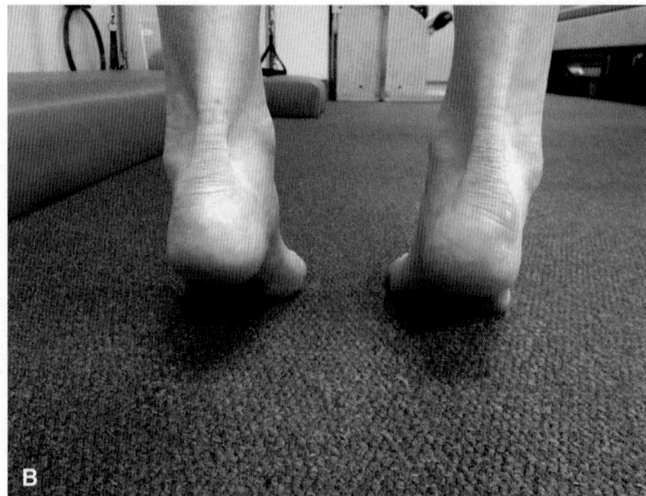

Figure 5.4. Double-limb heel rise test. Both heels are inverting properly. **A:** Double-limb heel rise test. **B:** Both heels are inverting properly.

forces. The longest toe is associated with increased load at its proximal metatarsal and metatarsal phalangeal joint, increasing the risk of arthritis in these structures (5).

GAIT

After observing the patient's arch and foot shape, you should watch the patient ambulate. An antalgic gait may be found in any condition that causes pain in the lower extremity. In an antalgic gait, the weight-bearing phase is shorter on the affected side, resulting in shorter stride length on the unaffected side and decreased velocity overall. An individual who has weak dorsiflexors may walk with a foot slap or steppage gait. A steppage gait involves excessive hip and knee flexion to give additional clearance for the foot and toes. This gait may also be seen with loss of ankle range of motion. Heel walking is a general test of ankle dorsiflexion strength, especially the tibialis anterior muscle. Dorsiflexion weakness should raise suspicion for a deep peroneal or common peroneal (L4, L5) nerve injury or an L4, L5 radiculopathy (6).

OTHER GAIT TESTS

Next, you can have the patient walk on their toes to test ankle plantar flexor strength, especially the gastrocnemius–soleus complex. A better test to detect subtle weakness of plantar flexor strength is to have the patient perform single-leg heel raises. Plantar flexor weakness is suspicious for injury to the Achilles tendon or dysfunction of either the sciatic or the tibial nerve, which supplies most of the main plantar flexors, or an S1 radiculopathy. The possibility of neurologic involvement is heightened if there is also toe flexion weakness. The examiner should also check for posterior tibial tendon dysfunction while the patient performs heel rises. While standing on one leg, the patient rises up on the forefoot. A normal posterior tibial tendon will bring the heel into varus, without pain. If the heel remains in valgus alignment, or if the patient feels pain along the medial hindfoot, then there is a likely dysfunction of the posterior tibial tendon (Fig. 5.4). Lateral foot walking is a test of inversion strength, which is primarily a function of the tibialis posterior muscle and tibial nerve; whereas medial foot walking tests eversion strength which is primarily a function of the peroneal muscles and the superficial peroneal nerve. This movement is rarely tested secondary to its difficulty for most patients. Apprehension with this test may suggest lateral ankle instability (7).

PALPATION

Most structures of the foot are fairly superficial and easy to palpate. When palpating the foot, you should describe any tenderness found in anatomical terms, and state exactly where the pain is located. The foot and ankle are usually composed of 26 primary bones, not including the tibia, fibula, accessory bones, and sesamoid bones (8). A good clinical examination can supplement the history and assist in making the correct diagnosis of any problem. Reproduction of the patient's symptoms is crucial and often key in making the correct diagnosis, as there are typical surface locations of injury symptoms in many diagnoses of the foot and ankle.

Tinel's sign over the medial ankle joint may suggest possible tarsal tunnel syndrome. A Thompson test should be performed to assess the integrity of the Achilles tendon. To perform the Thompson test, the patient should lie prone on the examination table. The patient's feet should extend farther than the end of the examination table. The examiner then squeezes the calf muscle. This motion, in a normal patient, should cause the toes to point downward as the Achilles pulls the foot. In a patient with a ruptured Achilles tendon, the foot will not move, which is a positive Thompson test (8).

MOTION

Assessment of motion is important when examining the foot and ankle and can give clues to certain overuse injuries. The examiner should first assess knee motion. Any misalignment or stiffness of the knee can overload the foot and cause pain. The examiner should also assess plantar flexion and dorsiflexion.

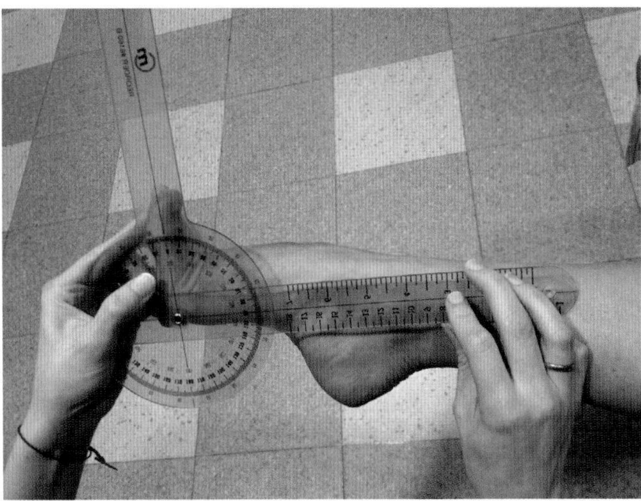

Figure 5.5. 90 degrees of dorsiflexion is demonstrated in the first MTP joint. Normal range is 45 to 90 degrees.

Normally, passive ankle dorsiflexion should be 10 degrees past neutral with the knee extended, with an additional 10 degrees with knee flexion. Limitation of ankle dorsiflexion with the knee extended that improves with the knee bent indicates gastrocnemius contracture. Limitations of motion with the knee extended and bent indicates contracture of both the soleus and gastrocnemius. In this position, the examiner may also check for dural tension if referred pain from the spine is suspected. This is done with the Slump Test or the Sitting Root Test. In this test, the patient is seated on the examination table with the neck flexed. The examiner extends the knee on the affected side up to 90 degrees. Low back pain and radiation of the pain indicate a positive test. This test places abnormal tension on the sciatic nerve and patients with a lumbar radiculopathy will tend to arch backward and complain of radicular pain.

Next, subtalar motion should be assessed. Subtalar motion is complex with contributions from the three hindfoot joints (talocalcaneal, talonavicular, and calcaneocuboid). The motion is described in terms of inversion and eversion. Subtalar motion can be assessed with the patient in a sitting position. The calcaneus is first placed in neutral, in line with the long axis of the tibia. With the examiner holding the calcaneus with one hand, a rotatory force is applied to the calcaneus, bringing the subtalar joint into eversion and inversion. Most individuals have at least double the degree of inversion compared to eversion. Lack of inversion should alert the examiner to a possible tarsal coalition or arthritic subtalar joint. Motion of the metatarsophalangeal (MTP) joints is highly variable. MTP dorsiflexion range of motion varies between 45 to 90 degrees, and plantar flexion varies from 10 to 40 degrees (Fig. 5.5) (9).

FOREFOOT–HINDFOOT RELATIONSHIP

When examining the foot and ankle, the relationship of the forefoot to the hindfoot should be determined. There are three possible forefoot positions: Neutral, varus, or valgus. This assessment is best performed with the patient prone or in a seated position with the knees flexed at 90 degrees. With the patient sitting, the examiner should grasp the patient's hindfoot, and place it in a neutral position (the calcaneus should be in line with the long axis of the leg). When examining the right foot, the heel should be grasped by the examiner's right hand, and the left hand should grasp the fifth metatarsal head. The examiner's right thumb should be placed over the talonavicular joint. Neutral position is obtained once the head of the talus is felt to be covered by the navicular. Once the subtalar joint is in neutral, a line perpendicular to a line bisecting the long axis of the calcaneus, along the inferior aspect of the calcaneus, is related to a line following the angle of the plantar aspect of the metatarsal heads (Fig. 5.6A).

In forefoot neutral, the metatarsal and calcaneal planes are perpendicular to each other. In the forefoot varus position, the fifth metatarsal is more plantar flexed than the first metatarsal, placing the forefoot in a supinated position. In forefoot valgus, the first metatarsal is more plantar flexed than the fifth metatarsal, placing the forefoot in a pronated position (Fig. 5.6) (9).

STABILITY

Assessing ankle stability is a crucial part of examining the foot and ankle. Stability of the lateral ankle ligaments are assessed with the anterior drawer and inversion stress test. The anterior drawer test is done by stabilizing the tibia with one hand and applying an anterior force to the hindfoot with the other hand. The normal ankle should have little translation with a solid end point felt by the examiner. The anterior drawer primarily tests the anterior

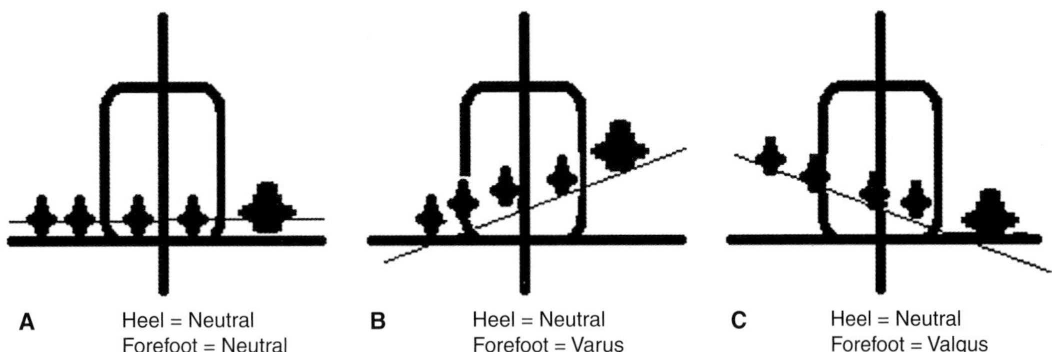

Figure 5.6. Relationship of forefoot to hindfoot. **A:** Normal alignment; forefoot perpendicular to calcaneus. **B:** Forefoot varus; lateral aspect of the forefoot is plantar flexed in relation to the medial aspect. **C:** Forefoot valgus; the medial aspect of the forefoot is plantar flexed in relation to the lateral aspect.

talofibular ligament. The inversion stress test primarily assesses the calcaneofibular ligament and is performed by tilting the talus into inversion. For each of the above tests, the results should be compared to that of the uninvolved side. In addition, an external rotation stress test can be performed to assess for a possible syndesmotic injury. This test is performed with the patient seated with the knee bent to 90 degrees and applying a passive external rotational stress to the foot and ankle. This is considered positive if pain is produced over the anterior or posterior tibiofibular ligaments and the interosseous membrane.

A patient may also have instability of the MTP joints, especially the second. This is checked by noting the inferior–superior motion of the phalanx on the metatarsal head with stressing. It is important to assess for any instability in the first ray since the human foot has evolved to have stability in the first ray, thus allowing for upright ambulation. Instability of the first metatarsocuneiform joint can lead to flatfoot deformity, transfer metatarsalgia, and hallux valgus deformity. To assess the stability of the first ray, the examiner should place one thumb under the lesser metatarsal heads and the other thumb under the first metatarsal head. Both thumbs should then apply an equal upward pressure to the forefoot. In a normal foot, the first metatarsal head will remain even with the second. If hypermobility of the first ray is present, the first metatarsal head will elevate above the second. A callus under the second metatarsal head is indirect evidence of first-ray instability (10).

STRENGTH

Strength of all of the muscle groups of the foot and ankle should be assessed and rated using the standard 1–5 scale of manual muscle testing. Grade 1 is a flicker of muscle movement, 2 is full range of muscle movement with gravity eliminated, 3 is full range of muscle movement again gravity only, 4 is full range of muscle movement with some resistance, 5 is full strength. Proximal strength testing of the major muscle groups is also important if distal weakness is noted, to detect the possibility of a lumbar radiculopathy.

VASCULAR EXAMINATION

Vascular health should be assessed when examining the foot and ankle. The examiner should check the dorsalis pedis and posterior tibial pulses, not just that they are present, but that they are strong and symmetric. The examiner should note any signs suggestive of vascular diseases such as hair loss, ischemic ulcers, or shiny skin. Additional symptoms of vascular diseases include color changes and/or a wooden skin surface appearance or texture.

SENSATION

When examining the foot and ankle, checking light touch sensation is easy to do and can help when defining previous traumatic nerve injures. The innervation of the foot and ankle is highly variable. The tibial nerve innervates the flexor digitorum longus, posterior tibialis, gastrocnemius, and soleus muscles, and provides the posterior calf with sensation. Branches of the tibial nerve include the medial and lateral plantar nerves, which supply the medial and lateral plantar surfaces, respectively, and the medial calcaneal nerve, which supplies the medial and plantar heels. The deep peroneal nerve supplies the tibialis anterior, extensor digitorum longus, and extensor hallucis longus muscles, and provides sensation to the first web space. The superficial peroneal nerve supplies the peroneal muscles and provides sensation to the dorsum of the foot. The sural nerve is formed from branches of both the tibial and common peroneal nerves, and supplies sensation to the lateral foot. The saphenous nerve provides sensation to the medial leg, ankle, and hindfoot (11).

It is important to check the skin sensitivity of the feet in diabetic patients. Since most diabetic patients with neuropathy will have intact light touch sensation, sensation should be assessed by pressing a 0.10 g, 5.07 diameter nylon monofilament over a representative sampling of points on the plantar surface. Lack of skin sensitivity at this level substantially increases the risk of a patient developing foot ulcers. The examiner can also check vibration sense with a tuning fork. Loss of vibration sense may be the earliest sign of peripheral neuropathy. The presence of allodynia may suggest sympathetically maintained pain.

CONCLUSION

As discussed in this chapter, a thorough and methodical history and physical examination is crucial in making the correct diagnosis during medical assessments of the foot and ankle. Following a systematic approach as outlined above will enable physicians to minimize incorrect diagnoses and maximize efficiency. Clinicians should also be cognizant of the fact that not all foot and ankle pain is intrinsic, and may be referred from more proximal body segments, particularly the spine.

REFERENCES

1. Goodwin R, Sferra J. Physical examination and orthotics. In: Thodarson D, Tornetta P, Einhorn T, eds. *Orthopaedic Surgery Essentials*. USA: Lippincott Williams & Wilkins; 2004:24–40.
2. Kannus VPA. Evaluation of abnormal biomechanics of the foot and ankle in athletes. *Br J Sports Med* 1992;26(2):83–89.
3. Roberts M, Greisberg J. Examination of the foot and ankle. In: Di Giovanni C, Greisberg C, eds. *Core Knowledge in Orthopaedics: Foot and Ankle*. USA: Mosby; 2007:10–15.
4. Wilder RP, Sethi S. Overuse injuries: Tendinopathies, stress fractures, compartment syndrome, and shin splints. *Clin Sports Med* 2004;23(1):55–81.
5. Hamilton W, Bauman P. Foot and Ankle Injuries in Dancers. In: Coughlin M, Mann R, Saltzman C, eds. *Surgery of the Foot and Ankle*. 8th ed. USA: Mosby; 2006:Chapter 26.
6. Sutherland DH. *Gait Disorders in Childhood and Adolescence*. Baltimore: Williams & Wilkins; 1984:51–64.
7. Jenkins DB. *Hollinshead's Functional Anatomy of the Limbs and Back*. 6th ed. Philadelphia, PA: W.B. Saunders; 1991.
8. Alexander IJ. *The Foot Examination and Diagnosis*. 2nd ed. New York, NY: Churchill Livingston; 1997.
9. Mann R, Davis H. Principles of Examination of the Foot and Ankle. In: Coughlin M, Mann R, Saltzman C, eds. *Surgery of the Foot and Ankle*. 8th ed. USA: Mosby; 2006:Chapter 2.
10. Morton DJ. Dorsal hypermobility of the first metatarsal segment: Part III. In: Morton DJ, ed. *The Human Foot: Its Evolution, Physiology, and Functional Disorders*. Morningside Heights, NY: Columbia University; 1935:187–195.
11. Pfeffer GB, Clain MR, Frey C, et al. Foot and ankle. In: Snider R, ed. *Essentials of Musculoskeletal Care*. 1st ed. Rosemont, IL: American Academy of Orthopaedic Surgeons; 1997:366–489.

Helene Pavlov
Carolyn M. Sofka
Gregory R. Saboeiro
Douglas N. Mintz

CHAPTER 6

Imaging of Foot and Ankle Athletic Injuries

Imaging of sports-related injuries to the foot and ankle require careful positioning and planning dependant on the mechanism of the injury and the resultant pain or limitation of function. Most injuries are predictable with specific radiographic and imaging patterns. The clinical history and thorough physical examination are essential parts in determining the appropriate imaging modality for the suspected injury or condition. Diagnostic confirmation may require the use of several imaging techniques, especially during the early onset of symptoms. Early diagnosis is critical to prevent prolonged immobilization which could devastate a professional athlete's career or inhibit a sports enthusiast's determination and regimen.

Communication of a suspected clinical condition to the radiologist optimizes the imaging examination. This consultation not only facilitates obtaining the appropriate modality (conventional x-ray, computed tomography [CT], magnetic resonance imaging [MRI], nuclear medicine scan [NM], or ultrasound [US]) for the suspected condition, but also ensures that the imaging examination will be obtained focused for a specific area and an optimal outcome.

Foot and ankle injuries include osseous injuries such as fractures, stress fractures, avulsion injuries, and also soft tissue injuries such as strains, sprains, inflammation, partial and complete tears of tendons and ligaments as well as neuromas, ganglions, bursitis, and formation of adventitial bursae. Cartilage injuries are also a significant source of both acute and chronic pain and eventual arthritis. Some injuries are very localized and the site of pathology very specific; while other injuries present with a more diffuse pain pattern rendering both the clinical and imaging diagnoses more elusive.

The initial imaging examination for all foot and ankle injuries that warrant objective documentation or confirmation is the conventional (x-ray) radiograph. The conventional x-ray will provide either a definitive confirmation or exclusion of a suspected diagnosis as well as an overview of the area. This initial imaging examination helps to determine if the acute focal site of pain is perhaps masking a more significant injury elsewhere in the foot or ankle. This initial study is essential in determining if further imaging is required and if so, the appropriate follow-up imaging examination. A CT examination is ideal for providing further information as to a suspected osseous lesion or to preoperatively validate in multiple planes, the position of fracture fragments or bony alignments. MR and CT both provide multiplanar imaging, but MR is more sensitive for detecting bone marrow edema patterns and soft tissue injuries including the status of the articular cartilage. US provides an excellent means to diagnose a localized injury or to follow a soft tissue injury during the healing process. In addition, US guidance is an excellent mechanism for targeted injections into an injured area (e.g., tendon sheath, bursae, etc.).

In order to focus an imaging examination on the area in question, it is ideal to categorize the clinical symptomatology by area. For the purpose of this chapter, we have categorized foot and ankle pain as follows: Posterior heel pain, plantar pain, midfoot pain, forefoot pain, diffuse foot and ankle pain, and ankle pain.

Posterior heel pain includes stress fractures, bursitis, Haglund's complex, Achilles tendon injuries, os trigonum (posterior impingement) syndrome and fractures of the posterior medial talar process (Figs. 6.1–6.8).

Plantar heel pain includes plantar fasciitis and fractures of the plantar calcaneal spur (Figs. 6.9–6.11).

Midfoot pain results from Lisfranc injuries, stress fracture of the cuboid or navicular, distraction/fracture of the accessory navicular (os tibialis externa), posterior tibial tendon injuries, distraction/fracture of the os peroneum and peroneal tendon injuries. Dorsal midfoot pain can present secondary to an os supranaviculare injury or a dorsal ganglion (Figs. 6.12–6.25).

Forefoot pain includes stress fractures of the metatarsals, Freiberg's infraction, neuromas, and/or sesamoid fractures and dislocations including turf toe with soft tissue injuries plantar to the metatarsal phalangeal joint of the great toe (Figs. 6.26–6.30).

Diffuse foot and ankle pain results from several injuries for which determining the best imaging examination can be confusing. Patients who present with diffuse pain commonly have either an avulsion fracture of the anterior calcaneal process; an avulsion injury of the lateral aspect of the talus where the extensor digitorum brevis inserts; a fracture of the base of the tuberosity of the fifth metatarsal; or a stress fracture of the fifth metatarsal distal to the tuberosity. All of these injuries are best identified on the routine conventional radiographs of the ankle, provided the frontal view of the ankle includes the inferior aspect of the talus and that the soft tissue in this area

(*Text continues on page 61*)

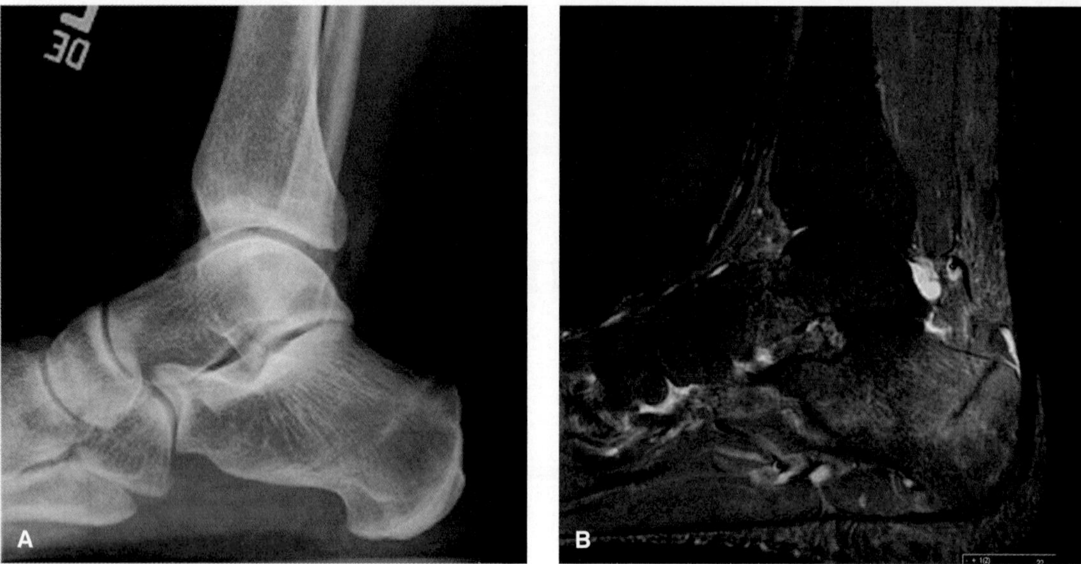

Figure 6.1. **A:** Standing lateral conventional radiograph of the ankle demonstrates characteristic cancellous stress fracture of the calcaneus with linear band of sclerosis oriented perpendicular to flow of trabeculae. **B:** Sagittal STIR MR image depicts calcaneal stress fracture with reactive bone marrow edema pattern surrounding the fracture. © Hospital for Special Surgery, New York, New York.

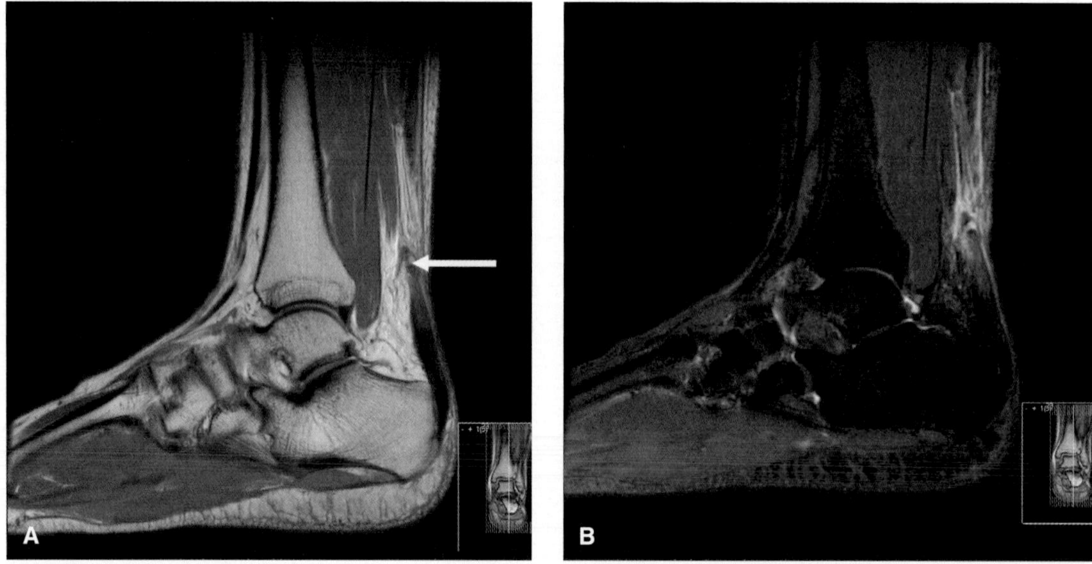

Figure 6.2. Sagittal FSE PD MR image **(A)** of the ankle demonstrates complete disruption of the Achilles tendon with a 5 cm gap (*arrow*). Sagittal STIR MR image **(B)** demonstrates that the injury is acute with hyperintensity and fluid filling the tendon gap. © Hospital for Special Surgery, New York, New York.

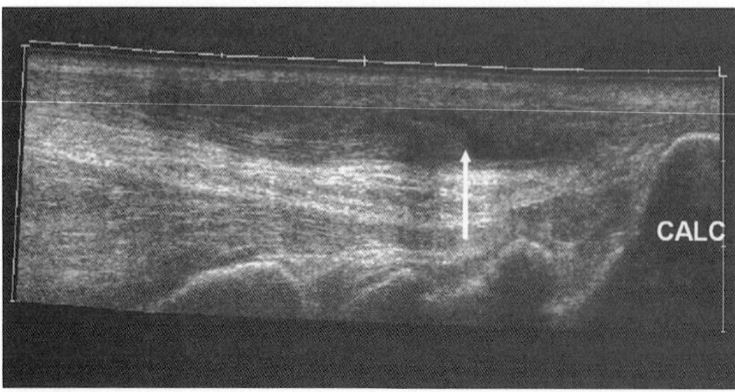

Figure 6.3. Long-axis ultrasound image of the Achilles tendon demonstrating a partial-thickness tear (*arrow*) in the setting of advanced tendinosis, with diffuse decreased echogenicity and thickening of the tendon. © Hospital for Special Surgery, New York, New York.

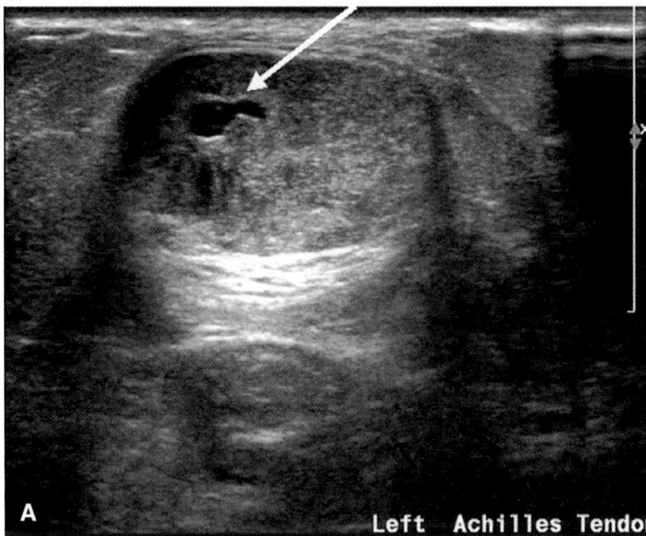

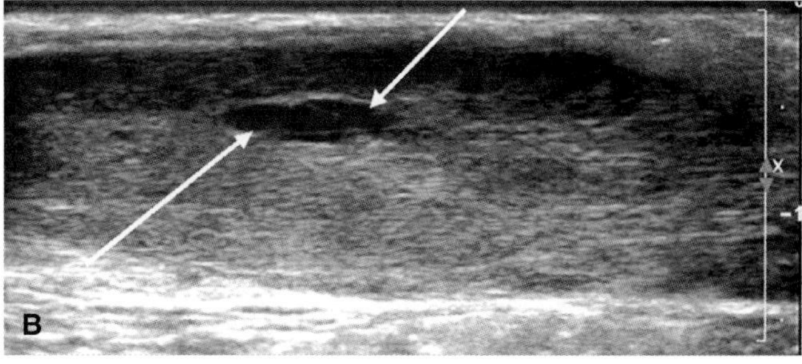

Figure 6.4. Short-axis (transverse) **(A)** and long-axis **(B)** ultrasound images demonstrating a small intrasubstance tear (*arrows*) of the Achilles tendon. © Hospital for Special Surgery, New York, New York.

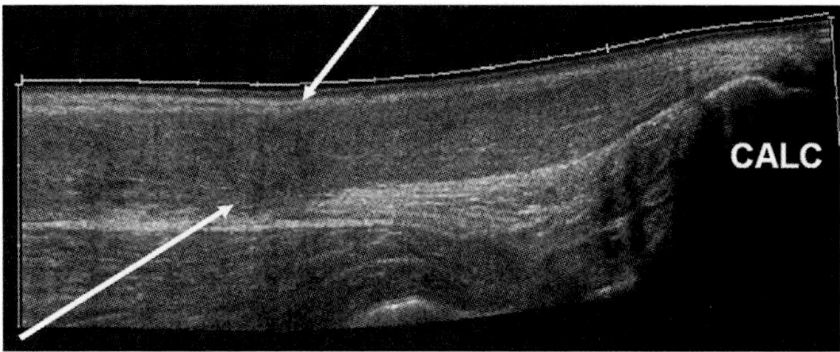

Figure 6.5. Long-axis ultrasound image demonstrating thickening of the Achilles tendon (*arrows*) consistent with tendinosis without tear. © Hospital for Special Surgery, New York, New York.

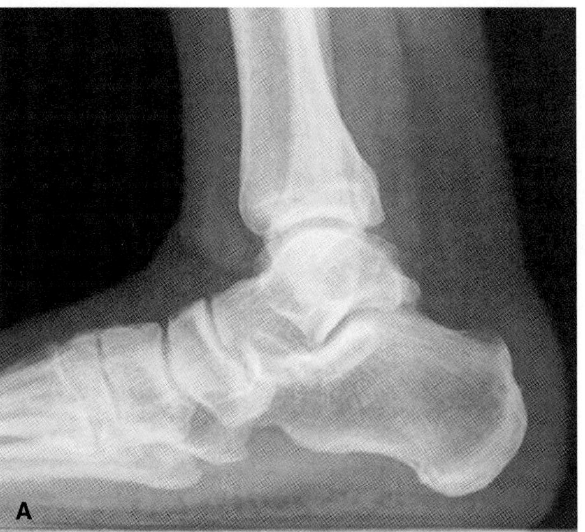

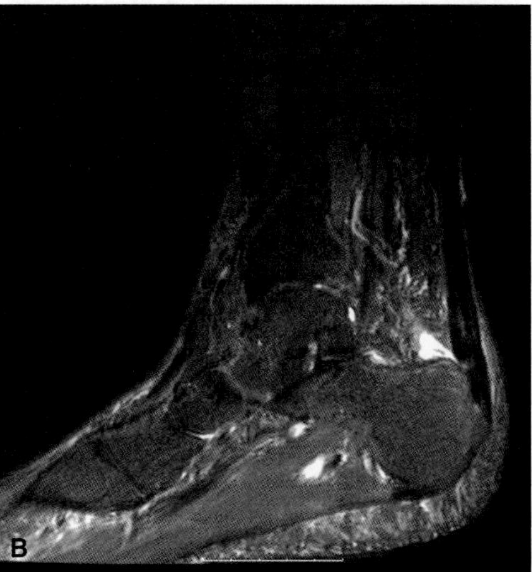

Figure 6.6. **A:** Standing lateral view of the foot demonstrates Haglund's disease with thickening of the Achilles tendon at its insertion, convexity of the soft tissues dorsal to the Achilles tendon indicating superficial tendo Achilles bursitis, soft tissue density in the retrocalcaneal bursae indicating retrocalcaneal bursitis and calcaneal prominence of the dorsal posterior calcaneus. **B:** Sagittal STIR MR image of the hindfoot demonstrates the characteristic findings of Haglund's disease with fluid in the deep retrocalcaneal bursa, moderate insertional tendinosis of the Achilles tendon, hyperintensity and thickening of the superficial tendo Achilles bursa and prominence of the posterior superior aspect of the calcaneus with mild reactive bone marrow edema pattern. © Hospital for Special Surgery, New York, New York.

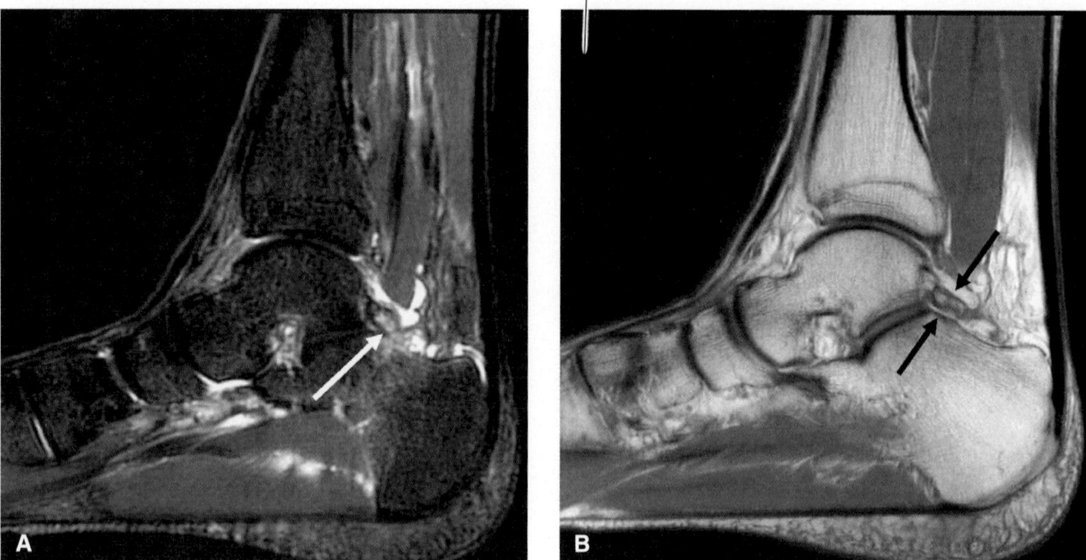

Figure 6.7. **A:** Sagittal STIR image of the ankle demonstrates posterior ankle impingement (os trigonum syndrome). Hyperintensity is seen within the os trigonum (*arrow*) and the posterior calcaneus with fluid surrounding the os. **B:** Sagittal FSE image of the ankle in the same patient demonstrates sclerosis from chronic remodeling and impaction in both the os trigonum and the calcaneus (*arrows*). © Hospital for Special Surgery, New York, New York.

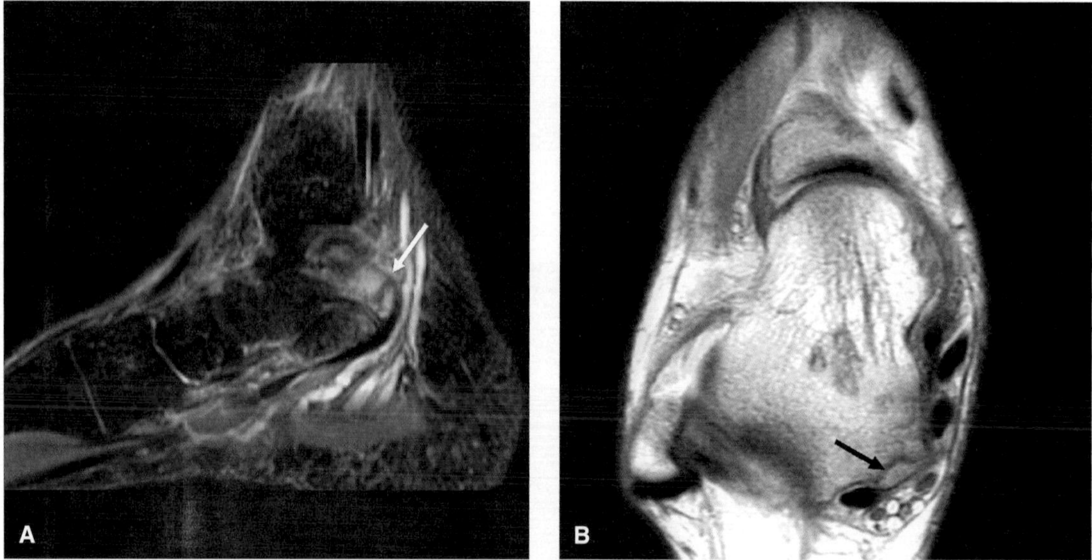

Figure 6.8. **A:** Sagittal STIR image demonstrates an acute fracture of the posterior aspect of the medial facet of the talus with bone marrow edema pattern surrounding the fracture (*arrow*). **B:** Axial FSE image in the same patient demonstrates a nondisplaced fracture (*arrow*). Note the proximity of the fracture to the posterior tibial neurovascular bundle and the flexor hallucis longus tendons. © Hospital for Special Surgery, New York, New York.

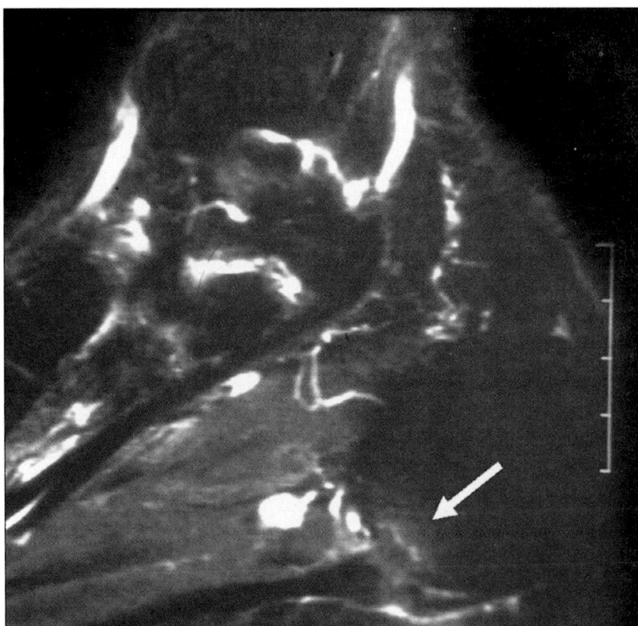

Figure 6.9. Sagittal fat-suppressed MR image of the ankle demonstrates moderate thickening and hyperintensity of the origin of the plantar fascia with reactive bone marrow edema (*arrow*) in the medial calcaneal tubercle. © Hospital for Special Surgery, New York, New York.

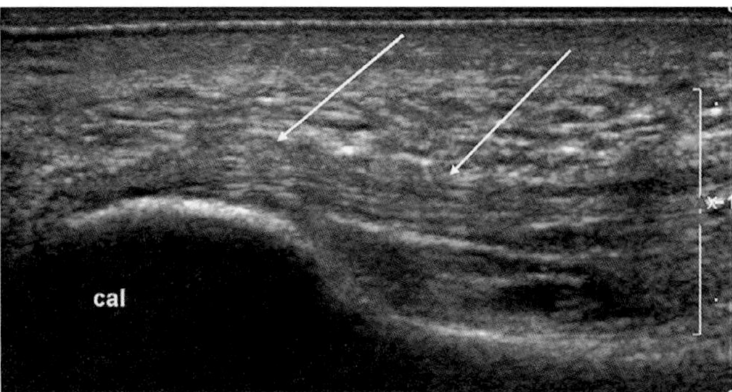

Figure 6.10. Long-axis ultrasound image of the plantar fascia (*arrows*) demonstrating normal echogenicity and thickness (<3.5 mm). © Hospital for Special Surgery, New York, New York.

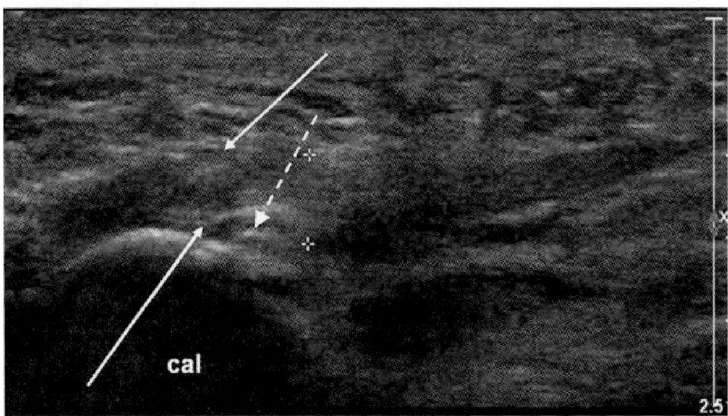

Figure 6.11. Long-axis ultrasound image demonstrating abnormal thickening (8 mm between the markers) and inhomogeneity of the plantar fascia reflecting plantar fasciitis (*arrows*) with a small deep surface partial-thickness tear (*dashed arrow*). © Hospital for Special Surgery, New York, New York.

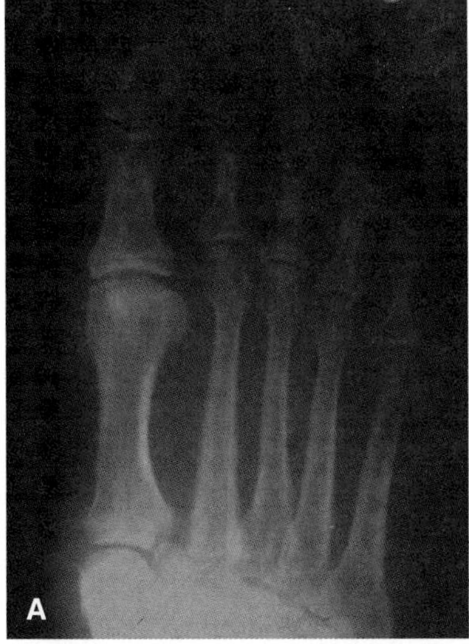

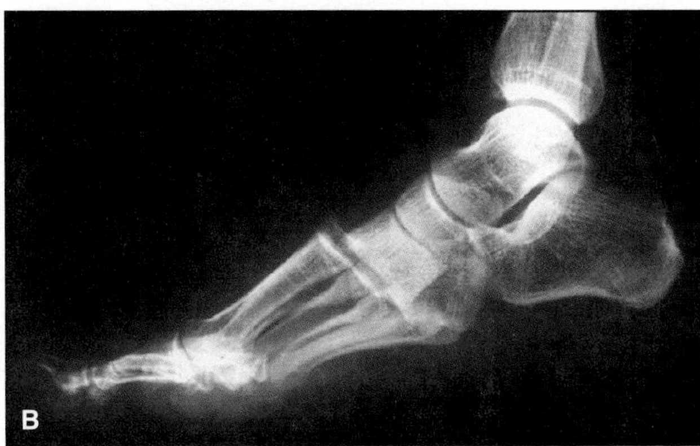

Figure 6.12. **(A/B)** Frontal and lateral views of the foot demonstrate Lisfranc plantar lateral dislocation of the second metatarsal–tarsal joint. © Hospital for Special Surgery, New York, New York.

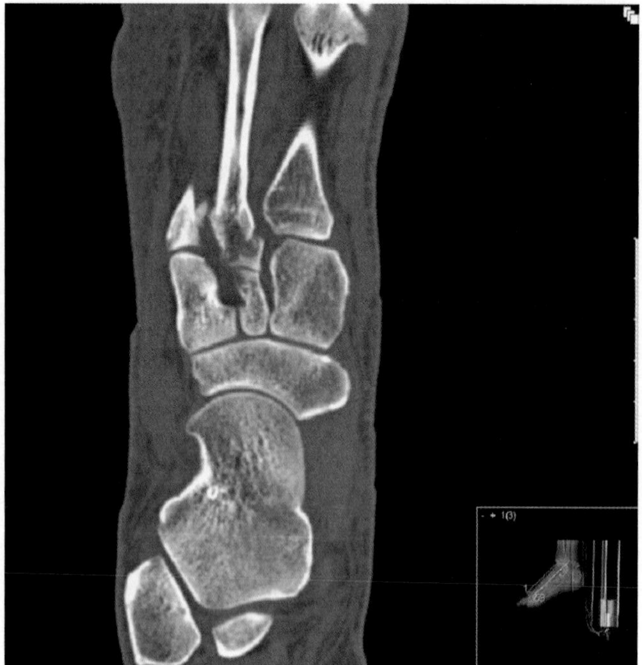

Figure 6.13. Coronal reformatted CT image demonstrates a comminuted fracture at the base of the second metatarsal with mild widening of the proximal first web space consistent with a Lisfranc fracture dislocation. © Hospital for Special Surgery, New York, New York.

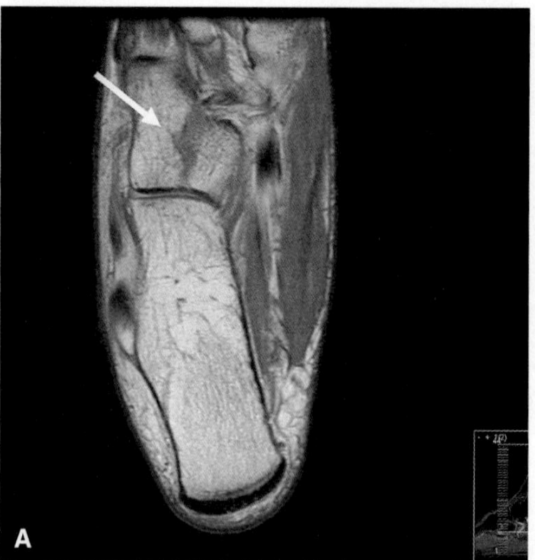

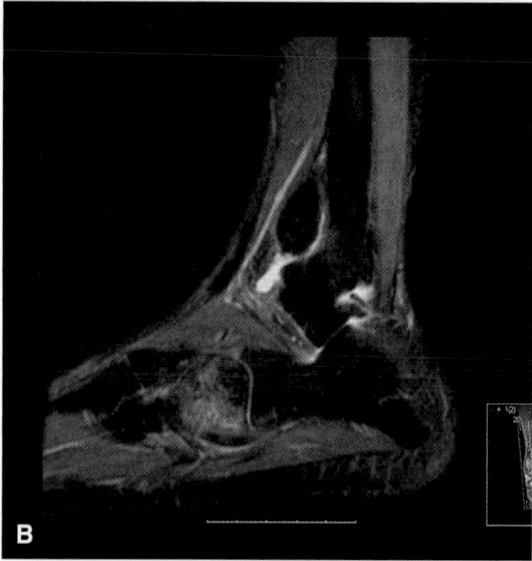

Figure 6.14. **A:** Axial FSE PD MR image of the midfoot demonstrates a complete fracture through the cuboid (*arrow*). **B:** Sagittal STIR MR image demonstrates intense bone marrow edema pattern in the cuboid. © Hospital for Special Surgery, New York, New York.

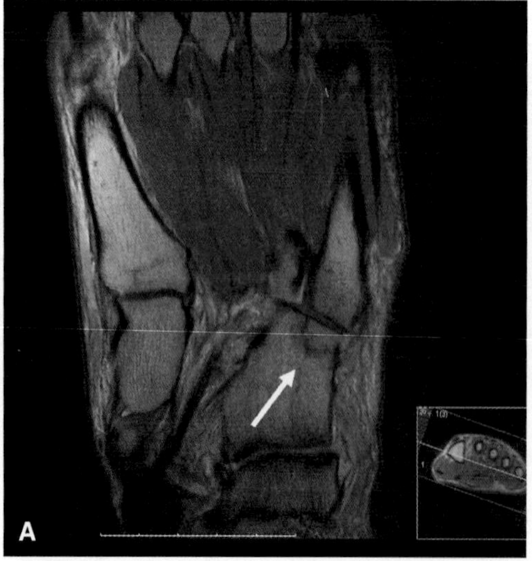

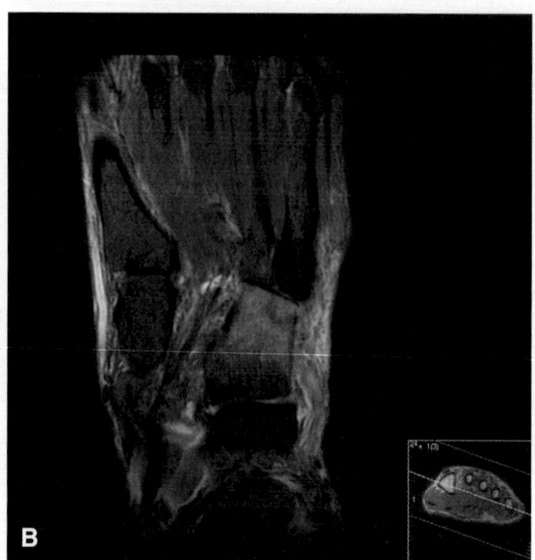

Figure 6.15. Coronal (to the plane of the foot) FSE PD (**A**) and STIR (**B**) MR images demonstrate an acute impacted intraarticular fracture (*arrow*) of the distal cuboid which extend into the tarsal–metatarsal joint. There is intense bone marrow edema pattern around the fracture. © Hospital for Special Surgery, New York, New York.

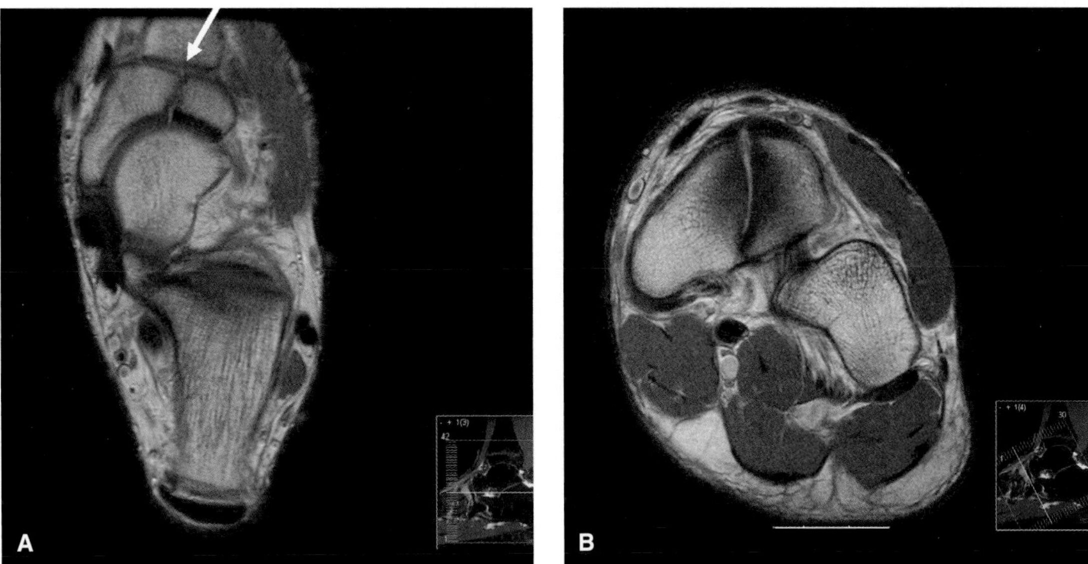

Figure 6.16. **(A/B)** Axial and coronal (to the plane of the ankle) FSE PD MR images demonstrate a complete fracture (*arrow*) through the body of the navicular at the junction of the medial and lateral third. Low signal intensity along the fracture margins suggests sclerosis and nonunion. © Hospital for Special Surgery, New York, New York.

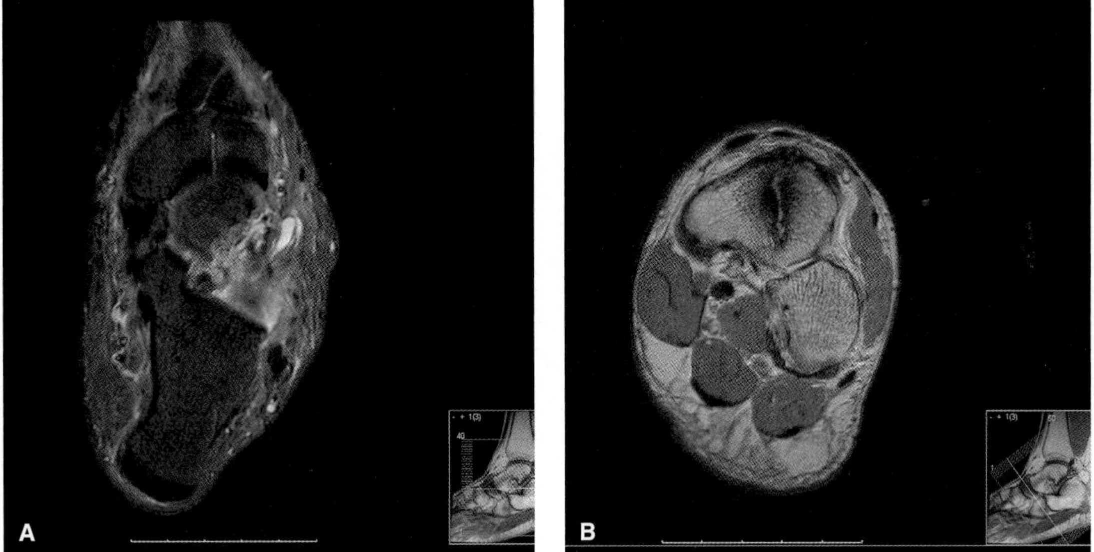

Figure 6.17. Axial STIR **(A)** image through the midfoot and coronal FSE PD **(B)** MR image demonstrate an incomplete fracture through the navicular with sclerotic margins consistent with nonunion. The absence of reactive bone marrow edema pattern further indicates that the fracture is not acute. © Hospital for Special Surgery, New York, New York.

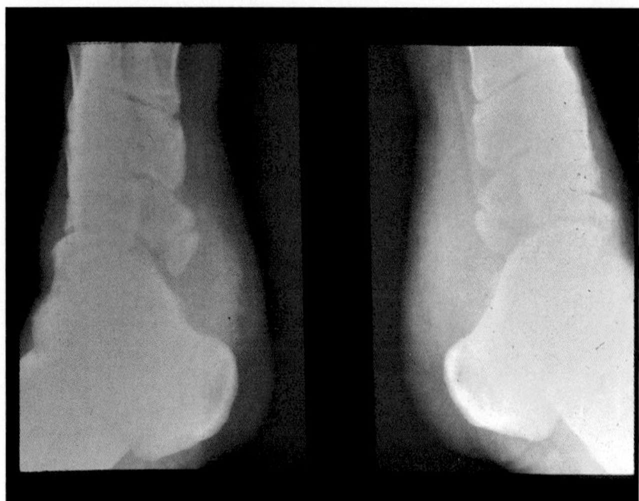

Figure 6.18. Oblique views of both feet obtained with maximum supination optimally demonstrates bilateral large accessory navicular bones (os tibialis externa). © Hospital for Special Surgery, New York, New York.

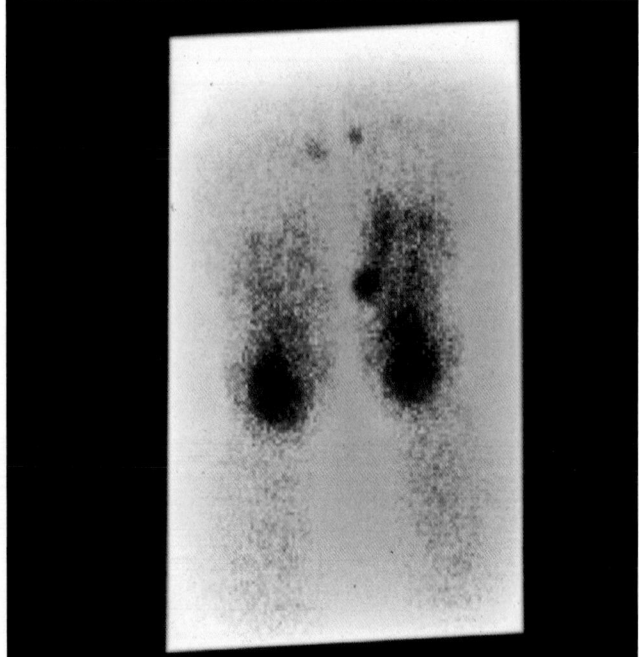

Figure 6.19. Radionuclide Technicium-99m bone scan of both feet obtained in the plantar position demonstrates augmented isotope uptake localized to the left os tibialis externa. © Hospital for Special Surgery, New York, New York.

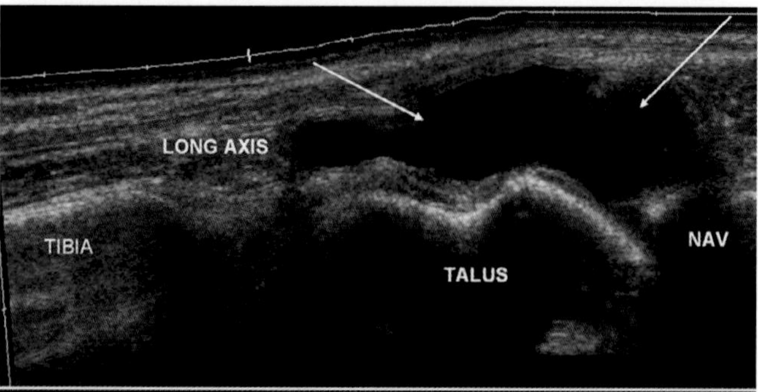

Figure 6.20. Long-axis ultrasound image demonstrates a large ganglion cyst (*arrows*) at the dorsal aspect of the midfoot arising from the talonavicular joint. © Hospital for Special Surgery, New York, New York.

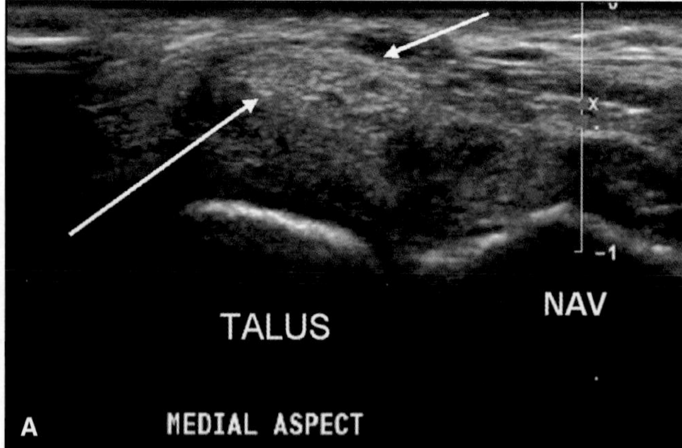

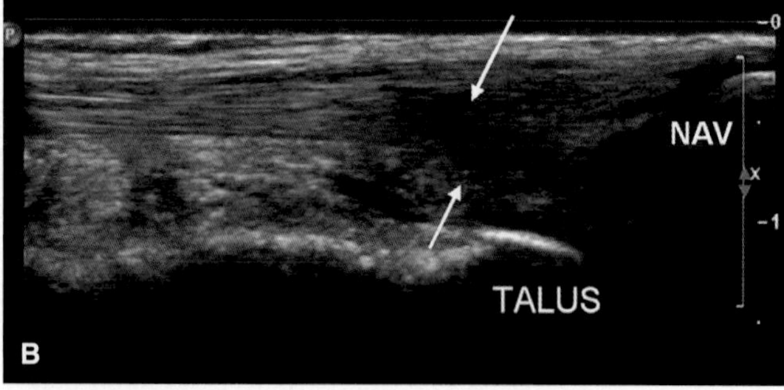

Figure 6.21. Short-axis (**A**) and long-axis (**B**) ultrasound images demonstrate insertional posterior tibial tendinosis with partial-thickness deep surface tear (*arrows*). © Hospital for Special Surgery, New York, New York.

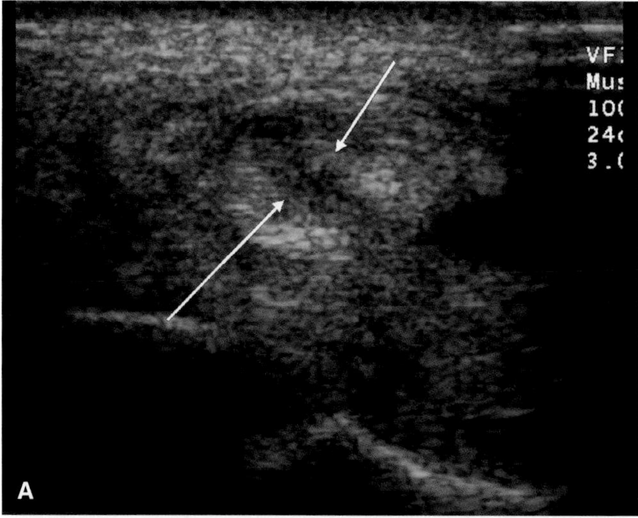

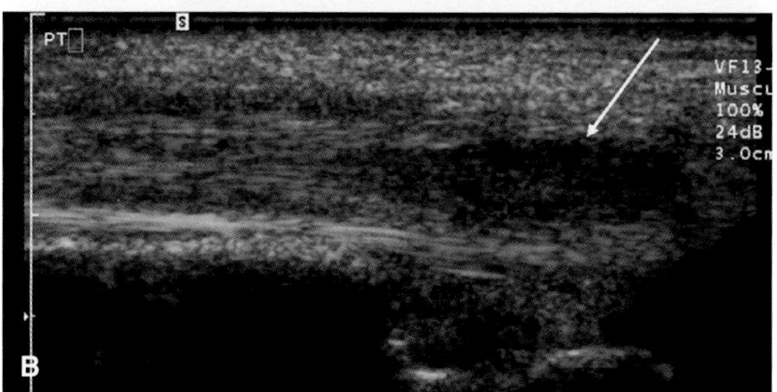

Figure 6.22. Short-axis (**A**) and long-axis (**B**) ultrasound images demonstrate an obliquely oriented full-thickness tear of the distal posterior tibial tendon (*arrows*). © Hospital for Special Surgery, New York, New York.

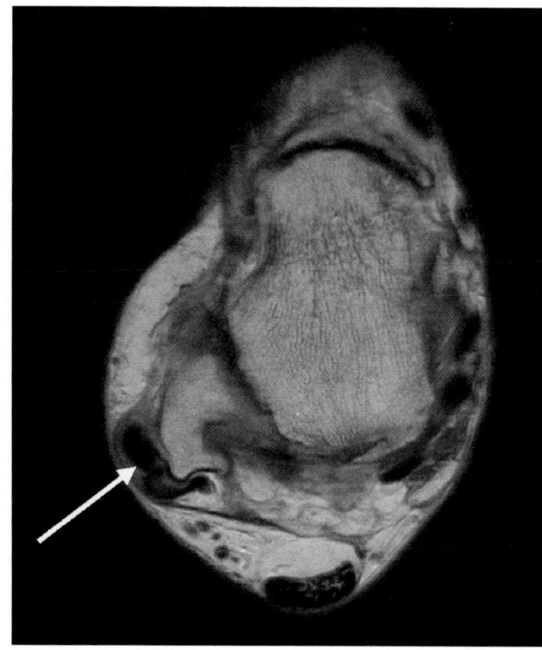

Figure 6.24. Axial FSE PD MR image demonstrates lateral dislocation of the peroneal tendons (*arrow*) from a relatively shallow fibular groove. © Hospital for Special Surgery, New York, New York.

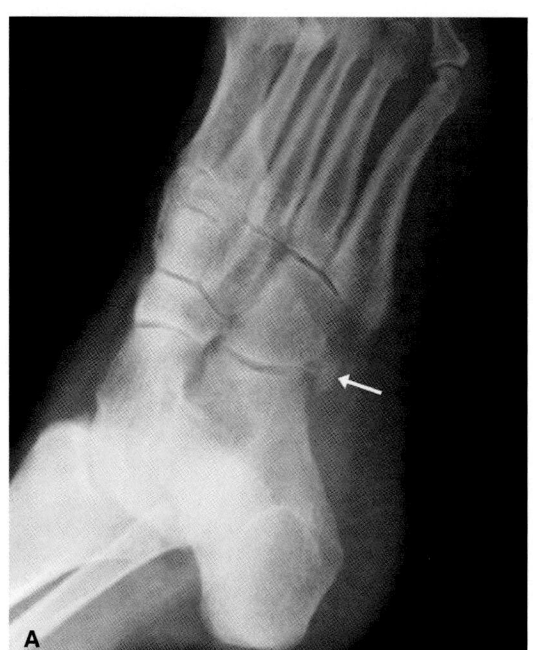

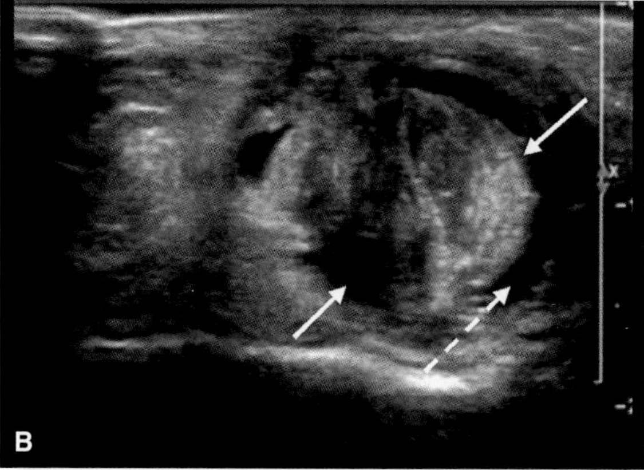

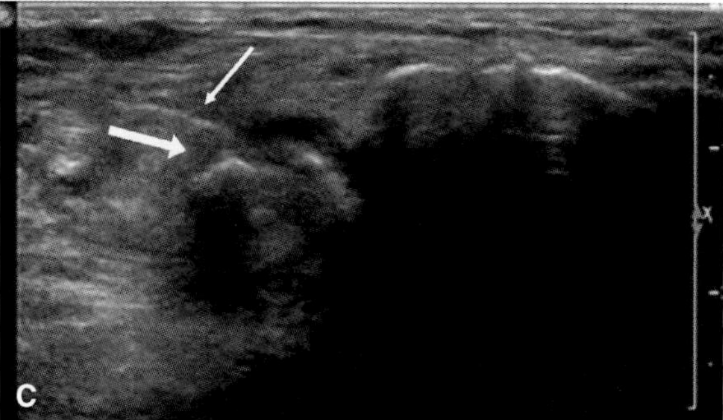

Figure 6.23. **A:** Oblique view of the foot demonstrates a large normally positioned os peroneum (*arrow*). **B:** Short-axis ultrasound image demonstrates marked tendinosis and degeneration of the peroneal tendons (*arrows*) with tendon sheath effusion (*dashed arrow*). **C:** Short-axis ultrasound image demonstrates a needle (*thin arrow*) directed toward the os peroneum (*thick arrow*) for a therapeutic injection procedure. © Hospital for Special Surgery, New York, New York.

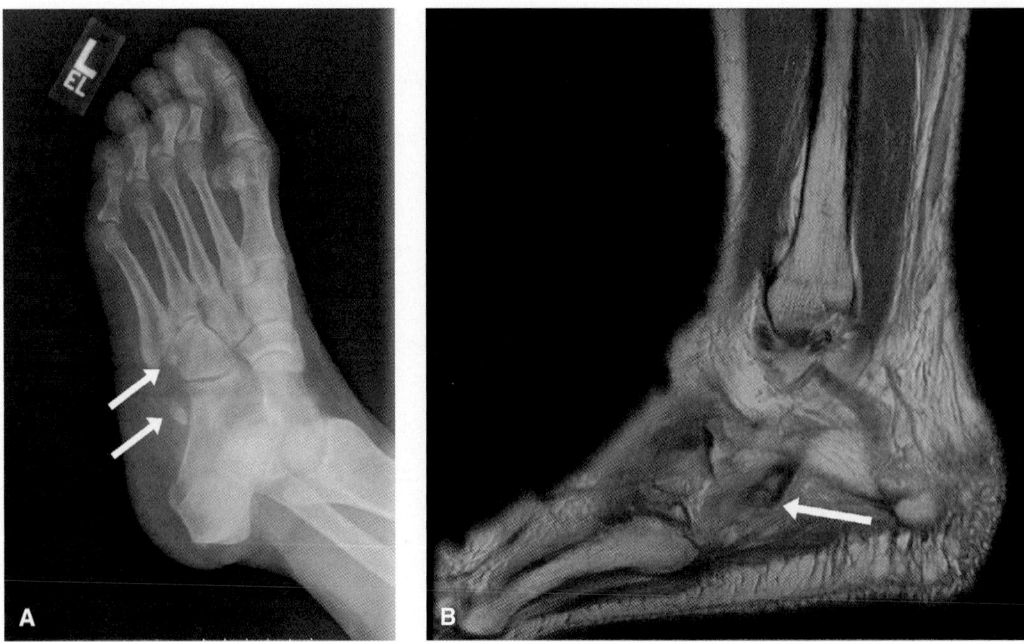

Figure 6.25. **A:** Oblique conventional x-ray of the foot demonstrates a fractured os peroneum with distraction of the fragments (*arrows*). **B:** Sagittal FSE PD MR image through the far lateral aspect of the midfoot demonstrates a fracture (*arrows*) of the proximally distracted os peroneum fragment. © Hospital for Special Surgery, New York, New York.

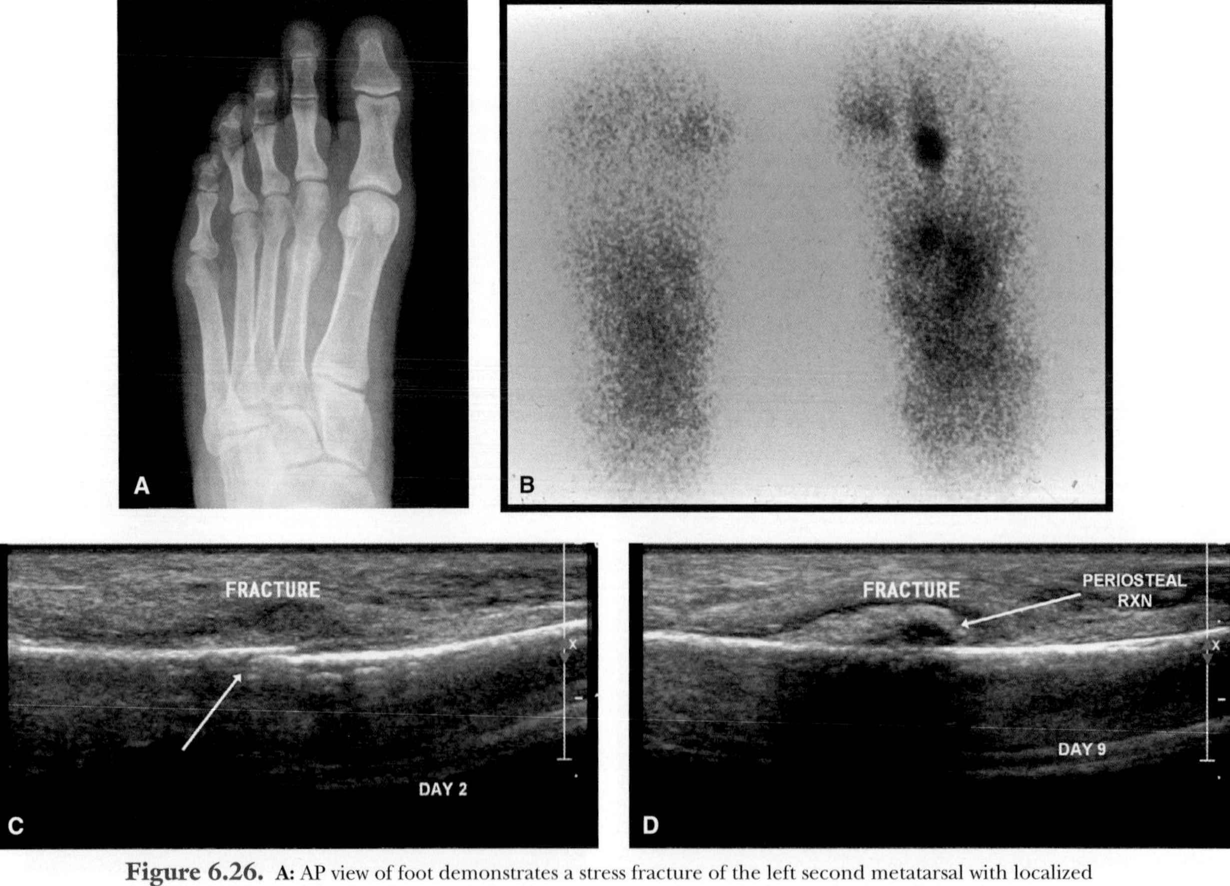

Figure 6.26. **A:** AP view of foot demonstrates a stress fracture of the left second metatarsal with localized area of callus at the neck. **B:** Radionuclide Technicium-99m bone scan demonstrates focused increased uptake of the left second metatarsal consistent with a stress fracture. **C:** Long-axis ultrasound image demonstrates cortical disruption of the third metatarsal (*arrow*) reflecting an acute stress fracture. **D:** Long-axis ultrasound on day 9 after the fracture demonstrates periosteal elevation and early callus formation at the fracture site. © Hospital for Special Surgery, New York, New York.

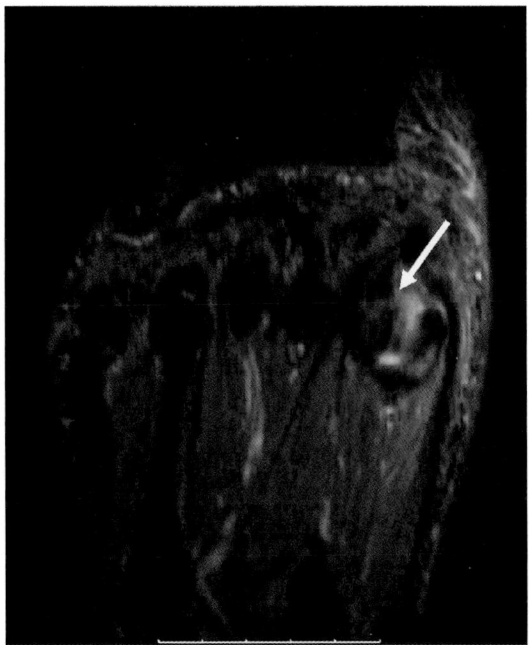

Figure 6.27. Coronal IR MR image through the plantar aspect of the foot demonstrates hyperintensity at the plantar margin of the first MTP joint with a subtle fracture of the distal pole of the lateral hallux sesamoid (*arrow*). © Hospital for Special Surgery, New York, New York.

are adequately penetrated and the lateral view of the ankle includes the base of the fifth metatarsal (Figs. 6.31–6.36).

Ankle pain results from tears of the deltoid, anterior talofibular. and calcaneofibular ligaments and osteochondral injuries. More proximally, cortical and cancellous stress fractures of the distal tibia and fibula can occur (Figs. 6.37–6.43).

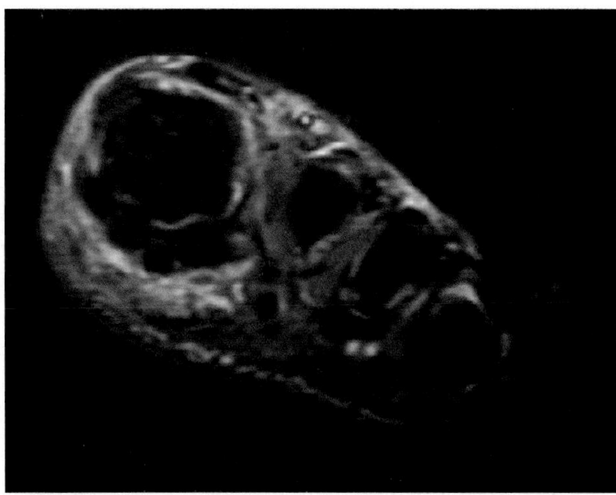

Figure 6.28. Axial IR images through the forefoot demonstrate extensive extra capsular soft tissue edema concentrated plantarly secondary to disruption of the plantar plate. © Hospital for Special Surgery, New York, New York.

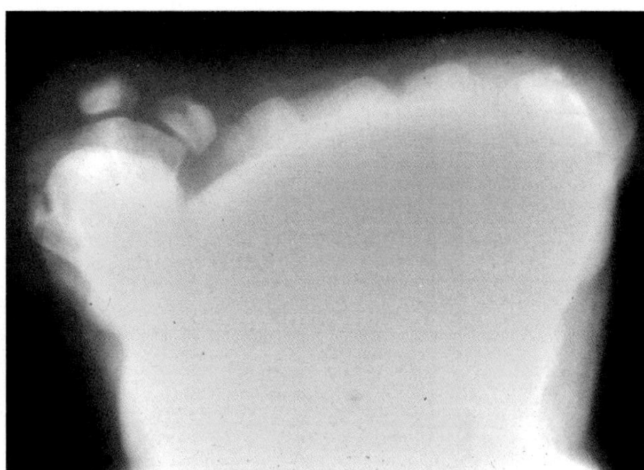

Figure 6.29. Axial view of the metatarsal sesamoid joints on conventional x-ray demonstrates lateral subluxation of both sesamoids from their respective metatarsal sulci. © Hospital for Special Surgery, New York, New York.

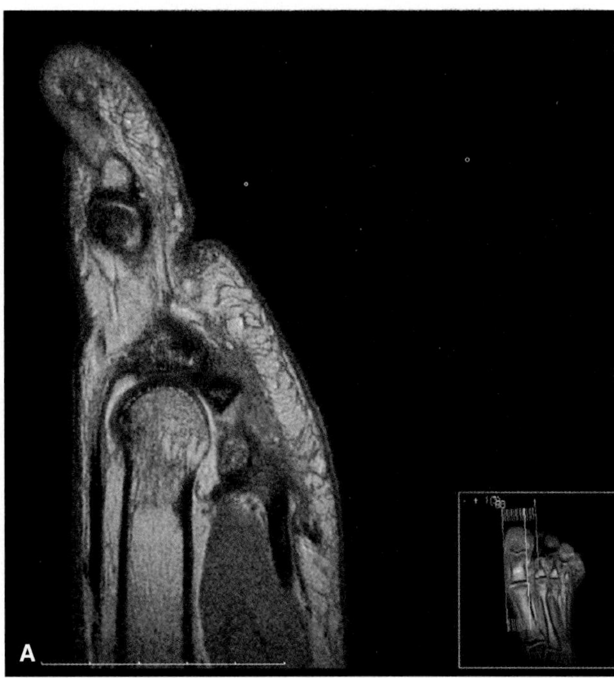

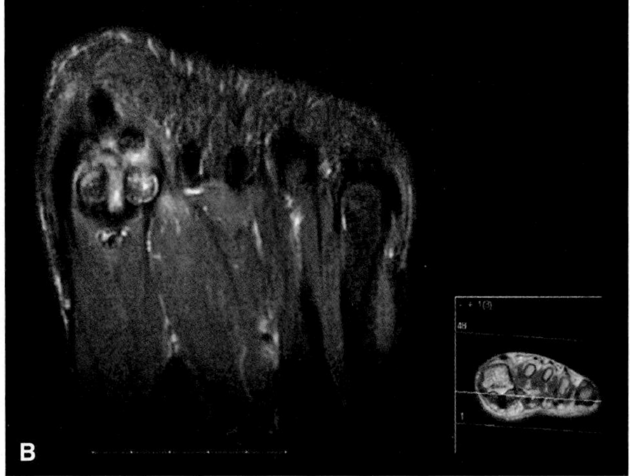

Figure 6.30. **A:** High-resolution sagittal FSE PD image through the great toe demonstrates an acute facture of the lateral hallux sesamoid with distraction of the fragments, disruption of the plantar plate and reactive synovitis in the first MTP joint. **B:** Coronal STIR image through the forefoot demonstrates fractures of the medial and lateral hallux sesamoids with reactive bone marrow edema pattern. (*continued*)

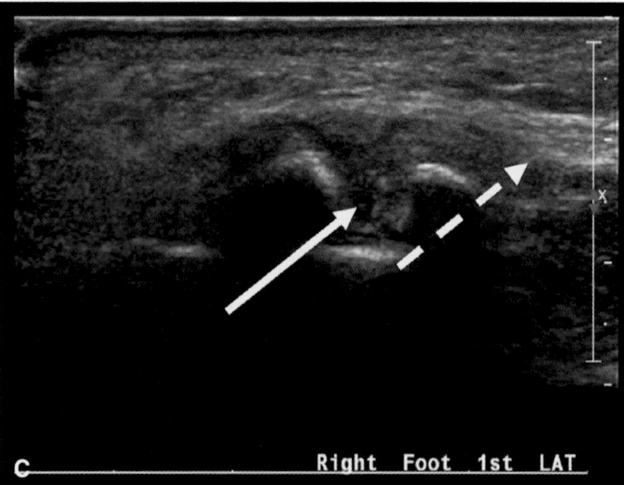

Figure 6.30. (*continued*) **C:** Longitudinal ultrasound image of the plantar aspect of the first MTP joint demonstrates a fracture of the lateral hallux sesamoid with distraction of the distal and proximal poles (*arrow*). The overlying lateral head of the flexor hallucis brevis tendon is identified (*dashed arrow*). © Hospital for Special Surgery, New York, New York.

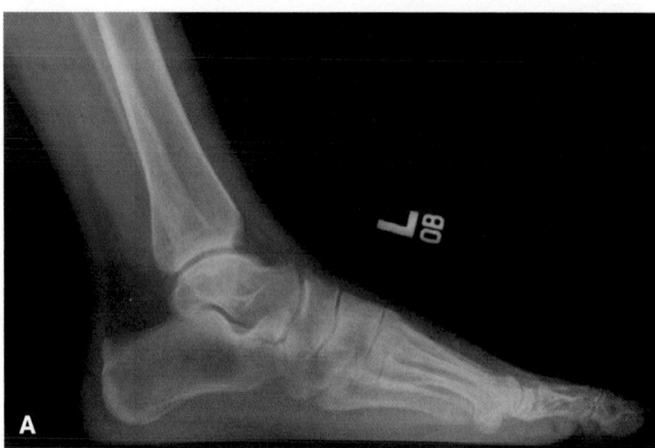

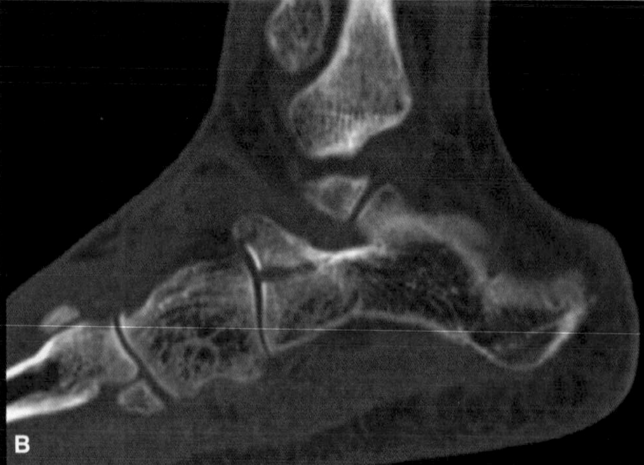

Figure 6.31. **A:** Lateral conventional radiograph of the foot demonstrates a fracture of the anterior calcaneal process. **B:** Sagittal reformatted CT image of the ankle in a different patient demonstrates a mildly comminuted horizontal fracture at the base of the anterior process of the calcaneus. © Hospital for Special Surgery, New York, New York.

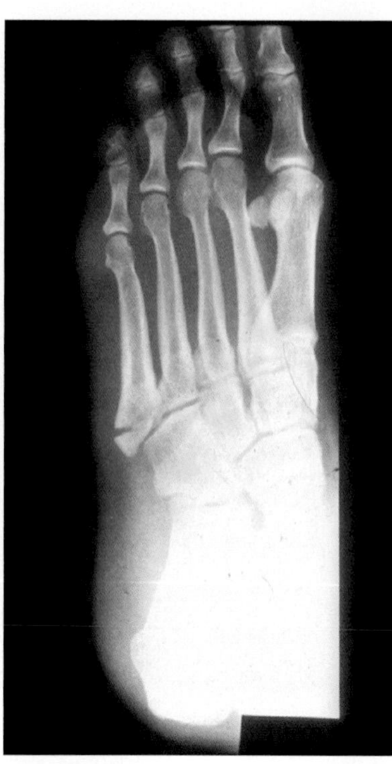

Figure 6.32. Oblique view of the foot demonstrates an avulsion fracture of the tuberosity at the base of the fifth metatarsal. © Hospital for Special Surgery, New York, New York.

Appropriate imaging and careful image acquisition is essential for the imaging examination to be diagnostic and not a waste of your patient's money. Utilizing appropriate positioning and/or protocols and/or technique in addition to optimal equipment that can best capture the information is a mandate. Once the

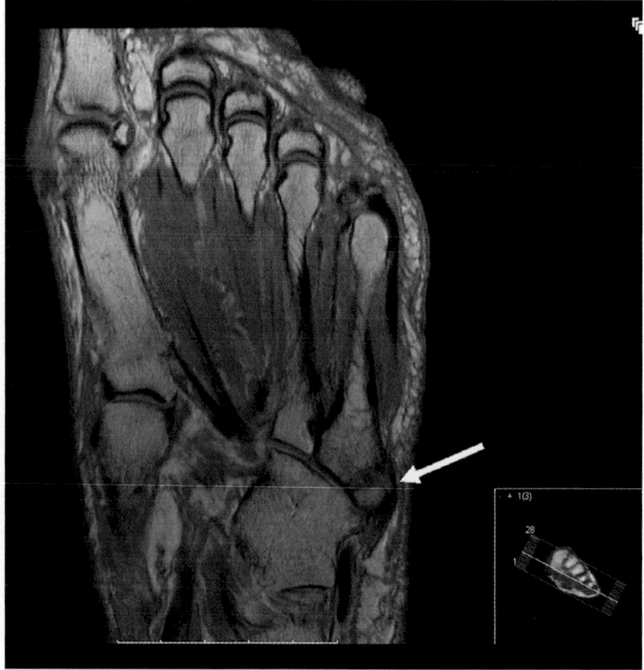

Figure 6.33. Coronal FSE PD MR image demonstrates a subacute nondisplaced fracture at the base of the fifth metatarsal (*arrow*). There is fibrous matrix bridging the fracture. © Hospital for Special Surgery, New York, New York.

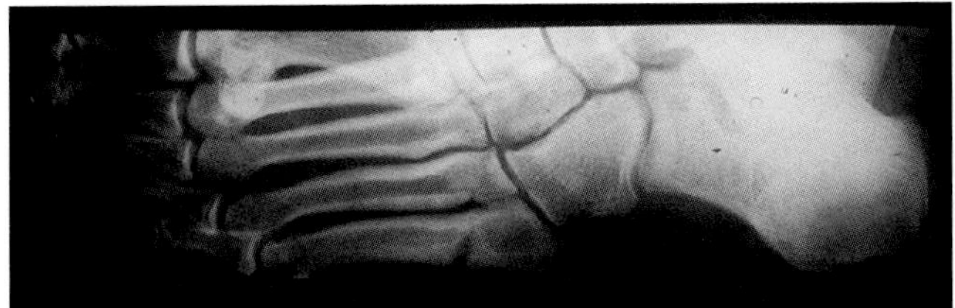

Figure 6.34. Lateral view of the foot demonstrates a stress fracture of the fifth metatarsal distal to the tuberosity. © Hospital for Special Surgery, New York, New York.

image is acquired, familiarity with common and uncommon entities, recognition of normal variants and distinguishing subtle abnormalities are essential for optimal patient care, justification for obtaining the imaging examination, and for planning and following management and treatment options.

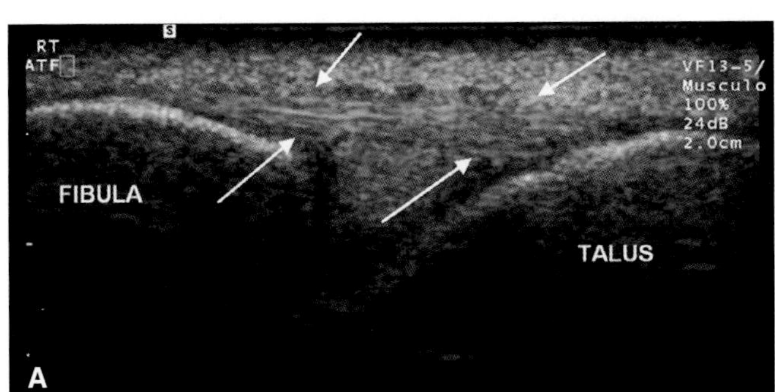

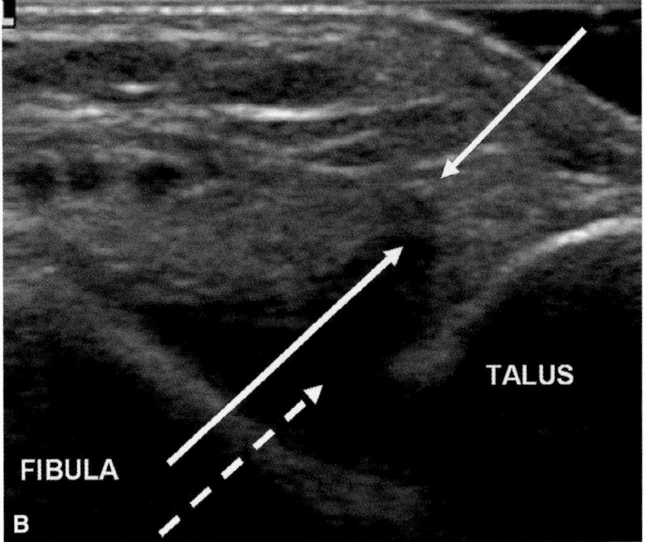

Figure 6.35. **A:** Long-axis ultrasound demonstrates a normal anterior talofibular ligament (*arrows*). **B:** Long-axis ultrasound demonstrates a partial-thickness tear of the anterior talofibular ligament (*arrows*) with fluid deep to the ligament (*dashed arrow*). © Hospital for Special Surgery, New York, New York.

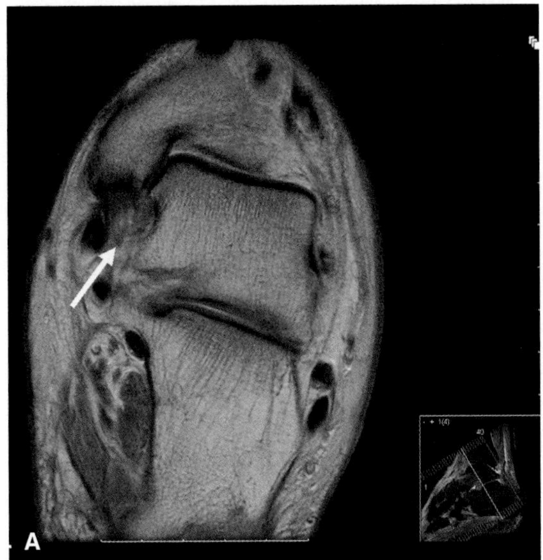

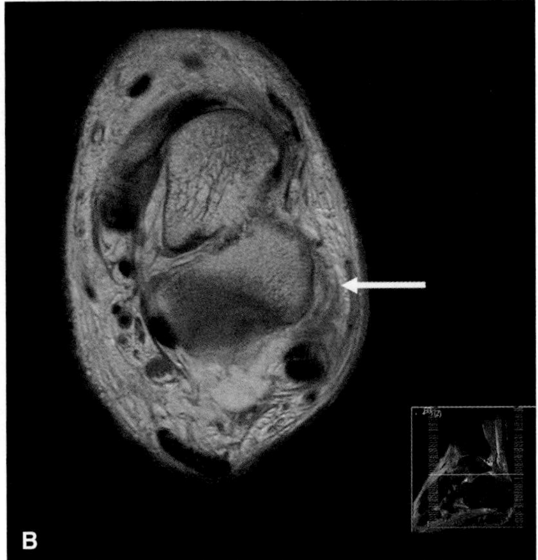

Figure 6.36. **A:** Coronal FSE PD MR image demonstrates complete disruption of the deep fibers of the deltoid near the talar insertion (*arrow*). **B:** Axial FSE PD MR image demonstrates focal complete disruption of the anterior talofibular ligament (*arrow*). © Hospital for Special Surgery, New York, New York.

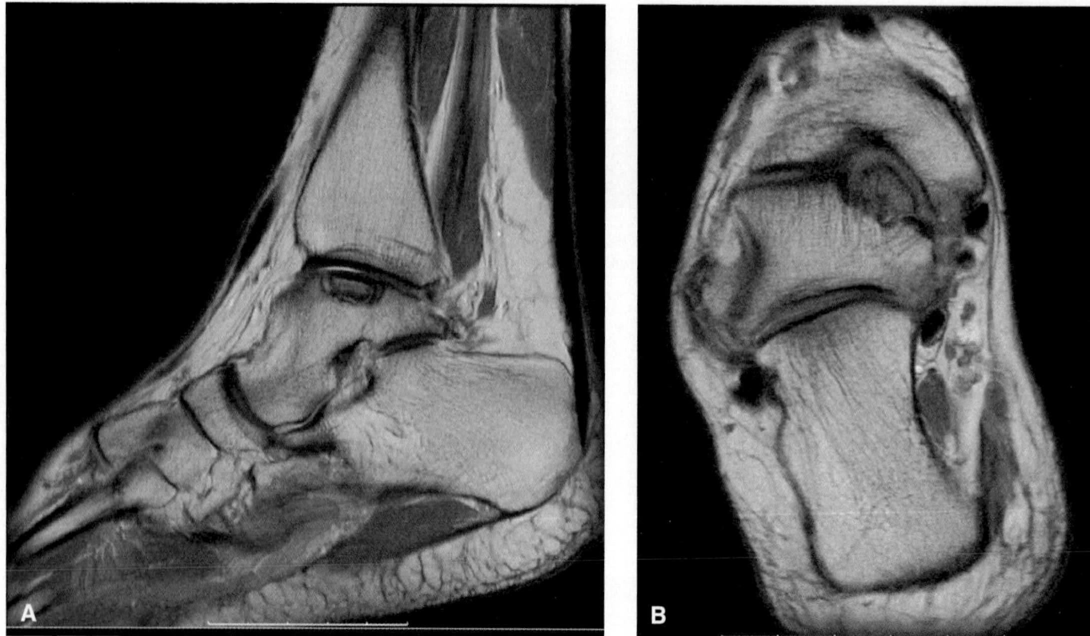

Figure 6.37. Sagittal **(A)** and coronal FSE PD **(B)** MR images through the ankle demonstrate osteochondritis dissecans in the medial aspect of the talar dome extending into the medial gutter. Hyperintense fluid partially surrounds the lesion, but does not extend through the subchondral plate, suggesting that it is not loose in situ. © Hospital for Special Surgery, New York, New York.

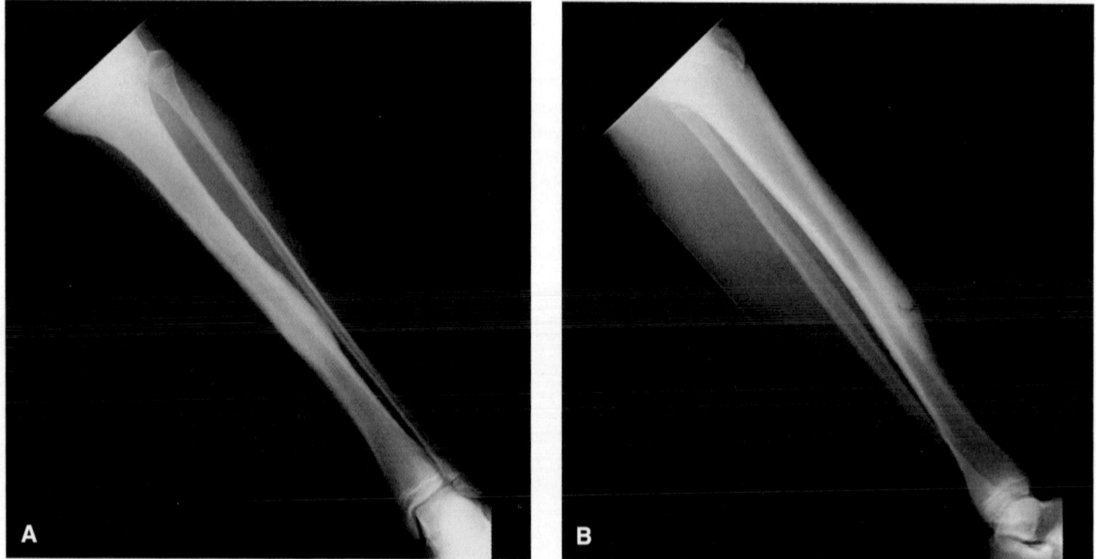

Figure 6.38. **(A/B)** Frontal and lateral views of the lower leg demonstrates a horizontal radiolucent fracture line within a focal cortical hyperostosis (thickening) of the anterior midtibial shaft, "the dreaded black line". © Hospital for Special Surgery, New York, New York.

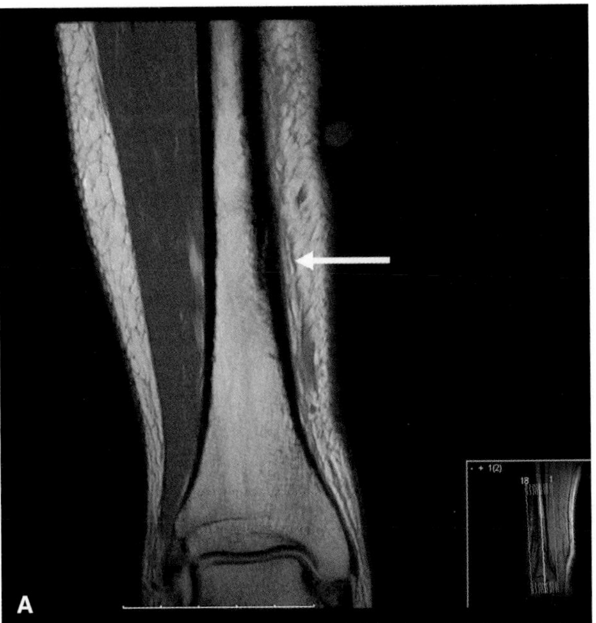

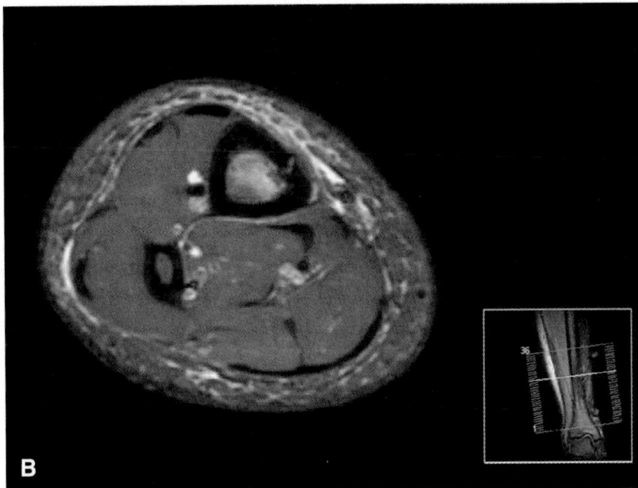

Figure 6.39. **A:** Coronal FSE PD MR image through the leg demonstrates hypointense medial cortical thickening and chronic remodeling of the endosteum consistent with a tibial stress fracture. **B:** Axial STIR MR image through the level of the midcalf demonstrates intense bone marrow edema pattern within the tibial medullary cavity and a cortical stress fracture. There is overlying soft tissue edema. © Hospital for Special Surgery, New York, New York.

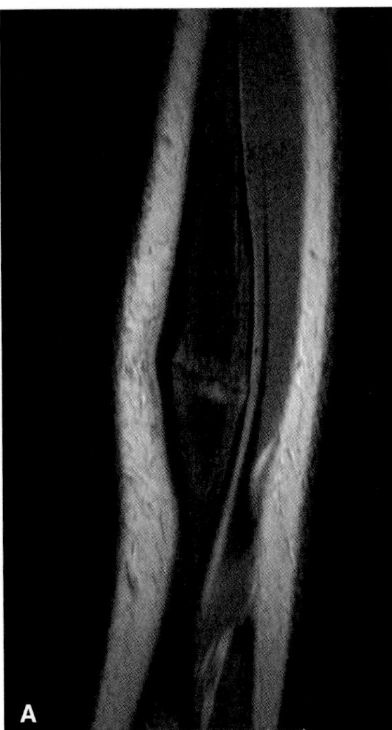

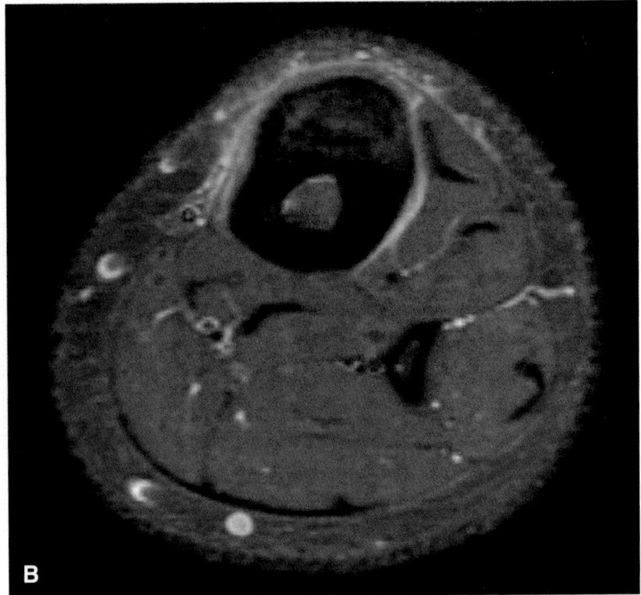

Figure 6.40. **A:** High-resolution coronal FSE MR image through the anterior tibial cortex demonstrates exuberant callous, cortical thickening and remodeling in the setting of a chronic nonacute stress fracture. **B:** Axial IR MR image demonstrates the exuberant cortical thickening and callous with mild reactive bone marrow edema pattern and soft tissue periostitis associated with the chronic stress fracture. © Hospital for Special Surgery, New York, New York.

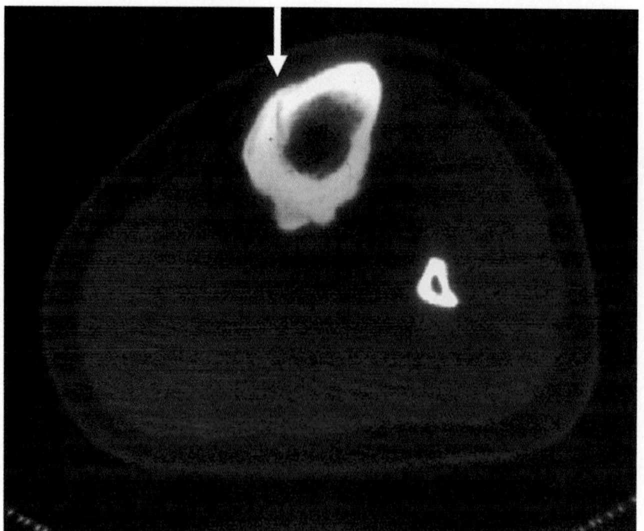

Figure 6.41. Axial CT image demonstrates a stress fracture (*arrow*) embedded within the thickened hyperostosis of the mid to posterior tibial cortex. © Hospital for Special Surgery, New York, New York.

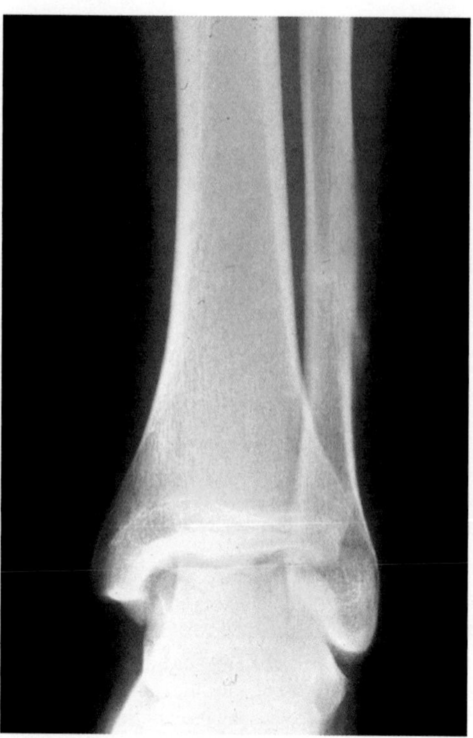

Figure 6.43. Frontal view of the ankle demonstrates a classic fibular stress fracture proximal to the fibular tip. © Hospital for Special Surgery, New York, New York.

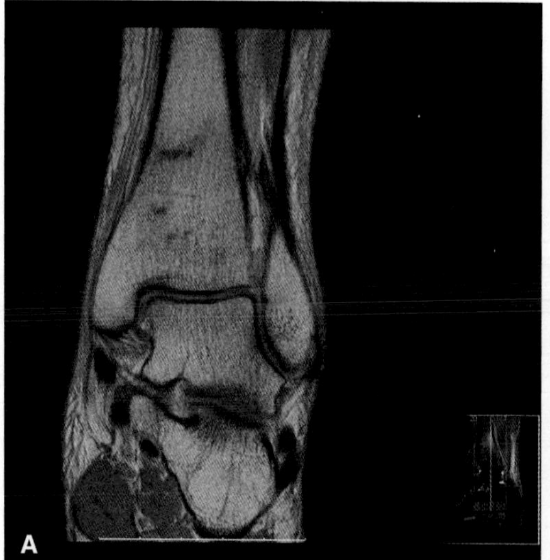

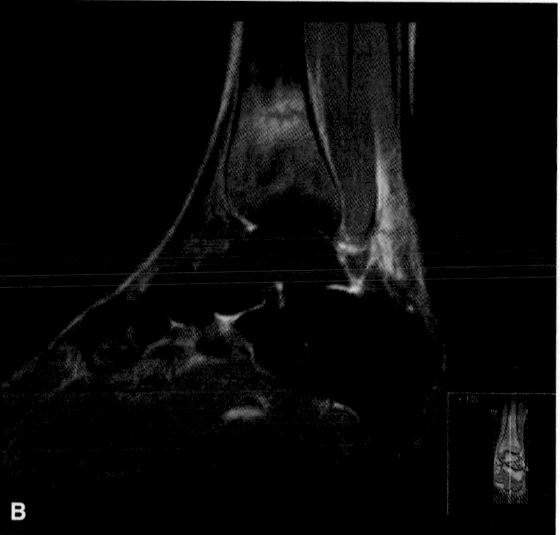

Figure 6.42. **A:** Coronal FSE PD MR image centered over the distal tibia demonstrates a hypointense sclerotic cancellous stress fracture line. **B:** Sagittal STIR MR image through the posterior distal tibia demonstrates the sclerotic low signal intensity band of an insufficiency fracture with reactive bone marrow edema pattern and periosteal reaction. © Hospital for Special Surgery, New York, New York.

Michael K. Ryan
Sepp Braun
Peter J. Millett

CHAPTER 7

Surgical Approaches to the Foot and Ankle

INTRODUCTION

Surgical approaches to the foot and ankle are generally straightforward, discounting any technical difficulties of the surgery itself. Many of the bony landmarks are easily palpable, lying superficially or subcutaneously, making access reasonably uncomplicated. The greatest complication associated with ankle and foot surgery is wound healing. The delicate nature of the thin skin in the ankle and foot requires careful incisions that provide the greatest chance of complete healing. Thus, incisions should maximize skin flap thickness and minimize the amount of forceful retraction required—longer incisions tend to favor better healing while providing greater exposure. This chapter will focus on the most important approaches used for sports-related ankle and foot injuries.

THE ANKLE

APPLIED SURGICAL ANATOMY

There are three specific categories of key structures crossing the ankle.

1. Tendons:
   a. Flexor tendons: tibialis posterior, flexor digitorum longus and flexor hallucis longus (Fig. 7.1).
   b. Extensor tendons: tibialis anterior, extensor digitorum longus, extensor hallucis longus and peroneus tertius (Fig. 7.2).
   c. Evertor tendons: peroneus longus and peroneus (Fig. 7.3).
   Planes exist medially, between the flexors (tibialis posterior) and extensors (tibialis anterior); posterolaterally, between flexors (flexor hallucis longus) and evertors (peroneus brevis); and laterally between extensors (peroneus tertius) and evertors (peroneus brevis).
2. Neurovascular bundles: There are two major neurovascular bundles that cross the joint to supply the foot.
   a. *Anterior neurovascular bundle* (Fig. 7.2): It crosses the central front of the ankle.
      • Anterior tibial artery
      • Deep peroneal nerve
   b. *Posterior neurovascular bundle* (Fig. 7.1): Located right behind the medial malleolus.
      • Posterior tibial artery
      • Tibial nerve
3. Superficial sensory nerves: Knowledge of the three major superficial sensory nerves that cross the ankle joint and innervate the dorsal aspect of the foot is vital in planning skin incisions.
   • *Saphenous nerve*
   • *Superficial peroneal nerve*
   • *Sural nerve*

Bony landmarks:
• Medial and lateral malleoli.

Medial approaches (Fig. 7.1)

Two groups of flexors lie on the medial side of the ankle:

1. The tibialis posterior, the flexor digitorum longus and the flexor hallucis longus muscles plantarflex the foot and ankle. The tibialis posterior is closest to the medial malleolus; the flexor digitorum longus is behind it; and the flexor hallucis longus is most posterior. Importantly, the posterior neurovascular bundle runs with these muscles.
2. The gastrocnemius, soleus and plantaris muscles insert into the posterosuperior part of the calcaneus as the common Achilles tendon. These three muscles are the most powerful plantarflexors of the ankle. They also invert the heel.

A fat pad and bursa lay between the Achilles tendon and the bone. Another bursa lies between the insertion of the tendon into the calcaneus and the skin.

Thickened fascia forms the *flexor retinaculum* that stretches from the medial malleolus to the back of the calcaneus

Anterior approach (Fig. 7.2)

Extensor muscles

The anterior aspect of the joint is crossed by four extensor muscles. From medial to lateral, they are the tibialis anterior, extensor hallucis longus, extensor digitorum longus and peroneus tertius.

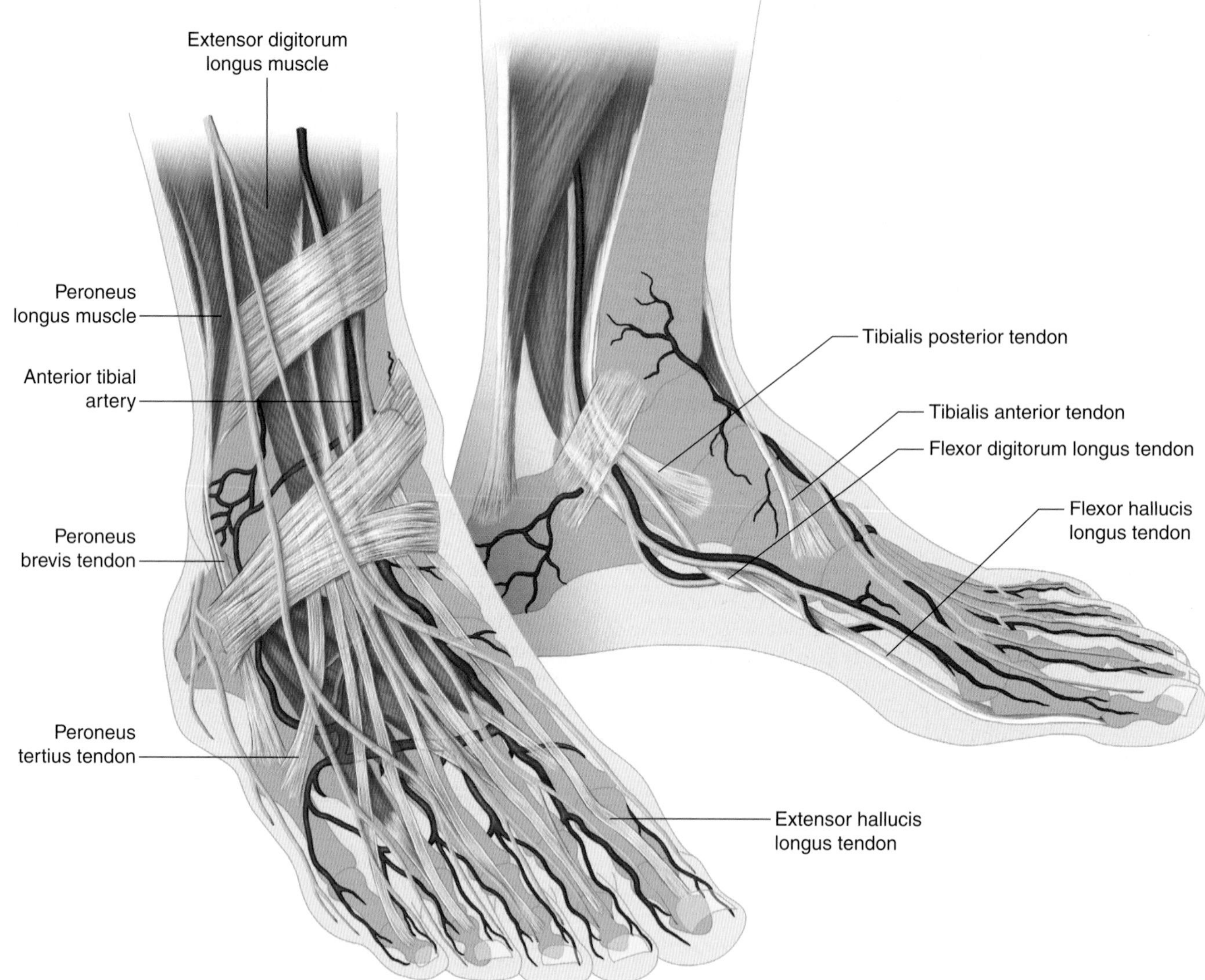

Figure 7.1. The Flexor tendons: The tibialis posterior, the flexor digitorum longus and the flexor hallucis longus.

The anterior neurovascular bundle crosses the front of the ankle directly under the tendon of the extensor hallucis longus (Fig. 7.2).

Extensor retinacula

- *Superior extensor retinaculum* (Fig. 7.2)
- *Inferior extensor retinaculum* (Fig. 7.2)

Lateral approach (Fig. 7.3)

The peroneal tendons run behind the lateral malleolus to reach the foot. The peroneus brevis tendon lies immediately behind the lateral malleolus and inserts at the styloid process of the fifth metatarsal. Both the peroneus longus and brevis are enclosed in one synovial sheath down to the peroneal tubercle.

Retinacula

- *Superior peroneal retinaculum*
- *Inferior peroneal retinaculum*

ANTERIOR APPROACH

Position of the Patient

The patient is placed supine on the operating table. Partially exsanguinate the foot, and then apply a thigh tourniquet.

Landmarks and Incision

1. Landmarks
   - Medial malleolus
   - Lateral malleolus
2. Incision

   Beginning 10 cm proximal to the joint, make a 15 cm longitudinal incision over the anterior aspect of the ankle joint. Extend the incision across the joint midway between the malleoli, terminating on the dorsum of the foot. Cut only the skin

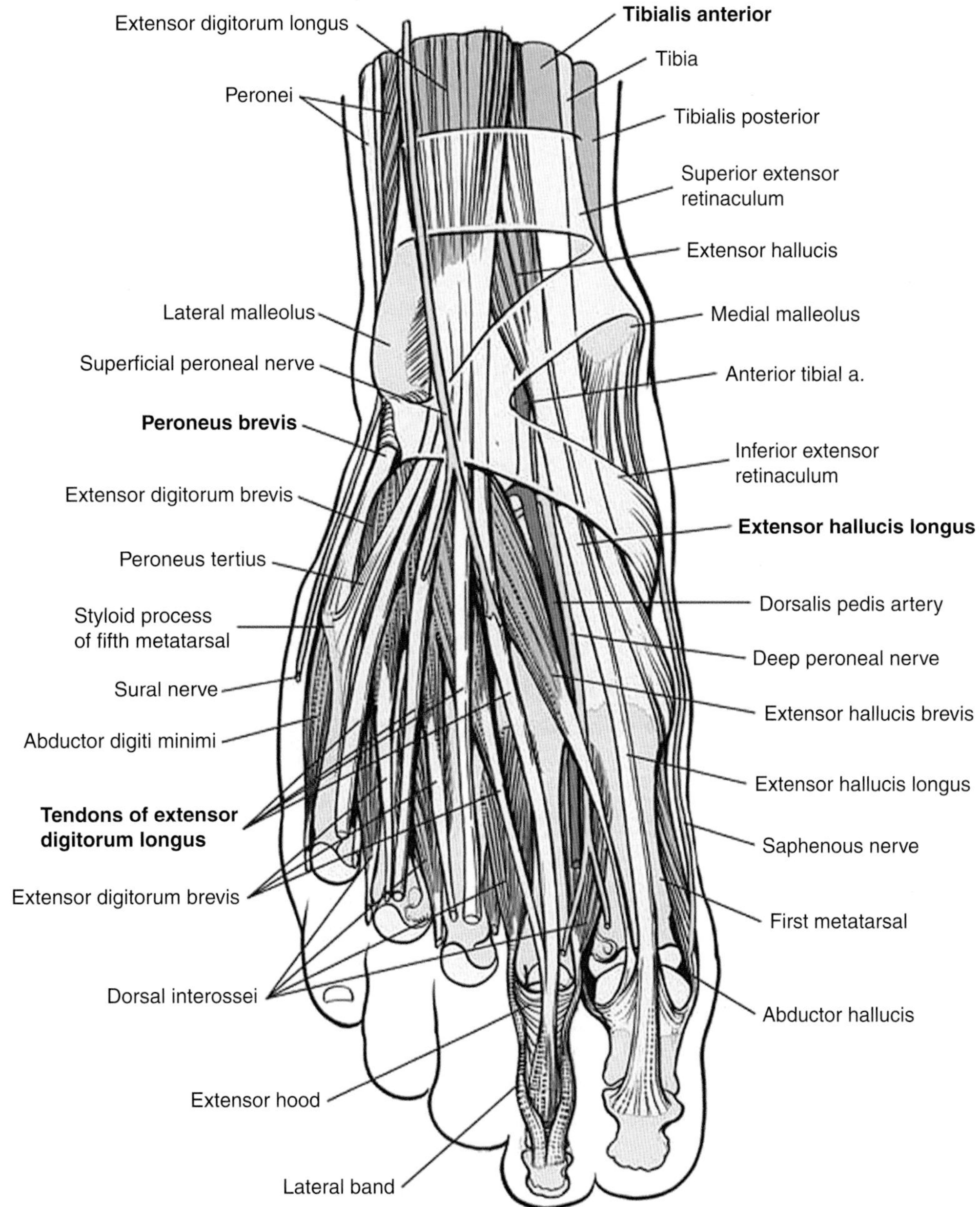

Figure 7.2. The extensor tendons: The tibialis anterior, the extensor digitorum longus, the extensor hallucis longus and peroneus tertius.

because the anterior neurovascular bundle and the superficial peroneal nerve cross the joint very near the incision (Fig. 7.4).

Internervous Plane

Although no true internervous plane exists, the *extensor hallucis longus* and *extensor digitorum longus* muscles provide a clear intermuscular plane.

Superficial Surgical Dissection

The deep fascia and extensor retinaculum are incised in line with the skin incision. A few centimeters above the ankle joint in the plane between the extensor hallucis longus and extensor digitorum longus muscles sits the anterior neurovascular bundle. Medially retract the extensor hallucis longus and the bundle together, and retract the extensor digitorum tendon laterally. Cutting the retinaculum releases the tendons, but the neurovascular bundle requires mobilization.

Alternatively, make the incision medial to the tibialis anterior tendon to expose the distal tibia and anteromedial ankle joint capsule (Fig. 7.4).

Deep Surgical Dissection

Incise the underlying soft tissues longitudinally, exposing the anterior surface of the distal tibia, down to the ankle

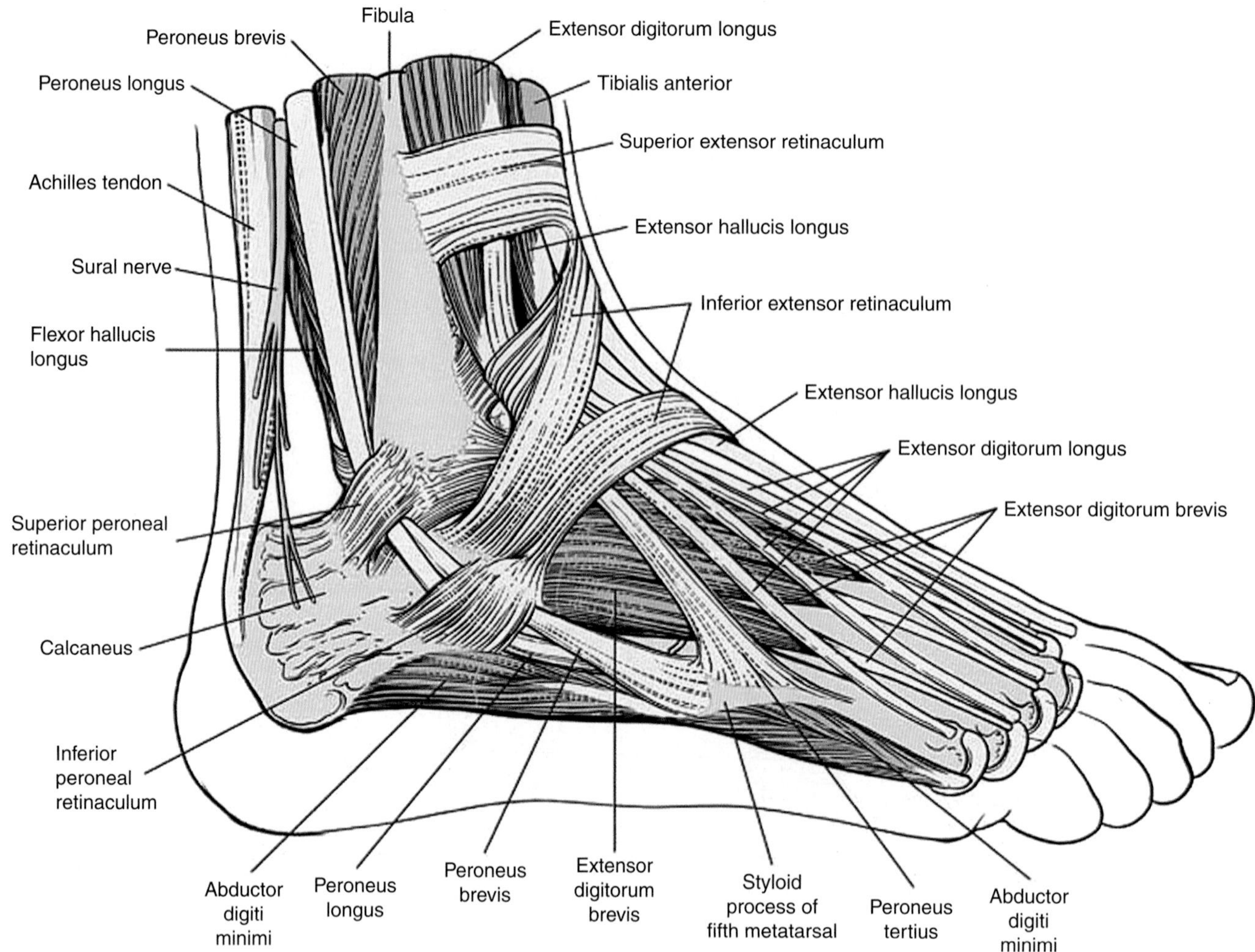

Figure 7.3. The evertor tendons: The peroneus longus and the peroneus.

joint. Cut the anterior joint capsule, and expose the joint by detaching the anterior capsule from the tibia or talus by sharp dissection. The distal tibia may require some periosteal stripping (Fig. 7.5).

Dangers

- Superficial peroneal nerve
- Anterior neurovascular bundle

How to Enlarge the Approach

This approach can be extended proximally to expose structures of the anterior compartment. The proximal tibia may be exposed using the plane between the tibia and the tibialis anterior muscle. Distal extension is possible but rarely used.

MEDIAL APPROACHES

Position of the Patient

Place the patient supine on the operating table allowing the natural external rotation of the legs to expose the medial malleolus. Partially exsanguinate the limb, then inflate a tourniquet.

Landmark and Incision

1. Landmark
   - The medial malleolus is the bony landmark for the medial approaches.
2. Incision

   Beginning over the medial surface of the tibia, approximately 5 cm proximal to the medial malleolus, make a 10 cm longitudinal incision centered over the tip of the malleolus. Below the malleolus curve, the incision forward along the medial side of the mid-foot ending some 5 cm anterior and distal (Fig. 7.6).

Superficial Surgical Dissection

Carefully mobilize the skin flaps without damaging the long saphenous vein and associated saphenous nerve, which run together along the anterior edge of the medial malleolus (Fig. 7.6).

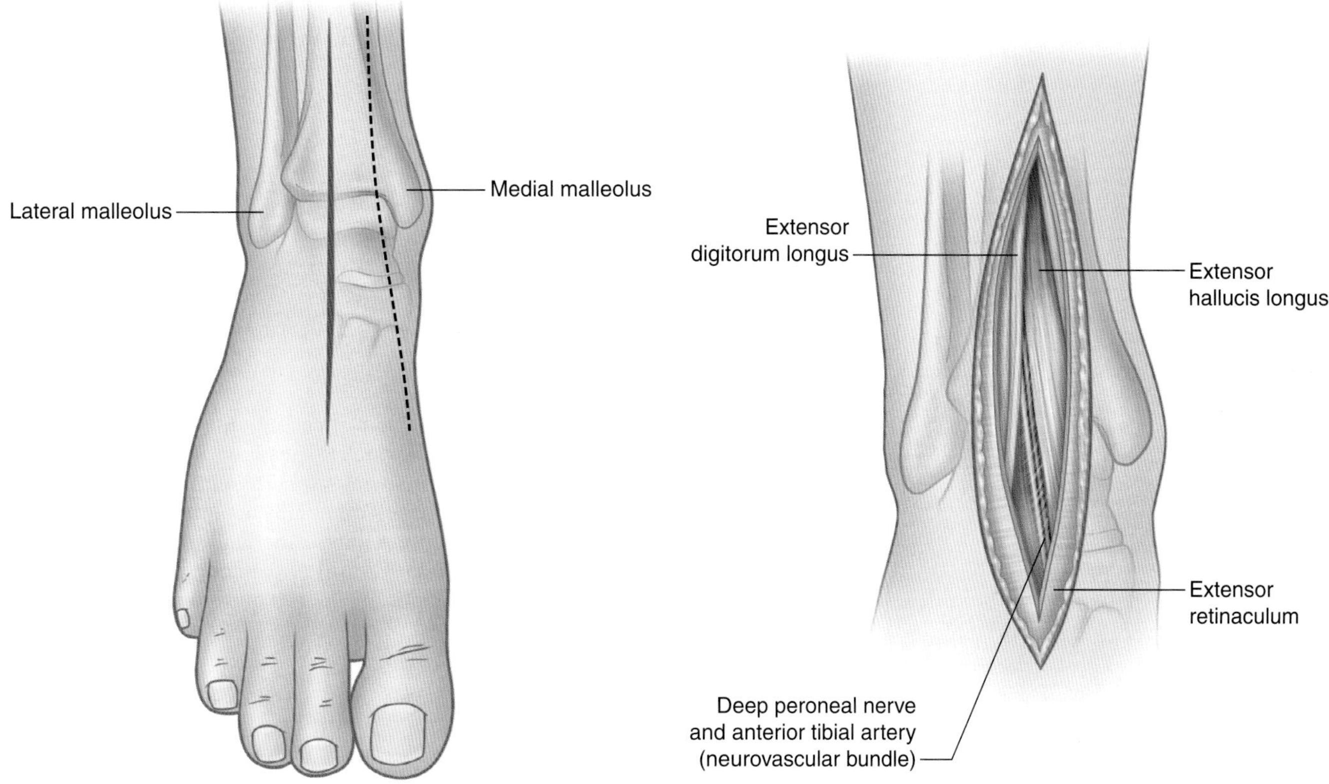

Figure 7.4. Superficial surgical dissection. Anterior aproach.

Deep Surgical Dissection

Make a small longitudinal incision in the anterior part of the joint capsule to locate the point at which the medial malleolus joins the shaft of the tibia.

To expose the posterior aspect of the medial malleolus, divide the flexor retinaculum and identify the tibialis posterior tendon, then retract it posteriorly.

Mark the bone longitudinally to facilitate correct alignment during closure. Drill and tap the medial malleolus so that it can be reattached with one or two screws.

Use an osteotome or/and oscillating saw to make a lateral cut obliquely from top to bottom at the junction of the malleolus and the shaft of the tibia. Check the position of the cut using the incision in the anterior capsule. A triangular osteotomy will help to reattach the malleolus.

Retract the medial malleolus and attached deltoid ligaments downward and forcibly evert the foot to expose the dome of the talus and the inferior articular surface of the tibia. The intact fibula limits eversion (Fig. 7.7).

Dangers

- Saphenous nerve
- Long saphenous vein
- Tibialis posterior tendon

There are two alternative approaches to the medial malleolus that are utilized primarily for open reduction and internal fixation of distal tibial fractures. The anterior approach to the medial malleolus enters the field over the anterior borders of the tibia and malleolus, while the posterior approach enters along the posterior border of the tibia and malleolus. For the anterior approach, take care not to damage the long saphenous vein and associated nerve, and for the posterior approach, avoid damaging the posterior neurovascular bundle.

Another alternative approach to the back of the ankle joint is the posteromedial approach, which enters midway between the medial malleolus and the Achilles tendon to explore the soft tissues of the back of the ankle joint.

POSTEROLATERAL APPROACHES

Position of the Patient

The patient is placed prone on the operating table with longitudinal pads below the pelvis and chest to allow full respiration. Place a sandbag under the affected ankle to allow full extension. Partially exsanguinate the limb and inflate a tourniquet.

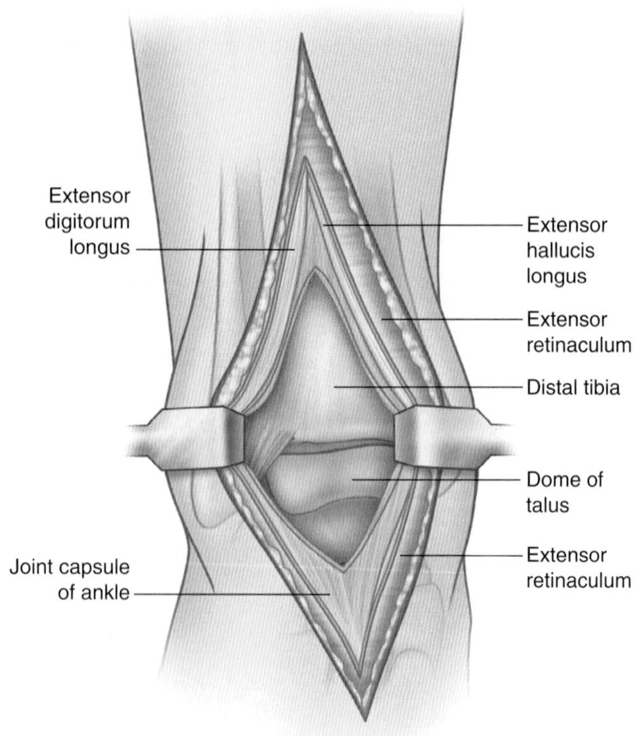

Figure 7.5. Deep surgical dissection.

Landmarks and Incision

1. Landmarks
   - Lateral malleolus
   - Achilles tendon
2. Incision
   Starting even with the malleolar tip, midway between the Achilles tendon and the posterior edge of the lateral malleolus, make a 10 to 15 cm incision, proximally.

Internervous plane

The internervous plane lies between the peroneus brevis muscle and the flexor hallucis longus muscle.

Superficial Surgical Dissection

Skin flaps are mobilized. The sural nerve and are short saphenous vein running just behind the lateral malleolus and anterior to the incision. Incise the deep fascia of the leg in line and identify the peroneal tendons. Cut the peroneal retinaculum to release the tendons, and retract them laterally and anteriorly, exposing the flexor hallucis longus muscle.

Deep Surgical Dissection

Incise the lateral fibers of the flexor hallucis longus muscle as they arise from the fibula, and retract it medially to expose the periosteum of the posterior tibia. Longitudinally cut the periosteum and strip it medially and laterally to reach the distal tibia. Enter the ankle joint by following the posterior tibia down to the posterior joint capsule and incise it transversely.

Dangers

- Sural nerve
- Short saphenous vein

How to Enlarge the Approach

Proximally, extend the skin incision superiorly and identify the plane between the lateral head of the gastrocnemius muscle and the peroneus muscles. Deepen the plane to the soleus muscle, and retract it medially with the gastrocnemius. Reflect the flexor hallucis longus medially, detaching it from its origin on the fibula. Continue dissecting medially across the interosseous membrane to the posterior aspect of the tibia.

APPROACH TO THE LATERAL MALLEOLUS

Position of the Patient

Place the patient supine on the operating table with a sandbag under the buttock of the affected leg to internally rotate the limb. The alternative lateral decubitus position provides excellent exposure to the lateral malleolus, but renders the medial malleolus unreachable in the case of bimalleolar fractures. Partially exsanguinate the limb and inflate a tourniquet.

Landmarks and Incision

1. Landmarks
   - Subcutaneous fibula and the lateral malleolus
   - The short saphenous vein
2. Incision
   Along the posterior margin of the fibula to its distal end, make a 10 to 15 cm longitudinal incision and continue 2 cm beyond the distal tip (Fig. 7.8).

Superficial Surgical Dissection

While elevating the skin flaps, take care not to damage the short saphenous vein or the sural nerve.

Deep Surgical Dissection

Incise the subcutaneous periosteum longitudinally, stripping only enough to expose the fibula below. Keep all dissection strictly subperiosteal to avoid damaging terminal branches of the peroneal artery, which lie near the lateral malleolus. Limit periosteal stripping as needed to prevent ischemia. Deflate the tourniquet prior to closure to ensure hemostasis (Fig. 7.8).

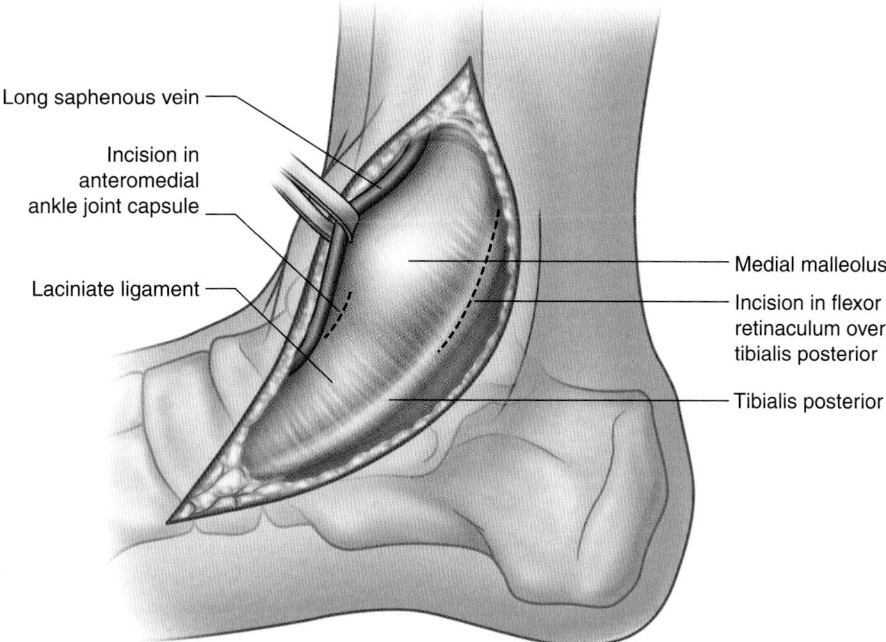

Figure 7.6. Incision.

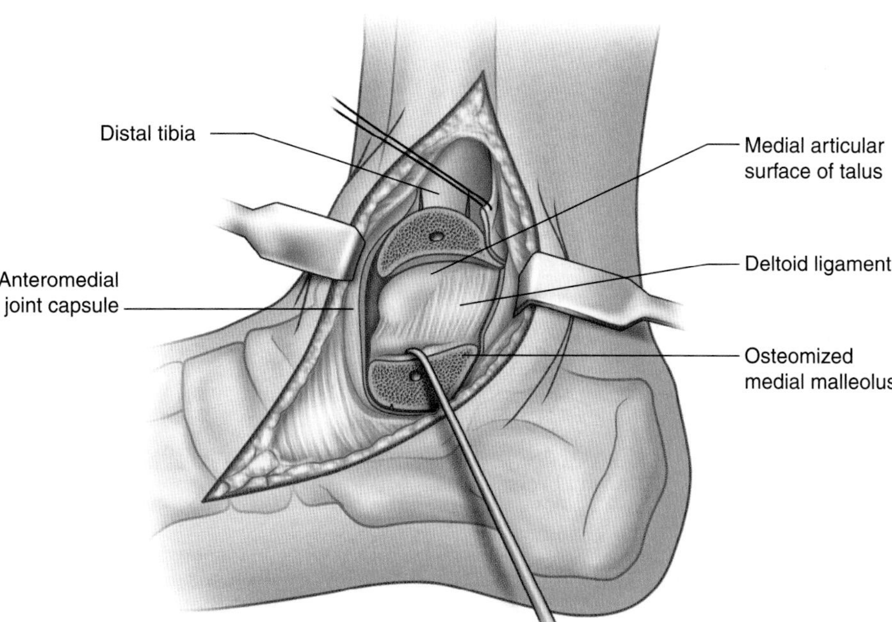

Figure 7.7. The intact fibula limits eversion.

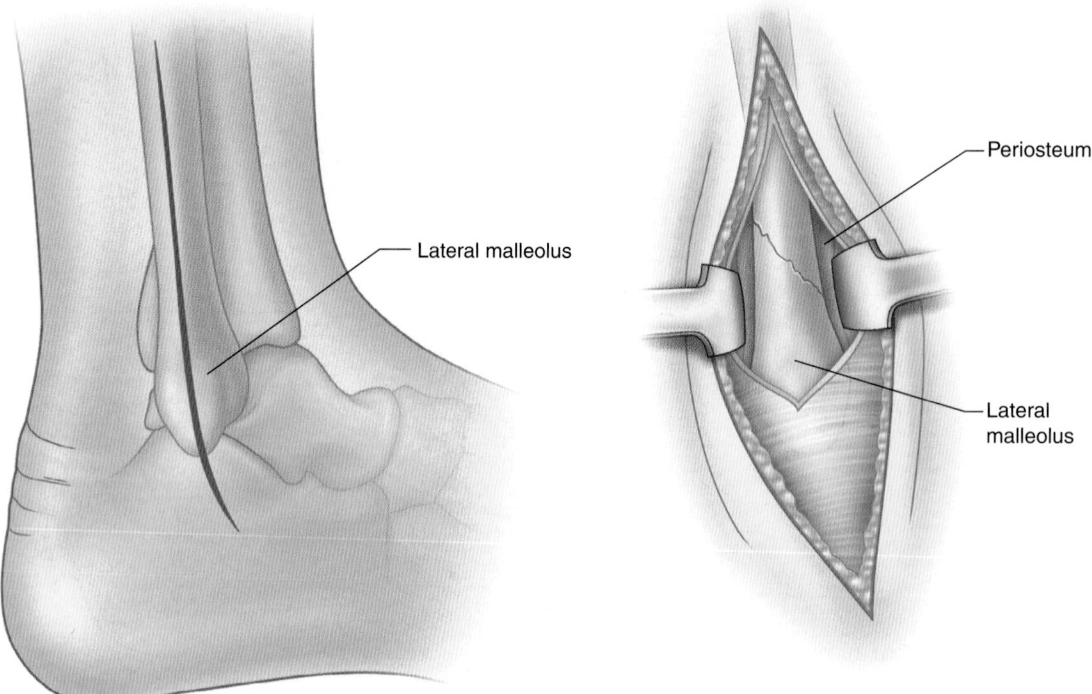

Figure 7.8. Along the posterior margin of the fibula to its distal end, make a 10 to 15 cm longitudinal incision and continue 2 cm beyond the distal tip.

Dangers

- Sural nerve
- Terminal branches of the peroneal artery

How to Enlarge the Approach

Proximal Extension. The incision is extended along the posterior border of the fibula, and the deep fascia is incised in line with the skin incision. A new plane is developed between the peroneal muscles and the flexor muscles. Exposure of the upper third of the fibula is possible if the common peroneal nerve is identified and traced down to the ankle.

Distal Extension. Curve the incision down the lateral side of the foot. Identify the peroneal tendons and cut the peroneal retinacula. Expose the calcaneocuboid joint on the lateral side of the tarsus by detaching the fat pad in the sinus tarsi and the origin of the extensor digitorum brevis.

THE HINDFOOT

APPLIED SURGICAL ANATOMY OF THE APPROACHES (FIGS. 7.9, 7.10)

The tarsal canal, formed by grooves on the inferior surface of the talus and the superior surface of the calcaneus, runs obliquely across the foot and is key to the anatomy of the hindfoot. It separates the talocalcaneonavicular and talocalcaneal joints and serves as a landmark for surgical access to the two joints. Laterally, the canal widens into the sinus tarsi.

The ligamentum cervicis tali and a large fat pat reside in the sinus tarsi. To access the joints, the ligamentum must be divided and the fat pad mobilized. Access to the calcaneocuboid joint is gained by detaching the extensor digitorum brevis tendon, which originates from the top of the anterior wall of the sinus.

The posterior aspect of the subtalar joint is behind the tarsal canal. The subtalar joint is oblique and is viewed best by retracting the overlying peroneal tendons anteriorly.

The talocalcaneonavicular joint lies distal to the tarsal canal, as does the calcaneocuboid joint.

Defining the sinus tarsi provides access to all of the joints provided that the different planes of the joints are identified.

ANTEROLATERAL APPROACH

Position of the Patient

The patient is positioned supine on the operating table with a sandbag below the affected buttock to internally rotate the limb, exposing the lateral malleolus. Partially exsanguinate the limb and inflate a tourniquet.

Landmarks and Incision

1. Landmarks
   - Lateral malleolus
   - Base of the fifth metatarsal

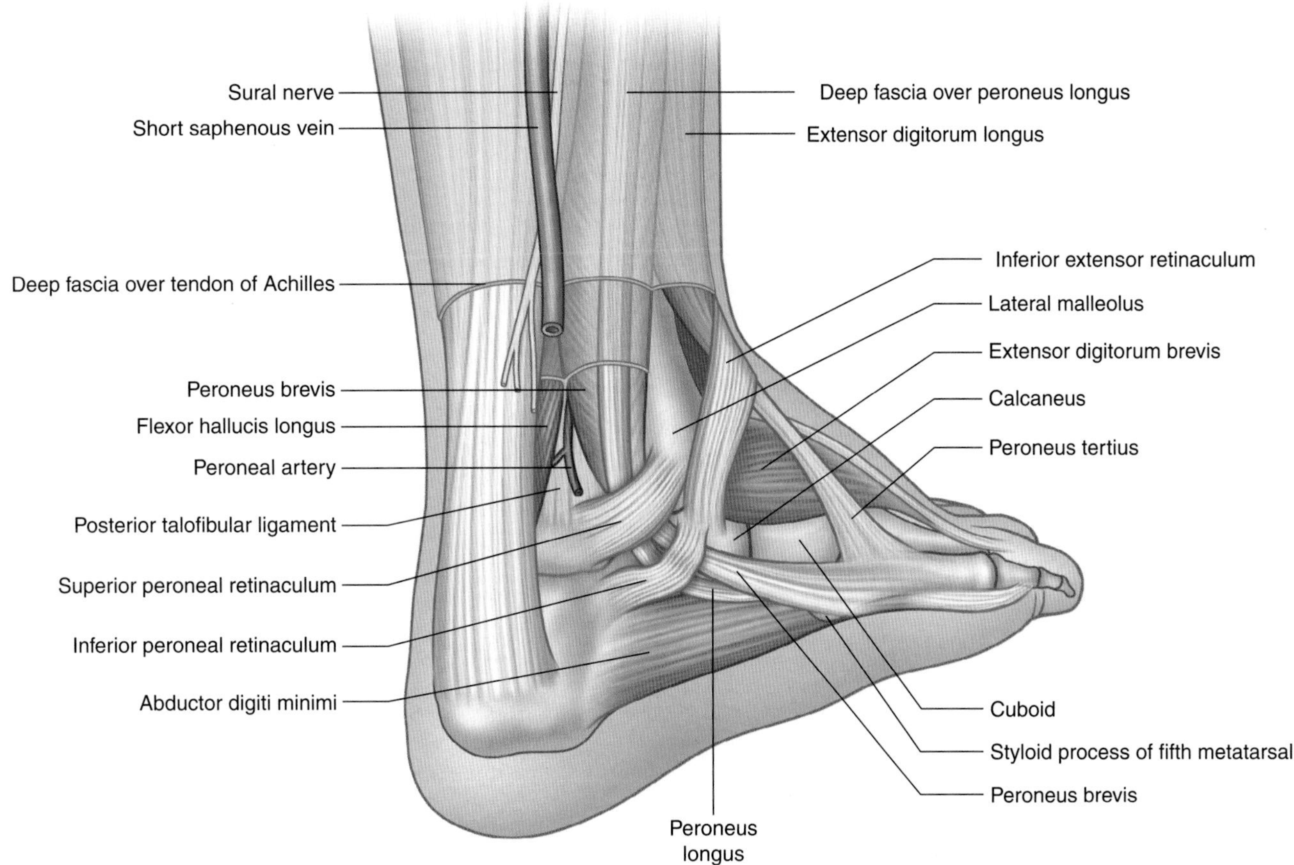

Figure 7.9. Applied surgical anatomy of the approaches to the hindfoot (Lateral).

2. Incision
   Beginning 5 cm proximal to the ankle joint and 2 cm anterior to the anterior border of the fibula make a 15 cm longitudinal incision on the anterolateral aspect of the ankle. Curve the incision down across the ankle joint 2 cm medial to the tip of the lateral malleolus onto the foot, ending 2 cm medial to the base of the fifth metatarsal over the base of the fourth metatarsal (Fig. 7.11).

Internervous Plane

Internervous plane is located between the peroneal muscles and the extensor muscles.

Superficial Surgical Dissection

The deep fascia and the superior and inferior extensor retinacula are incised in line with the incision. Identify and preserve any dorsal cutaneous branches of the superficial peroneal nerve. Therefore avoid developing skin flaps. In the upper half of the wound, lateral to the peroneus tertius and extensor digitorum longus, incise down to the bone laterally (Fig. 7.11).

Deep Surgical Dissection

Reflect the extensor musculature medially to expose the anterior aspect of the distal tibia and the ankle joint. Distally, detach the extensor digitorum brevis at its origin from the calcaneus. Cauterize branches of the lateral tarsal artery that will be cut during dissection to prevent postoperative hematoma. Retract the extensor digitorum brevis muscle fascia distally and medially as one flap with the subcutaneous fat and skin. Identify the clinical midtarsal joint composed of the dorsal capsules of the calcaneocuboid and talonavicular joints. Mobilize the fat in the sinus tarsi to expose the talocalcaneal joint. Preserving the fat pad will prevent a dimple and will aid wound healing.

Incise all the capsules that have been exposed, and open them by forcefully flexing and inverting the foot in the plantar direction (Fig. 7.12).

Dangers

- Anterior neurovascular bundle

How to Enlarge the Approach

Proximally, extend the incision over the anterior compartment of the leg, and incise the deep fascia along the same line to explore structures of the anterior compartment.

Distally, continue the incision over the fourth metatarsal to expose the tarsometatarsal joint on the lateral half of the foot.

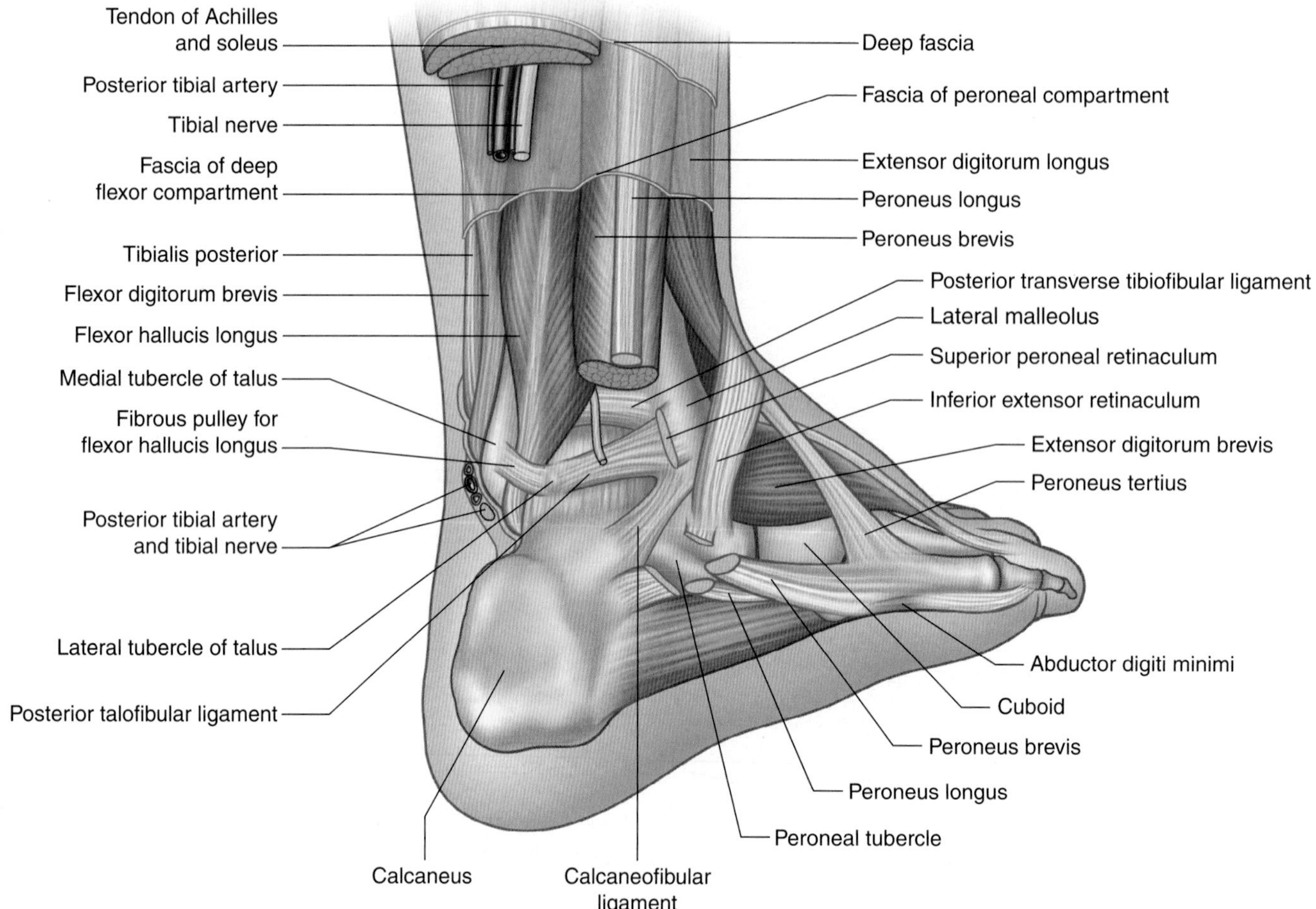

Figure 7.10. Applied surgical anatomy of the approaches to the hindfoot (Lateral).

LATERAL APPROACH

Position of the Patient

Place the patient supine on the operating table with a sandbag below the affected side's buttock to internally rotate the limb, exposing the lateral aspect of the ankle and foot. Partially exsanguinate the limb and inflate a tourniquet.

Landmarks and Incision

1. Landmarks
   - Lateral malleolus
   - Lateral wall of the calcaneus
   - Sinus tarsi
2. Incision
   Beginning just distal and slightly posterior to the tip of the lateral malleolus, make a curved incision that continues distally over the lateral side of the hind part of the foot and over the sinus tarsi. Curve the incision medially, ending over the talocalcaneonavicular joint (Fig. 7.13).

Internervous Plane

The internervous plane exists between the peroneus tertius tendon and the peroneal tendons.

Superficial Surgical Dissection

Avoid to mobilize skin flaps. Ligate any veins crossing the operative field. Without damaging the underlying tendons of the peroneus tertius and extensor digitorum longus, cut the deep fascia in line with the incision. Retract these tendons medially. Do not retract the peroneal tendons at this point (Fig. 7.13).

Deep Surgical Dissection

By sharp dissection partially detach the sinus tarsi fat pad, leaving it attached to the skin flap, and detach the extensor digitorum brevis at its origin. Retract the muscle distally to expose the dorsal capsules of the more distal talocalcaneonavicular and more lateral calcaneocuboid joints. Incise

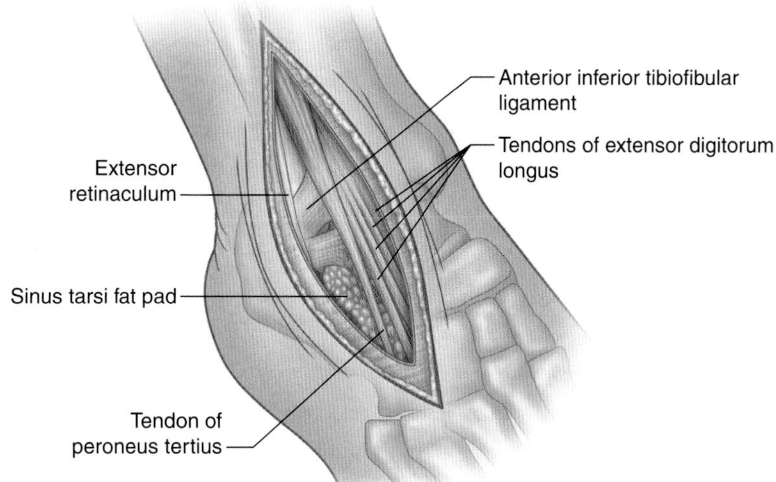

Figure 7.11. Curve the incision down across the ankle joint 2 cm medial to the tip of the lateral malleolus onto the foot, ending 2 cm medial to the base of the fifth metatarsal over the base of the fourth metatarsal.

these capsules and open the joints by forceful inversion of the foot. Now, incise the peroneal retinacula and reflect the peroneal tendons anteriorly to expose the talocalcaneal joint. Incise the capsule and open the joint by inverting the heel (Fig. 7.14).

Dangers

- Minimize retraction of skin flaps and periosteal stripping

How to Enlarge the Approach

STEP 1: Incise the calcaneocuboid, talocalcaneonavicular and posterior subtalar joints and invert the foot to open and expose the joints.

STEP 2: Proximally, curve the incision along the posterior border of the fibula, and develop a plane between the peroneal muscles and the extensor muscles to expose the entire length of the fibula.

Posterior and proximal extension of the incision can help to expose the Achilles tendon.

LATERAL APPROACH TO THE POSTERIOR TALOCALCANEAL JOINT

Position of the Patient

The patient is placed supine on the operating table with a sandbag under the buttock, to internally rotate the limb.

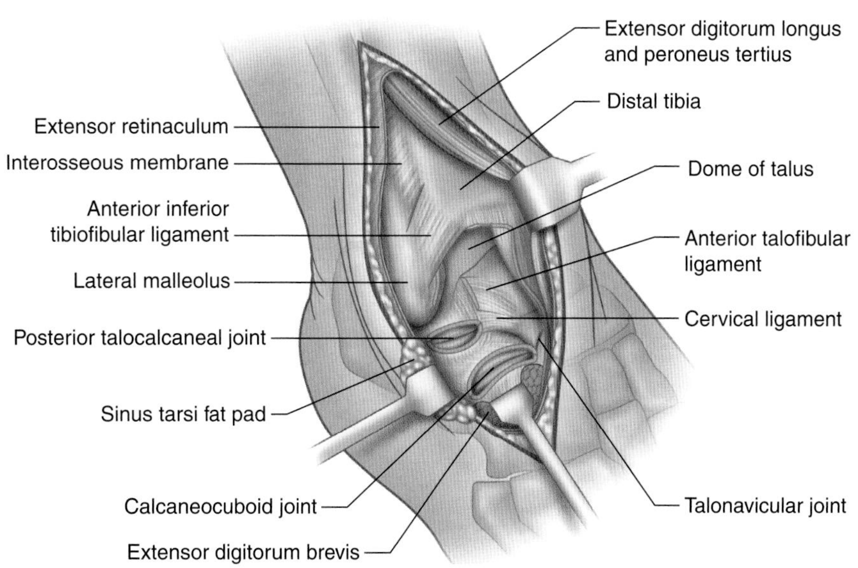

Figure 7.12. Incise any or all of the capsules that have been exposed, and open them by forcefully flexing and inverting the foot in the plantar direction.

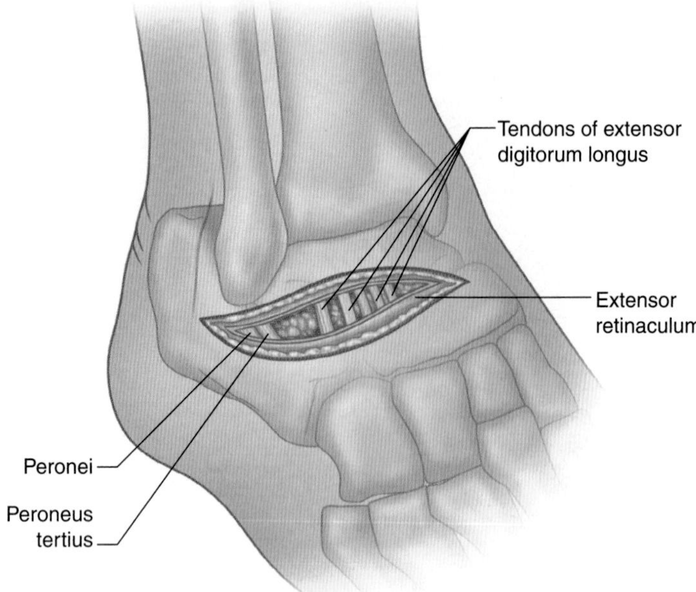

Figure 7.13. Beginning just distal and slightly posterior to the tip of the lateral malleolus, make a curved incision that continues distally over the lateral side of the hind part of the foot and over the sinus tarsi. Curve the incision medially, ending over the talocalcaneonavicular joint.

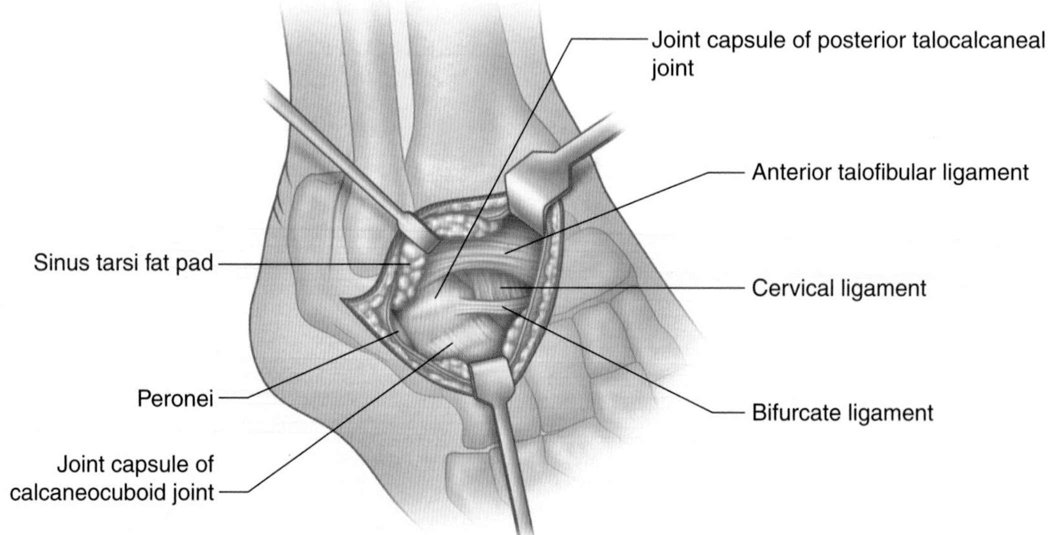

Figure 7.14. Incise the capsule and open the joint by inverting the heel.

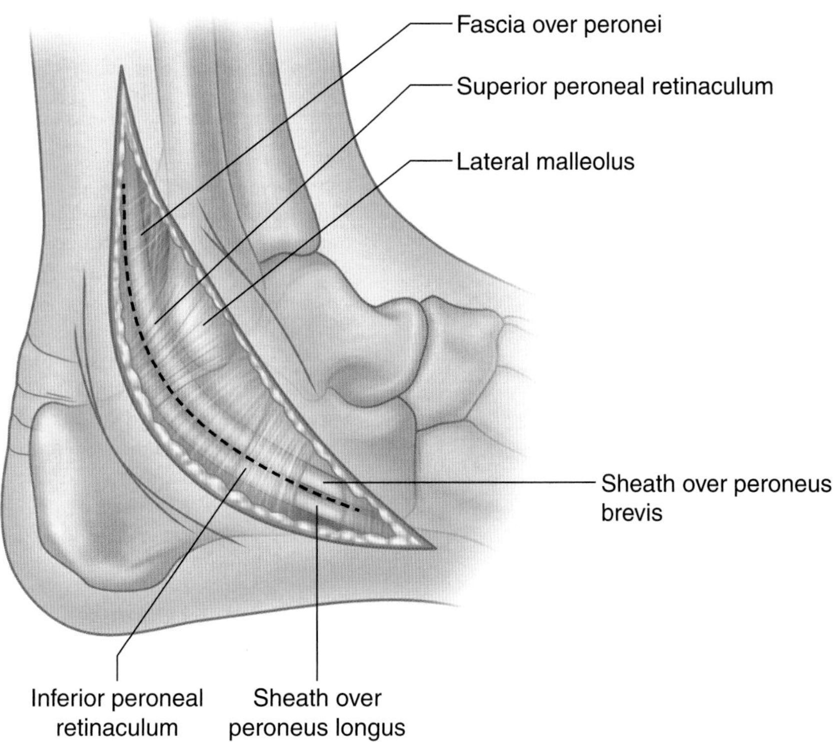

Figure 7.15. Make a 10 to 13 cm incision following the posterior border of the fibula to the tip of the lateral malleolus, and then curve forward over the peroneal tubercle parallel to the course of the peroneal tendons.

With a support on the opposite iliac crest, tilt the table about 30 degrees away from the surgeon. Partially exsanguinate the limb and inflate a tourniquet.

Landmarks and Incision

1. Landmarks
   - Lateral malleolus
   - Peroneal tubercle
2. Incision
   Begin on the posterior border of the fibula 4 cm above the lateral malleolus. Make a 10 to 13 cm incision following the posterior border of the fibula to the tip of the lateral malleolus, and then curve forward over the peroneal tubercle parallel to the course of the peroneal tendons (Fig. 7.15).

Superficial Surgical Dissection

Mobilize the skin flaps minimally without damaging the sural nerve or short saphenous vein. Uncover the peroneal tendons by incising the deep fascia in line with the skin incision.

In line with the peroneus brevis, incise the inferior peroneal retinaculum. A similar fibrous sheath covers the peroneus longus; incise the sheath in line with the tendon. These ligaments must be repaired during closure to prevent tendon dislocation. Anteriorly retract both tendons over the distal tip of the fibula (Fig. 7.15).

Deep Surgical Dissection

Locate the calcaneofibular ligament, which is closely bound to the talocalcaneal joint capsule. Some subperiosteal dissection along the lateral aspect of the calcaneus is usually necessary to locate the joint. Once located, incise the capsule transversely to open the joint (Fig. 7.16).

Dangers

- Sural nerve
- Short saphenous vein

How to Enlarge the Approach

To expose the bare lateral surface of the calcaneus, incise and use sharp dissection to strip the lateral peritoneum. View the talus better by incising the calcaneofibular ligament and joint capsule superiorly.

Inversion of the foot will expose the articular surfaces of the joint, but forceful inversion is ineffective if the anterior portion of the talocalcaneal (talocalcaneonavicular) joint remains intact.

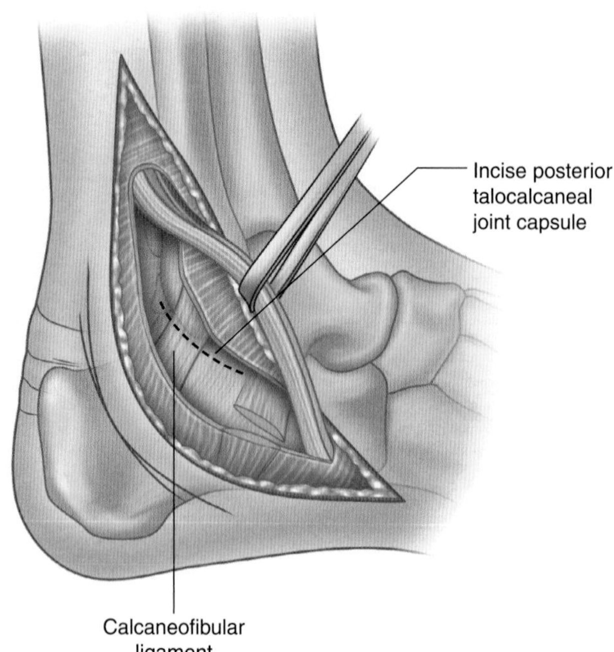

Figure 7.16. Once located, incise the capsule transversely to open the joint.

THE MID-FOOT AND FOREFOOT

APPLIED SURGICAL ANATOMY

Overview

All bones of the foot can be approached dorsally, and this approach is preferred over a plantar approach for two major reasons: First, critical neurovascular structures sit on the plantar side in the forepart of the foot; second, dorsal approaches avoid damaging weight-bearing skin on the plantar side of the foot.

Anatomy of the Dorsum of the Foot

The thin and loose skin of the dorsum of the foot facilitates retraction and accounts for the enormous amount of dorsal swelling following foot trauma. Distally, the lines of cleavage run roughly transversely.

1. Nerve supply
   - Cutaneous branches of the saphenous, superficial peroneal and sural nerves
   - Branches of the deep peroneal nerve
2. Superficial veins
   - Superficial veins form a dorsal venous arch that drains medially into the long saphenous vein and laterally into the short saphenous vein.
3. Tendons
   - Extensor digitorum longus, extensor digitorum brevis, extensor hallucis longus and extensor hallucis brevis tendons.
4. Deep artery
   - Dorsalis pedis artery

Anatomy of the Sole of the Foot

1. Skin
   The skin of the sole of the foot must endure enormous stress, thus it is tough, resilient and highly specialized with callosities formed by hypertrophy of the keratinized layer.
2. Deep fascia
   The thicker central portion, the plantar aponeurosis, originates from the medial tubercle of the calcaneus and runs forward, becoming thinner, and attaches to the proximal phalanges of each toe.
3. First muscular layer
   The superficial layer consists of the flexor digitorum brevis, abductor hallucis and abductor digiti minimi.
4. Superficial nerves and vessels
   The medial and lateral plantar arteries and nerves lie between the first and second layers of muscle.
5. Second muscular layer
   This layer consists of the long flexor tendons (the flexor hallucis longus, the flexor digitorum longus and flexor accessorius).
6. Third muscular layer
   The flexor hallucis brevis, adductor hallucis and flexor digiti minimi compose this layer.
7. Fourth muscular layer
   The deepest layer contains the interosseous muscles, the tibialis posterior tendon and the peroneus longus tendon.

DORSAL APPROACHES TO THE MID-FOOT

Position of the Patient

Place the patient supine on the operating table with the leg in natural external rotation for a dorsomedial approach. Place a sandbag under the buttock to internally rotate the limb for a dorsolateral approach. Partially exsanguinate the limb and inflate a tourniquet.

Landmarks and Incisions

1. Landmarks
   - First metatarsal cuneiform joint
   - Tubercle of the navicular
   - Talar head
   - Base of the fifth metatarsal
2. Incisions
   Make a longitudinal, dorsomedial incision directly over the area to be explored (Fig. 7.17). This will expose the talonavicular joint, the navicular-medial cuneiform joint and the first metatarsocuneiform joint, along with the insertions of the tibialis anterior and tibialis posterior tendons. To expose the calcaneocuboid joint and the base of the fifth metatarsal, make a dorsolateral incision directly over the area to be explored (Fig. 7.18).

   Two separate incisions are necessary if access to both the medial and lateral sides of the tarsus is required, such as an open reduction of fractures of Lisfranc's joint.

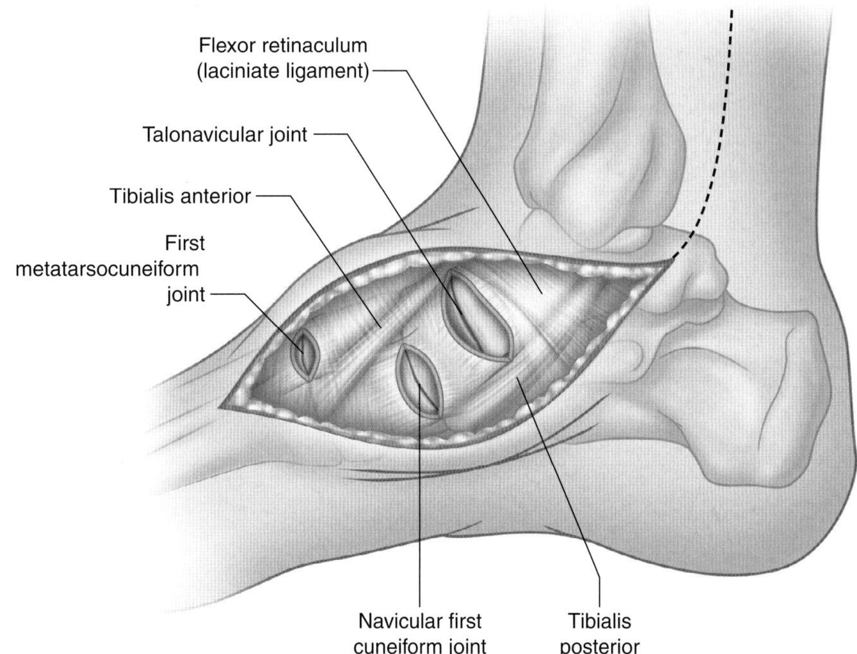

Figure 7.17. Make a longitudinal, dorsomedial incision directly over the area to be explored.

Surgical Dissection (Figs. 7.17, 7.18)

Avoiding cutaneous nerves incise directly over the area to be explored. Maximize skin flap thickness and minimize retraction to promote wound healing. Most dorsal structures are subcutaneous, so take care not to damage the insertions of the four invertors and evertors of the foot.

How to Enlarge the Approach

Both approaches can be extended proximally. Laterally, extend the incision posteriorly and up behind the posterior border of the lateral malleolus. Medially, extend the incision up behind the medial malleolus staying midway between the malleolus and the Achilles tendon.

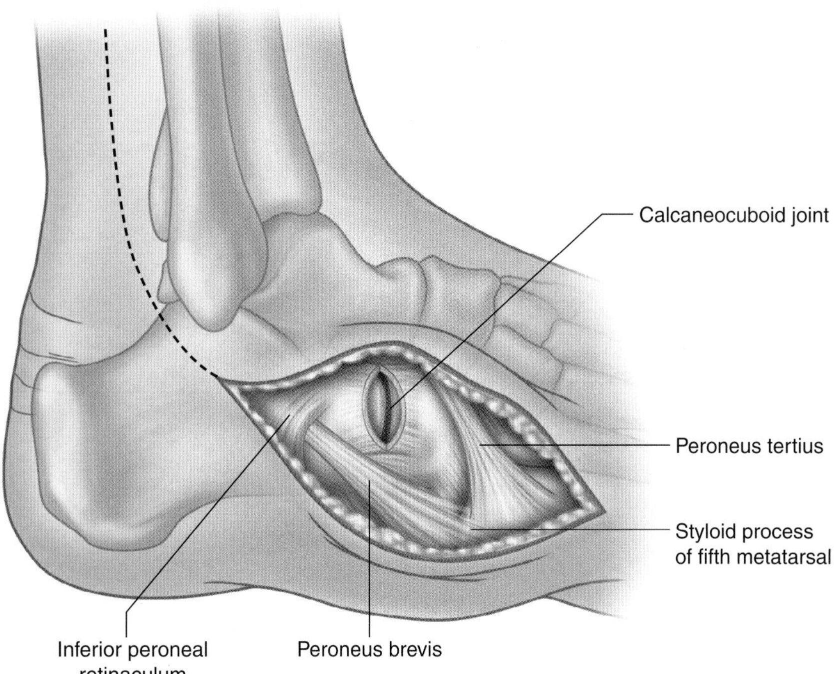

Figure 7.18. After separating the two adjacent toes of the affected web space, make a 2 to 3 cm longitudinal incision over the center of the web space, beginning distally and ending proximally.

DORSAL APPROACH TO THE METATARSOPHALANGEAL JOINTS OF THE SECOND, THIRD, FOURTH AND FIFTH TOES

Position of the Patient

Position the patient supine on the operating table, and place a bolster under the thigh to flex the knee, allowing the plantar surface of the foot to lie flat on the table.

Landmarks and Incisions

1. Landmarks
   - Metatarsal heads
   - The tendon of the extensor digitorum longus
2. Incision
   Make a 2 to 3 cm longitudinal incision parallel and just lateral to the long extensor tendon of the affected metatarsophalangeal joint.

Superficial Surgical Dissection

In line with the skin incision cut the deep fascia on the medial side of the long extensor tendon to expose the dorsal aspect of the metatarsophalangeal joint. Retract the tendon laterally.

Deep Surgical Dissection

Enter the metatarsophalangeal joint by incising the capsule longitudinally.

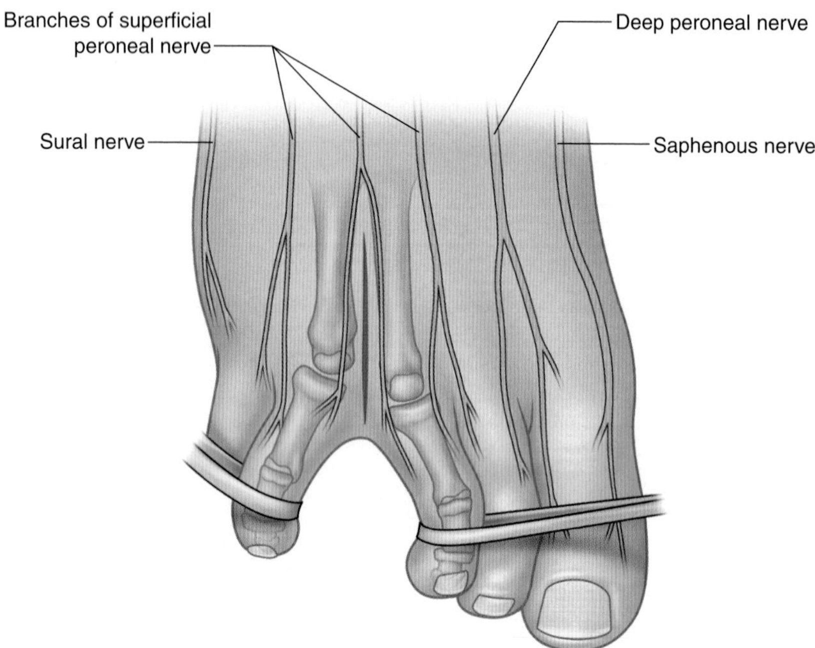

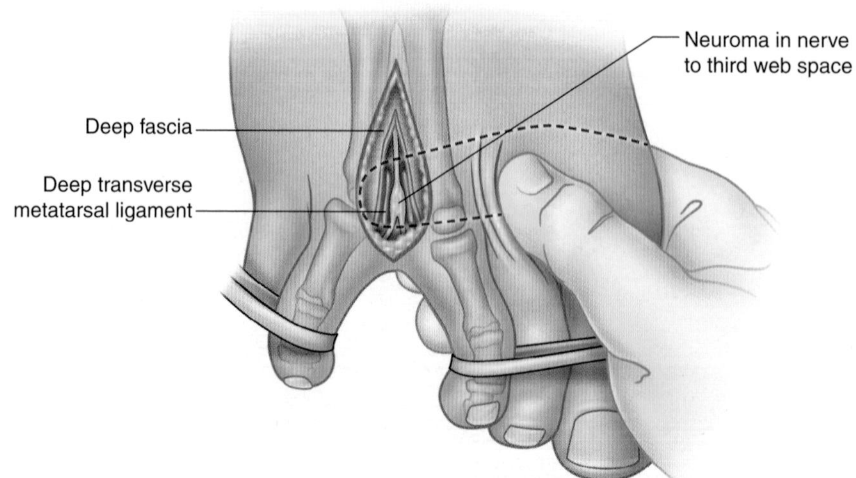

Figure 7.19. The longitudinal incision is centered over the web space.

Dangers

- Plantar nerves
- Plantar vessels
- Long extensor tendon

APPROACH TO THE DORSAL WEB SPACES

Position of the Patient

Position the patient supine on the operating table, and place a pillow under the patient's thigh to flex the knee, allowing the plantar surface of the foot to lie flat on the table. Partially exsanguinate the limb and inflate a tourniquet.

Landmarks and Incision

After separating the two adjacent toes of the affected web space, make a 2 to 3 cm longitudinal incision over the center of the web space, beginning distally and ending proximally (Fig. 7.19).

Superficial Surgical Dissection

Bluntly dissect the deep transverse metatarsal ligament in line with the skin incision. Longitudinally open the blades of a pair of scissors to expose the neurovascular bundle (Fig. 7.19).

Dangers

- The digital nerve; dorsal cutaneous nerves
- The digital vessels
  Take care not to cut the digital arteries; one damaged artery will not render a toe ischemic, but a second damaged artery will cause ischemia.

RECOMMENDED READINGS

Grose A, Gardner MJ, Hettrich C, et al. Open reduction and internal fixation of tibial pilon fractures using a lateral approach. *J Orthop Trauma* 2007;21(8):530–537.

Herscovici D, Sanders RW, Infante A, et al. Böhler incision: An extensile anterolateral approach to the foot and ankle. *J Orthop Trauma* 2000;14(6):429–432.

Hoppenfeld S, Deboer P. *Surgical Exposures in Orthopaedics: The Anatomic Approach.* 3rd ed. Philadelphia, Lippincott Williams & Wilkins; 2003.

Huene DB, Bunnell WP. Operative anatomy of nerves encountered in the lateral approach to the distal part of the fibula. *J Bone Joint Surg Am* 1995;77-A(7):1021–1024.

Mann RA. *Surgery of the Foot.* 5th ed. St. Louis, MO: C.V. Mosby Company; 1986:273–283.

Shereff M. *Atlas of Foot and Ankle Surgery.* Philadelphia, PA: W.B. Saunders Company; 1993.

Yablon IG, Segal P, Leach RE, eds. *Ankle Injuries.* New York, NY: Churchill Livingstone Inc; 1983.

CHAPTER

8

Andrew J. Rosenbaum
Rock CJ. Positano
Meaghan M. Colletti
Joshua Dines

Ankle Arthroscopy

INTRODUCTION

Ankle arthroscopy has been documented as early as 1931, when Burman reported a study on cadaveric ankle joints in New York, in which he explained that the ankle was unsuitable for such techniques due to the narrowness of the joint and inability to enter posteriorly with an arthroscope (1). However, this notion was refuted by Watanabe, who described ankle arthroscopy in a study of 28 patients in 1972 (2). In 1976, Chen described the operative anatomy of the ankle based on 67 arthroscopies of the joint (3). While these were some of the initial attempts to understand the role of arthroscopy in the ankle, ankle arthroscopy continues to evolve. Major technological advances in cameras, fiber optic light sources, and smaller instrumentation, coupled with improved distraction technique, have increased the indications for and improved the outcomes of ankle arthroscopy (4).

This chapter will explore ankle arthroscopy as a valuable tool in the treatment of many disorders, specifically elucidating the indications, contraindications, relevant anatomy, surgical technique, treatment and results, postoperative management and the complications and limitations of this procedure.

INDICATIONS AND CONTRAINDICATIONS

There is an increasing number of studies supporting the use of arthroscopy for myriad indications (4–7). Proper indications depend on a thorough history, physical examination, the use of diagnostic injections and the use of relevant imaging studies including radiographs, CT scans and magnetic resonance imaging (MRI). For most indications, only after nonoperative management fails, should arthroscopy of the ankle be performed.

Diagnostic indications for ankle arthroscopy include unexplained pain, swelling, stiffness, instability, hemarthrosis, locking and popping. Additionally, it can be performed in the setting of a negative workup in a patient with significant symptoms refractory to conservative management. In such patients, an underlying soft-tissue lesion or chondral fracture undetected via physician examination or imaging may be apparent on arthroscopic examination.

Once a diagnosis is made, nonoperative management strategies should be applied. While a patient's occupation, activity level and expectations must be considered when formulating the specifics of a treatment program, the common conservative measures include immobilization, bracing, anti-inflammatory measures and physical therapy.

For those patients with intra-articular pathology that fails conservative treatment, arthroscopy is a viable option. When used appropriately and for the proper indications, it leads to less morbidity, lower costs and more rapid return to physical activity than open surgery (4,8). Additionally, this minimally invasive technique allows direct visualization of intra-articular structures without arthrotomy or malleolar osteotomy (6). Despite the increasing body of data in favor of arthroscopy, a surgeon must understand that simply because indications are present for a procedure to be performed arthroscopically, better outcome and technical results are not guaranteed; such success largely depends on one's experience and confidence with the arthroscopic technique and instrumentation (4).

The current generally accepted therapeutic indications include repair of osteochondral lesions (OCLs), debridement of injuries to articular cartilage and soft tissue, loose-body removal, bony and soft-tissue impingement, ankle fractures and some conditions of the subtalar joint. Arthroscopy may also be indicated in instability, arthrofibrosis, osteoarthritis, irrigation and debridement of septic arthritis and arthrodesis (4–7).

Absolute contraindications to arthroscopy of the ankle are severe degenerative joint disease (DJD) and localized soft-tissue infection. Relative contraindications include moderate DJD with a restricted range of motion, severe edema, and a tenuous vascular supply (5).

ARTHROSCOPIC ANATOMY OF THE ANKLE

A thorough understanding of surface anatomy will guide portal placement and minimize risk of damaging tendinous and neurovascular structures (9). The skin overlying the joint line, the superficial peroneal nerve, the dorsalis pedis artery, the greater saphenous vein, the anterior tibial tendon, and the peroneus tertius tendon should be demarcated prior to any incisions (2,8). Note that some of these structures may take variable courses, making it impossible to identify them before portal placement.

The superficial peroneal nerve and its branches must be protected because they can be easily damaged, causing postoperative pain or numbness. The nerve divides into intermediate and medial dorsal cutaneous branches approximately 6.5 cm proximal to the tip of the fibula (10). With the fourth toe grasped and the forefoot pulled into plantar flexion and adduction, these branches can be seen as they are pulled taut beneath the skin. The intermediate dorsal cutaneous nerve passes superficial to the inferior extensor retinaculum. It crosses anterior to the common extensor tendons of the fourth and fifth toes and begins to travel towards the space between the third and fourth metatarsals before it divides into dorsal digital branches. The medial dorsal cutaneous branch crosses the anterior aspect of the ankle superficial to the common extensor tendons. It runs just lateral to the extensor hallucis longus tendon, dividing distal to the inferior extensor retinaculum into its dorsal digital branches.

Although as many as 14 ankle arthroscopy portals have been described, the majority of patients can be treated via anteromedial, anterolateral and posterolateral portals only (4) (Fig. 8.1). In an anatomic study by Feiwell and Frey (1993), these portals were found to be safest, allowing no penetration of neurovascular structures (11).

We first establish the anteromedial portal, which is placed just medial to the tendon of the anterior tibialis at or just proximal to the level of the joint line. Many advocate that this portal be placed first, as it is the least dangerous and most reproducible (2). The greater saphenous vein and nerve are most threatened when establishing this portal, respectively, lying approximately 9 mm medial to and 7.4 mm medial to the portal (11).

Placement of the anterolateral portal is made just lateral to the peroneus tertius tendon at or just proximal to the level of the joint line. Most at risk during creation of this portal are branches of the superficial peroneal nerve, of which its intermediate branch lies approximately 6.2 mm away (11). If established following the anteromedial portal, the appropriate location for the anterolateral portal can be determined via direct visualization with the use of a 25 gauge 1.5 inch needle. Transillumination of the overlying skin with the arthroscope can also be performed to aid in avoiding tendons and neurovascular structures during portal placement (8).

The posterolateral portal is produced approximately 1.0 to 1.5 cm proximal to the distal tip of the fibula, just lateral to the Achilles tendon. With the assistance of the arthroscope, which has been placed in the anteromedial portal inferior to the medial tibial notch and aimed posterolaterally, the posterolateral portal is established through direct visualization via insertion of an 18 gauge spinal needle just lateral to the Achilles tendon at a 45-degree angle toward the medial malleolus. With this technique, the posterior

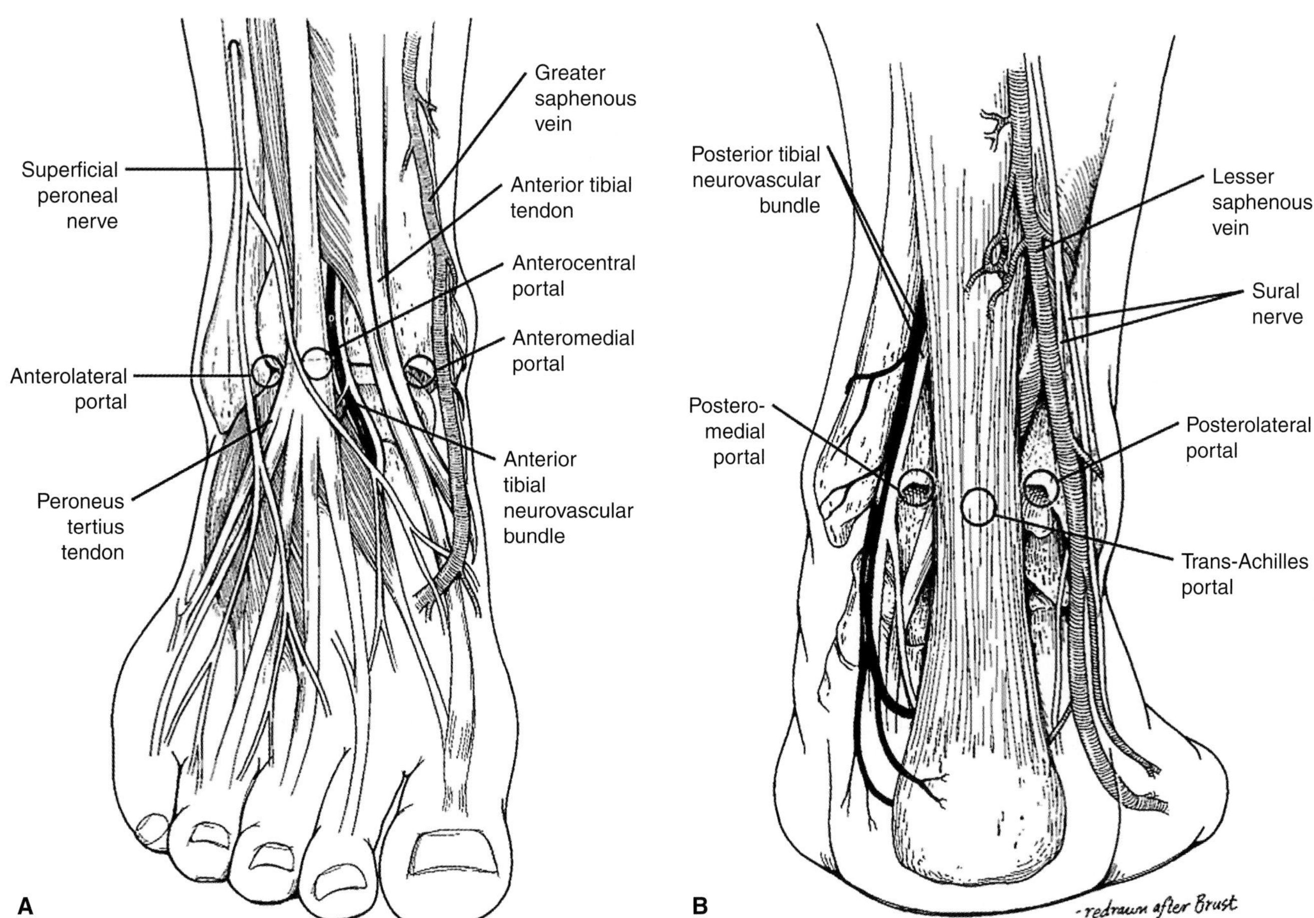

Figure 8.1. Appropriate portal placement of most commonly used portals.

aspect of the capsule is usually punctured just medial to the transverse tibiofibular ligament (8). At risk when establishing this portal are the lesser saphenous vein and the sural nerve, which run parallel to each other, about 3.5 mm apart, along the posterolateral aspect of the ankle joint. On average, the sural nerve and lesser saphenous vein lie 6.0 mm and 9.5 mm anterior to the portal, respectively (11).

An alternative approach for posterolateral portal placement is to use a switching stick through the anteromedial or anterolateral portal. The stick, which is a smooth metal rod, is inserted through the cannula and pushed out through the skin in the region of the posterolateral portal. The cannula is then switched to the new portal and the arthroscope is introduced. Marked distraction of the joint is required for this technique. Without sufficient distraction, the portal may be established too far proximally (2,4,8).

Production of other portals has been described (2,4,8). However, their use is often discouraged due to inherent neurovascular risks. An anterocentral portal, which is established between the tendons of the extensor digitorum communis, poses great risk to the peroneal nerve, dorsalis pedis artery and vein, which lie as a bundle approximately 3.3 mm from the portal (2,11). Posteriorly, a portal can be established centrally just below the joint line and through the middle of the Achilles tendon. Such iatrogenic injury to the Achilles is not advised. A portal can also be developed posteromedially, but is contraindicated due to the proximity of the posterior tibial artery and nerve as well as risk to the tendons of the flexor hallucis and flexor digitorum longus, and to branches of the calcaneal nerve (8). Lastly, transmalleolar portals and transtalar portals have been reported for Kirschner-wire drilling of defects of the talar dome (2,8).

Prior to portal placement, the ankle joint should be distended with 10 mL of lactated ringer's solution via 18 to 20 gauge needle injection just medial to the anterior tibialis tendon. The provided distention will help determine appropriate portal location (8).

ARTHROSCOPIC TECHNIQUE: INSTRUMENTS, SETUP, DISTRACTION, INSPECTION

INSTRUMENTS

The 2.7 mm, 30-degree short arthroscope is most commonly used during arthroscopy of the ankle as opposed to a standard 4.0 mm arthroscope. The former provides easier maneuverability, reduced risk of damage to the articular surface, availability of interchangeable cannulae, and a shorter lever arm enabling easier accessibility to the joint. We have a low-threshold to switch to a 70-degree arthroscope to improve visualization. Small-joint arthroscopic instruments, including 2.0 and 2.7 mm burrs and shavers, miniprobes, 2.7 mm graspers, 4.5 and 7.0 mm curettes, pituitary rongeurs, and small-joint osteotomes and rasps, are essential for performing safe arthroscopy in the ankle joint (4,8). Adequate inflow of lactated ringer's solution can be ensured via gravity drainage or use of a pressure-sensitive arthroscopic pump to be inserted through the same cannula in which the arthroscope is placed. When relying on gravity, a larger cannula (3.7 mm cannula for a 2.7 mm scope) is required, or a dedicated inflow portal can be established. Insertion of a spinal needle into the joint can be used to produce additional outflow of solution (4,8).

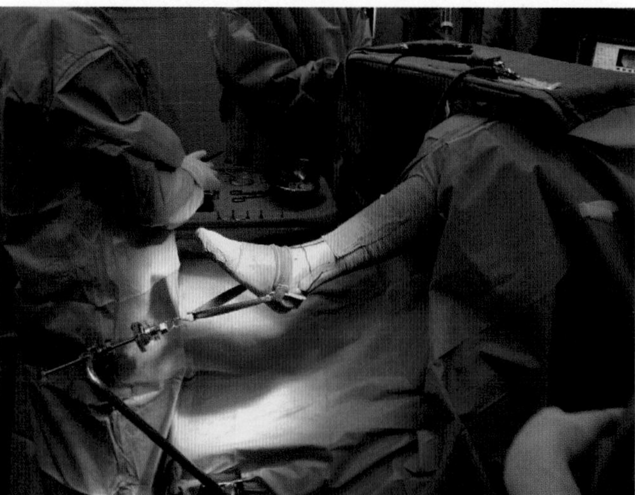

Figure 8.2. Operative setup with patient supine, hip and knee flexed and the use of an external distraction device.

SETUP

General, regional, or local anesthesia can be used during arthroscopy of the ankle. The position of the patient is dependent of the surgeon's preference. We prefer that the patient is supine with the hip and knee flexed over a non-sterile support and the foot supported with a sterile holder (9) (Fig. 8.2). When supporting the flexed hip, adequate padding is needed on the thigh support to prevent injury to the sciatic nerve.

Alternative positioning includes flexion of the knee over the end of the operating table with the patient supine, or placement of the patient in the lateral decubitus position with a beanbag support under the trunk. When the knee is flexed over the end of the table, some distraction by gravity occurs. However, this positioning limits access to posterior portals.

The ipsilateral hip should be externally rotated for access to anterior portals; for posterior portals, the hip must be internally rotated. A tourniquet can be applied if so desired by the surgeon (8).

DISTRACTION

We routinely use an external distraction device to aid with visualization during the arthroscopy. Noninvasive distraction can be accomplished with a strap wrapped over the foot and behind the heel, as well as through several other methods and commercial products. Figure 8.2 While some critics believe that noninvasive distraction can at times fail to provide sufficient visualization of the ankle joint, it has fewer associated complications and should always be used in athletes as it will not cause pin-induced stress risers.

Invasive distraction has been used, but as the name implies, it is more invasive necessitating the use of tibial and calcaneal pins (12). The superficial peroneal nerve is at risk near the tibial pin and has been found on average to reside 7 mm posterior to the pin (11). The peroneal tendon sheath, sural nerve and lesser saphenous vein travel anterior to the distal pin. Compromise of these structures during calcaneal pin placement is less likely than damage to the superficial peroneal nerve during proximal pin placement (11). It has also been shown that distraction forces greater than 90 N while the ankle is in the 20-degree dorsiflexion position produce injury to the calcaneofibular ligament (13). Further, invasive distraction of greater than 7 or 8 mm should not be performed for greater than 1.5 hours (8).

INSPECTION

A thorough, systemic evaluation of the ankle joint after appropriate joint distention and debridement of hypertrophic synovium should be performed by the surgeon. Such a meticulous assessment of the entire joint assures the surgeon of a complete and accurate diagnosis of ankle pathology, while providing a complete photographic or videotape record that can be reviewed at a future time for clinical studies and improvements to patient care.

The normal intra-articular anatomy, as visualized through an arthroscope, has been well described (3,14). The 21-point arthroscopic examination evaluates the significant intra-articular structures and is initially done through the anteromedial portal with subsequent examination through anterolateral and posterolateral portals (8). During anterior inspection, structures to be identified are the deltoid ligament, medial gutter, medial talus Figure 8.3, central talus and overhang, Figure 8.4 lateral talus, trifurcation of the talus, tibia and fibula, Figure 8.5 lateral gutter, anterior gutter. Centrally, identification of the following structures is crucial the medial tibia and talus, central tibia and talus, lateral tibiofibular or talofibular articulation, posterior inferior tibiofibular ligament, transverse ligament, reflection of the flexor hallucis longus. During posterior evaluation, anatomy to be assessed includes posteromedial gutter, posteromedial talus, posterocentral talus, posterolateral talus, posterior talofibular articulation, posterolateral gutter, posterior gutter (8).

Extreme caution must be taken when in the posterior capsule to not damage the sheath of the flexor hallucis longus tendon as it travels in its groove on the posterior talus. The surgeon can look down this sheath by carefully slipping out of the posterior capsule during inspection. The surgeon must recognize the inherent risks when trying to visualize this tendon sheath.

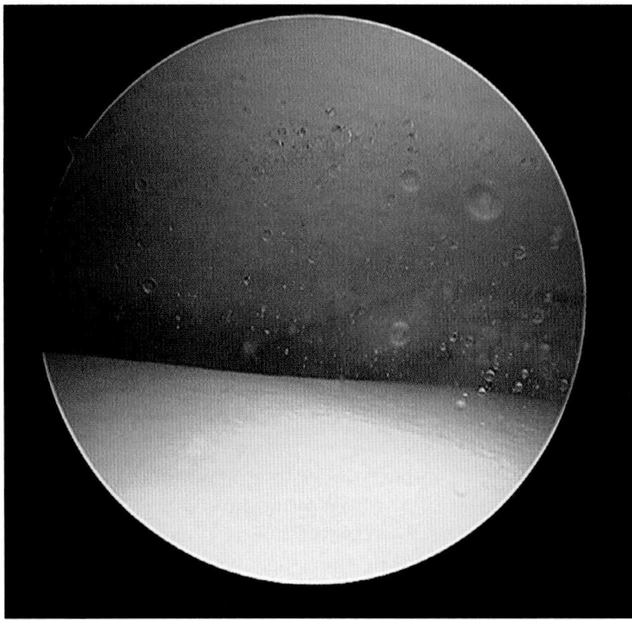

Figure 8.4. Arthroscopic view of central talus and tibia.

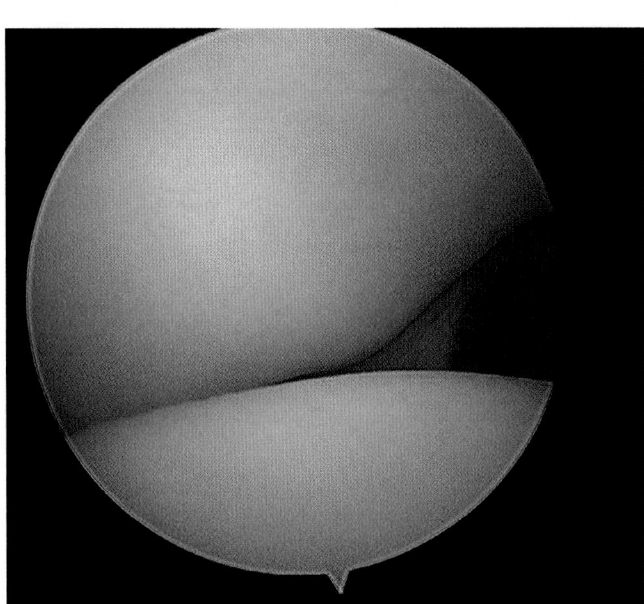

Figure 8.3. View of medial malleolus from anterolateral viewing portal.

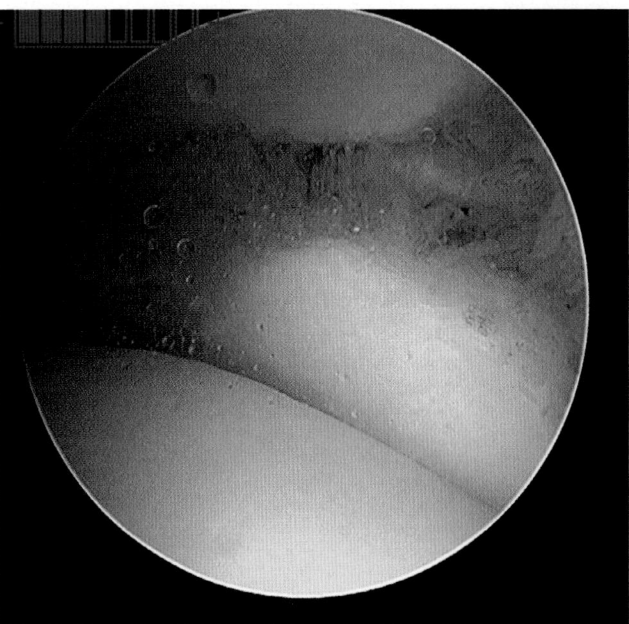

Figure 8.5. Arthroscopic view from anteromedial portal of trifurcation of tibia, talus and fibula.

INDICATIONS AND RESULTS

OSTEOCHONDRAL LESIONS OF THE TALUS

Osteochondral lesions of the talar dome are commonly encountered when evaluating chronic pain after an ankle sprain (4). These chondral lesions have also been attributed to degenerative changes following repetitive microtrauma and have also been described as idiopathic, in patients without a history of trauma (5).

Medial lesions, which are more common than lateral lesions, typically occur in the middle or posterior thirds of the talar body and tend to be deeper, nondisplaced and cup shaped. Lateral lesions, which are more commonly acute traumatic injuries requiring more aggressive treatment, are shallow, displaced and wafer shaped (5).

A patient may complain of swelling, pain, catching or locking as well as decreased range of motion or medial or lateral pain and tenderness. Such symptoms are nondescript, making diagnosis difficult. Further, there may be a lack of correlation between radiographic appearance of these lesions and the findings at arthroscopy. For this reason, diagnosing and staging these lesions should be performed based on CT or MR appearance.

Most intact, nondisplaced lesions are treated conservatively with casting for a minimum of 4 to 6 weeks. Surgical treatment is recommended for patients who fail conservative measures, and for displaced fractures.

Arthroscopy has eliminated much of the morbidity associated with open repair, including stiffness and atrophy of the ankle, as well as malleolar malunion or nonunion from the transmalleolar osteotomies performed during open surgery. The specific arthroscopic procedures to be performed are based on the location, extent and chronicity of osteochondral injury Figure 8.6A, B. When the lesion is acute, displaced and primarily chondral, fragment excision with subsequent debridement and drilling of the base is done. If the lesion is less than 1 cm, abrasion can be performed instead of drilling. When enough underlying bone remains attached to the chondral fragment, it should be reattached via absorbable pins, Kirschner wires or Herbert screws. Most commonly, chronic lesions must be excised as they are loose and nonviable. Curettage and drilling or abrasion proceed fragment removal (5).

In a study of 59 patients who received arthroscopic treatment of osteochondral lesions, 84% had good to excellent results at the 40 month follow-up (15). In a systematic review by Glazebrook et al. (2009), it was determined that fair evidence exists in support of treatment of osteochondral lesions of the talus with arthroscopic debridement and any form of subchondral bone penetration (curettage, drilling, microfracture) in lesions under 15 mm in diameter (6). In regard to lesions greater than 15 mm, the authors believe that there is insufficient evidence-based literature to evaluate arthroscopic effectiveness (6).

SOFT-TISSUE LESIONS

Soft-tissue lesions of the ankle are secondary to many conditions, including congenital bands, posttraumatic or postoperative scar tissues, synovitis, rheumatoid arthritis, gouty arthritis, synovial chondromatosis, infection, ganglions and arthrofibrosis (16). Although these lesions account for approximately 30% to 50% of ankle joint lesions, diagnosis is often difficult due to vague symptoms and inconclusive imaging. MRI is the most helpful in uncovering soft-tissue pathology. However, arthroscopy is the principle and most effective means by which to confirm diagnosis and treat these lesions (5).

LOOSE BODIES

Comprised of chondral or osteochondral fragments, loose bodies result from trauma, synovial chondromatosis or synovial osteochondromatosis, amongst other conditions. Symptoms vary but usually include catching, locking, swelling, pain and decreased range of motion. Often these are visualized on standard radiographs, but occasionally, advanced imaging can help (5).

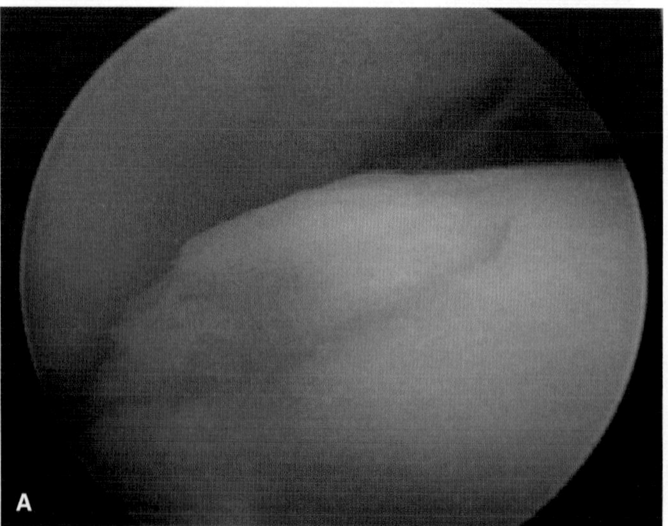

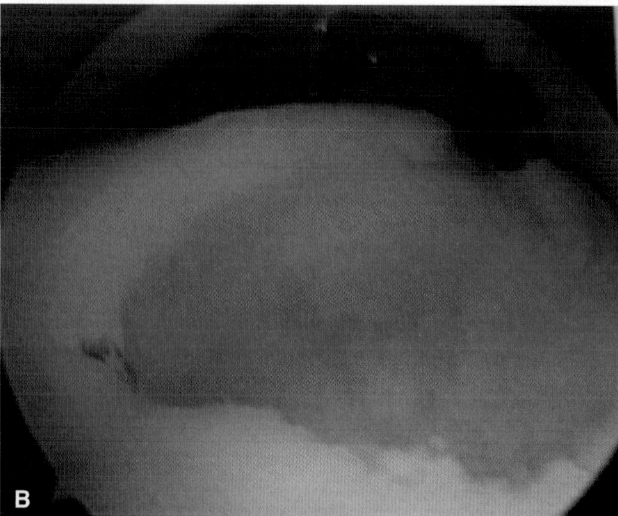

Figure 8.6. **A:** Osteochondral lesion viewed from anteromedial portal. **B:** Same lesion after debridement as viewed from the posterolateral portal.

In the systematic review by Glazebrook et al. (2009), it was determined that poor-quality evidence exists in support of arthroscopic intervention for loose-body removal (6). The authors cite a lack of evidence-based literature for this procedure, explaining that most loose-body removal occurs in conjunction with procedures for other pathology, such as fractures or osteochondral lesions (6). In patients undergoing arthroscopy for loose-body removal and an additional diagnosis, good results are present when the associated pathology has a good prognosis (6).

IMPINGEMENT (BONY AND SOFT TISSUE)

Bony impingement most commonly involves the anterior distal lip of the tibia and commonly has a corresponding lesion on the dorsal aspect of the talar neck (17). Rapid plantarflexion of the foot, as seen when kicking a ball, and repetitive forced dorsiflexion, as seen in football players and dancers, are thought to cause osteophyte formation and subsequent bony impingement.

Arthroscopic osteophyte resection is performed following debridement of surrounding soft tissue, hypertrophied synovium and adhesions which are frequently present (4). Unlike the distal tibia, osteophytes on the talar neck are more commonly missed, leading to a poor outcome for some patients.

Soft-tissue impingement is thought to be caused by multiple inversion injuries to the ankle and is a source of prolonged pain following a sprain. The patient may localize his or her pain anterolaterally, suggesting a tear of the anterior talofibular ligament. Included in the differential for anterior soft-tissue impingement are subtalar instability and a tear of the interosseous ligament. Careful history and physical examination are crucial for diagnosis, as studies have shown MRI to be positive in only 40% of patients (4).

Prior to arthroscopic debridement of the inflamed synovium and ligamentous tissue seen with this pathology, 4 to 6 months of conservative treatment should be completed. When performing the arthroscopy, the shaver's cutting blade must always be visible and the mouth must never be turned dorsally and anteriorly, where neurovascular structures such as the superficial peroneal nerve lie. Several authors have documented good to excellent results in 75% to 96% of patients treated with arthroscopy (18–22).

Less commonly, posterior impingement may occur as a result of synovitis, fibrosis or capsulitis leading to hypertrophy or tearing of the posterior inferior tibiofibular ligament, transverse tibiofibular ligament, tibial slip or pathologic labrum of the posterior ankle joint (5). Management is similar to that of anterior soft-tissue impingement.

In the absence of concurrent osteoarthritis of the ankle, Glazebrook et al. (2009) believe that fair evidence exists in support of arthroscopy for the treatment of soft-tissue or bony-ankle impingement (6).

ANKLE FRACTURES

Arthroscopy in the setting of acute ankle fractures has gained popularity due to the high prevalence of concurrent pathology amenable to arthroscopic treatment. Both osteochondral lesions and loose bodies have been found to be strongly associated with ankle fractures (79% and 55%, respectively) (23).

Arthroscopic evacuation of fracture hematoma and debris are performed first, followed by reduction of fracture fragments via a Freer elevator or percutaneous K-wire insertion. Permanent fixation based on the surgeon's preference is then performed. One concern with this procedure is extravasation of fluid through the fracture and into surrounding tissue. However, with sufficient inflow and outflow, this does not appear to be problematic (4).

POSTOPERATIVE MANAGEMENT

The ankle endures greater hydrostatic pressures than other joints that are commonly treated with arthroscopy, such as the knee, wrist, elbow and shoulder. Further, the wound-sealing effects of soft tissue are absent at the ankle, predisposing the joint to edema, intra-articular hemorrhage and effusion. Thus, the surgeon must pay careful attention to wound closure and apply a compression dressing over the wound site. For the first 3 to 5 days postoperatively, rest with limb elevation and ankle immobilization are needed.

COMPLICATIONS

The complications of ankle arthroscopy include neurologic, tendon, and ligament injuries, infections, wound complications, instrument breakage, effusions, stress fractures secondary to invasive distraction and reflex sympathetic dystrophy (8). These complications can be minimized with a thorough knowledge of surface and intra-articular ankle anatomy. Meticulous preoperative planning coupled with the use of appropriate instruments and distraction techniques will also help curb complications.

The overall complication rate is 9% (24). Neurologic injury has been found to be the most common, comprising 49% of the complications in a study by Ferkel et al. that included 612 cases (8). The superficial peroneal nerve was most commonly involved (56%), followed by the sural nerve (22%) and the deep peroneal nerve (4%) (8).

Most of the complications associated with ankle arthroscopy are transient and resolve within 6 months. The only complication to persist at 10 years follow-up was numbness at the incision site (24). However, as the difficulty and breadth of procedures being performed arthroscopically increases, greater measures will need to be taken to prevent complications and ensure satisfactory outcomes.

CONCLUSION

Ankle arthroscopy is a dynamic, minimally invasive technique that permits direct visualization of intra-articular structures without arthrotomy or malleolar osteotomy. When used appropriately, it gives a high percentage of good results, decreasing morbidity and leading to faster recovery times. However, this procedure should not replace a thorough history, physical examination, diagnostic workup and conservative management. Instead, it should be applied as an alternative strategy to certain open procedures. Although ankle arthroscopy has immensely evolved over the last several decades, additional research must be conducted to ensure further development of this procedure in the treatment of diverse ankle pathology.

REFERENCES

1. Burman MS. Arthroscopy of direct visualization of joints: An experimental cadaver study. *J Bone Joint Surg* 1931;13:669–695.
2. Ferkel RD, Scranton PE. Arthroscopy of the ankle and foot. *J Bone Joint Surg* 1993;75:1233–1242.
3. Chen YC. Clinical and cadaver studies on the ankle joint arthroscopy. *J Japanese Orthop Assn* 1976;50:631.
4. Stephenson KA, Raines RA, Brodsky JW. Ankle arthroscopy: current applications and techniques. *Oper Tech Sports Med* 1999;7:20–27.
5. Stetson WB, Ferkel RD. Ankle arthroscopy: II. Indications and Results. *J Am Acad Orthop Surg* 1996;4:24–34.
6. Glazebrook MA, Ganapathy V, Bridge MA, et al. Evidence-based indications for ankle arthroscopy. *Arthroscopy* 2009;25:1478–1490.
7. Lui TH. Arthroscopy and endoscopy of the foot and ankle: indications for new techniques. *Arthroscopy* 2007;23:889–902.
8. Stetson WB, Ferkel RD. Ankle arthroscopy: I. Technique and complications. *J Am Acad Orthop Surg* 1996;4:17–23.
9. Ferkel RD. Arthroscopy of the ankle and foot. In: Mann RA, Coughlin MJ, eds. *Surgery of the Foot and Ankle*. 6th ed. St Louis, MO: Mosby; 1993:1277–1310.
10. Adkison DP, Bosse MJ, Gaccione DR, et al. Anatomic variations in the course of the superficial peroneal nerve. *J Bone Joint Surg Am* 1991;73:112–114.
11. Feiwell LA, Frey C. Anatomic study of arthroscopic portal sites of the ankle. *Foot Ankle* 1993;14:142–147.
12. Guhl JF. New concepts (distraction) in ankle arthroscopy. *Arthroscopy* 1988;4:160–167.
13. Albert J, Reiman P, Njus G, et al. Ligament strain and ankle joint opening during ankle distraction. *Arthroscopy* 1992;8:469–473.
14. Drez D Jr, Guhl JF, Gollehon DF. Ankle arthroscopy: technique and indications. *Foot Ankle* 1981;2:138–143.
15. Ferkel RD, Sgaglione NA, Del Pizzo W, et al. Arthroscopic treatment of osteochondral lesions of the talus: technique and results. *Orthop Trans* 1990;14:172–173.
16. Ferkel RD. Soft tissue pathology of the ankle. In: McGinty JB, ed. *Operative Arthroscopy*. New York, NY: Raven Press; 1991:713–725.
17. Ogilvie-Harris DJ, Mahomed N, Demazière A. Anterior impingement of the ankle treated by arthroscopic removal of bony spurs. *J Bone Joint Surg Br* 1993;75:437–440.
18. DeBerardino TM, Arciero RA, Taylor DC. Arthroscopic treatment of soft-tissue impingement of the ankle in athletes. *Arthroscopy* 1997;13:492–498.
19. Martin DF, Curl WW, Baker CL. Arthroscopic treatment of chronic synovitis of the ankle. *Arthroscopy* 1989;5:110–114.
20. Ferkel RD, Karzel RP, Del Pizzo W, et al. Arthroscopic treatment of anterolateral impingement of the ankle. *Am J Sports Med* 1991;19:440–446.
21. Liu SH, Raskin A, Osti L, et al. Arthroscopic treatment of anterolateral ankle impingement. *Arthroscopy* 1994;10:215–218.
22. Meslin RJ, Rose DJ, Parisien JS. Arthroscopic treatment of synovial impingement of the ankle. *Am J Sports Med* 1993;17:16–23.
23. Ferkel RD, Orwin JF. Arthroscopic treatment of acute ankle fractures and postfracture defects. In: Ferkel RD, ed. *Arthroscopic Surgery: the Ankle and Foot*. Philadelphia, PA: Lippincott-Raven; 1995:185–200.
24. Ferkel RD, Small HN, Gittins JE. Complications in foot and ankle arthroscopy. *Clin Orthop Relat Res* 2001;391:89–104.

CHAPTER

9

Lauren Turteltaub
Christopher Cook

Principles of Anesthesia for Foot and Ankle Surgery

INTRODUCTION

Foot and ankle procedures are commonly performed orthopedic surgeries. From an anesthetic perspective, these procedures can be managed with a multitude of techniques. An overview of anesthetic techniques will be covered in this chapter, with a discussion of the benefits, indications, contraindications, and complications for each (1). Local infiltration, peripheral nerve blocks, neuraxial techniques (including spinal anesthesia, epidural anesthesia, and combined spinal-epidural [CSE] anesthesia), and general anesthesia have all been used effectively for operations on the foot and ankle. The choice of anesthetic is based on many factors: Location of the surgery (forefoot vs. hindfoot), length of surgery, the patient's postoperative disposition, and factors related to the individual patient's medical history. Another important factor is the experience and skill of the anesthesiologist with the various techniques, a factor that varies widely by practice.

The ideal anesthetic for foot and ankle surgery would confer both intraoperative and postoperative benefits. It would render patients insensible to pain and immobile during the operation to allow for optimal surgical conditions. It would allow for amnesia based on the patient's desires, and allow maximal hemodynamic stability. Postoperatively, an ideal anesthetic should provide excellent pain control, and provide rapid recovery of motor function to allow for appropriate discharge home and assess neurologic function (2). The overall goal is to limit postoperative sedation, nausea, or other untoward side effects facilitating fast tracking through the recovery room. Unfortunately, many of these ideal characteristics are in opposition to each other. Therefore, a balanced approach, utilizing a combination of anesthetic techniques, is often best for patient care and resource management.

ANESTHETIC TECHNIQUES FOR FOOT AND ANKLE SURGERY

GENERAL ANESTHESIA

General anesthesia (GA) has a long history as the anesthetic of choice for many orthopedic procedures. It may be used for foot and ankle surgery, and is considered reliable, quick, and safe in a wide variety of patients. It does have several disadvantages which diminish its appeal for the foot and ankle patient and the ambulatory surgery patient in particular.

Airway manipulation, either with a traditional endotracheal tube or the newer laryngeal mask airway, results in potential risk. This risk can range from mild issues, such as sore throat and damage to dentition, to much more serious complications. Some of the most dreaded and life-threatening complications of anesthesia can occur, such as failure to intubate or ventilate a patient after induction of general anesthesia, laryngospasm, bronchospasm, and aspiration of gastric contents. During GA, systemic use of medication can also cause perturbations of the major organ systems, including cardiovascular, pulmonary, neurologic, renal, and gastrointestinal.

Fortunately, the most common adverse effects of GA are not life threatening, but still can significantly complicate perioperative management. These complications include postoperative nausea and vomiting, and increased postoperative pain compared to regional anesthesia. Although less serious, these are important concerns, as they are the most common reason ambulatory patients are unexpectedly admitted, and can have an impact on patient satisfaction and cost containment (3,4).

It is difficult to discuss GA in the context of foot and ankle surgery without comparing it with regional anesthesia. The question of the "best" anesthetic for ambulatory surgery patients is controversial, and varies significantly with the type of surgery. The benefits of neuraxial anesthesia in the ambulatory population is a debatable topic, and many institutions safely utilize GA for ambulatory lower-extremity surgery. Liu et al, in their meta-analysis on the subject, found that neuraxial blocks (while they decreased pain scores and the need for analgesics in the PACU) did not decrease total time in the ambulatory surgery unit. The relative importance of this issue is institution specific.

In his commentary regarding Liu's study, Hadzic said that fast tracking through postoperative recovery can be accomplished with general anesthesia, but it must be coupled with state-of-the-art "multimodal" anesthetic techniques consisting of nonsteroidal anti-inflammatory drugs, local infiltration of the surgical site, routine antiemetic prophylaxis, and rapid emergence anesthetics. However, despite the faster, early recovery profile of "high-tech" GA techniques, actual cost savings have been difficult to establish. In fact, the current impetus to discharge patients quickly may not result in tangible financial savings (5). This highlights the fact that the "best" anesthetic may be different for various institutions. At our institution, for a variety of reasons, we prefer neuraxial anesthesia to general anesthesia for ambulatory lower-extremity operations.

REGIONAL ANESTHESIA

Regional Anesthesia (RA) is a broad term, defined as "loss of sensation in a circumscribed region of the body, produced by application of local anesthetic by injection" (6). The techniques defined here may be used alone, in conjunction with other regional techniques, or in conjunction with general anesthesia. Perhaps most importantly, these techniques provide a unique bridge into the postoperative period. With the use of long-acting local anesthetics and catheters, the benefits seen in the operating room can extend to the recovery room and beyond. RA encompasses both neuraxial and peripheral techniques. An overview of RA as a whole will be provided, and each technique will be described in detail as it pertains to foot and ankle surgery.

RA is particularly well suited to lower-extremity surgery, and is clearly the anesthetic of choice at our institution for foot and ankle surgery. We believe that in experienced hands, it is the best anesthetic for these procedures. The major absolute contraindication is patient refusal. Other contraindications include infection or distortion at the site of the block, coagulopathy (particularly for neuraxial techniques), preexisting nerve damage in the extremity of interest, and the need for prompt neurologic evaluation of the extremity postoperatively. Often, practical barriers prevent the use of RA, including patient acceptance, surgeon's support of regional techniques, and availability of necessary equipment, and trained perioperative staff.

A discussion of contraindications would be incomplete without considering the patient's desires. A significant barrier is created by patients' fears regarding these techniques, many of which are unfounded. A large survey by Shevde et al revealed that 69% of patients prefer general anesthesia to RA (7). The most common reason was a fear of pain during block placement or surgery. These results highlight the importance of educating the patient during the preoperative visit about the availability and use of sedative hypnotic drugs and/or analgesics during the placement of regional anesthetics. Appropriate sedation has been shown to increase patient satisfaction with regional anesthesia. In another survey by Matthey et al showed that the complications most feared by patients are those which almost never occur (paralysis and back injury) (8). Similarly, the most common complications (spinal headache) were of little concern to the patients surveyed. On speaking to patients, it becomes obvious that many have irrational fears of serious complications despite evidence to the contrary. It is the role of the anesthesiologist to educate patients about the data in this regard. A partnership between surgeons and anesthesiologists provides immeasurable help in this educational process. At our institution, the orthopedic surgeons act as powerful advocates for our techniques weeks before we meet the patient. This preoperative preparation expedites the anesthetic evaluation process on the day of surgery and provides a comfort level for patients regarding techniques that may otherwise seem foreign.

Block failure is a valid concern among surgeons and patients. We recognize this issue, but advocate regional anesthesia and aim to use it both as the intraoperative anesthetic and postoperative analgesic. A regional technique is used for over 90% of approximately 31,000 orthopedic anesthetics per year at our institution (9). This model functions because we enjoy success rates that are acceptable to ourselves and our surgical colleagues. Success rates vary widely by institution and practitioner and depend on many factors, including how "success" is defined. It is important to recognize that neither GA nor RA is an all or none phenomenon, but a continuum, flexible and adaptable. Success rates can be improved tremendously by judicious use of sedatives and communication between anesthesiologists and surgeons.

NEURAXIAL BLOCKADE

Neuraxial anesthesia (NA), including both spinal and epidural techniques are utilized more than any other regional anesthetic. Neuraxial anesthesia has been used for surgical procedures for over 100 years and more recent developments such as continuous catheter techniques, CSE anesthesia and adjuvants can provide patients with expanded benefits of regional anesthesia. When compared with peripheral nerve blocks, some anesthesiologists find spinal and epidural anesthesia more familiar and technically easier to perform. The benefits of both epidural and spinal anesthesia include the avoidance of general anesthesia and its associated complications of airway management. A common concern with NA is hemodynamic instability in moderate to high-risk patients. Even in seemingly high-risk cardiac patients NA can be used safely with careful titration of local anesthetic, and judicious use of fluids and vasopressors (10). In general, hemodynamic stability with NA is not maintained as consistently as with peripheral nerve blockade. Neuraxial anesthesia has been demonstrated to provide better postoperative analgesia and reduce opioid consumption as compared with general anesthesia, and provide greater patient satisfaction (3). However, anesthesia induction time (which vary by institution) and PACU time may be prolonged with neuraxial techniques compared to general anesthesia (3).

EPIDURAL ANESTHESIA

Epidural anesthesia involves injecting local anesthetics and adjunctive medications into the potential space around the dura. There are multiple benefits of epidural anesthesia including segmental spread, titratability, longer duration of anesthesia, and generally greater hemodynamic stability compared to spinal anesthesia. Currently the two most commonly used medications in the epidural space for surgical anesthesia are local anesthetics and opioids. To understand how an epidural anesthetic functions, a general understanding of the pharmacodynamics of local anesthetics must be appreciated. When local anesthetics are administered into the epidural space, they exert their initial effects on spinal nerve roots and dorsal-root ganglia as they exit the intervertebral foramina. Neural blockade may also take place at the paravertebral level, implying both peripheral and central nervous system target sites. Individual nerve target sites are responsible for the segmental nature of the epidural block when local anesthetics are employed (11,12). For our discussion, as it pertains to foot and ankle surgery, we will focus on two approaches to the epidural space, the lumbar and caudal approaches.

Lumbar epidural anesthesia is an excellent choice for patients undergoing foot and ankle surgery. This technique is typically accompanied by a catheter allowing for both continuous and intermittent bolusing of epidural medications. The presence of the catheter is particularly useful in long cases, where the surgical level can be maintained almost indefinitely. Therefore epidural anesthesia as a sole technique allows for greater control and titratability of analgesia, anesthesia, and the associated sympathectomy when compared with spinal anesthesia (13).

Caudal epidural anesthesia in surgery of the foot and ankle is used primarily for postoperative analgesia in pediatric patients. Because of the risk of infection, this technique is typically a single-shot technique. In the past, caudal anesthesia was used more frequently in adults, but because of the anatomic variability of the sacrum, and decreased training in this technique, it has fallen out of vogue in many institutions.

Complications of epidural anesthesia can range from minor to life threatening. While serious complications are infrequent, it must be emphasized that wherever these blocks are performed, an anesthesiologist should be present to perform or supervise these techniques. To ensure patient safety, adequate equipment and personnel should be available for performing advanced airway management and cardiovascular resuscitation. The complications of epidural anesthesia include cardiovascular compromise, accidental high epidural levels, unintended spinal anesthesia, neurologic injury, bleeding, and infectious complications.

Cardiovascular complications related to epidural anesthesia can occur from intravascular injection, from delayed systemic uptake of local anesthetic or indirectly from sympathectomy associated with the blockade of sympathetic nerve fibers.

Intravascular injection can result in local anesthetic toxicity manifesting in minor symptoms including tinnitus and circumoral numbness to serious signs such as seizures and cardiovascular collapse. The incidence of these complications can be reduced by routinely administering epidural test doses and incremental injections. Compared to peripheral nerve blocks of the lower-extremity and spinal anesthetics, lumbar and caudal epidural anesthetics result in greater plasma levels of local anesthetics.

High epidural levels can severely compromise cardiovascular status by causing significant hypotension, bradycardia, and in extreme cases, apnea. Fortunately, this rarely occurs if placed in the lumbar and caudal regions.

Unintended spinal anesthesia is another complication that can be reduced by careful technique. To help prevent unintended subarachnoid injection, one should always aspirate from the needle or catheter prior to injection ensuring that no CSF is present. Complications of unintended spinal anesthesia result from large volumes of local anesthetic being placed in the subarachnoid space resulting in a rapidly occurring, high, and dense spinal blockade which can lead to cardiovascular and respiratory collapse.

SPINAL ANESTHESIA

Spinal anesthesia is an excellent choice for procedures on the foot and ankle. It is an excellent primary anesthetic, particularly when a thigh tourniquet is utilized and tourniquet times are anticipated to be long. The advantages of spinal blockade include rapid onset, reliably dense sensory/motor blockade of the lower extremities, and avoidance of airway manipulation. In general, compared to an epidural technique, spinal blockade has a more rapid onset, is technically easier to perform, and provides a more intense motor and sensory blockade. It is often utilized in conjunction with a peripheral block for postoperative pain, and is the most common technique utilized at our institution for foot and ankle surgery.

Spinal blockade occurs when local anesthetic is deposited in the subarachnoid space, thus preventing the propagation of neural impulses by blocking sodium channels. Spinal anesthesia appears to exert its activity directly on the spinal cord compared to epidural anesthesia which exerts its effects both within the subarachnoid and epidural spaces. Spinal anesthesia is characterized by rapid onset of dense motor and sensory blocks, but onset and duration vary by the local anesthetic injected into the subarachnoid space. Local anesthetics of varying duration of activity are available for use. Lidocaine and mepivacaine are the most common short- to intermediate-acting LAs utilized, while intermediate to long-acting medications include tetracaine, bupivacaine, and ropivacaine. These medications can be prepared as hypobaric, isobaric and hyperbaric solutions. The baricity of the solutions can impact the behavior of the block and the optimal patient positioning for the procedure. For example, using a hypobaric lumbar spinal blockade performed on a patient in the left lateral decubitus position would provide anesthesia for the right lower extremity greater than the left. Since the solution is hypobaric, the local anesthetic would rise in the subarachnoid space to block nerve roots innervating the right leg located in a nondependent position. At our institution, however, we most commonly utilize isobaric local anesthetics for spinal techniques (Table 9.1).

COMBINED SPINAL EPIDURAL

The combined spinal epidural (CSE) is a relatively new technique. It allows for an initial subarachnoid injection, followed by epidural catheter placement. It is superior to an epidural in its rapidity of onset, saving 15 to 20 minutes compared with epidural alone (14). It also decreases local anesthetic dosage, decreasing the risk of toxicity. CSEs provide the benefit of block supplementation as needed, and extension of the block indefinitely, should the procedure outlast the spinal. For foot and ankle procedures expected to last more than 3 hours, the CSE is our technique of choice as the primary anesthetic.

COMPLICATIONS OF NEURAXIAL ANESTHESIA

POSTDURAL PUNCTURE HEADACHE (PDPH)

PDPH is defined as a headache following dural puncture, resulting from leakage of cerebrospinal fluid. It is characterized by its positional nature, worsening in the sitting or standing position and improving in the supine position. The headache is usually located in the occipital and frontal regions. There

TABLE 9.1 Dose Response Effects of Spinal Local Anesthetics

Local Anesthetic	Dose (mg)	Duration of Sensory Block (min)	Duration of Motor Block (min)
Lidocaine	40	130 (26)	93 (24)
	60	162 (32)	128 (31)
	80	170 (24)	142 (32)
Bupivacaine	7.5	144 (25)	75 (24)
	10	194 (26)	100 (24)
	15	343 (28)	150 (24)
Mepivacaine	45	182 (38)	142 (37)
	60	203 (36)	168 (36)
Ropivacaine	12	176 (42)	162 (37)
	14	192 (48)	189 (44)

Modified from Liu SS, McDonald SB. Current issues in spinal anesthesia. *Anesthesiology* 2001;94:888–906.

can be associated tinnitus, photophobia, and diplopia. PDPH is a well-known complication of neuraxial anesthesia, but current practice techniques of using smaller gauge pencil-point needles for spinal anesthesia has reduced the risk of PDPH to approximately 1% (15). The risk varies by institution, and is estimated to be higher in teaching hospitals where anesthesia trainees perform NA techniques under supervision. The incidence of PDPH following epidural anesthesia is also around 1%. The traditional pathophysiologic mechanism described since this complication was first observed stems from stretching and irritation of the meninges secondary to CSF volume changes. Conservative treatment of PDPH includes bed rest, oral analgesics, hydration, and caffeine. If these measures are insufficient, an epidural blood patch should be performed. The efficacy of a blood patch for PDPH secondary to small gauge spinal needle puncture (95% or greater) is much greater than a 16 to 18 gauge epidural needle puncture (30% to 75%) (16–18).

EPIDURAL ABSCESS AND MENINGITIS

Infectious complications are extremely rare, but can be severe. Moen et al estimated the incidence of meningitis to be 1 in 50,000 following spinal anesthesia and 1 in 90,000 after epidural anesthesia (19). Epidural abscess occurred 1 in 37,000 following epidural blocks. Sources of infection following neuraxial anesthesia include patients' skin, blood secondary to bacteremia, contaminated equipment, and prolonged indwelling catheters. Indwelling epidural catheters should be monitored daily for signs of erythema, edema, induration or symptoms like tenderness around the catheter site. If such signs or symptoms are present, removal of catheter should be considered, with continued monitoring of the site after catheter removal. If a superficial infection is suspected, culturing of the epidural catheter tip and implementation of an antibiotic regimen should occur. Severe back pain or a new neurologic deficit not consistent with the epidural infusion should prompt consideration of an epidural abscess with subsequent MRI or CT imaging along with neurosurgical consultation for incision and drainage. Of course, a high index of suspicion is crucial when evaluating patients with possibly severe complications (11).

HEMORRHAGIC COMPLICATIONS

The risk for hemorrhagic complications associated with neuraxial blockade is low in the general patient population. Because of the noncompressible nature of the tissue surrounding the spinal cord, a high index of suspicion must be given to the possibility of hematoma formation which can lead to spinal-cord or nerve-root compression and injury. Horlocker et al estimated the incidence of spinal hematoma in the absence of anticoagulant and antiplatelet medications to be less than 1 in 150,000 neuraxial blocks (20). Patients at increased risk include those on antiplatelet medications, anticoagulants, or have a coexisting disease inducing a coagulopathy or thrombocytopenia.

PERIPHERAL NERVE BLOCKS

Lower-extremity peripheral nerve blocks are advantageous because they can provide excellent surgical anesthesia and postoperative analgesia. When compared with neuraxial blockade, there are fewer hemodynamic changes, less postoperative nausea and vomiting, less urinary retention, and earlier discharge from the PACU (3) Unfortunately, because of the increased skill level and equipment required to perform lower-extremity blocks, peripheral nerve blocks are arguably not performed as often as they should be in the foot and ankle patient.

SCIATIC AND FEMORAL BLOCKS

The sciatic nerve provides all of the motor functions of the foot and ankle and a majority of the sensory functions. The blockade of the sciatic nerve in the popliteal fossa provides sensory blockade to most of the ankle and foot, but surgery on the medial aspect requires a supplemental saphenous nerve block. Both lateral and posterior approaches to this block are well described. The saphenous nerve is a purely sensory branch of the femoral nerve, innervating the medial aspect of the ankle and foot. At our institution, these peripheral blocks are rarely used as the sole anesthetic. They are used quite commonly for postoperative pain control.

Nerve localization of the sciatic nerve in the popliteal fossa can be accomplished by neurostimulation or ultrasound guidance. In some studies, the combination of the two techniques has improved success rates and decreased needle passes. (21) Duration of analgesia for a single injection of 20 mL of bupivacaine 0.5% can extend a popliteal block beyond 18 hours (22). The saphenous nerve is only a sensory division and is typically localized by surface landmarks and by ultrasound guidance.

Complications from the popliteal block are rare but include intravascular injection, local anesthetic toxicity, or nerve injury. Complications from saphenous nerve blockade are also rare. Intravascular injection is a concern due to proximity to the saphenous vein.

ANKLE BLOCK

The ankle block is an excellent choice for surgery of the foot that does not require a tourniquet above the ankle. Although ultrasound and neurostimulation can be used, the ankle block requires no expensive equipment or patient cooperation for placement. It is a field block, targeting the 5 terminal nerves to the foot. Its simplicity, safety, reliability, and high success rate (noted to be anywhere from 94% to 98%) make it an appealing anesthetic for a wide variety of clinical scenarios (23,24). The ankle block meets the overall goal of performing a regional anesthetic with minimal hemodynamic perturbation, and has the added advantage of potential prolonged postoperative analgesia. Also, the lack of significant motor blockade makes it an ideal choice for ambulatory surgery.

Contraindications to the ankle block are few; it is in fact a good choice for patients with coagulopathies, or serious cardiopulmonary conditions. With the possible exception of infection, scarring, or anatomical distortion at the injection site, it may be used safely in nearly any patient.

The technique involves blocking the sural, posterior tibial, deep peroneal, and superficial peroneal nerves (all branches of the sciatic) plus the saphenous nerve (which arises from the femoral nerve). In broad terms, 2 techniques have been described: The classic perimalleolar approach, and the more distal midtarsal approach, commonly used at our institution. The midtarsal approach has been found to have a higher success rate, likely because of the more superficial location of the nerves at this level (24). Sharrock et al also found the ankle tourniquet to be well tolerated, despite the distal placement of the block. The choice of local anesthetic depends largely on the duration of surgery and need for abrupt onset. To tap into the benefits of both prompt onset and longevity, at our institution, a mixture of 2% lidocaine and 0.75% marcaine (without epinephrine) is routinely utilized.

Duration of the ankle block has been found to be anywhere from 6 to 25 hours (25). The length of the block likely depends on technique, volume of local anesthetic, and specific mixture of local anesthetics. This very wide range of duration should be considered when evaluating patients with "prolonged" blocks.

Complications from ankle blocks are actually extremely rare. Patients can have discomfort during the performance of this block because of the multiple injections required, but titrated intravenous sedation can improve patient satisfaction significantly. Serious complications such as compartment syndrome have only been reported in patients with severely altered anatomy (26). Similarly, infection, hematoma, and local anesthetic toxicity are possible, but incidence is extremely low; less than one in a thousand (25–27) Many studies in fact found zero complications after ankle block (28).

CONTINUOUS PERIPHERAL NERVE BLOCKS

Single-shot peripheral nerve blocks are limited by the duration of action of the chosen local anesthetic. Continuous perineural infusions overcome this limitation and help us provide postoperative analgesia well beyond the 16 hours single-shot blocks may provide. Although continuous nerve blocks have been described since 1946 by Ansbro et al, continuous popliteal blocks have only recently been prospectively evaluated both on an inpatient and outpatient basis. In both patient populations improved analgesia, decreased opioid consumption, and improved patient satisfaction were demonstrated using continuous catheters. Optimal local anesthetic dosing regimen via patient controlled regional anesthesia (PCRA) for popliteal infusions has been studied prospectively, and studies revealed that basal rate infusions were superior for preventing sleep disturbance, improving analgesia, and providing for high patient satisfaction compared to the bolus-only method (29).

HOME CATHETERS

At our institution, a home catheter program is in its early stages, and perineural catheters are still primarily reserved for inpatients. Nationally, outpatient perineural catheter placement is on the rise. Careful patient selection and education must be advised. It must be kept in mind that postoperative cognitive dysfunction (from residual anesthetic agents) may prevent a patient from understanding and following instructions and an educated caretaker can be a useful asset in assisting with home catheter management. In addition, an appropriate follow-up system should be in place to evaluate the patient and catheter.

Complications associated with perineural catheters include infection, catheter migration, myonecrosis, pump malfunction or misuse, and local anesthetic toxicity. Many of these complications are still theoretical in nature. In a prospective study by Borgeat et al of over 1000 patients receiving popliteal catheters, no patients experienced infection or neuropathy (30). Despite the successful track record of popliteal catheters, placement of such catheters should not be taken lightly. Organized, systematic followup and management is a necessity when undertaking these techniques.

ROLE OF ULTRASOUND

Ting et al first published the usage of ultrasound for regional anesthesia in 1989 (31). Since that publication, ultrasound has emerged as an integral tool in the modern practice of regional anesthesia. This technique allows an anesthesiologist to visualize in real time vascular, muscular, bony, and visceral structures. The real time footage allows the physician to navigate a needle towards its target nerve(s) and away from undesirable structures. In addition, it provides the ability to observe local anesthetic spread around target nerves and the ability to adjust needle position to provide a more optimal delivery position for medication depositions. Some studies have shown ultrasound to improve the quality of sensory blockade, onset time, and the success rate compared to nerve stimulation Ultrasound-guided nerve blocks can be used with and without neurostimulation (32). Its application for anesthesia for foot and ankle surgery involves its use in spinal and epidural blockade, saphenous nerve blockade, popliteal blockade of the sciatic nerve, as well as blockade of the posterior tibial nerve in the ankle block.

POSTOPERATIVE PAIN MANAGEMENT

A discussion of regional anesthesia for foot and ankle surgery would be incomplete without reference to the significant contribution these techniques add to the management of acute postoperative pain. The choice for pain management after foot and ankle surgery is complex but crucial to the patient's well being. The possible modalities are many and the "best choice" depends on many factors: Site of surgery, length of procedure, discharge plans, and factors specific to the patient's history. Foot and ankle surgery can be fraught with some of the most challenging postoperative pain treatment decisions. Large bony surgery often requires large doses of opioids for prolonged periods of time, particularly if the modality is utilized alone. Opioids can cause various well-described side effects including pruritus, postoperative nausea and vomiting, urinary retention, ileus, and respiratory depression. These unpleasant occurrences and the quality of postoperative pain control have a significant effect on patient satisfaction. They can also have an impact on timely discharge for both ambulatory and same-day patients.

The distal site of foot and ankle operations makes them particularly amenable to both prolonged regional block and peripheral catheter techniques. These techniques are clearly ideal for a situation where minimizing both pain and systemic narcotic side effects are priorities.

Single-shot peripheral nerve blocks performed preoperatively are an excellent choice for postoperative pain. It is clear that lower-extremity blocks provide superior pain control compared with traditional parenteral opioids.

Ankle blocks have a long safety history and may be the analgesic technique of choice for surgery of the forefoot. When compared with popliteal blocks, they are more distal and superficial, intuitively conferring a better safety profile (22). As outlined earlier, the simplicity of this block, along with the fact that it needs no expensive or complicated equipment, make it extremely appealing in a wide variety of practices. For many operations, an ankle block may be used as the primary anesthetic. Utilizing enough long-acting local anesthetics will extend the block well into the postoperative period.

Single-shot popliteal blocks are also an excellent choice for postoperative pain control. The analgesia provided is more extensive in coverage than that of the ankle block (particularly in conjunction with a saphenous nerve block), and it is the single-shot analgesic block of choice for surgery involving the hindfoot at our institution. Klein et al looked at 1781 ambulatory patients after various peripheral nerve blocks. Their findings for long-acting popliteal fossa blocks showed very high efficacy, safety, and patient satisfaction (33). There is evidence that the analgesia from a popliteal block exceeds that of an ankle block. Macleod et al prospectively compared the two using the same dose of bupivacaine 0.5%, and found that the popliteal block significantly outlasted the ankle block (18 hours vs. 11 hours) (22). Another study by Migues et al found a less impressive difference, with ankle blocks lasting 11 hours and popliteal blocks 14 hours, on average (34). Both techniques in this study provided an excellent safety profile and high patient satisfaction. The use of ultrasound has made the popliteal block more appealing, providing direct visualization of the nerve during needle placement and injection.

Extensive foot and ankle surgery, as noted earlier, may involve several days of significant pain. The use of continuous peripheral catheters can extend the analgesia as long as the catheter may safely be left in place. The greatest barrier for catheter use is availability of relatively complex equipment for placement and infusion. In recent years, the availability of lightweight, reliable infusion pumps has made it possible to send patients home with a peripheral infusion. Much has been written recently about the benefits of continuous peripheral nerve blocks. Studies found excellent analgesia and a very acceptable side-effect profile for peripheral catheters. Ilfeld et al looked at postoperative analgesia in 30 foot and ankle patients in a randomized, controlled, double-blinded study. The study found excellent analgesia in the study group, with decreased opioid use and side effects, increased patient satisfaction, and no catheter or local anesthetic-related complications in any patient (35). A large meta-analysis by Richman found that continuous peripheral nerve blocks, regardless of catheter site, provided superior analgesia and fewer side effects compared to opioids (36). In fact, the data is clear that popliteal catheters are superior to both IV narcotics and placebo infusions (37).

REFERENCES

1. Fisher L, Gordon M. *Anesthesia for Hand Surgery.* Publication Pending.
2. Shah S, Tsai T, Iwata T, et al. Outpatient regional anesthesia for foot and ankle surgery. *Int Anesthesiol Clin* 2005;43(3):143–151.
3. Liu SS, Strodtbeck WM, Richman JM, et al. A comparison of regional versus general anesthesia for ambulatory anesthesia: A meta-analysis of randomized controlled trials. *Anesth Analg* 2005;101:1634–1642.
4. Hill RP, Lubarsky DA, Phillips-Bute B, et al. Cost-effectiveness of prophylactic antiemetic therapy with ondansetron, droperidol, or placebo. *Anesthesiology* 2000;92:958–967.
5. Hadzic A. Is regional anesthesia really better than general anesthesia? *Anesth Analg* 2005; 101:1631–1633.
6. American heritage dictionary of the English language. 4th ed.
7. Shevde K, Panagopoulos G. A survey of 800 patients' knowledge, attitudes, and concerns regarding anesthesia. *Anesth Analg* 1991;73:190–198.
8. Mattey PW, Finegan BA, Finucane BT. The public's fears about and perceptions of regional anesthesia. *Reg Anesth Pain Med* 2004;29(2):96–101.
9. HSS Website www.hss.edu
10. Ho MC, Beathe JC, Sharrock NE. Hypotensive epidural anesthesia in patients with aortic stenosis undergoing total hip replacement. *Reg Anesth Pain Med* 2008;33(2):129–133.
11. Warren DT, Liu SS. Neuraxial anesthesia. In: Longnecker DE, ed. *Anesthesiology.* McGraw-Hill Co.; 2008.
12. Hines RL, Rathmell JP, Neal JM, et al. Regional anesthesia: The Requisites in Anesthesiology. Mosby; 2004.
13. Liu SS, McDonald SB. Current issues in spinal anesthesia. *Anesthesiology* 2001;94: 888–906.
14. Holmstrom B, Laugaland K, Rawal N, et al. Combined spinal epidural block vs spinal and epidural block for orthopedic surgery. *Can J Anesth* 1993;40:606–609.
15. Lambert DH, Hurley RJ, Hertwig L, et al. Role of needle gauge and tip configuration in the production of lumbar puncture headache. *Reg Anesth* 1997;22:66–72.
16. Bart AJ, Wheeler AS. Comparison of epidural saline placement and epidural blood placement in the treatment of post-lumbar-puncture headache. *Anesthesiology* 1978;48:221–223.
17. Safa-Tisseront V, Thormann F, Malassine P, et al. Effectiveness of epidural blood patch in the management of post-dural puncture headache. *Anesthesiology* 2001;95:334–349.
18. Paech M. Epidural blood patch - myths and legends. Can *J Anesth* 2005.
19. Moen V, Dahlgren N, Irestedt L. Severe neurological complications after central neuraxial blockades in Sweden 1990–1999. *Anesthesiology* 2004;101:950–959.
20. Horlocker TT, Wedel DJ, Benzon HT, et al. Regional anesthesia in the anticoagulated patient: defining the risks (the Second ASARA Consensus Conference on Neuraxial Anesthesia and Anticoagulation). *Reg Anesth Pain Med* 2003;28:172–197.

21. Vicente Domingo-Triadó, Salvador Selfa, Francisco Martínez, et al. Ultrasound guidance for lateral midfemoral sciatic nerve block: A prospective, comparative, randomized study. *Anesth Analg* 2007;104:1270–1274.
22. Macleod DH, Wong DH, Vaghadia H, et al. Lateral popliteal sciatic nerve block compared with ankle block for analgesia following foot surgery. *Can J Anesth* 1995;42(9):765–769.
23. Rudkin GE, Rudkin AK, Dracopoulos GC. Ankle block success rate: A prospective analysis of 1000 patients. *Can J Anesth* 2005;52:209–210.
24. Sharrock NE, Waller JF, Fierro LE. Midtarsal block for surgery of the forefoot. *Br J Anaesth* 1996;58:37–40.
25. Myerson MS, Ruland CM, Allon SM. Regional anesthesia for foot and ankle surgery. *Foot Ankle* 1992 13(5):282–288.
26. Noorpuri BS, Shahane SA, Getty CJ. Acute compartment syndrome following revisional arthroplasty of the forefoot: The dangers of ankle block. *Foot Ankle Int* 2000;21:680–687.
27. Frederic A, Bouchon Y. Analgesia in Surgery of the Foot. *Can Anesthesiol* 1996;44:115–118.
28. Hadzik A. *Textbook of Regional Anesthesia and Pain Medicine.* McGraw Hill.
29. Ilfeld BM, Enneking FK. Continuous peripheral nerve blocks at home: A review. *Anesth Analg* 2005;100:1822–1833.
30. Borgeat A, Blumenthal S, Lambert M, et al. The feasibility and complications of the continuous popliteal nerve block: 1001-case study. Anesth Analg. 2006;103(1):229–233.
31. Ting PL, Sivagnanaratnam V. Ultrasonographic study of the spread of local anesthetic during axillary brachial plexus block. *Br J Anaesth* 1989;63:326–329.
32. Chan VW, Perlas A, McCarney CJ, et al. Ultrasound guidance improves success rate of axillary brachial plexus block. *Can J Anaesth* 2007;54:176–182.
33. Klein SM, Neilsen KC, Greengrass RA, et al. Ambulatory discharge after long acting peripheral nerve blockade: 2382 blocks with ropivacaine. *Anesth Analg* 2002;94(1):65–70.
34. Migues A, Gaston S, Vescove A, et al. Peripheral Foot Blockade vs Popliteal Fossa Nerve Block: A Prospective Randomized Trial in 51 Patients. American College of Foot and Ankle Surgeons Elsevier Ltd; 2005.
35. Ilfeld BM, Morey TE, Wang RD, et al. Continuous popliteal sciatic nerve block for postoperative pain control at home: A randomized double blinded placebo controlled study. *Anesthesiology* 2002;97(4):959–965.
36. Richman J, Liu S, Courpas B, et al. Does continuous peripheral nerve block provide superior pain control to opioids? A meta-analysis. *Anesth Analg* 2006;102:248–257.
37. Singelyn FJ, Aye F, Gouverneur JM. Continuous popliteal sciatic nerve block: An origin technique to provide postoperative analgesia after foot surgery. *Anesth Analg* 1997;84(2):383–386.

CHAPTER

10

Mark Drakos
Edward Chang
Russell F. Warren

Acute Ankle Instability

INTRODUCTION

Ankle sprains are the single most common acute orthopedic pathology seen by physicians. They account for almost a quarter of all musculoskeletal injuries (1). More than 23,000 patients are diagnosed daily in the United States (2). In a population of high level athletes ankle injuries accounted for 21% of all injuries in professional basketball players (3). Similarly, in a cohort of professional football players, ankle sprains had the highest injury incidence at 29.1 per 100 players (4). Risk factors include ligamentous laxity, increased baseline talar tilt, inappropriate shoe wear, irregular playing surface, cutting activities, and history of previous ankle sprain. The lateral ligaments are involved in up to 85% of cases (1,5). These injuries typically occur from an inversion and/or internal rotation force. Accurate diagnosis of ankle injuries requires an understanding of the anatomy and biomechanics of this joint. Following a detailed history and physical examination, radiographic imaging can help rule out fractures and associated pathology. Because of its weight-bearing function and narrow articulation, trauma to the ankle joint is a frequent cause of morbidity in the general population. Early diagnosis along with appropriate treatment and rehabilitation is essential in allowing a timely return to normal activities.

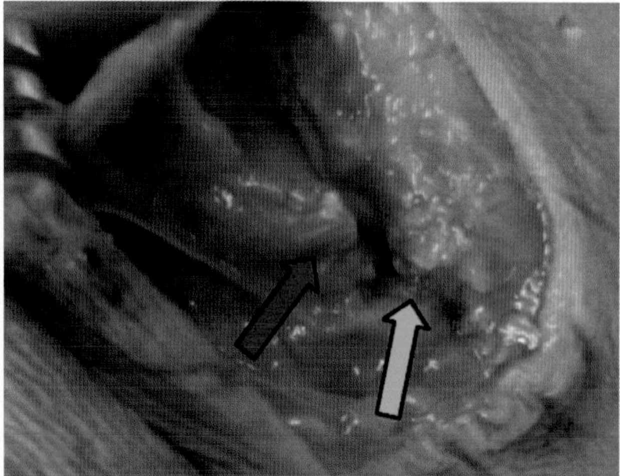

Figure 10.1. Cadeveric left ankle with both the ATFL (*red arrow*) and CFL sectioned from the fibula. Note that these 2 ligaments are thickenings of the lateral ankle joint capsule.

The injury pattern is dictated by the anatomy and foot position (6). The lateral ankle complex consists of three distinct bands: The anterior talofibular ligament (ATFL), posterior talofibular ligament (PTFL) and the calcaneofibular ligament (CFL). The ATFL is a thickening of the ankle capsule that extends a short distance from the anterior edge of the distal fibula to the talar neck (7). In plantarflexion, the ligament is parallel to the long axis of the foot in contrast to being aligned with the tibial and fibular shafts in dorsiflexion (8). A cadaveric biomechanical study measuring strain on the ATFL showed that strain is minimal in dorsiflexion and increases as the ankle is moved progressively through plantarflexion along with internal rotation and inversion (9). The CFL is a discrete ligament that courses from the inferior tip of the distal fibula and inserts on the mid-posterolateral part of the calcaneus. This ligament is considered extra-articular. Strain is minimal at plantarflexion and maximal at dorsiflexion and inversion (10,11). Due to its anatomical location, the CFL also plays a role in subtalar joint stabilization (10,11). The PTFL runs from the posterior border of the lateral malleolus to the posterolateral tubercle of the talus. Maximal strain of the PTFL occurs when the ankle is dorsiflexed and externally rotated (12). The authors concluded that the ATFL and the CFL function together and are most important in providing lateral stability at all positions of ankle flexion (10,11).

The two other areas which may lead to ankle instability and may be associated with lateral ankle sprains or occur in isolation are injuries to the deltoid and syndesmosis. The deltoid ligament is a strong, flat, triangular band that originates from the medial malleolus and consists of superficial and deep components. The deep fibers originate from the medial malleolus and insert at the medial border of the talus. The superficial ligament has three distinct fiber patterns: The tibionavicular fiber, the most anterior, inserts at the tuberosity of the navicular bone; the tibiocalcaneal fiber, the middle fiber, descends and inserts at the sustentaculum tali of the calcaneus; the posterior tibiotalar passes posteriorly and inserts at the talus. Studies of the deltoid ligament show that it primarily acts to resist external rotation and abduction of the talus. It is also a less frequently disrupted ankle ligament, with an isolated deltoid injury reported in approximately 2.5% of all ankle sprains (11). This may be attributed to the inherent strength of the deltoid which requires the highest load to failure of all ligaments (13). Also, persistent symptoms are usually related to chronic anteromedial pain rather than instability.

The distal tibiofibular syndesmosis consists of the inferior potions of the anterior tibiofibular and posterior tibiofibular ligaments, the interosseous membrane, and the inferior transverse ligament. The anterior tibiofibular ligament originates from Chaput's tubercle of the tibia and inserts on Wagstaffe's tubercle of the fibula. The posterior tibiofibular originates from Volkmann's tubercle of the tibia and inserts into the posterolateral malleolus. The inferior transverse ligament consists of the distal portion of the posterior tibiofibular ligament. The interosseous ligament is the thickened part of the distal interosseous membrane. Strain increases with dorsiflexion and external rotation which is also the most commonly reported injury mechanism (14,15). However, the incidence of this specific injury is relatively low as well only occurring in approximately 1% to 5% of patients after severe inversion trauma (10).

MECHANISM

Ankle instability usually occurs following severe sprains. The most common mechanism of a sprain is ankle inversion and/or internal rotational force applied to the foot when the ankle is plantarflexed, placing maximal strain on the lateral ligaments (16). In this position the ATFL acts as the intra-articular reinforcement of the capsule and is the main stabilizer on the lateral ankle. Furthermore, it courses within the plane of plantar and dorsiflexion making it effectively the lateral collateral ligament of the ankle. Thus, it is a restraint to both varus and rotational forces. In the plantarflexed position the dome of the talus is the most narrow which in turn allows for the greatest osseous excursion medially and laterally of the tibiotalar joint. The combination of this positional laxity and function of the ATFL contribute to the high incidence of injury (7). The ATFL is the first ligament to rupture in anterior instability. Rupture of the ATFL occurs as an isolated injury in 50% to 75% of cases (13,17,18).

Higher-energy mechanisms can lead to CFL injury. Biomechanical studies of isolated CFL injuries demonstrated isolated varus instability (2). It may also function as a lateral collateral ligament of the ankle joint. Rupture of the ATFL and CFL occurs in 15% to 25% of cases (8). Clinically, however, isolated rupture of the ligament is unlikely. More commonly it represents a continuum of increased severity of a lateral-sided injury. PTFL ligament injury is usually seen in severe ankle sprains with associated fractures. Like isolated injury to the CFL, an isolated PTFL injury is a rare finding occurring in less than 1% of cases (2,9).

The role of the biomechanics of these ligaments is critical to understanding the potential for instability. When the ATFL is sectioned there is an increase in the talar tilt in plantarflexion and no change in dorsiflexion. When the CFL is sectioned there is an increase in the talar tilt in dorsiflexion and no change in plantarflexion. When both of these two ligaments are divided the talar tilt increases by an average of 20 degree. Sectioning of the PTFL allows increased ankle dorsiflexion but has no effect on lateral instability (17,19,20).

CLASSIFICATION

Given the frequency of lateral ligament injuries we will focus on this region for the remainder of the chapter. A classification scheme was developed and later modified to organize these injuries based on ligament integrity (14,18,21,22). A grade 1 injury represents a stretch of the ATFL and the anterior without frank ligamentous disruption. Patients complain of mild swelling and occasionally difficulty with full weight bearing. Physical examination reveals little or no ecchymosis, point tenderness on the ATFL and mild or no restriction of active range of motion (ROM). No laxity is elicited on examination.

A grade 2 injury is associated with moderate injury to the ATFL and occasionally the CFL. There is marked swelling and ecchymosis as compared to grade 1 injury. There is tenderness over the anterolateral aspect of the ankle and laxity may or may not be elicited.

A grade 3 injury occurs when there is a complete disruption of the ATFL and CFL. There is diffuse swelling over the lateral ankle and heel and marked tenderness over the ligaments and anterolateral capsule. Malliaropoulos further subclassified grade 3 injuries based on anterior drawer stress radiographs (23,24). Grade 3A injuries have normal stress radiographs with a decrease in ROM >10 degree and edema greater than 2 cm. Grade 3B injuries have more than 3 mm difference in distance between the posterior articular surface of the tibia and the nearest point of the talus on comparison of the injured versus uninjured ankle.

ASSESSMENT

A thorough history and physical examination is helpful to making the diagnosis. Often patients will report an inversion type injury, classically landing on someone's foot after jumping. This is usually followed by pain, swelling, ecchymosis on the lateral ankle. Examination should include palpation of all ligaments including the ATFL, CFL, PTFL, syndesmosis, and deltoid. Range of motion and ability to bear weight should also be evaluated. The patient may or may not be able to walk. This in itself may occur in either the severe sprain or broken ankle and may require further work-up. Laxity of the ligament can be assessed by comparing the amount of anterior subluxation of the talus on the injured with the contralateral side. This can be done by performing the anterior drawer test with the hindfoot in neutral, allowing the ATFL to be the primary restraint to anterior talar displacement (24). The inversion test is another examination performed to assess the amount of talar tilt present when the hind foot is inverted. However, the reliability and accuracy of these tools have been debated. The sensitivity and specificity of these examinations are increased when repeated 5 days after the injury (5). At that time point the anterior drawer test is more likely to be more accurate due to the decrease in pain which should become more localized. Pain upon palpation of the ATFL combined with ecchymosis is indicative of an ATFL rupture in 90% of cases. A positive anterior drawer examination is 73% sensitive and 97% specific. However, when these three tests are combined the resulting sensitivity is 100% and specificity is 77% (2).

X-rays are useful particularly if there is a question of fracture. Emergency room physicians have used the "Ottawa criteria" to determine the likelihood of fracture to reduce the costs due to unnecessary tests (9,25,26). Some authors even advocate the use of stress radiographs to determine competency of the ligaments (27,28). However, we do not recommend routine use of stress radiographs to assess ligamentous capacity. While this imaging as well as magnetic resonance imaging (MRI), ultrasound (US), and other modalities may provide the treating personnel with more information regarding the extent of the injury, the frequency of these injuries virtually precludes an extensive work-up for everyone with ankle pain.

NON-OPERATIVE MANAGEMENT

Conservative treatment options are usually divided into cast immobilization and functional management. Patients treated with cast immobilization are given the knee walking cast for 3 weeks followed by proprioceptive rehabilitation. This allows rapid return to activity in the weight-bearing cast. This plays a role in the low-demand patient who cannot bear weight due to pain (24). Furthermore, this may reduce swelling which some authors espouse may not only hasten recovery, but promote healing in a more anatomic position. To optimize healing the ankle is usually casted in 5 to 15 degree of dorsiflexion and slight eversion. This is somewhat theoretical. As Ruth reported, the ligament ends were never opposed regardless of foot position when an open evaluation was performed (5).

In a complete rupture, the presence of excessive soft tissue edema may cause the ATFL to heal in a "stretched" position. Elimination of this swelling by immobilization may allow ligament ends to become more opposed and promote anatomic healing. Furthermore, the cast provides effective protection against re-injury in the acute period which will also help to minimize swelling and exacerbation of the initial injury. However, some authors contend that this likely delays recovery for the period of time the cast is in place.

In contrast, functional management refers to early mobilization with external support followed by rigorous rehabilitation, including proprioceptive training. A short period of rest is combined with rest, ice, compression, elevation, nonsteroidal anti-inflammatory medications (RICEN) in the first few days. Early weight bearing without crutches is advocated with gradual return to full activity. In addition, active and passive ROM, neuromuscular training, proprioceptive exercises, and peroneal strengthening are encouraged. In order to avoid complete immobilization but still provide protection lace up ankle braces, ankle taping, and elastic bandages can give the ankle support. People usually return to their normal activities in 1 to 3 weeks depending on the extent of the injury and the demands placed on the ankle.

Clinical studies and literature reviews have supported the idea that functional management allows patients to return to normal activities sooner than immobilization. A randomized controlled trial was done to compare plaster cast immobilization for 21 days with functional management in athletic adults less than 35 years of age suffering a grade 3 tear for the first time (29). It was concluded that functional management showed significant earlier and better return to physical activity, fewer symptoms, and better decrease in joint laxity on radiographic examination. There was no difference in re-injury rate. This was supported by Eiff and colleagues who performed a study looking at military recruits and randomized them into two groups (30). They found that patients in the early mobilization group were more likely to be back to full work (54% vs. 13%) 10 days after injury. However, no difference was appreciated at 1-year follow-up between cast treatment and early mobilization.

A meta-analysis of randomized controlled trials comparing cast immobilization and functional management found that in all analyses performed, no results were significantly in favor of cast immobilization (31). Functional management held significant advantages in time to return to sports, time to return to work, number of patients with persistent pain, and amount of laxity in the joint. The authors concluded that functional management is superior when compared to cast immobilization.

OPERATIVE MANAGEMENT

Several authors advocate early acute repair of the disrupted lateral ligaments (32). The most common tear is usually midsubstance. Early intervention allows anatomic repair before scar, which may make the identification of ligament ends difficult, is formed.

Brostrom was the first to report his result using this technique in 1966 (5,6,32). He found that in 105 acute sprains the ATFL was completely torn in 65 and the CFL was partially or completely torn in 23. In cases of complete tear the adjacent capsule was always torn. Also, torn ends of ligaments and capsule could be well opposed in almost all cases. The advantages of his procedure include no normal tissue sacrificed, no tenodesis effect restricting motion, no donor site morbidity, no loss of eversion strength, preservation of tibiotalar and subtalar motion and less pain compared to reconstruction. The disadvantages are that frayed ligaments are often difficult to find and when found they are often stretched, not simply torn. Despite these pitfalls, he had excellent results and over 90% return to prior activity.

The operative alternative is to perform a reconstruction such as the Chrisman–Snook procedure with either autologous or allograft tissue. Many of these are non-anatomic by design and utilize local tendon (peroneus brevis or plantaris), fascia lata, or allograft in reconstruction. The advantage of this procedure is that it involves a graft to re-establish the appropriate restraints when no local tissue is available. Its disadvantages include donor site morbidity, especially eversion weakness when the peroneals are harvested.

Given that these two operative approaches have consistently shown good outcomes it remains a challenge to appropriately select patients for operative intervention. Although it is widely accepted that functional management is the treatment of choice in patients with grade 1 and 2 injuries, the treatment in grade 3 injuries remains controversial. In 1986, Eggert et al. reported better results in patients treated with functional management when compared to operative intervention (33,34). This was supported by a randomized prospective trial comparing 3 weeks plaster immobilization with and without a prior surgical repair (35). At 2 years follow-up the authors found similar radiographic results, but slightly worse functional results as many patients in the operative group gave up physical activity.

Recent studies have shown statistically significant differences in favor of surgical intervention. Pijnenburg et al. conducted a randomized controlled trial comparing functional and surgical management in adult patients less than 45 years of age presenting with a primary acute ankle injury (<48 hours) (36). The authors found statistically significant differences in favor of surgical intervention with regard to pain, instability, and recurrent sprains. They therefore concluded that operative treatment led to better results at short- and long-term follow-up, but suggested that surgery be reserved in selected cases when higher functional demands are preferred due to cost, risks of complications, and similar results with delayed and acute repair.

ANKLE INSTABILITY

The most common failure of the ATFL and CFL is by midsubstance rupture. Ruth reported that the ligament ends were never approximated during exploration during primary repair (37). Moreover, manipulation had no effect. One might surmise that closed treatment would almost always result in non-anatomic healing with potential clinical sequelae. This is further complicated by the associated injuries which occur at the time of initial injury. These may include disruption of normal capsular mechanoreceptors, loss of afferent fibers, loss of proprioceptive feedback, and loss of effective motor coordination. Each of these is a potential major contributor to recurrent instability and possible target of any proposed treatment.

The so-called "functional ankle instability" is the most common adverse sequelae of an acute lateral ligament rupture. Clinically, the patient may report pain and episodes of "giving way". However, this may or may not correlate with the clinical measurement of ankle stability indicated by the anterior drawer and talar tilt (29). Thus, the other factors such as proprioception and peroneal strength may play as important a role as the laxity or competence of the lateral ligament complex. This was demonstrated in a study which looked at the EMG activity of the peroneal muscles in unstable ankles (19,32). The authors found that the reaction time was significantly lower in the muscles in the affected group when subjected to an inversion moment than the control group. The authors assert that a delayed proprioceptive response to a sudden angular displacement of the ankle may be an important cause of the instability. Most authors agree that it is often a combination of these issues that are present and must be addressed individually.

DISCUSSION

Severe injuries of the soft tissues may lead to acute instability. A small percentage goes on to chronic ankle instability. However, most studies have demonstrated good medium- and long-term outcomes regardless of primary choice of treatment (cast, functional mobilization, surgery). More than 90% of patients have been reported to regain functional ankle stability after non-operative treatment. The case for early operative intervention is further hampered by the good outcomes with delayed reconstruction. Studies have shown no difference in objective and subjective findings when compared to acute repair (38).

It should be noted that many of these outcomes have not been examined as critically with current physical examination and radiographic modalities to assess subtle changes. Moreover, when closely investigated (33,34,39,40) authors have reported that patients can have long-term residual symptoms, including chronic instability, in more than 30% to 40% of the cases (20). Moreover, to date the diagnostic tools we have at our disposal (radiographic laxity and severity of injury) have yet to reliably predict which ankle sprains will ultimately fall into this category.

When chronic instability is evaluated there is a high incidence of associated pathology, particularly lesions of the talar dome (2,5,8,9,22,24,41,42). This may help explain the persistent symptoms which may not be related to the initial ligamentous injury. However, due to the high level of return to sport and the minimal impact of symptoms when they do persist our approach to these injuries has yet to change in years. If high-quality imaging such as MRI were performed after every ankle sprain or even just the more severe injuries, it is likely that these associated pathologies might be addressed at an earlier time point. However, given the raw frequency of these injuries this plan is flawed by the cost effectiveness of such a paradigm. If acute ligamentous reconstruction is advocated, it is still hard to determine which patients would benefit from this versus those which would have healed with conservative measures alone. Moreover, in the case of chronic instability, there are several procedures with good long-term follow-up data which can adequately address this problem making the urgency of these injuries less clear. More research is needed to help delineate which patients may benefit from early operative intervention and those who would benefit from a more aggressive work-up in the acute phase of injury.

REFERENCES

1. Klenerman L. The management of sprained ankle. *J Bone Joint Surg Br* 1998;80(1):11–12.
2. Krips R, de Vries J, van Dijk CN. Ankle instability. *Foot Ankle Clin* 2006;11(2):311–329, vi.
3. Deitch JR, Starkey C, Walters SL, et al. Injury risk in professional basketball players: a comparison of Women's National Basketball Association and National Basketball Association athletes. *Am J Sports Med* 2006;34(7):1077–1083.
4. Brophy RH, Barnes R, Rodeo SA, et al. Prevalence of musculoskeletal disorders at the NFL Combine–trends from 1987 to 2000. *Med Sci Sports Exerc* 2007;39(1):22–27.
5. Maffulli N, Ferran NA. Management of acute and chronic ankle instability. *J Am Acad Orthop Surg* 2008;16(10):608–615.
6. Kannus P, Renstrom P. Treatment for acute tears of the lateral ligaments of the ankle. Operation, cast, or early controlled mobilization. *J Bone Joint Surg Am* 1991;73(2):305–312.
7. Wright IC, Neptune RR, van den Bogert AJ, et al. The influence of foot positioning on ankle sprains. *J Biomech* 2000;33(5):513–519.
8. Glasgow M, Jackson A, Jamieson AM. Instability of the ankle after injury to the lateral ligament. *J Bone Joint Surg Br* 1980;62-B(2):196–200.
9. Boruta PM, Bishop JO, Braly WG, et al. Acute lateral ankle ligament injuries: a literature review. *Foot Ankle* 1990;11(2):107–113.
10. Colville MR, Marder RA, Boyle JJ, et al. Strain measurement in lateral ankle ligaments. *Am J Sports Med* 1990;18(2):196–200.
11. Renstrom P, Wertz M, Incavo S, et al. Strain in the lateral ligaments of the ankle. *Foot Ankle* 1988;9(2):59–63.
12. Heilman AE, Braly WG, Bishop JO, et al. An anatomic study of subtalar instability. *Foot Ankle* 1990;10(4):224–228.
13. Fallat L, Grimm DJ, Saracco JA. Sprained ankle syndrome: prevalence and analysis of 639 acute injuries. *J Foot Ankle Surg* 1998;37(4):280–285.
14. Attarian DE, McCrackin HJ, DeVito DP, et al. Biomechanical characteristics of human ankle ligaments. *Foot Ankle* 1985;6(2):54–58.
15. Rasmussen O. Stability of the ankle joint. Analysis of the function and traumatology of the ankle ligaments. *Acta Orthop Scand Suppl* 1985;211:1–75.
16. Hopkinson WJ, St Pierre P, Ryan JB, et al. Syndesmosis sprains of the ankle. *Foot Ankle* 1990;10(6):325–330.
17. Brostrom L. Sprained ankles. 3. Clinical observations in recent ligament ruptures. *Acta Chir Scand* 1965;130(6):560–569.
18. Rasmussen O, Kromann-Andersen C. Experimental ankle injuries. Analysis of the traumatology of the ankle ligaments. *Acta Orthop Scand* 1983;54(3):356–362.

19. Karlsson J, Andreasson GO. The effect of external ankle support in chronic lateral ankle joint instability. An electromyographic study. *Am J Sports Med* 1992;20(3):257–261.
20. Karlsson J, Lansinger O. Lateral instability of the ankle joint. *Clin Orthop Relat Res* 1992;(276):253–261.
21. Cass JR, Morrey BF, Chao EY. Three-dimensional kinematics of ankle instability following serial sectioning of lateral collateral ligaments. *Foot Ankle* 1984;5(3):142–149.
22. Hertel J. Functional Anatomy, Pathomechanics, and Pathophysiology of Lateral Ankle Instability. *J Athl Train* 2002;37(4):364–375.
23. Chorley JN, Hergenroeder AC. Management of ankle sprains. *Pediatr Ann* 1997;26(1):56–64.
24. Malliaropoulos N, Papacostas E, Papalada A, et al. Acute lateral ankle sprains in track and field athletes: an expanded classification. *Foot Ankle Clin* 2006;11(3):497–507.
25. van Dijk CN, Lim LS, Bossuyt PM, et al. Physical examination is sufficient for the diagnosis of sprained ankles. *J Bone Joint Surg Br* 1996;78(6):958–962.
26. van Dijk CN, Mol BW, Lim LS, et al. Diagnosis of ligament rupture of the ankle joint. Physical examination, arthrography, stress radiography and sonography compared in 160 patients after inversion trauma. *Acta Orthop Scand* 1996;67(6):566–570.
27. Pigman EC, Klug RK, Sanford S, et al. Evaluation of the Ottawa clinical decision rules for the use of radiography in acute ankle and midfoot injuries in the emergency department: an independent site assessment. *Ann Emerg Med* 1994;24(1):41–45.
28. Stiell IG, Greenberg GH, McKnight RD, et al. A study to develop clinical decision rules for the use of radiography in acute ankle injuries. *Ann Emerg Med* 1992;21(4):384–390.
29. Ruth CJ. The surgical treatment of the fibular collateral ligament of the ankle. *J Bone Joint Surg Am* 1961;43A:229.
30. Ardevol J, Bolibar I, Belda V, et al. Treatment of complete rupture of the lateral ligaments of the ankle: a randomized clinical trial comparing cast immobilization with functional treatment. *Knee Surg Sports Traumatol Arthrosc* 2002;10(6):371–377.
31. Eiff MP, Smith AT, Smith GE. Early mobilization versus immobilization in the treatment of lateral ankle sprains. *Am J Sports Med* 1994;22(1):83–88.
32. Kerkhoffs GM, Handoll HH, de Bie R, et al. Surgical versus conservative treatment for acute injuries of the lateral ligament complex of the ankle in adults. *Cochrane Database Syst Rev* 2007;2(2):CD000380.
33. Brostrom L. Sprained ankles. V. Treatment and prognosis in recent ligament ruptures. *Acta Chir Scand* 1966;132(5):537–550.
34. Brostrom L. Sprained ankles. VI. Surgical treatment of "chronic" ligament ruptures. *Acta Chir Scand* 1966;132(5):551–565.
35. Eggert A, Gruber J, Darda L. Therapy of injuries of the exterior ankle joint ligaments. Randomized study of postoperative therapy and early functional treatment tactics. *Unfallchirurg* 1986;89(7):316–320.
36. Evans GA, Hardcastle P, Frenyo AD. Acute rupture of the lateral ligament of the ankle. To suture or not to suture? *J Bone Joint Surg Br* 1984;66(2):209–212.
37. Pijnenburg AC, Bogaard K, Krips R, et al. Operative and functional treatment of rupture of the lateral ligament of the ankle. A randomised, prospective trial. *J Bone Joint Surg Br* 2003;85(4):525–530.
38. Karlsson J, Peterson L, Andreasson G. The unstable ankle: a combined EMG and biomechanical modeling study. *Int J Sports Biomechanics* 1992;8:129–134.
39. Brostrom L, Sundelin P. Sprained ankles. IV. Histologic changes in recent and "chronic" ligament ruptures. *Acta Chir Scand* 1966;132(3):248–253.
40. Takao M, Uchio Y, Naito K, et al. Arthroscopic assessment for intra-articular disorders in residual ankle disability after sprain. *Am J Sports Med* 2005;33(5):686–692.
41. DiGiovanni BF, Partal G, Baumhauer JF. Acute ankle injury and chronic lateral instability in the athlete. *Clin Sports Med* 2004;23(1):1–19, v.
42. van Rijn RM, van Os AG, Bernsen RM, et al. What is the clinical course of acute ankle sprains? A systematic literature review. *Am J Med* 2008;121(4):324–331.e6.

David I. Pedowitz
Justin M. Kane
David N. Garras
Christopher C. Dodson

CHAPTER 11

Chronic Ankle Instability

INTRODUCTION AND EPIDEMIOLOGY

Ankle sprains are one of the most common orthopedic injuries encountered by healthcare professionals and over 80% are injuries to the lateral ankle ligamentous complex. They comprise nearly one in every ten visits to the emergency room and have an incidence of 2.15 per 1000 persons per year (1,2). During the second decade of life, the rate jumps to 7.2 per 1000 persons per year, and those participating in sports are thought to be at an even higher risk (1,3,4). Sporting activities are thought to be responsible for up to half of all ankle sprains with basketball (41.1%), American football (9.3%), and soccer (7.9%) being associated with the highest percentage of ankle sprains (4). The socioeconomic implications of ankle sprains are also massive, with estimated aggregate healthcare costs thought to be in excess of two billion dollars annually. One compounding factor in consideration of ankle sprains is that these injuries tend to be undertreated and over time may lead to recurrent sprains, chronic pain, muscular weakness as well as the feeling of instability about the ankle. It has been estimated that only 26% of athletes treated for ankle sprains achieve a full recovery (no pain, weakness, or instability) (3,5). In fact, the most predictive risk factor for an ankle sprain is a previous sprain in the same ankle (6). With this in mind, the importance of a systematic approach to the diagnosis and treatment of lateral ankle sprains cannot be overstated. For the purposes of this chapter, however, we will focus on the treatment of ankle sprains that have not improved over time, with or without adequate treatment, and have evolved into cases of chronic ankle instability. Chronic lateral ankle instability is present when there is a pattern of repeated clinical symptomatic laxity (giving way) which interferes with normal function.

ANATOMY AND BIOMECHANICS

The ankle joint has three categories of stabilizers; the bony architecture itself, the capsuloligamentous connections around the joints and between the bones, and the dynamic muscular stabilizers surrounding the ankle.

The ankle joint consists of the articulations between the talus and the distal tibial plafond, the medial malleolus and the lateral malleolus, often referred to as the ankle mortise. Its unique shape allows for efficient transfer of torque to be transmitted from the lower leg to the foot during weight bearing. The mortise is primarily stabilized by the bony interface of the tibia, fibula and talus. In addition to bony stability, additional stability is provided by the joint capsule and the lateral and medial ligament complexes. The lateral ankle ligament complex consists of three ligaments: The anterior talofibular ligament (ATFL); the calcaneofibular ligament (CFL); and the posterior talofibular ligament (PTFL).

The ATFL extends from the anterior-inferior border of the lateral malleolus to the neck of the talus. It is the most commonly injured ligament of the lateral ankle ligament complex and this can be attributed to it having the lowest threshold for failure under loading in cadaveric studies (7,8). It lies on the dorsolateral aspect of the foot and travels at a 45 degree angle anteromedially from its fibular origin to its talar insertion. On average, the ATFL is 7.2 mm wide and 24.8 mm long (9). It is tensioned as the foot progresses from dorsiflexion into plantarflexion and functions as a restraint to anterior translation of the tibiotalar joint (10). This explains why those patients with acute tears of the ATFL become incre asingly symptomatic as their ankles are brought into plantarflexion.

The CFL extends from the tip of the lateral malleolus to the lateral tubercle of the calcaneus. It travels at 133 degrees posteriorly from the long axis of the fibula as it reaches its insertion point on the calcaneus (9). The orientation of the CFL confers resistance to excessive inversion at both the mortise and distally at the subtalar joint. It is tensioned as the foot is placed into dorsiflexion (10). After the ATFL, it is the most commonly injured lateral ankle ligament (7,8).

The PTFL extends from the digital fossa on the posterior border of the lateral malleolus to the posterolateral aspect of the talus on the lateral tubercle (9). It travels in a posterior direction and at both its origin and insertion has a broad surface conferring it an inherently high tensile strength. It provides resistance to inversion and internal rotation to the mortise and is the least likely to be injured of the lateral ankle ligaments (7,8).

Dynamic stabilizers are those structures which confer stability by being activated. In the ankle, the lateral dynamic stabilizers consist primarily of the peroneal tendons. The peroneus longus and brevis muscles originate on the lateral aspect of the leg, hug the posterior border of the fibula, and insert on the plantar aspect of the medial midfoot and base of the fifth metatarsal respectively. While the peroneus longus muscle is responsible for ankle plantarflexion, subtalar eversion and midfoot pronation and abduction, along with the peroneus brevis, these two tendons play a major role in ankle stability due to their strength in eversion. Conversely, this can also be viewed as their ability to resist inversion.

MECHANISM OF INJURY

The mechanism by which chronic ankle instability occurs is the same as that seen with an acute inversion ankle injury. The main difference is that these episodes of inversion occur on a regular basis and are often recalcitrant to traditional conservative treatment. The clinical entity of chronic ankle instability has its foundation in both the functional and mechanical changes produced by repeated acute ankle injuries (11).

The vast majority of ankle instability involves failure of the lateral stabilizers under forced inversion. The tendency for injury to involve inversion of the hindfoot at the mortise is due to both the bony anatomy as well as the ligamentous structures that stabilize the ankle. When comparing the medial and the lateral malleolus, the lateral malleolus extends further distally conferring an intrinsic osseous block to eversion. The deltoid ligament on the medial aspect of the ankle is significantly stronger than that of the lateral ligament complex thus offering another stabilizer against medial ankle injury.

Sprains about the lateral ankle have been classified into three grades based on the mechanical integrity of the injured ligaments as well as the clinical presentation accompanying the injury. Table 11.1 summarizes this classification that largely applies to the acute setting (12,13). Since chronic instability often presents with acute-on-chronic symptoms, this classification remains useful for the chronic setting as well.

TABLE 11.1 Classification of Lateral Ankle Sprains (11)

	Ligaments Affected	Clinical Findings
Grade I	ATFL stretched with some fibers torn (no frank disruption of ATFL)	Mild swelling, minimal ecchymosis, point tenderness over ATFL. Little difficulty with ROM or weight bearing.
Grade II	Moderate injury to the lateral ankle ligament complex; ATFL tear with frequent involvement of CFL.	Moderate swelling and ecchymosis. Tenderness over anterolateral ankle. Mild ligament laxity. Difficulty with weight bearing and ROM. Acutely may be indiscernible from grade III injury.
Grade III	Complete tear of ATFL and CFL often involving the PTFL and joint capsule.	Diffuse swelling and ecchymosis. Tenderness over anterolateral ankle, ATFL, and CFL. Inability to bear weight.
Grade IIIa (13)		ROM decreased by >10 degrees, edema >2 cm. Normal stress radiographs.
Grade IIIb (13)		ROM decreased by >10 degrees, edema >2 cm. >3 mm difference in the distance between the posterior articular surface of the tibia to the nearest point of the talus on radiographic comparison with the contralateral ankle.

The etiology of chronic lateral instability of the ankle lies in both the structural and functional changes that occur as the result of repeated inversion injuries without appropriate healing. Exploring them in detail is essential for one to fully appreciate how to make an accurate diagnosis. However, it is more important to be able to assess the effectiveness of conservative treatment and how to decide when reconstructive options are most appropriate.

MECHANICAL CHANGES IN CHRONIC INSTABILITY

The structural changes that accompany acute ankle injuries change the biomechanics of the ankle such that they result in instability. As the lateral ligament complex becomes attenuated, its decreased resting tension affords the ankle a greater degree of hypermobility.

As the various stabilizers of the ankle become weak, stretched out, or fail, necessary changes occur in the joint mechanics in and around the ankle. Subsequently, as the ankle attempts to undergo its normal range of motion during the stance phase, ligaments fail to provide adequate restrain to what is now abnormal bony movement.

In addition to bony and ligamentous changes, the trauma experienced by the soft tissue surrounding the ankle during ankle sprains can add to the pathology seen in chronic instability. Synovial inflammation and hypertrophy often results in anterior and anterolateral impingement as well as the development of chondral lesions in the joint (11,14). In fact, in patients undergoing surgery for lateral ankle instability, it has been found that 67% had anterolateral impingement syndrome and an additional 49% had hypertrophic synovitis (14).

Changes also occur within the joint surfaces due to the repeated trauma experienced with chronic lateral instability. In patients requiring surgery for ankle ligament reconstruction, a 3-fold increase in the presence of osteophytes and loose bodies has been found when compared to healthy controls (15).

FUNCTIONAL CHANGES

Functional instability refers to instability related to neuromuscular factors. Rather than a single abnormality, there seem to be a spectrum of neuromuscular derangements that are responsible for chronic functional instability (11). Disruptions in proprioception, the ability to sense joint position, have been highly implicated in this process. Patients who experience recurrent ankle sprains and chronic instability have been shown to have impaired proprioception and replication of joint angles (16–18) compared with healthy controls on kinesthetic measures (19–21). While conflicting studies exist regarding the true etiology of impaired neuromuscular firing, there is evidence that suggests a definitive role played by impairment of neuromuscular recruitment (11,22). In one study, bilateral gluteus medius recruitment deficits were noted in patients with a history of severe ankle sprains. That impairment exists across multiple pathways in multiple joints is suggestive of central neural changes affecting peripheral joint conditions (23). More research is needed however, to clearly define the role neuromuscular firing plays in functional instability.

Impairment of postural control has also been demonstrated in patients with a history of repetitive ankle sprains. The modified Romberg test allows for subjective measurement of a patient's postural control. The patient is asked to stand on a single limb for a period of 10 to 30 seconds. Both the affected and unaffected limbs are tested with both patient and examiner assessing which limb appears to cause a greater postural instability. In patients with chronic instability, there is functional instability demonstrated with the affected extremity. Deficits are likely due to a combination of impaired proprioception and neuromuscular control (11,19,20,24,25,26). During a single-leg stance, the foot pronates and supinates to keep the body's center of gravity above the base of support. This is referred to as the "ankle strategy" of postural control. In patients suffering from chronic instability, there is a tendency to use a "hip strategy" of postural control. This tends to be a less efficient modality to maintain balance (27).

In patients with chronic ankle instability, there is ample evidence to also implicate the role of strength deficits. Both eversion and inversion deficits have been reported. Whether this is due to intrinsic weakness in the muscles surrounding the ankle or if it is an impairment in neuromuscular recruitment has yet to be delineated and further studies are needed to explore this topic (11,28–30).

Evaluation of the patient with lateral ankle instability

PHYSICAL EXAMINATION

In the case of chronic ankle instability, there are two general presentations. One, is the patient who has had repeated episodes of instability and presents with an acutely painful injury. The second is the patient who complains largely of the ankle giving way on a regular basis. This second presentation is often devoid of pain. Lateral ankle sprains are almost always the result of excessive inversion, often described as a "rolling in" of the ankle. While 80% of ankle sprains occur at the lateral ligament complex, only 4.8% of these are thought to be first time sprains (31). This is suggestive that recurrent ankle sprains are extremely prevalent and the acute injury should also warrant an evaluation for chronic instability.

Chronic ankle instability is characterized primarily by repeated episodes of the ankle giving way, often without any preceding trauma. Symptoms are generally described as a feeling of weakness, looseness, and the inability to control the ankle on the slightest uneven surface. Pain is infrequently the primary complaint. While it may occasionally accompany chronic instability, if instability episodes are accompanied by pain, this should alert the examining physician to look for additional causes of pathology.

It is important to note that it is the patient's history and symptoms which define instability about the ankle and not the clinical or radiographic findings. This is underscored by recent estimates that as much as 11% of healthy subjects have hypermobility about the ankle joint without accompanying symptoms (15).

Once an acute fracture has been ruled out with standard weight-bearing radiographs, and instability is suspected, a focused examination is undertaken. Thorough physical examination has been shown to have a 96% sensitivity and 84% specificity in the diagnosis of chronic instability (32). Tenderness over the lateral ankle is commonly seen in those with instability and ranges from isolated tenderness over the ATFL to generalized joint line tenderness with a discernible effusion and palpable synovium.

Assessment for peroneal tendon tears and instability is necessary as an association often exists with instability. This is particularly important in cases where patients present with chronic instability and pain. Pain overlying the course of the peroneal tendons is characteristic of tenosynovitis and split tears of the peroneal tendons. Taking the ankle through a range of motion and exaggerating plantarflexion and eversion may result in a palpable snapping of the peroneal tendons. This can be either intrasheath subluxation of the tendons or frank dislocation of the tendons anterior to the fibula. Resisted eversion and dorsiflexion is another way to produce subluxation/dislocation.

The anterior drawer test assesses anterior translation of the talus under the mortise in the sagittal plane. The test is done with the examiner placing one hand on the distal tibia and using the other hand to apply an anterior force to the calcaneus while the patient keeps their ankle at a position of rest (20 degrees of plantarflexion). The characteristic suction sign is seen with a drawing in of the skin at the lateral gutter and is a result of the synovium being sucked into the joint (33). Attention should not only be paid to the amount of translation present when compared to the contralateral ankle, but should also focus on the end-point of translation. A soft or painful end-point could be indicative of ligament injury.

The talar tilt test is performed by tilting the hindfoot and looking for a suction sign or asymmetric movement. The ankle should be placed into plantarflexion during the examination (33). Care must be taken in discerning true movement at the ankle joint from that at the subtalar joint. Palpating the talar neck can help in this differentiation.

Along with a focused examination about the lateral ankle, assessment of the overall shape of the foot as well as a thorough neurovascular examination should be performed. This can help in identifying the underlying cause of chronic instability.

Pain along the ankle joint line can be seen in chronic instability. Aside from the pathology seen at lateral ankle, there is often a proliferative synovium, spurring of the tibia and talus, or osteochondral lesions of the talus. These findings can be demonstrated with the Malloy impingement test. Pain with palpation of the anterior joint line or the lateral and medial gutters rather than the motion of dorsiflexion

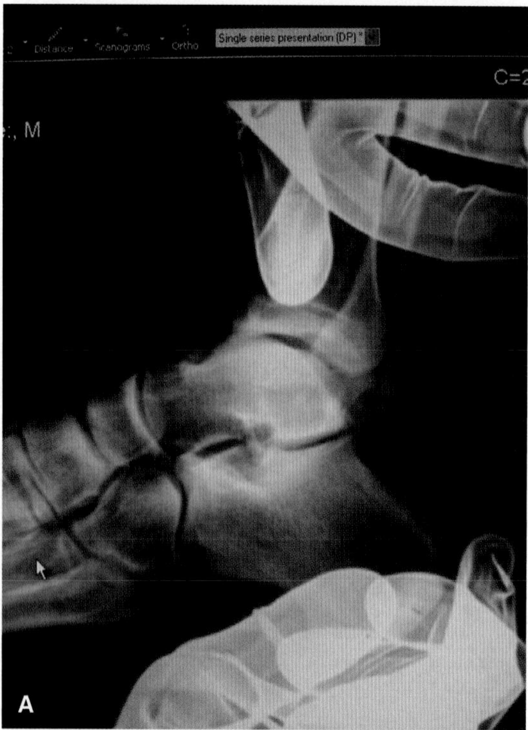

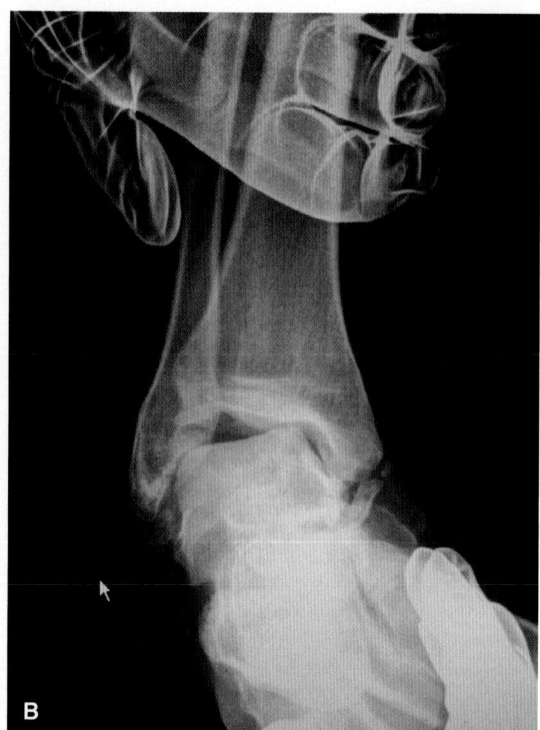

Figure 11.1. Stress radiographs. **(A)** anterior drawer and **(B)** talar tilt x-rays should be obtained and compared to the unaffected side. The examiner should wear lead-lined gloves during the examination for protection.

denotes a positive test and is suggestive of an osteochondral lesion (34).

Proprioception is tested with the Romberg test. Assessment begins with the unaffected ankle and is executed by having the patient stand on the limb first with the eyes open and then again with the eyes closed assessing the patient's ability to balance on the foot. This is then repeated for the affected limb. It is important to assess the patient for a functional instability as studies suggest that conservative management for these patients is more successful (35).

RADIOGRAPHIC ASSESSMENT

Plain Radiography

When obtaining plain films to assess the ankle, it is important to use weight-bearing films. While plain films are not helpful for assessing soft tissue structures, they may help with the diagnosis of concomitant injury. Stress radiographs are valuable in detecting mechanical instability but are not a prerequisite for making the diagnosis (36). Across the literature, there is wide variation in the criteria used for diagnosing instability. Karlsson et al. have the most comprehensive data series. Their criteria for radiographic evidence of ankle instability was an anterior drawer test of >10 mm or a talar tilt of >9 degrees (Fig. 11.1). When comparison of the contralateral ankle was possible, a difference of >3 mm on anterior drawer test or >3 degrees on talar tilt was significant for instability (37).

Ultrasound

It has been demonstrated that in the hands of a skilled ultrasonographer, acute tears of the ATFL and CFL can be diagnosed (32,38). However, the same study shows superiority of physical examination in both specificity and sensitivity (32).

Magnetic Resonance Imaging

MRI is a useful adjunct to plain films as it allows for assessment of ligaments, tendons, muscles, bones, chondral surfaces, the synovium, and the joint space. Without dynamic imaging studies, MRI cannot demonstrate ankle instability. While its use as a modality in the diagnosis of instability is questionable, it has utility in preoperative planning for patients who fail conservative management. The diagnosis of concomitant injury may alter surgical planning for ligament reconstruction. Of note, it has been demonstrated that MR arthrogram is superior to both MRI and plain films for the detection of ATFL and CFL tears (39). Most importantly, in the evaluation of chronic instability in the presence of pain, MRI is particularly useful in identifying osteochondral lesions of the talus and peroneal tendon pathology which may need to be assessed separately.

CONSERVATIVE MANAGEMENT

After a diagnosis of lateral ankle instability is made, treatment begins in the same manner as with any soft tissue injury.

Particularly for the acute episode, rest, ice, compression and elevation are initiated. Once swelling and pain have subsided and protected weight bearing has been initiated, physical therapy should be started. While conventional wisdom would suggest that a course of nonoperative management should be attempted prior to progressing to surgical repair, only one series exists examining the effect of functional rehabilitation on chronic instability. In the series, half of all patients benefited from a structured rehabilitation program. Those with functional instability tended to have greater results with nonoperative treatment modalities (40).

Peroneal strengthening and proprioceptive training are initiated in two consecutive phases. Initially, a functional phase is utilized. All exercises and activities should be pain-free. Multidirectional and weight-bearing exercises about the ankle are initiated, focusing on taking the ankle through a full range of normal motion. After the functional phase is completed, patients undergo a prophylactic phase in which strengthening of the muscle groups around the ankle is implemented. The activities place an emphasis on performing exercises that place the ankle in plantarflexion and inversion with a gradual increase in the stresses experienced across the joint and an increase in the demand imposed on it (6,41).

While various external bracing methods exist, none address the underlying pathology that contributes to chronic instability. Nevertheless, there may be a role for ankle bracing during the prophylactic phase of rehabilitation, as functional demands are increased on the ankle (42). Taping and a variety of braces exist for ankle instability. While taping seems to confer more stability to the ankle joint, braces have been proven effective in preventing, decreasing, or slowing the motions considered "at risk" for causing lateral ankle injuries (42,43). The advantage of bracing is that unlike taping, it can be removable and reusable and are easily adjusted when support becomes compromised (43).

SURGICAL MANAGEMENT

The primary indication for surgical intervention for lateral ankle instability is the failure of a nonoperative treatment course. An adequate rehabilitation course is generally felt to be 2 to 3 months of treatment—*not* of symptoms alone. If patients present with 6 months of symptoms without an adequate trial of supervised conservative treatment (which is not uncommon), that patient still requires an attempt to succeed with nonoperative care. If a patient fails to have symptomatic relief or has recurrent symptoms, they may be candidates for a surgical intervention (44). While a multitude of surgical interventions have been described, all can either be categorized as either an anatomic repair, or tenodesis stabilization (Table 11.2).

TABLE 11.2 Surgical Techniques for Chronic Instability

Anatomic repair	Tenodesis stabilization
Brostrom repair (45)	Watson-Jones (46)
Modified Brostrom repair (47)	Evans (48)
	Chrisman—Snook (49)

Anatomic Repair

The goal of anatomic repair is to restore the normal anatomy and joint mechanics while maintaining physiologic motion at the ankle and subtalar joints.

The modified Brostrom repair is the cornerstone for anatomic repair techniques. Originally described by Brostrom as a midsubstance imbrication and suturing of the ruptured ligaments (45), Gould et al. offered a modification of the Brostrom repair with a mobilized portion of the lateral extensor retinaculum (47). After imbrication of the ATFL and CFL, the mobilized retinaculum is attached to the fibula (47). It is important to note that the ATFL and CFL are more often scarred, stretched out and attenuated rather than disrupted (50). The recommendation is to shorten the ligaments amputating the pathologic tissue and then reattaching them at their anatomic origins through drill holes (see Fig. 11.2).

Tenodesis Stabilization

The goal of tenodesis is to restrict pathologic ankle motion but ignores the injured lateral ankle ligaments. As a result, biomechanics of the ankle and hindfoot are altered. Watson-Jones first described a nonanatomic stabilization procedure in 1952. He weaved the peroneus brevis tendon through the calcaneus and the talus (46). Evans simplified this procedure passing the distally attached peroneus brevis through an oblique posterior-superior drill hole in the distal fibula. Rather than replicating the ATFL or CFL, the pathway taken by the peroneus brevis is midway between the normal course of the two (48). Chrisman and Snook attempted to more closely replicate the path of the ATFL and CFL. It incorporates a split peroneus brevis tendon thus maintaining some peroneus brevis function (49).

While tendon transfers are anatomically convenient, they sacrifice an important dynamic stabilizer of the ankle in the process of attempted stabilization. In an effort to avoid taking valuable functional stabilizers, autograft and allograft reconstructions have become more popular. The authors' preferred method for reconstruction of chronic instability in the setting of a large body habitus, or excessive functional demands, is a hamstring autograft reconstruction (Fig. 11.2). The patient is positioned laterally and the doubled over tendon graft is secured both in the talus and the calcaneus with an absorbable tenodesis and interference screw respectively. This technique has the benefit of low morbidity, anatomic reconstruction, and avoids any compromise to the surrounding musculotendinous envelope of the ankle. It is supplemented with a modified Brostrom procedure (Fig. 11.3).

Arthroscopy

Chronic ankle instability is associated with several intra-articular conditions. Osteochondral lesions of the talus, impingement, loose bodies, adhesions, chondromalacia, and osteophytes have all been described in association with chronic ankle instability. Addressing these pathologies at the time of surgery is vital in maximizing the patient's recovery. In addition, the role of arthroscopy is expanding. The authors prefer to arthroscope the ankle at the time of ligament reconstruction when there is

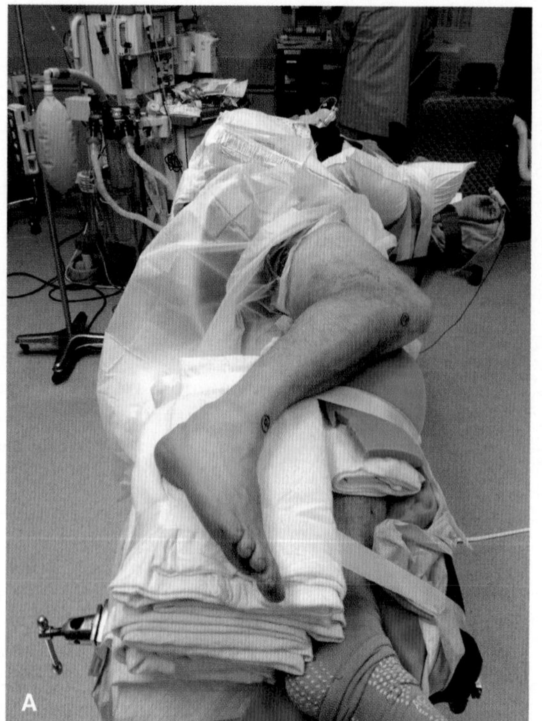

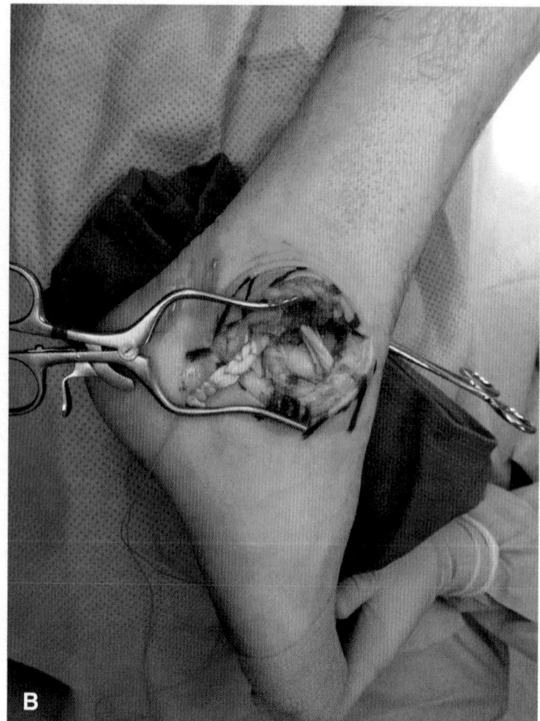

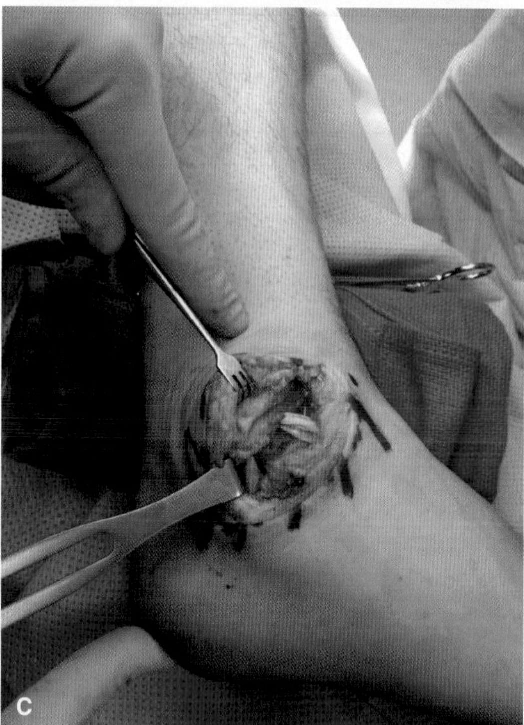

Figure 11.2. Hamstring autograft procedure. **A:** The patient is positioned in the lateral position with a large bolster supporting the ankle. **B:** The hamstring autograft is docked in the talus with a tenodesis screw and brought through drill holes in the fibula. **C:** It is then secured under tension into the calcaneus deep to the overlying peroneal tendons (retracted in this photograph).

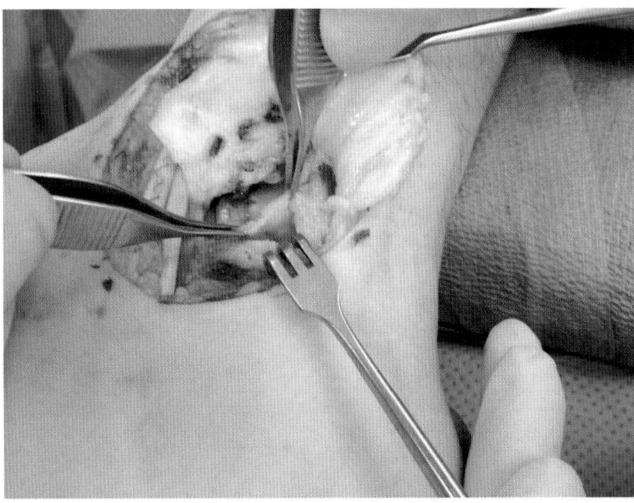

Figure 11.3. Modified Brostrom ligament reconstruction. Three drill holes have been made in the anterolateral fibula for reattachment of the ATFL being held by the forceps. Repaired split tear in the peroneus longus can be seen posterior to the fibula.

unexplained pain, or intra-articular abnormalities have been identified preoperatively with MRI. Preoperatively, pain which can be addressed with arthroscopy should be relieved with an intra-articular injection of anesthetic. If the pain is not relieved, even temporarily with an injection, the surgeon should be wary that there is an additional source of pain that may not be adequately dealt with at the time of surgery.

While no results have been reported to date, arthroscopically assisted repair of both the ATFL and CFL has recently been described and the technique continues to evolve (51).

In summary, lateral ankle sprains are a common orthopedic injury well recognized by all who care for the musculoskeletally injured patient. Unfortunately, once a patient has had a sprain of the lateral ligament complex, many experience further recurrences, residual pain, and the feeling of giving way. Chronic ankle instability is the result of both mechanical and functional factors that contributes to the symptomatology experienced by patients and requires attention to a complex nuance of findings. Conservative management of instability should be initiated and 2 to 3 months of a functional rehabilitation program should be completed before considering operative intervention. Half of these patients will typically have relief of their symptoms with rehabilitation. For those patients who fail conservative management, surgery is an option with good long-term results provided that concomitant diagnoses are recognized and addressed.

REFERENCES

1. Ferran NA, Maffulli N. Epidemiology of sprains of the lateral ankle ligament complex. *Foot Ankle Clin* 2006;11(3):659–662.
2. Garrick JG. The frequency of injury, mechanism of injury, and epidemiology of ankle sprains. *Am J Sports Med* 1977;5(6):241–242.
3. Cameron KL, Owens BD, DeBerardino TM. Incidence of ankle sprains among active-duty members of the United States Armed Services from 1998 through 2006. *J Athl Train* 2010;45(1):29–38.
4. Waterman BR, Belmont PJ Jr, Cameron KL, et al. Epidemiology of ankle sprain at the United States Military Academy. *Am J Sports Med* 2010;38(4):797–803.
5. Anandacoomarasamy A, Barnsley L. Long term outcomes of inversion ankle injuries. *Br J Sports Med* 2005:39;e14.
6. Smith RW, Reischl SF. Treatment of ankle sprains in young athletes. *Am J Sports Med* 1986;14(6):465–471.
7. Bahr R, Pena F, Shine J, et al. Ligament force and joint motion in the intact ankle: a cadaveric study. *Knee Surg Sports Traumatol Arthrosc* 1998;6(2):115–121.
8. Kjaersgaard-Andersen P, Wethelund JO, Helmig P, et al. The stabilizing effect of the ligamentous structures in the sinus and canalis tarsi on movements in the hindfoot. An experimental study. *Am J Sports Med* 1988;16(5):512–516.
9. Burks RT, Morgan J. Anatomy of the lateral ankle ligaments. *Am J Sports Med* 1994;22(1):72–77.
10. Renstrom P, Wertz M, Incavo S, et al. Strain in the lateral ligaments of the ankle. *Foot Ankle* 1988;9(2):59–63.
11. Hertel J. Functional anatomy, pathomechanics, and pathophysiology of lateral ankle instability. *J Athl Train* 2002;37(4):364–375.
12. Chorley JN, Hergenroeder AC. Management of ankle sprains. *Pediatr Ann* 1997;26(1): 56–64.
13. Malliaropoulos N, Papacostas E, Papalada A, et al. Acute lateral ankle sprains in track and field athletes: an expanded classification. *Foot Ankle Clin* 2006;11(3):497–507.
14. DiGiovanni B, Fraga CJ, Cohen BE, et al. Associated injuries found in chronic lateral ankle instability. *Foot Ankle Int* 2000;21(10):809–815.
15. Scranton PE Jr, McDermott JE, Rogers JV. The relationship between chronic ankle instability and variations in mortise anatomy and impingement spurs. *Foot Ankle Int* 2000;21(8):657–664.
16. Docherty CL, Moore JH, Arnold BL. Effects of strength training on strength development and joint position sense in functionally unstable ankles. *J Athl Train* 1998;33(4): 310–314.
17. Glencross D, Thornton E. Position sense following joint injury. *J Sports Med Phys Fitness* 1981;21(1):23–27.
18. Konradsen L, Magnusson P. Increased inversion angle replication error in functional ankle instability. *Knee Surg Sports Traumatol Arthrosc* 2000;8(4):246–251.
19. Forkin DM, Koczur C, Battle R, et al. Evaluation of kinesthetic deficits indicative of balance control in gymnasts with unilateral chronic ankle sprains. *J Orthop Sports Phys Ther* 1996;23(4):245–250.
20. Garn SN, Newton RA. Kinesthetic awareness in subjects with multiple ankle sprains. *Phys Ther* 1988;68(11):1667–1671.
21. Lentell G, Baas B, Lopez D, et al. The contributions of proprioceptive deficits, muscle function, and anatomic laxity to functional instability of the ankle. *J Orthop Sports Phys Ther* 1995;21(4):206–215.
22. Isakov E, Mizrahi J, Solzi P, et al. Response of the peroneal muscles to sudden inversion of the ankle during standing. *Int J Sport Biomech* 1986;2:100–109.
23. Bullock-Saxton JE, Janda V, Bullock MI. The influence of ankle sprain injury on muscle activation during hip extension. *Int J Sports Med* 1994;15(6):330–334.
24. Freeman MA. Instability of the foot after injuries to the lateral ligament of the ankle. *J Bone Joint Surg Br* 1965;47(4):669–677.
25. Freeman MA, Dean MR, Hanham IW. The etiology and prevention of functional instability of the foot. *J Bone Joint Surg Br* 1965;47(4):678–685.
26. Lentell G, Katzman LL, Walters MR. The relationship between muscle function and ankle stability. *J Orthop Sports Phys Ther* 1990;11(12):605–611.
27. Pintsaar A, Brynhildsen J, Tropp H. Postural corrections after standardised perturbations of single limb stance: effect of training and orthotic devices in patients with ankle instability. *Br J Sports Med* 1996;30(2):151–155.
28. Bush K. Predicting ankle sprain. *J Manual Manip Ther* 1996;4(2):54–58.
29. Hartsell HD, Spaulding SJ. Eccentric/concentric ratios at selected velocities for the invertor and evertor muscles of the chronically unstable ankle. *Br J Sports Med* 1999;33(4): 255–258.
30. Tropp H. Pronator muscle weakness in functional instability of the ankle joint. *Int J Sports Med* 1986;7(5):291–294.
31. Beynnon BD, Vacek PM, Murphy D, et al. First-time inversion ankle ligament trauma: the effects of sex, level of competition, and sport on the incidence of injury. *Am J Sports Med* 2005;33(10):1485–1491.
32. van Dijk CN, Mol BW, Lim LS, et al. Diagnosis of ligament rupture of the ankle joint. Physical examination, arthrography, stress radiography and sonography compared in 160 patients after inversion trauma. *Acta Orthop Scand* 1996;67(6):566–570.
33. Bahr R, Pena F, Shine J, et al. Mechanics of the anterior drawer and talar tilt tests. A cadaveric study of lateral ligament injuries of the ankle. *Acta Orthop Scand* 1997;68(5): 435–441.
34. Molloy S, Solan MC, Bendall SP. Synovial impingement in the ankle. A new physical sign. *J Bone Joint Surg Br* 2003;85(3):330–333.
35. McKeon PO, Hertel J. Systematic review of postural control and lateral ankle instability, part I: can deficits be detected with instrumented testing. *J Athl Train* 2008;43(3): 293–304.
36. Frost SC, Amendola A. Is stress radiography necessary in the diagnosis of acute or chronic ankle instability? *Clin J Sport Med* 1999;9(1):40–45.
37. Karlsson J, Lansinger O, Faxen E. [Lateral instability of the ankle joint (2). Active training programs can prevent surgery]. *Lakartidningen* 1991;88(15):1404–1407.
38. Campbell DG, Menz A, Isaacs J. Dynamic ankle ultrasonography. A new imaging technique for acute ankle ligament injuries. *Am J Sports Med* 1994;22(6):855–858.
39. Chandnani VP, Harper MT, Ficke JR, et al. Chronic ankle instability: evaluation with MR arthrography, MR imaging, and stress radiography. *Radiol* 1994;192(1):189–194.
40. Karlsson J, Lansinger O. [Lateral instability of the ankle joint (1). Non-surgical treatment is the first choice-20 per cent may need ligament surgery]. *Lakartidningen* 1991; 88(15):1399–1402.
41. Drez D Jr, Young JC, Waldman D, et al. Nonoperative treatment of double lateral ligament tears of the ankle. *Am J Sports Med* 1982;10(4):197–200.

42. Shapiro MS, Kabo JM, Mitchell PW, et al. Ankle sprain prophylaxis: an analysis of the stabilizing effects of braces and tape. *Am J Sports Med* 1994;22(1):78–82.
43. Ajis A, Maffulli N. Conservative management of chronic ankle instability. *Foot Ankle Clin* 2006;11(3):531–537.
44. Trevino SG, Davis P, Hecht PJ. Management of acute and chronic lateral ligament injuries of the ankle. *Orthop Clin North Am* 1994;25(1):1–16.
45. Brostrom L. Sprained ankles. VI. Surgical treatment of "chronic" ligament ruptures. *Acta Chir Scand* 1966;132(5):551–565.
46. Watson-Jones R. Recurrent forward dislocation of the ankle joint. *J Bone Joint Surg Br* 1952;34(3):519.
47. Gould N, Seligson D, Gassman J. Early and late repair of lateral ligament of the ankle. *Foot Ankle* 1980;1(2):84–89.
48. Evans DL. Recurrent instability of the ankle; a method of surgical treatment. *Proc R Soc Med* 1953;46(5):343–344.
49. Chrisman OD, Snook GA. Reconstruction of lateral ligament tears of the ankle. An experimental study and clinical evaluation of seven patients treated by a new modification of the Elmslie procedure. *J Bone Joint Surg Am* 1969;51(5):904–912.
50. Karlsson J, Bergsten T, Lansinger O, et al. Reconstruction of the lateral ligaments of the ankle for chronic lateral instability. *J Bone Joint Surg Am* 1988;70(4):581–588.
51. Maffulli N, Ferran NA. Management of acute and chronic ankle instability. *J Am Acad Orthop Surg* 2008;16(10):608–615.

CHAPTER

12

Kaj TA. Lambers
Anne H. Johnson

Ankle Impingement

ANTERIOR ANKLE IMPINGEMENT

The anterior ankle impingement syndrome is a common cause of chronic ankle pain, especially seen in athletes. Morris was the first to describe this condition in 1943, naming it the "athlete's ankle". Later, in 1950, McMurray renamed it the "footballer's ankle" (1,2). Since then, more cases of this condition have been described and although it is classically associated with soccer players (1), anterior ankle impingement can be found in numerous other sports and is also found in many nonathletes. Symptoms accompanying this syndrome are painful restriction of movement caused by hypertrophied soft tissue or bony spurs within the anterior ankle joint. Differentiation, therefore, is now made between soft tissue impingement and osseous impingement. An anatomical differentiation can also be made, as many describe impingement as either anterior, anteromedial or anterolateral. Clinical findings and etiologic factors often overlap and the authors think it is more useful to discuss differences in etiologic existence rather than anatomical localization. Therefore, we will indicate anterior ankle impingement from now on as either osseous or soft tissue.

ETIOLOGY/ANATOMY

Traditionally, anterior ankle impingement is associated with osseous changes. The first cases in the literature described athletes who complained of increasing pain in their anterior ankle due to extensive bony outgrowths. More recently, ankle impingement is simply defined as entrapment of an anatomic structure; in addition to osseous impingement, soft tissue impingement is now also widely described (3–6). The entrapment itself leads to the specific symptoms belonging to this syndrome, namely pain, decreased dorsiflexion, and sometimes swelling after activity (4).

Where osseous spurs are more common in the anterior and anteromedial parts of the ankle (7), soft tissue impingement most often occurs in the anterolateral ankle, especially in the anterolateral recess (8–10).

Osseous Impingement

In up to 60% of professional soccer players, the presence of tibial and talar spurs have been reported (11). The bony protuberances do not always yield symptoms but do form a significant component in the pathology of anterior ankle impingement and are often used to confirm the diagnosis (7,12,13). Bony spurs that form along the anterior aspect of the tibia and opposing talus can often be seen on a simple lateral x-ray (8,12). Different hypotheses about the origin of these bony spurs exist. McMurray first described the mechanism of bone spur formation. He attributed the development of spurs to repeated capsular and ligamentous traction during plantarflexion (1). According to his hypothesis, the outgrowths, or enthesophytes, are located precisely at the site of capsular attachment. More recent literature, however, shows outgrowths at the site of this attachment on the lateral site of the talus (14). Others show no relationship to the anterior ankle joint capsule at all (15). The spurs are considered to develop within the joint capsule, at the margin of the articular cartilage rim, through a process called osteophytosis, the formation of osteophytes (16,17). Chronic damage of the cartilage rim results in cartilage proliferation, scar tissue formation, and eventually the formation of these osteophytes. Damage of the cartilage rim may be due to different types of injuries. For instance, in most supination traumas, damage to the cartilage rim is known to occur during the impact of the tibia and talus at the time of injury; this may lead to proliferation of osteophytes, especially if the injury is recurrent (16,18). Forced dorsiflexion and repeated direct microtrauma are also causes of damage to the cartilage rim (3,13,19).

The bony spurs also have a relatively consistent pattern of formation. The talar spur is mostly present medial to the midline while the tibial spurs typically occur more lateral to the midline. The spurs typically do not overlap each other (20).

The pain accompanying osseous impingement, however, is thought not to be secondary to the bony spur itself, but rather due to the soft tissue impingement that occurs between the bony spurs (13,15). This soft tissue component gets compressed between the anterior distal tibia and the talus during dorsiflexion, described as the nutcracker effect (3). As a result, this may lead to hypertrophy of the synovial layer, subsynovial fibrotic tissue formation, and infiltration of inflammatory cells (12,21).

The presence of anteromedial bone spurs have also been reported, although medial impingement is a more uncommon cause of chronic ankle pain. The spurs originate in the anteromedial recess, located anterior to the medial malleolus and medial to the anteromedial margin of the talar dome, body, and neck. Superficially, this recess is bounded by the anteromedial ankle capsule (22). Chronic instability leads to recurrent inversion trauma and is therefore correlated with anteromedial spur development. The inversion traumas will weaken the cartilage on the medial side causing degenerative changes, the formation of scar tissue, and eventually osteophyte formation (17,23,24).

Soft Tissue Impingement

Soft tissue impingement occurs as a result from scarring and fibrosis, associated with synovial, capsular or ligamentous injury (7,9). The injured soft tissue hypertrophies, and becomes entrapped most commonly in the anterolateral recess.

Anatomically, the anterolateral recess of the ankle is bounded posteriorly by the anterolateral tibia and the anteromedial fibula, the anterior boundary is formed by the joint capsule, which is reinforced by the anterior tibiofibular, anterior talofibular, and calcaneofibular ligaments (7,8,21,25). It is thought that relatively minor injury can cause anterolateral impingement. Either a single inversion injury or repetitive plantarflexion and inversion (21,26) can result in tearing of the anterolateral ankle ligaments or joint capsule without clinically significant mechanical instability (5,21). Initially, this may not cause any symptoms, but because of the subsequent functional instability and the associated repeated microtrauma, this may lead to intra-articular and soft tissue hemorrhage, hypertrophy and synovial scarring. Compression of this abnormal soft tissue during dorsiflexion or eversion is the cause of anterolateral impingement.

Bony spurs or additional hypertrophy of the inferior portion of the anterior tibiofibular ligament are also considered contributors to anterolateral impingement, but these are rarely predominant factors (21,25,27).

CLINICAL FEATURES

Ankle impingement is usually diagnosed clinically. The typical patients are young athletes, particularly soccer players and ballet dancers, presenting with chronic anterior ankle pain that is activity related (19,27–29). The pain described is vague, mainly exacerbated during exercise but can often occur in activities of daily living. Pain is often accompanied by swelling and limited dorsiflexion (4), symptoms that can be confirmed at physical examination (Fig. 12.1). There will be recognizable local tenderness to palpation anteriorly and bony spurs along the anterior tibia and dorsal talus may be palpable with the ankle in slight plantarflexion (8,18). It is important to differentiate where the pain is located anteriorly in order to diagnose which type of impingement is present. While the central anterior area between the tibialis anterior muscle and the extensor digitorum longus muscle may be difficult to assess by palpation due to the covering tendons and neurovascular structures (12), the anteromedial and anterolateral aspects of the ankle have less soft tissue covering and the joint is easier to palpate. If the pain is predominantly present during anteromedial palpation, the impingement is present more medially. If the pain is located more anterolaterally, the impingement will be present more anterolaterally. Lateral impingement also gives local tenderness at the site of the anterolateral recess. Forced dorsiflexion can provoke the pain but is often not positive (12).

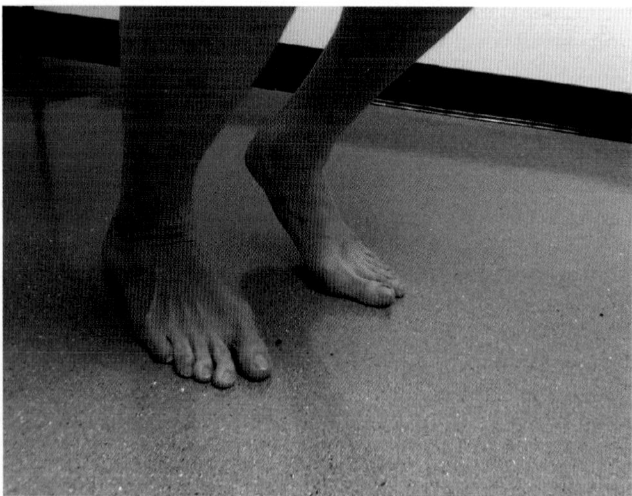

Figure 12.1. Clinical image of a 25-year-old soccer player with significantly restricted dorsiflexion in his left ankle compared with his right side.

A helpful tool in the diagnosis of synovial (soft tissue) impingement is described by Molloy et al. (30). First, the examiner manually dorsiflexes the ankle in a standard way. Then he or she passively dorsiflexes the ankle while applying pressure with the thumb over the lateral gutter. If the hypertrophic synovium resides in the ankle, it will be forced into the joint by the examiner's thumb and will impinge between the neck of the talus and the distal tibia in full dorsiflexion. If the second maneuver intensifies the pain, it is a positive impingement sign. This test was found to have a sensitivity of 94.8% and a specificity of 88% in a study involving 73 patients.

IMAGING

Standard ankle radiographs, consisting of lateral and anteroposterior views, are often the only imaging necessary to assess and diagnose osseous ankle impingement (31). The detection of spurs correlates with the outcome of surgery, and is therefore important for preoperative planning since classification of spur formation (5,16,32). These radiographs better delineate the size and location of the spurs and also give information about the tibiotalar joint space, and whether joint degeneration exists (16,17,33). The signs of osseous impingement on these radiographs vary and are often directly related to the duration of the symptoms. Slight periosteal roughening is seen in the early stages on the anterior aspect of the lower end of the tibia. Later on, a bony ridge may be seen extending forward from the surface of the tibia with an occasionally similar bony outgrowth projecting upward and slightly backward from the neck of the talus (1,12,34) (Fig. 12.2).

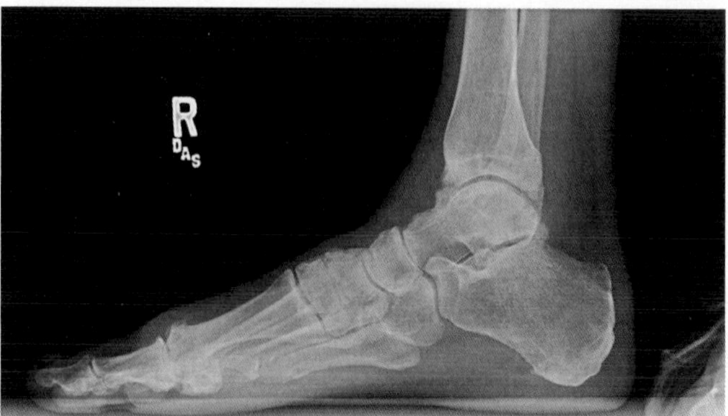

Figure 12.2. Lateral ankle weight-bearing radiograph demonstrates anterior bony impingement.

Anteromedial spurs are more difficult to detect on a lateral ankle radiograph because of the anterotibial notch. The anteromedial tibial spurs remain undetected because of superposition or over-projection of the more prominent anterolateral border of the distal tibia. Similarly, anteromedial talar spurs remain undetected because of superposition or overprojection of the lateral part of the talar neck and body (35). In these cases, an oblique radiograph as described by Tol et al. can be useful (Fig. 12.1) (35,36). The use of this additional anteromedial impingement view in combination with a standard lateral view increased the sensitivity (from 0.40 to 0.85 for tibial osteophytes, and from 0.32 to 0.73 for talar osteophytes), but specificity however simultaneously decreased (from 0.70 to 0.45 for tibial osteophytes, and from 0.82 to 0.68 for talar osteophytes) (36).

With soft tissue impingement, radiographs show no specific abnormalities but they can be useful in excluding coexisting osseous abnormalities, such as a fracture, osteochondral lesion of the talus or associated anterior tibial spurs (9). To demonstrate soft tissue impingement, other imaging studies are required.

MR imaging for soft tissue impingement can be useful but is also still controversial. In different studies about the assessment of soft tissue abnormality, sensitivity ranged from 39% to 100%, and specificity ranged from 50% to 100% (37–39). It is also stated that MR imaging is only accurate when a significant joint effusion is present (39). MR imaging findings that can be seen at lateral soft tissue impingement are fullness in the anterolateral recess, a focal mass within the recess demonstrating intensity on T1- and T2-weighted sequences and replacement of the normal fat signal within the anterolateral recess by scar tissue or edema (9) (Fig. 12.3).

Direct MR arthrography is highly successful in demonstrating the presence of anterolateral impingement. A sensitivity of 96% and specificity of 100% was found with an accuracy of 100% when clinical signs of anterolateral impingement are present (40). For instance, a very specific but insensitive finding is the absence of a normal fluid-filled recess between the anterolateral soft tissues and anterior surface of the fibula. Adhesions and scar tissue may be present that impair the entrance of fluid into the normal recess. However, these findings should be clinically correlated since abnormal soft tissue scarring, with or without synovitis, are also seen in asymptomatic patients (31,40,41). With articular distension, diagnosis of syndesmotic impingement will be more precise. Often-observed changes in syndesmotic impingement are fibrosis and focal synovitis surrounding the anteroinferior tibiotalar ligament (42,43). MR arthrography of the more uncommon anteromedial impingement may reveal medial meniscoid lesions, capsular abnormalities and synovial soft-tissue thickening anterior to the tibiotalar ligaments as well as any associated osseous abnormality (31,41,44,45). With osseous impingement, MR arthrography is not necessary, as conventional radiography imaging is sufficient. It may be utilized to assess cartilage damage, demonstrate loose bodies and detect capsular thickening and synovitis in the anterior capsular recess (31,44).

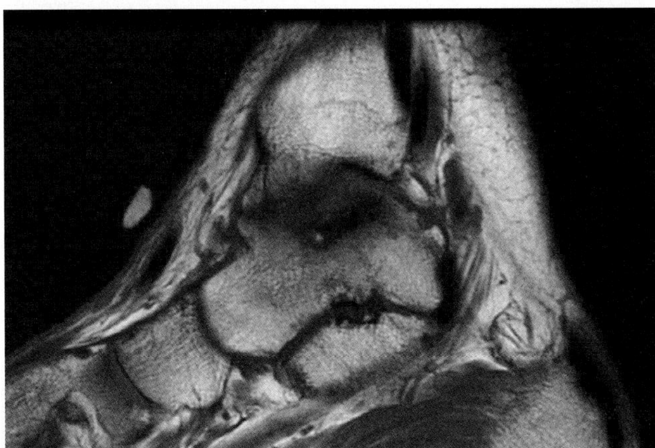

Figure 12.3. MRI T2-weighted image demonstrating anterior bony impingement with surrounding edema, effusion, and synovitis.

Recently, the use of ultrasound assessment in patients with clinical anterolateral soft tissue impingement has shown to be a useful tool in identifying synovitic lesions within the anterolateral recess. In one study by McCarthy et al., a synovitic mass was identified in 100% of all the eight patients with anterolateral ankle impingement. Similar findings, however, were found in two of the control groups without any accompanying symptoms (22%). Ultrasound imaging was also able to demonstrate any associated ligamentous injuries and differentiate between soft tissue and osseous impingement (46).

Findings were not dependent on the presence of an ankle joint effusion, this is in contrast to MR imaging (39).

TREATMENT

Initially, non-operative treatment, consisting of activity modification, intra-articular injections and non-steroidal anti-inflammatory medication can offer short-term, or in some cases, permanent relief of symptoms. Injections are more effective in soft tissue impingement as the steroid can decrease the inflammation in the synovium and capsule. A small heel lift, usually about 3/8 inch or less, can offload the front of the ankle and reduce symptoms of both bony and soft tissue impingement (4,47). However, once the lift is discontinued, the pain often returns. In addition, using a heel lift can exacerbate issues in other joints and may not be well tolerated (48).

Surgery is indicated when symptoms persist despite conservative treatment. Depending on the patient's goals, surgical intervention is indicated. Recovery goals may vary, and the risks and benefits of surgery must be weighed in each individual case. Resection of bony spurs and soft tissue abnormalities within the joint have demonstrated good to excellent results. Resection may be performed by classical open arthrotomy or the now widely used arthroscopy.

Open arthrotomy of osseous ankle impingement was initially described by Mcmurray in 1950 (1). He described three cases of professional soccer players who, returned to full sport, are being treated successfully by open removal of anterior bony spurs. After that, more cases of open arthrotomy are reported, all showing good results (28,49–51). Currently, minimally invasive arthroscopic debridement is the preferred way of treatment, and studies have shown that it can be highly successful (13,17,33). If the spurs are quite large, or loose bodies are encountered, often a small arthrotomy may also be needed for full debridement, however.

SURGICAL TECHNIQUE

1. Anesthesia should include either general, spinal, or spinal-epidural, with or without a lower extremity block for postoperative pain relief.

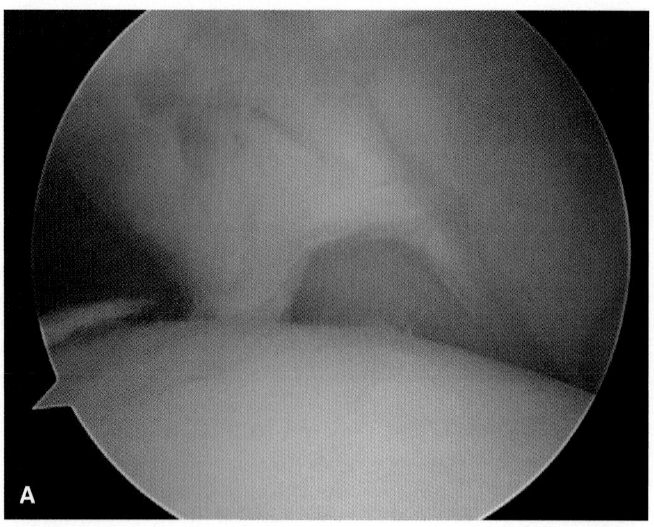

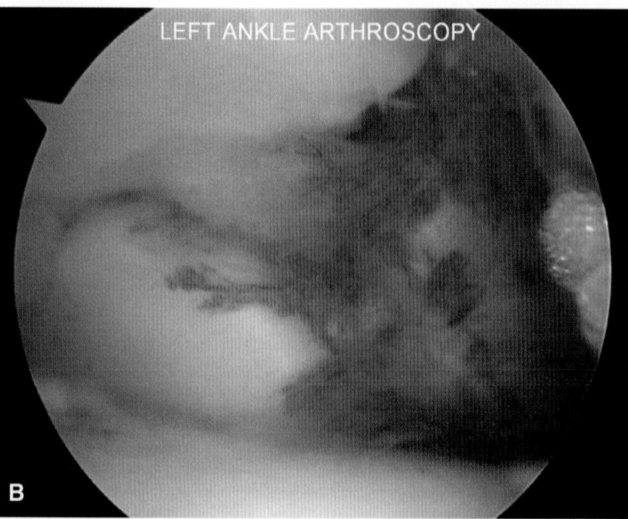

Figure 12.4. **A:** Arthroscopic image of anteromedial soft tissue impingement lesion, capsular thickening. **B:** Arthroscopic image of anterior soft tissue impingement, synovitis.

2. The patient is placed in supine position with a roll underneath the ipsilateral hip to maintain the ankle in neutral rotation.
3. The ankle may be placed in gentle traction using an external ankle distractor device. The amount of traction needed will vary depending on the location and accessibility of the osseous spurs. Often distraction tightens the anterior joint capsule, making it more difficult to identify and debride osteophytes.
4. Standard anteromedial and anterolateral ports should be established for both osseous and soft tissue impingement. Additional portals, anterior to the tip of the medial or lateral malleolus portal, are occasionally necessary.
5. A 2.7 mm, 30 degree arthroscope is used. After the rest of the joint is inspected, attention is turned to the anterior aspect of the joint.
6. To address anterior osteophytes, a 2.9 or 3.5 burr device is utilized. Spurs can be easily identified when the ankle is in a slightly or even fully dorsiflexed position. This gives the additional advantage that the weight-bearing cartilage of the talus is concealed in the joint and protected from any iatrogenic damage. Care must be taken to carefully contour the front of the ankle without resecting too much bone.
7. For resection of soft tissue as scar tissue, hypertrophic synovium, and any impinging distal fascicle of the antero-inferior tibiofibular ligament, a full-radius shaver 2.9 can be used. If the tissue is especially tenacious, a 3.5 shaver tip can be utilized for a speedier resection (Fig. 12.4A, B).
8. Resection of tissue is complete when there is complete removal of the impinging soft tissue at the tibiotalar joint as in the anteromedial and anterolateral recesses. All bony outgrowths should be removed until normal tibial and talus contours are replicated. The ankle should be placed in full dorsiflexion and assessed to be sure that no impingement lesions remain anteriorly (Fig. 12.5A, B).
9. Other joint pathology should be addressed, and then the joint should be carefully irrigated to ensure that no debris remains. The arthroscopic instruments are then removed, and the portals are closed with nylon sutures on the skin.

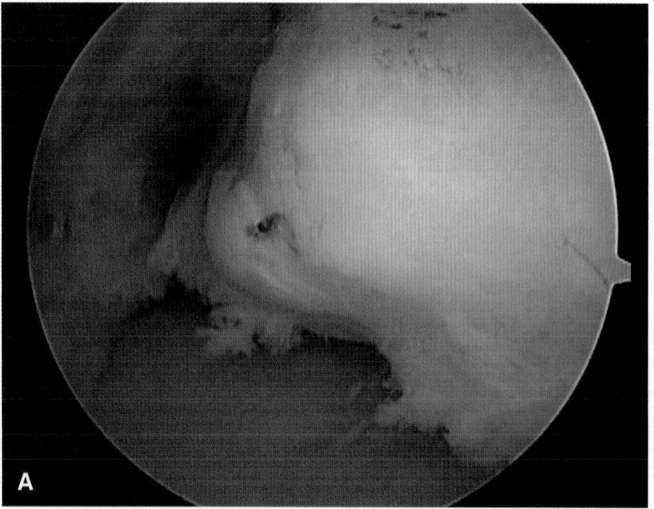

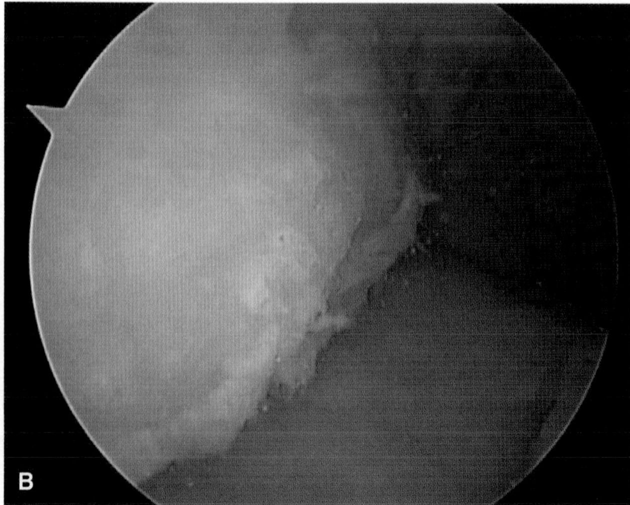

Figure 12.5. **A:** Arthroscopic image of anterior tibial osseous impingement lesion. **B:** Arthroscopic image of ankle in full dorsiflexion after anterior osseous spurs have been resected. No further anterior impingement is seen.

Postoperatively, a compressive bandage or AO splint is applied. The postoperative protocol depends on whether or not other procedures were performed on the ankle at the same time. For isolated treatment of anterior impingement, this author prefers immobilization for 1 week. Gentle, active range of motion exercises commence after 1 week, progressing with more aggressive motion and weight bearing as soon as the wounds are healed. Return to sport in these cases can be anticipated in 6 weeks (12,16,26,33,52).

RESULTS

McMurray already stated in 1950, that his open surgical treatment of ankle impingement proved to be successful (1). The three soccer players he reported on were all able to get back to professional level. Currently, arthroscopic debridement is the preferred method of treatment, and the good results have supported the technique. One of the first follow-up series after arthroscopy by Martin et al. described the outcome on 58 arthroscopic-treated ankles (53). Of that group, 26 were preoperatively diagnosed as synovitis, 17 with transchondral defects, 8 with degenerative joint disease and 7 with osteophytes or loose bodies. He showed good to excellent results in 64% overall, but the success rate for the degenerative joint disease was far lower. Only 12% showed good to excellent results and 43% resulted in a subsequent fusion.

Biedert showed good or very good results in about two-third of his 21 patients, but he also reported about different diagnoses. He did however come to the same conclusion as Martin et al. that degenerative changes mainly resulted in an unsatisfactory outcome (3). Specific reports about arthroscopic-treated soft tissue impingent of the ankle started about 20 years ago and mainly show a good outcome. One of the first studies by Martin et al. showed 75% of good to excellent results in their cohort of 16 patients (54). A series of 31 patients with soft tissue impingement described by Ferkel et al. showed 26 good to excellent results (84%) (5). One of the larger studies round that time, that of a large group of 60 athletes with chronic soft tissue impingement after a previous injury reviewed by DeBardino gave an almost perfect outcome with 58 patients showing good or excellent results at an average followup of 27 months (55). Other arthroscopic-treated soft tissue impingement studies in that period showed similar good results (56–60).

One report by Jerosch et al. demonstrated only 9 of the 35 treated athletes returned to their pre-injury level of athletics at an average followup of 32 months. This study may be considered an outlier as the majority of studies have shown much more positive results (61).

More recent articles about arthroscopic-treated soft tissue impingement continue to demonstrate satisfactory to perfect results. For example, mostly good to excellent results were found by Urguden et al. (90% of 41 patients), Hassan (91% of 23 patients), and Moustafa El-Sayed (85% of 20 patients) (52,62,63). They all reported similar factors and associated lesions that negatively affected the final outcome, including chondral lesions of the talus, syndesmotic lesions, and new inversion injuries afterward.

Ogilvie-Harris et al. was the first to report about isolated anterior osseous impingement. From a group of 17 treated patients, 15 (88%) reported substantial improvement at an average followup of 39 months. They excluded patients with obvious osteoarthritis.

A year later, Reynaert et al. showed good to excellent results in 12 (92%) of their 13 treated soccer players (64). Out of these 13 patients, 10 (77%) went back to their preoperative sports after a mean of 4 months. In a following study, Amendola et al. described a large group of arthroscopically treated ankles, of which 14 had anterior bony impingement (65). Another 15 were diagnosed with anterolateral soft tissue impingement. In both of these groups, 12 patients showed benefits from the treatment (86% and 80% respectively). He also showed that patients with associated osteoarthritis had poor results. A prospective study by van Dijk et al. described the outcome of 62 patients with anterior ankle impingement (16). In 52 patients a bony obstruction was present. Two years after surgical treatment, the overall rate of excellent or good results was 73%. However, they also made a comparison between patients without joint space narrowing and those with joint space narrowing. Excellent or good results were obtained with 90% of the patients without against 50% of the patients with joint space narrowing. There was a significant difference between those two groups. Also, the patients who had experienced pain for less than 2 years before surgery showed a better satisfaction rate than those with longer preoperative pain. Same was found for patients with more anteromedial-located bony spurs, they showed a better satisfaction rate than patients whose spurs were found anterolateral. In this study, patients who showed loose bodies, osteochondritis dissecans, or severe osteoarthritic changes with strong reduction of motion were excluded. A recent study by Bauer et al. does report about outcome on patients with anterior bony impingement with joint motion loss, and at a mean of 15 months, 10 out of the 13 patients were satisfied or very satisfied with the result (66). Anterior impingement symptoms had disappeared in 12 of the 13 patients and mean plantar and dorsiflexion improved significantly.

CONCLUSION

Anterior ankle impingement, secondary to inversion injuries, chronic instability, and overuse can cause debilitating pain in the athlete. Non-operative treatment including rest, activity modification, and selective injections may alleviate symptoms. Arthroscopic debridement of both soft tissue and osseous lesions in the ankle offers good to excellent results in the majority of cases, and typically allows athletes a chance to get back to their pre-injury level of activity. However, results decline when osteoarthritic changes are present already.

POSTERIOR ANKLE IMPINGEMENT

Posterior ankle impingement is characterized by provoked pain in the posterior aspect of the ankle during forced plantarflexion. This clinical syndrome, like anterior ankle impingement, is recognized in dancing, especially ballet, and numerous sports that emphasize plantarflexion at the ankle, such as gymnastics, football, soccer, cricket, and high jumping. Pain is often accompanied by restricted range of motion at the ankle. The consequences for professional dancers and athletes suffering from this syndrome may be significant as performance is impaired. Even for the recreational athlete, pain from posterior impingement may be severely limiting.

PATHOGENESIS

Etiology and Epidemiology

Distinguishing the etiology of posterior impingement is important, as different causes carry a different prognosis. Authors have found that symptoms that arise following overuse, as opposed to trauma, have a better prognosis (67). Impingement secondary to overuse is seen after forceful and repetitive plantarflexion. This motion is seen frequently in many sports, but has classically been described in ballet dancers by Hamilton and others (68–71). The typical ballet dancers load the ankle and foot during plantarflexion of the ankle frequently, especially in the *demi-pointe* and *en pointe* positions (72–74). In the *en pointe* position, the vertical alignment of the tibial and metatarsal shafts results in directing the full body weight onto the forefoot, and specifically the distal phalanx of the great toe. As for the *demi-pointe* position, the foot and ankle are aligned in a similar fashion except that the toes are hyperextended and the weight of the body is directed onto the heads of the metatarsals. Both of these positions bring the posterior edge of the distal tibia, posterior aspect of the talus, and superior surface of the calcaneus together, producing compression at the posterior aspect of the ankle joint (67,73,75) (Fig. 12.6).

As for other sports, the mechanism stays the same. When the sport involves repetitive ankle plantarflexion, posterior ankle impingement syndrome may arise. The forced plantarflexion imposes repetitive stress on the posterior aspect of the ankle (67,69). As joint mobility and range of motion gradually increase during the activity, the distance between the calcaneus and the posterior portion of the distal tibia decreases. Runners may develop complaints after exercising with forced plantarflexion, such as during downhill running. In horizontal-jump athletes, the repetitive, rapid, and high-force plantarflexion in the take-off phase often predisposes the athlete for posterior ankle impingement (76).

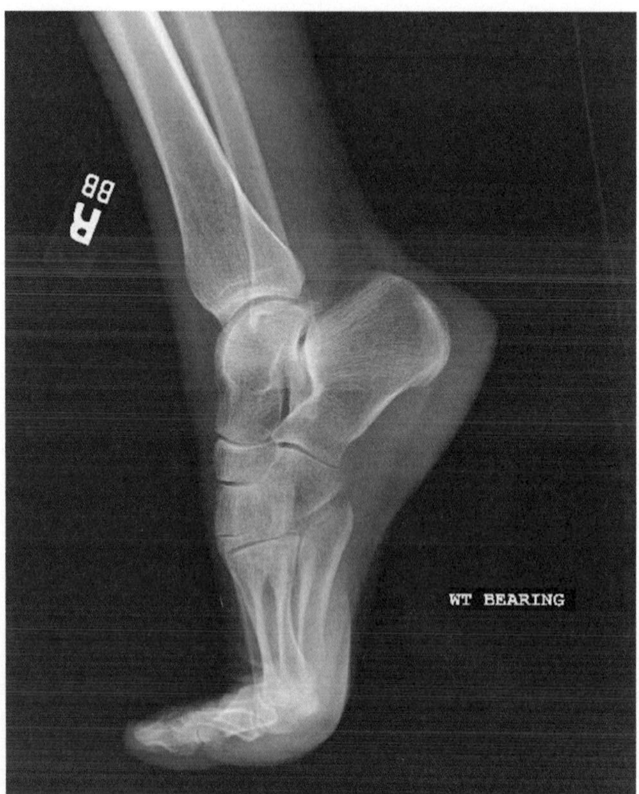

Figure 12.6. Lateral radiograph of a patient in the demi-pointe position. Note the proximity of the posterior bony structures at the ankle and the hindfoot.

Pathophysiology

The pathophysiology of posterior ankle impingement is essentially the same as with anterior impingement. There is entrapment of an anatomic structure that can be defined as either osseous impingement or soft tissue impingement. While impingement involving osseous structures is the most commonly seen, soft tissue impingement may be closely related. Often determining the etiology is challenging due to the anatomical location of the structures, and a diagnosis is often confirmed only after radiography or arthroscopy.

Osseous Impingement

In osseous impingement, individual ankle plays an important role. Several possible anatomic variations exist which can contribute to an osseous posterior impingement syndrome, including an os trigonum, a Stieda process, a prominent posterior calcaneal tuberosity and a downward-sloping tibia (77,78).

A Stieda process is an elongated extension of the lateral tubercle of the talus, an anatomic variation first identified by Stieda himself (79) (Fig. 12.7). It can cause considerable pain and a posterior block to plantarflexion when it comes into contact with posterior soft tissue structures or when it compresses against the posterior lip of the tibial plafond (70,73). During repetitive and/or forceful plantarflexion, recurrent small traumas result in chronic inflammation and disability (70). A Stieda process may be fractured by tibial compression only because of its position (73,77,80,81). An avulsion fracture of the process, a Shepherd fracture, may also occur due to the tension forces which are created by the fibers of the posterior talofibular ligament (73,80). Symptoms related to the Stieda process are similar to those of the os trigonum, and may be confused. Even with complex imaging techniques, it can be hard to differentiate between the two (8,77).

The os trigonum is a prominent lateral talar tubercle that remains disjoined and non-ossified from the rest of the talus

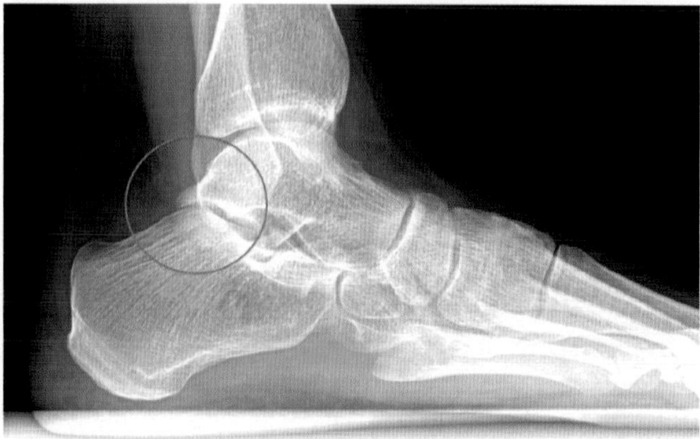

Figure 12.7. Lateral ankle radiograph demonstrating a Stieda process.

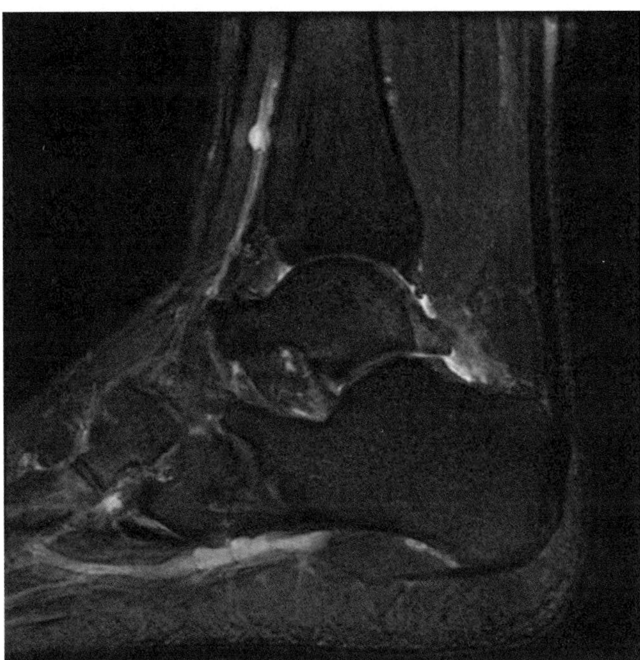

Figure 12.8. Lateral ankle radiograph demonstrating an os trigonum.

(5,82–84) (Fig. 12.8). While 7% of the population have an os trigonum, most clinicians agree that it is a separate bone, and see it as a remnant of ossification remaining posterior to the lateral talar tubercle at teen years (73). As with the Stieda process, the os trigonum creates the same problems with repeated plantarflexion, namely irritation of the surrounding soft tissue, resulting in chronic inflammation (70). The anatomic alignment of the foot with an ostrigonum may predispose the patient to symptoms (78). With pes planus, the everted hindfoot causes the talus to be anatomically plantarflexed and adducted, creating an additional force applied to the os trigonum during each plantarflexion. In pes cavus, the inverted hindfoot structure incurs additional impingement on the os trigonum as the supination of the talus forces the posterior surface of the tibia medially and inferiorly (78).

Other less common osseous prominences may exist that can create an impingement syndrome. A prominent posterior calcaneal tuberosity can cause problems during repetitive plantarflexion leading to inflammation of the surrounding soft tissue (70,78). In addition, a prominent downslope in posterior tibial articular surface may act like an additional ankle malleolus located posteriorly (70,77,85,86). In plantarflexion, it can contact the calcaneus or talus and entraps the posterior soft tissue. If an opposite process is present, such as an os trigonum, Stieda process or posterior calcaneal tuberosity, the posterior joint space decreases, and the patient is more susceptible to impingement. The mere presence of a prominent posterior talar process or os trigonum in and of itself, however, is not sufficient to produce the posterior impingement; anatomic predisposition combined with an additional traumatic event or repetitive and forced plantarflexion will create the setup for symptoms (87).

Soft Tissue Impingement

Soft tissue structures in both the posteromedial and posterolateral aspects of the ankle and hindfoot have the potential to become sources of impingement. Medially, the flexor hallucis longus tendon (FHL) and the deltoid ligament may be the offending structures, whereas laterally, the peroneal tendon, the posteroinferior tibiofibular ligament and the posterior talofibular ligament can become the source of pain (82,88). In addition, the intermalleolar ligament of the posterior ankle or the joint capsule can become involved. Traumatic inversion is often identified as the underlying cause for entrapment of the soft tissue structures posteriorly. Stenosing tenosynovitis of the FHL may develop, and the tissue inflammatory response may progress to a calcifying state (78). Repetitive plantarflexion and inversion will potentially entrap the tendon on a regular basis, which will reinforce the effect.

Another posteromedial impingement lesion is caused by a crush injury to the deep posterior fibers of the deltoid ligament, also secondary to a severe inversion injury (88). The ligamentous fibers are crushed between the medial malleolus and medial talar wall when heavy weight bearing is added to an already plantarflexed and internally rotated talus. This kind of lesion usually resolves spontaneously or with non-operative treatment. However, if inadequate healing of the contused structures occurs, chronic inflammation and hypertrophic fibrosis and metaplasia may develop (88). In this case, the fibers remain disorganized and impinge between the medial wall of the talus and the medial malleolus.

On the lateral side, similar to the FHL tendon, the peroneal tendons, sheath, or posterolateral ligaments can also impinge after traumatic or repetitive ankle plantarflexion and eversion. Injury and subsequent hypertrophy of these structures, just like with the medial structures, may result in the formation of accessory masses that create the impingement feeling at full plantarflexion (70,80,89). Repetitive plantarflexion combined with eversion can exacerbate pain and disability since the structures become further irritated and impinged between the posterior corner of the fibula and the talus (70).

DIAGNOSIS

Posterior ankle impingement is often more difficult to diagnose clinically than anterior impingement, as the offending structures are deeper within the ankle with more overlying soft tissue support structures. The typical patient with posterior ankle impingement complains of pain over the posterior aspect of the ankle that is provoked during sports, downhill walking or running, and descending stairs. There may be a history of an acute or remote ankle injury, or the pain began insidiously. Another complaint is limited and painful plantarflexion of the ankle, also mostly during sports activity.

Clinical Features

Determining the cause of posterior ankle pain may be challenging, and it is critical to be as specific as possible when palpating and examining each anatomic structure. Patients may exhibit tenderness or pain on palpation in the region of the posterior ankle joint and most posterior aspect of the subtalar joint. The posterior talar process can be best palpated posterolaterally between the peroneal tendons and the Achilles tendon (67). If the pain is located posteromedially, the overlying neurovascular bundle and flexor tendons covering the talus may be the offending structures, and symptoms in this area do not automatically imply impingement (76). Sometimes patients also experience pain during dorsiflexion as traction is applied to the posterior joint capsule and posterior talofibular ligament, both attaching to the posterior talar process (67).

With posteromedial impingement secondary to an os trigonum or Stieda process, symptoms are typically exacerbated with forceful plantarflexion. With the knee flexed at 90 degree (preferably in a relaxed prone position), a repetitive, quick passive hyper-plantarflexion movement should be performed. This test can be repeated with either slight internal rotation or external rotation of the foot and on the point of maximal plantarflexion, a rotational movement can be applied. A positive test should be followed by further investigation to the origin of the pain with the use of a local anesthetic (Xylocaine). In the office setting or under fluoroscopic guidance, the anesthetic should be injected from the posterolateral side, thereby infiltrating the capsule between the prominent posterior talar process and the posterior edge of the tibia. If the patients' symptoms are alleviated during the offending activity, the diagnosis posterior ankle impingement is confirmed.

Due to its anatomic position in the posterior ankle, the FHL is especially susceptible to injury secondary to overuse in activities that require excessive or repetitive plantarflexion. Involvement of the FHL tendon may be suspected if, in the previous described prone position with 90 degree flexion of the knee, resisted isometric plantarflexion of the first metatarsophalangeal joint results in posterior ankle pain. One of the most common pathologies of the FHL is stenosing tenosynovitis. This occurs at the tendon's fibro-osseous tunnel at the point where it passes the posterior aspect of the talus toward the medial ankle. Repeated pressure, such as during the *en pointe* position for dancers, causes irritation within this narrow channel. Hallux saltans occurs when a nodule may develop along the FHL tendon and/or its sheath may occur as well. Patients can experience a popping sensation during contraction and elongation as the nodule drags back and forth across through the tight tunnel and adjacent tissues. This can cause a pseudo–hallux rigidus at the MTP joint, termed hallux saltans.

Radiologic Features

Normal lateral radiographs of the ankle are usually insufficient in patients with posterior ankle impingement. It is sometimes possible to demonstrate a prominent os trigonum, Stieda process, other calcifications or, more rarely, a fracture or fragmentation of the process (9). Since a Stieda process or os trigonum is located posterolaterally, the medial talar tubercle is often overlying, leaving the abnormality undetectable. To prevent this superimposing effect, different projection types are used, either by holding the foot in plantarflexion or with the foot in 25 degree of external rotation (8,67,85). The anteroposterior ankle radiograph typically does not show abnormalities and is therefore not useful. Computed tomography (CT) can be very helpful in demonstrating the bony anatomy and fracture, as it can ascertain the extent of the injury and exact location of possible calcifications or bony fragments (68,90). However, CT is less usable for soft tissue impingement. Traditionally, bone scans were used to help rule in or out impingement, with a negative scan excluding a bony problem. If positive, however, the precise resolution of the bony abnormality is difficult and this technique is also relatively insensitive for soft tissue problems (7).

Conventional magnetic resonance imaging (MRI) with its multiplanar capabilities and soft tissue contrast typically overcomes the limitations of the other radiographic modalities (85). Active bony impingement typically presents with bone marrow edema, fracture line or disruption of the synchondrosis around an os trigonum, Stieda process, or posterior talus (7,77,90,91) (Fig. 12.9). Capsular abnormalities can also be assessed and the integrity of the ligaments can accurately be observed with MRI (77,92). Intravenous gadolinium given to athletes showed a potential highlight of small focal areas of synovitis around the posterior ligaments if edema is not a predominating feature (7). Furthermore, MRI provides an accurate anatomical assessment of all the surrounding structures which will aid surgical planning.

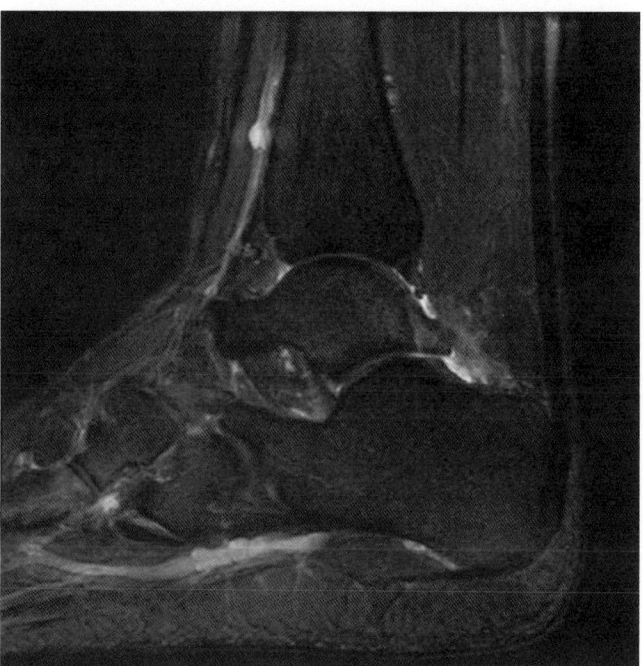

Figure 12.9. T2-weighted MRI image of symptomatic os trigonum, with local bony edema and an effusion.

Finally, in experienced hands, ultrasound is also a useful modality to detect impingement since the symptomatic area is usually focal and susceptive to visualization (7). After the lesion is identified, an ultrasound-guided injection of a local anesthetic and/or a very small amount of steroid can help solidify a diagnosis and provide patients with some symptomatic relief.

TREATMENT

Non-surgical Treatment

Conservative treatment of posterior ankle impingement such as rest, activity modification, and physiotherapy may give good results. Other therapy consists of intra-articular injections or injection into the os trigonum synchondrosis (image guided), steroidal and non-steroidal, can be very helpful. Ultrasound-guided injections into focal capsular thickening or the FHL or other tendon sheath can be used as a diagnostic tool and offer short-term relief of symptoms. For professional or other high-level athletes this is most useful to allow them to continue competition until the end of the season or, if necessary, until surgery may be performed.

Surgical Treatment

If non-surgical treatment fails or is insufficient, surgical intervention is advised. Traditional open excision or arthroscopic excision may be utilized depending on the surgeon's experience and the pathology present.

Open Excision

The outcome of open treatment of posterior ankle impingement is generally successful. The os trigonum may be accessed through either a medial or lateral approach, but if the FHL needs to be addressed, a medial approach should be utilized.

For the medial approach, the patient is positioned supine, and a thigh or high calf tourniquet used. The incision is made over the neurovascular bundle at the level of the superior border of the calcaneus. Since the bundle is quite superficial, care should be taken to incise through only the dermis first; the bundle is identified, then retracted posteriorly. The FHL tunnel can be identified by moving the great toe. Posteriorly, the entire fibro-osseous tunnel is released after which the FHL tendon can be inspected and any existing pathology can be addressed. Next, the FHL tendon is also retracted posteriorly together with the neurovascular bundle, and the os trigonum or Stieda process is excised. By placing the ankle in full plantarflexion, the posterior aspect of the ankle and subtalar joints may be inspected, and any additional osseous or soft tissue impingement excised. After the wound is closed, the ankle is splinted in neutral position.

For the lateral approach, the patient may be placed in a lateral decubitus position or with bump under the hip to provide the exposure for the lateral ankle. After the calf or thigh tourniquet is inflated, the incision is made just posterior to the peroneal tendons at the level of the posterior ankle. The sural nerve usually lies just posterior in the fatty tissue and should be avoided. Dissection proceeds through the fatty tissue to the posterior capsule. With the ankle in dorsiflexion, any osseous prominence is palpable and is excised. As a final inspection, the ankle is then ranged through neutral to full plantarflexion. Any remaining osseous and/or soft tissue impingement lesions are removed. After the wound is closed, the ankle is splinted in neutral position (93).

Arthroscopic Excision

Although open excision and debridement of posterior impingement lesions demonstrate good results in experienced hands, the arthroscopic approach has been shown to cause less morbidity and with a quicker return to previous activities and sports (94–98). Hindfoot arthroscopy was developed in the late 1990s when Bazaz and Ferkel reported on the results of arthroscopic plantar fascia release (99). Lombardi et al. published a new technique of arthroscopic excision of an os trigonum, also propagated and advanced by van Dijk (67,87,100,101).

The patient is positioned prone, and a tourniquet is not mandatory. The ankle is positioned slightly over the distal edge of the operating table allowing free ankle movement (Fig. 12.9). Posteromedial and posterolateral hindfoot portals provide good access to the posterior aspect of the ankle and subtalar joints. A 4.0 mm or 2.7 mm 30 degree arthroscope is used. The posterolateral portal has to be made at the level or slightly above the tip of the lateral malleolus lateral to the Achilles tendon. After a careful incision, the soft tissue is dissected with a small clamp and a blunt trocar is inserted. The arthroscope is introduced via the lateral portal aiming distally at the first intermetatarsal space. The posteromedial portal is made at the same level as the posterolateral portal on the medial side of the Achilles tendon. A clamp is introduced through the incision and is directed toward the arthroscope shaft at a right angle until the clamp contacts the arthroscope. The arthroscope shaft is used as a guide for the clamp to travel anteriorly toward the posterior edge of the subtalar joint. The soft tissue in front of the arthroscopic tip is spread with the clamp, and then the clamp is exchanged for a 5 mm or 2.9 mm full-radius shaver. The subtalar joint capsule and soft tissue are removed with the shaver. The joint may be easily entered by opening this thin joint capsule. Depending on the situation, an os trigonum, a hypertrophic posterior joint capsule or hypertrophic posterior talus process can be debrided. The FHL can also be released if necessary. After the debridement and excision are completed, the ankle should be ranged to ensure that all impingement lesions are gone. The portal incisions are closed, and the ankle is splinted in neutral (Figs. 12.10A, B, 12.11).

Whether open or arthroscopic excision has been performed, the ankle is immobilized for 7 to 10 days until the incisions are

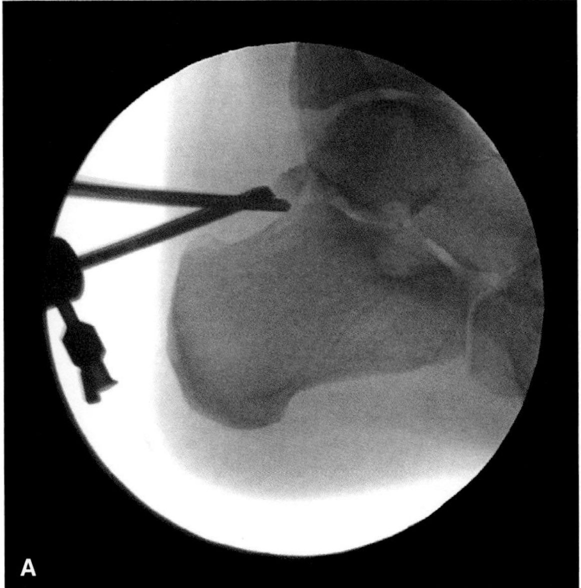

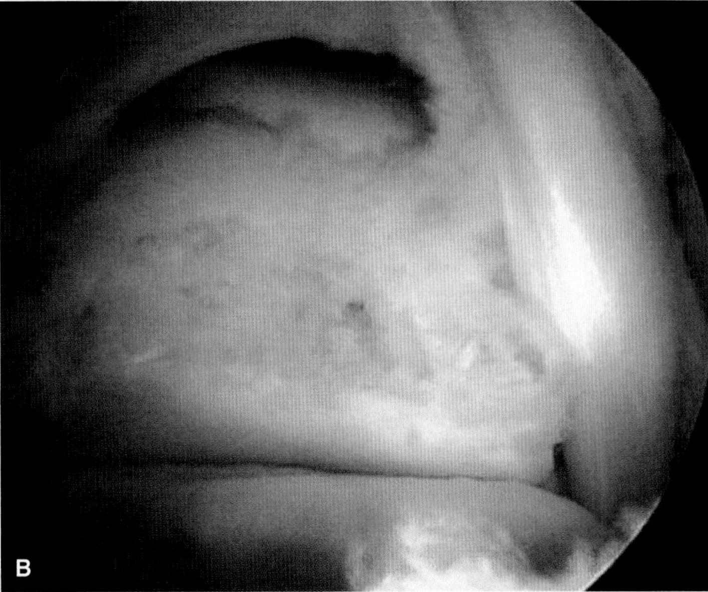

Figure 12.10. **A:** Arthroscopic image of an os trigonum. **B:** Arthroscopic image of the posterior ankle after excision of os trigonum.

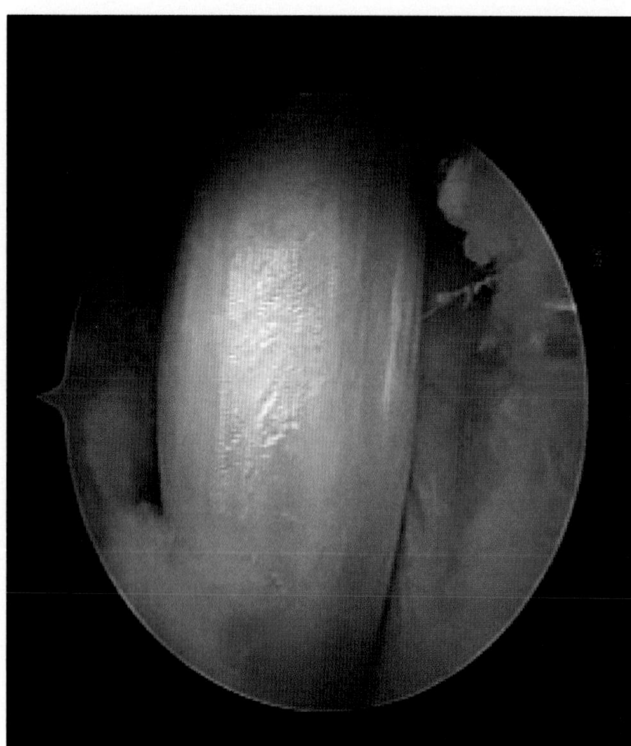

Figure 12.11. Arthroscopic image of the FHL tendon in the posterior ankle.

healed. Active range of motion and progressive weight bearing in a boot are then started. Care should be taken to address motion in the ankle, hindfoot, and the metatarsal–phalangeal joints. Physical therapy commences, and return to sport can be expected at 6 to 10 weeks, depending on the extent of debridement necessary.

RESULTS

When comparing both techniques, open versus arthroscopic approaches to the posterior ankle, arthroscopy tends to have lower complication rates and a shorter time to full recovery. The overall postoperative complication rate for the open procedure ranges from 12.5% to 24% (102–104). In contrast, the arthroscopic complication rate has been described as 0% to 4% (94,101,103). In a large study examining 146 patients who underwent hindfoot arthroscopy, the authors found a complication rate of 1.4% (101). Two patients had a small area of hypoesthesia on the lateral foot that was interpreted as sural nerve injury. In open procedures, sural nerve injury has been reported as high as 19.5% (102). However, these results can be misleading, as the cohorts are often very small. For instance, one study directly compares 16 patients who were treated with open excision of an os trigonum versus 25 patients who were treated arthroscopically. In each group, one patient suffered sensory loss from a presumed sural nerve injury (103). In the same study, the authors did find a difference for the time to return to previous sports level, with an average of 11.9 weeks for the open group and 6.0 weeks for the arthroscopic group ($P < 0.001$) (37). This trend of earlier recovery has been demonstrated in other studies, with an average of 8 to 9 weeks to return to sports after arthroscopic treatment versus an average of 4 to 6 months after open surgery (94,101,102,104).

CONCLUSION

Posterior ankle impingement commonly affects dancers and athletes who frequently load the foot and ankle in a plantarflexed position. Symptoms may be clinically diagnosed, and can be readily confirmed with conventional radiographs and more advanced imaging if necessary. Painful os trigonum and Stieda lesions may be excised in an open procedure or arthroscopically, and concomitant pathology may be addressed at the same time. Both techniques have shown good to excellent results, though arthroscopically treated patients have been shown to have a lower complication rate and a shorter recovery period before returning to sport.

REFERENCES

1. McMurray TP. Footballer's ankle. *J Bone Joint Surg Am* 1950;32:68–69.
2. Morris LH. Report of cases of athlete's ankle. *J Bone Joint Surg Am* 1943;25:220.
3. Biedert R. Anterior ankle pain in sports medicine: aetiology and indications for arthroscopy. *Arch Orthop Trauma Surg* 1991;110(6):293–297.
4. Cutsuries AM, Saltrick KR, Wagner J, et al. Arthroscopic arthroplasty of the ankle joint. *Clin Podiatr Med Surg* 1994;11(3):449–467.
5. Ferkel RD, Fasulo GJ. Arthroscopic treatment of ankle injuries. *Orthop Clin North Am* 1994;25(1):17–32.
6. van den Bekerom MP, Raven EE. The distal fascicle of the anterior inferior tibiofibular ligament as a cause of tibiotalar impingement syndrome: a current concepts review. *Knee Surg Sports Traumatol Arthrosc* 2007;15(4):465–471.
7. Robinson P. Impingement syndromes of the ankle. *Eur Radiol* 2007;17(12):3056–3065.
8. Hopper MA, Robinson P. Ankle impingement syndromes. *Radiol Clin North Am* 2008; 46(6):957–971, v.
9. Sanders TG, Rathur SK. Impingement syndromes of the ankle. *Magn Reson Imaging Clin N Am* 2008;16(1):29–38, v.
10. Watson AD. Ankle instability and impingement. *Foot Ankle Clin* 2007;12(1):177–195.
11. Massada JL. Ankle overuse injuries in soccer players. Morphological adaptation of the talus in the anterior impingement. *J Sports Med Phys Fitness* 1991;31(3):447–451.
12. Tol JL, van Dijk CN. Anterior ankle impingement. *Foot Ankle Clin* 2006;11(2):297–310, vi.
13. Tol JL, Verheyen CP, van Dijk CN. Arthroscopic treatment of anterior impingement in the ankle. *J Bone Joint Surg Br* 2001;83(1):9–13.
14. Hayeri MR, Trudell DJ, Resnick D. Anterior ankle impingement and talar bony outgrowths: osteophyte or enthesophyte? Paleopathologic and cadaveric study with imaging correlation. *AJR Am J Roentgenol* 2009;193(4):W334–W338.
15. Tol JL, van Dijk CN. Etiology of the anterior ankle impingement syndrome: a descriptive anatomical study. *Foot Ankle Int* 2004;25(6):382–386.
16. van Dijk CN, Tol JL, Verheyen CC. A prospective study of prognostic factors concerning the outcome of arthroscopic surgery for anterior ankle impingement. *Am J Sports Med* 1997; 25(6):737–745.
17. van Dijk CN, Verhagen RA, Tol JL. Arthroscopy for problems after ankle fracture. *J Bone Joint Surg Br* 1997;79(2):280–284.
18. van Dijk CN, Bossuyt PM, Marti RK. Medial ankle pain after lateral ligament rupture. *J Bone Joint Surg Br* 1996;78(4):562–567.
19. Tol JL, Slim E, van Soest AJ, et al. The relationship of the kicking action in soccer and anterior ankle impingement syndrome. A biomechanical analysis. *Am J Sports Med* 2002;30(1):45–50.
20. Berberian WS, Hecht PJ, Wapner KL, et al. Morphology of tibiotalar osteophytes in anterior ankle impingement. *Foot Ankle Int* 2001;22(4):313–317.
21. Ferkel RD, Karzel RP, Del Pizzo W, et al. Arthroscopic treatment of anterolateral impingement of the ankle. *Am J Sports Med* 1991;19(5):440–446.
22. Linklater J. MR imaging of ankle impingement lesions. *Magn Reson Imaging Clin N Am* 2009;17(4):775–800, vii–viii.
23. Krips R, Brandsson S, Swensson C, et al. Anatomical reconstruction and Evans tenodesis of the lateral ligaments of the ankle. Clinical and radiological findings after follow-up for 15 to 30 years. *J Bone Joint Surg Br* 2002;84(2):232–236.
24. Krips R, van Dijk CN, Halasi T, et al. Anatomical reconstruction versus tenodesis for the treatment of chronic anterolateral instability of the ankle joint: a 2- to 10-year follow-up, multicenter study. *Knee Surg Sports Traumatol Arthrosc* 2000;8(3):173–179.
25. Bassett FH 3rd, Gates HS 3rd, Billys JB, et al. Talar impingement by the anteroinferior tibiofibular ligament. A cause of chronic pain in the ankle after inversion sprain. *J Bone Joint Surg Am* 1990;72(1):55–59.
26. Kim SH, Ha KI. Arthroscopic treatment for impingement of the anterolateral soft tissues of the ankle. *J Bone Joint Surg Br* 2000;82(7):1019–1021.
27. Nihal A, Rose DJ, Trepman E. Arthroscopic treatment of anterior ankle impingement syndrome in dancers. *Foot Ankle Int* 2005;26(11):908–912.
28. O'Donoghue DH. Impingement exostoses of the talus and tibia. *J Bone Joint Surg Am* 1957;39-A(4):835–852; discussion, 52; passim.
29. O'Kane JW, Kadel N. Anterior impingement syndrome in dancers. *Curr Rev Musculoskelet Med* 2008;1(1):12–16.
30. Molloy S, Solan MC, Bendall SP. Synovial impingement in the ankle. A new physical sign. *J Bone Joint Surg Br* 2003;85(3):330–333.

31. Robinson P, White LM. Soft-tissue and osseous impingement syndromes of the ankle: role of imaging in diagnosis and management. *Radiographics* 2002;22(6):1457–1469; discussion 70–71.
32. Scranton PE Jr, McDermott JE. Anterior tibiotalar spurs: a comparison of open versus arthroscopic debridement. *Foot Ankle* 1992;13(3):125–129.
33. Ogilvie-Harris DJ, Mahomed N, Demaziere A. Anterior impingement of the ankle treated by arthroscopic removal of bony spurs. *J Bone Joint Surg Br* 1993;75(3):437–440.
34. McDougall A. Footballer's ankle. *Lancet* 1955;269(6902):1219–1220.
35. van Dijk CN, Wessel RN, Tol JL, et al. Oblique radiograph for the detection of bone spurs in anterior ankle impingement. *Skeletal Radiol* 2002;31(4):214–221.
36. Tol JL, Verhagen RA, Krips R, et al. The anterior ankle impingement syndrome: diagnostic value of oblique radiographs. *Foot Ankle Int* 2004;25(2):63–68.
37. Jordan LK 3rd, Helms CA, Cooperman AE, et al. Magnetic resonance imaging findings in anterolateral impingement of the ankle. *Skeletal Radiol* 2000;29(1):34–39.
38. Liu SH, Nuccion SL, Finerman G. Diagnosis of anterolateral ankle impingement. Comparison between magnetic resonance imaging and clinical examination. *Am J Sports Med* 1997;25(3):389–393.
39. Rubin DA, Tishkoff NW, Britton CA, et al. Anterolateral soft-tissue impingement in the ankle: diagnosis using MR imaging. *AJR Am J Roentgenol* 1997;169(3):829–835.
40. Robinson P, White LM, Salonen DC, et al. Anterolateral ankle impingement: mr arthrographic assessment of the anterolateral recess. *Radiology* 2001;221(1):186–190.
41. Cerezal L, Llopis E, Canga A, et al. MR arthrography of the ankle: indications and technique. *Radiol Clin North Am* 2008;46(6):973–994, v.
42. Cerezal L, Abascal F, Garcia-Valtuille R, et al. Ankle MR arthrography: how, why, when. *Radiol Clin North Am* 2005;43(4):693–707, viii.
43. Umans HR, Cerezal L. Anterior ankle impingement syndromes. *Semin Musculoskelet Radiol* 2008;12(2):146–153.
44. Cerezal L, Abascal F, Canga A, et al. MR imaging of ankle impingement syndromes. *AJR Am J Roentgenol* 2003;181(2):551–559.
45. Robinson P, White LM, Salonen D, et al. Anteromedial impingement of the ankle: using MR arthrography to assess the anteromedial recess. *AJR Am J Roentgenol* 2002;178(3): 601–604.
46. McCarthy CL, Wilson DJ, Coltman TP. Anterolateral ankle impingement: findings and diagnostic accuracy with ultrasound imaging. *Skeletal Radiol* 2008;37(3):209–216.
47. Ferkel RD, Scranton PE Jr. Arthroscopy of the ankle and foot. *J Bone Joint Surg Am* 1993;75(8):1233–1242.
48. Edmonds EW, Chambers R, Kaufman E, et al. Anterolateral ankle impingement in adolescents: outcomes of nonoperative and operative treatment. *J Pediatr Orthop* 2010;30(2): 186–191.
49. Coull R, Raffiq T, James LE, et al. Open treatment of anterior impingement of the ankle. *J Bone Joint Surg Br* 2003;85(4):550–553.
50. Hensley JP, Saltrick K, Le T. Anterior ankle arthroplasty: a retrospective study. *J Foot Surg* 1990;29(2):169–172.
51. Parkes JC 2nd, Hamilton WG, Patterson AH, et al. The anterior impingement syndrome of the ankle. *J Trauma* 1980;20(10):895–898.
52. Moustafa El-Sayed AM. Arthroscopic treatment of anterolateral impingement of the ankle. *J Foot Ankle Surg* 2010;49(3):219–223.
53. Martin DF, Baker CL, Curl WW, et al. Operative ankle arthroscopy. Long-term followup. *Am J Sports Med* 1989;17(1):16–23; discussion.
54. Martin DF, Curl WW, Baker CL. Arthroscopic treatment of chronic synovitis of the ankle. *Arthroscopy* 1989;5(2):110–114.
55. DeBerardino TM, Arciero RA, Taylor DC. Arthroscopic treatment of soft-tissue impingement of the ankle in athletes. *Arthroscopy* 1997;13(4):492–498.
56. Meislin RJ, Rose DJ, Parisien JS, et al. Arthroscopic treatment of synovial impingement of the ankle. *Am J Sports Med* 1993;21(2):186–189.
57. Thein R, Eichenblat M. Arthroscopic treatment of sports-related synovitis of the ankle. *Am J Sports Med* 1992;20(5):496–498.
58. Clasper JC, Pailthorpe CA. Chronic ankle pain in soldiers: the role of ankle arthroscopy and soft tissue excision. *J R Army Med Corps* 1996;142(3):107–109.
59. Cerulli G, Caraffa A, Buompadre V, et al. Operative arthroscopy of the ankle. *Arthroscopy* 1992;8(4):537–540.
60. Liu SH, Raskin A, Osti L, et al. Arthroscopic treatment of anterolateral ankle impingement. *Arthroscopy* 1994;10(2):215–218.
61. Jerosch J, Steinbeck J, Schroder M, et al. Arthroscopic treatment of anterior synovitis of the ankle in athletes. *Knee Surg Sports Traumatol Arthrosc* 1994;2(3):176–181.
62. Hassan AH. Treatment of anterolateral impingements of the ankle joint by arthroscopy. *Knee Surg Sports Traumatol Arthrosc* 2007;15(9):1150–1154.
63. Urguden M, Soyuncu Y, Ozdemir H, et al. Arthroscopic treatment of anterolateral soft tissue impingement of the ankle: evaluation of factors affecting outcome. *Arthroscopy* 2005; 21(3):317–322.
64. Reynaert P, Gelen G, Geens G. Arthroscopic treatment of anterior impingement of the ankle. *Acta Orthop Belg* 1994;60(4):384–388.
65. Amendola A, Petrik J, Webster-Bogaert S. Ankle arthroscopy: outcome in 79 consecutive patients. *Arthroscopy* 1996;12(5):565–573.
66. Bauer T, Breda R, Hardy P. Anterior ankle bony impingement with joint motion loss: the arthroscopic resection option. *Orthop Traumatol Surg Res* 2010;96(4):462–468.
67. van Dijk CN. Anterior and posterior ankle impingement. *Foot Ankle Clin* 2006;11(3):663–683.
68. Hamilton WG, Geppert MJ, Thompson FM. Pain in the posterior aspect of the ankle in dancers. Differential diagnosis and operative treatment. *J Bone Joint Surg Am* 1996; 78(10):1491–1500.
69. Hedrick MR, McBryde AM. Posterior ankle impingement. *Foot Ankle Int* 1994;15(1):2–8.
70. Hess GW. Ankle impingement syndromes: a review of etiology and related implications. *Foot Ankle Spec* 2011;4(5):290–297.
71. van Dijk CN, Lim LS, Poortman A, et al. Degenerative joint disease in female ballet dancers. *Am J Sports Med* 1995;23(3):295–300.
72. Hamilton WG, Hamilton LH, Marshall P, et al. A profile of the musculoskeletal characteristics of elite professional ballet dancers. *Am J Sports Med* 1992;20(3):267–273.
73. Russell JA, Kruse DW, Koutedakis Y, et al. Pathoanatomy of posterior ankle impingement in ballet dancers. *Clin Anat* 2010;23(6):613–621.
74. Stretanski MF, Weber GJ. Medical and rehabilitation issues in classical ballet. *Am J Phys Med Rehabil* 2002;81(5):383–391.
75. Macintyre J, Joy E. Foot and ankle injuries in dance. *Clin Sports Med* 2000;19(2):351–368.
76. Rogers J, Dijkstra P, McCourt P, et al. Posterior ankle impingement syndrome: a clinical review with reference to horizontal jump athletes. *Acta Orthop Belg* 2010;76(5):572–579.
77. Bureau NJ, Cardinal E, Hobden R, et al. Posterior ankle impingement syndrome: MR imaging findings in seven patients. *Radiology* 2000;215(2):497–503.
78. Maquirriain J. Posterior ankle impingement syndrome. *J Am Acad Orthop Surg* 2005; 13(6):365–371.
79. Stieda L. Ueber secundäre fusswerzelknochen. *Arch Anat Physiol Wiss Med* 1869;36:108–111.
80. Golano P, Vega J, Perez-Carro L, et al. Ankle anatomy for the arthroscopist. Part II: Role of the ankle ligaments in soft tissue impingement. *Foot Ankle Clin* 2006;11(2):275–296, v–vi.
81. Jourdel F, Tourne Y, Saragaglia D. Posterior ankle impingement syndrome: a retrospective study in 21 cases treated surgically. *Rev Chir Orthop Reparatrice Appar Mot* 2005;91(3):239–247.
82. Henderson I, La Valette D. Ankle impingement: combined anterior and posterior impingement syndrome of the ankle. *Foot Ankle Int* 2004;25(9):632–638.
83. McDougall A. The os trigonum. *J Bone Joint Surg Br* 1955;37-B(2):257–265.
84. Robinson P, Bollen SR. Posterior ankle impingement in professional soccer players: effectiveness of sonographically guided therapy. *AJR Am J Roentgenol* 2006;187(1):W53–W58.
85. Datir A, Connell D. Imaging of impingement lesions in the ankle. *Top Magn Reson Imaging* 2010;21(1):15–23.
86. Lee KB, Kim KH, Lee JJ. Posterior arthroscopic excision of bilateral posterior bony impingement syndrome of the ankle: a case report. *Knee Surg Sports Traumatol Arthrosc* 2008;16(4):396–399.
87. van Dijk CN, van Bergen CJ. Advancements in ankle arthroscopy. *J Am Acad Orthop Surg* 2008;16(11):635–646.
88. Paterson RS, Brown JN. The posteromedial impingement lesion of the ankle. A series of six cases. *Am J Sports Med* 2001;29(5):550–557.
89. Golano P, Mariani PP, Rodriguez-Niedenfuhr M, et al. Arthroscopic anatomy of the posterior ankle ligaments. *Arthroscopy* 2002;18(4):353–358.
90. Karasick D, Schweitzer ME. The os trigonum syndrome: imaging features. *AJR Am J Roentgenol* 1996;166(1):125–129.
91. Wakeley CJ, Johnson DP, Watt I. The value of MR imaging in the diagnosis of the os trigonum syndrome. *Skeletal Radiol* 1996;25(2):133–136.
92. Helgason JW, Chandnani VP. MR arthrography of the ankle. *Radiol Clin North Am* 1998; 36(4):729–738.
93. Chao W. Os trigonum. *Foot Ankle Clin* 2004;9(4):787–796, vii.
94. Jerosch J, Fadel M. Endoscopic resection of a symptomatic os trigonum. *Knee Surg Sports Traumatol Arthrosc* 2006;14(11):1188–1193.
95. Noguchi H, Ishii Y, Takeda M, et al. Arthroscopic excision of posterior ankle bony impingement for early return to the field: short-term results. *Foot Ankle Int* 2010;31(5):398–403.
96. Scholten PE, Sierevelt IN, van Dijk CN. Hindfoot endoscopy for posterior ankle impingement. *J Bone Joint Surg Am* 2008;90(12):2665–2672.
97. van Dijk CN, de Leeuw PA, Scholten PE. Hindfoot endoscopy for posterior ankle impingement. Surgical technique. *J Bone Joint Surg Am* 2009;91(Suppl 2):287–298.
98. Willits K, Sonneveld H, Amendola A, et al. Outcome of posterior ankle arthroscopy for hindfoot impingement. *Arthroscopy* 2008;24(2):196–202.
99. Bazaz R, Ferkel RD. Results of endoscopic plantar fascia release. *Foot Ankle Int* 2007; 28(5):549–556.
100. Lombardi CM, Silhanek AD, Connolly FG. Modified arthroscopic excision of the symptomatic os trigonum and release of the flexor hallucis longus tendon: operative technique and case study. *J Foot Ankle Surg* 1999;38(5):347–351.
101. van Dijk CN. Hindfoot endoscopy. *Foot Ankle Clin* 2006;11(2):391–414, vii.
102. Abramowitz Y, Wollstein R, Barzilay Y, et al. Outcome of resection of a symptomatic os trigonum. *J Bone Joint Surg Am* 2003;85-A(6):1051–1057.
103. Guo QW, Hu YL, Jiao C, et al. Open versus endoscopic excision of a symptomatic os trigonum: a comparative study of 41 cases. *Arthroscopy* 2010;26(3):384–390.
104. Marotta JJ, Micheli LJ. Os trigonum impingement in dancers. *Am J Sports Med* 1992; 20(5):533–536.

CHAPTER

13

Randall Farac
Michael Brage
Keri Reese
Eric Giza

Osteochondral Lesions of the Ankle

EPIDEMIOLOGY OF TALUS INJURY

Kappis was the first to apply the term osteochondritis dissecans to the talus in 1922. A number of etiologies have been suggested in the last century including acute and repetitive trauma, genetic predisposition, systemic metabolic disorders and abnormal vascularity. The damage articular cartilage experiences due to direct impact from ankle sprains and fractures is becoming recognized as a major etiology of cartilage lesions. The term osteochondritis dissecans should only be used for idiopathic causes and thus *osteochondral lesion or defect* is the preferred nomenclature.

Ankle sprains are common injuries with a daily incidence of 1 per 10,000 people per day. There are 23,000 ankle injuries each day in the US with basketball, soccer, and volleyball having the highest incidence per hour of play. Both acute injury and chronic lateral ligament insufficiency can lead to talar osteochondral lesions (1).

The incidence has been reported to be 0.09% of all fractures and 0.1% of all talar fractures, although these estimates were performed before modern imaging modalities became commonplace (2,3). When the degree of energy and severity of injury increases, chondral injury is more common. In the setting of unstable ankle fractures, Loren and Ferkel found that 63% of 48 ankles had chondral defects while Hintermann found 69% in 228 fractures at the time of arthroscopy and internal fixation (4,5).

TALUS ANATOMY

FUNCTION

The talus articulates with the tibia, fibula, calcaneus, and navicular and of its surface, 60% is covered in cartilage. It serves as a link to transmit load to the foot and experiences up to six times the body weight with each step. It affords pronation–supination and dorsiflexion–plantarflexion through multiple facets, a unique bony architecture and multiple ligament attachments. The talus has no tendinous attachments (Fig. 13.1).

CARTILAGE AND VASCULARITY

On a microscopic basis, talar articular cartilage is like other articular cartilage having superficial, middle, and deep calcified zones. The tidemark separates the deep from the calcified zone. Articular cartilage lacks neural structures and thus damage to cartilage should not cause pain. In addition, cartilage lacks vascular networks and sustenance is maintained by the surrounding synovial fluid (Fig. 13.2). The lack of vascular networks also limits the ability of partial thickness lesions to heal. Branches of the peroneal, posterior tibial, and anterior tibial arteries supply the talus. The extraosseous contributions of the arteries of the tarsal sinus and tarsal canal are particularly important (6).

Talar dome cartilage is thickest on the medial side and ranges from 0.8 to 2 mm on average. It thins at the proximal and distal portions of the curved dome. The talus radius of curvature is flattest in the center and matches the radius of curvature and cartilage thickness of the medial and lateral edges of the femoral trochlea (7).

The talar articular cartilage is hyaline in nature and has a similar collagen orientation to other weight-bearing joints. It is thought that the ankle joint's propensity for degenerative arthrosis is less than that for the hip due to its resistance to tensile forces over time. Talar articular injury is the major cause of advanced joint disease in the ankle (8,9). It is more resilient in the aging patient by exhibiting a fracture stress decrease of 20% compared to a 67% decrease in femoral head articular cartilage. Tensile stiffness of femoral head articular cartilage decreases 45% compared to 20% in the talus.

The chondrocytes have a limited capacity for intrinsic repair due to encasement in matrix proteins and limited vascularity. Full thickness injuries below the subchondral bone allow recruitment of marrow elements but injuries greater than 2 to 4 mm have a poor potential to heal with normal-appearing cartilage. A chondrocyte's biosynthetic machinery is impaired with senescence and further hampers healing of defects regardless of technique.

CAUSE OF INJURY

IDIOPATHIC

The incidence of idiopathic osteochondral lesions of the talus is unknown. Descriptions of knee osteochondritis dissecans by Konig have provided an analogue for the discussion of talar lesions. Patients without a specific traumatic event with a history and examination that reveal a stable ankle are

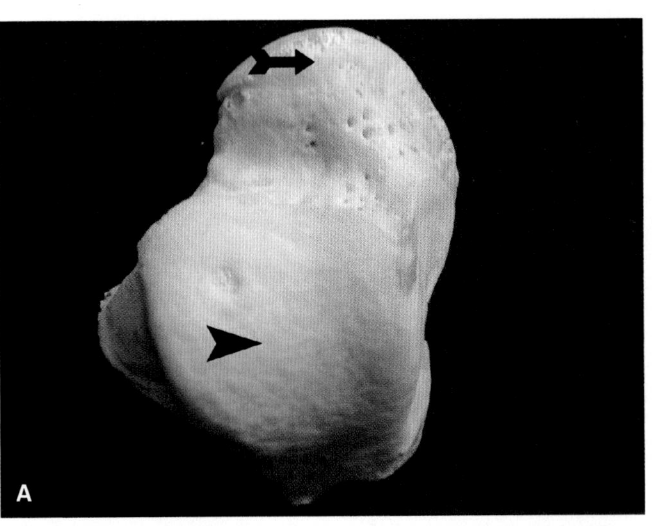

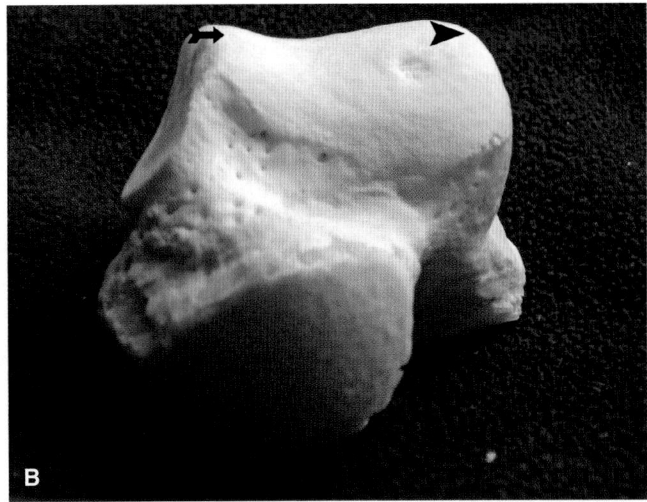

Figure 13.1. Photograph of the talus demonstrating the talar head (*arrow*) and dome of the talus (*arrowhead*) (**A**). Photograph demonstrating the medial (*arrow*) and lateral (*arrowhead*) dome as commonly seen on the mortise-view radiograph (**B**).

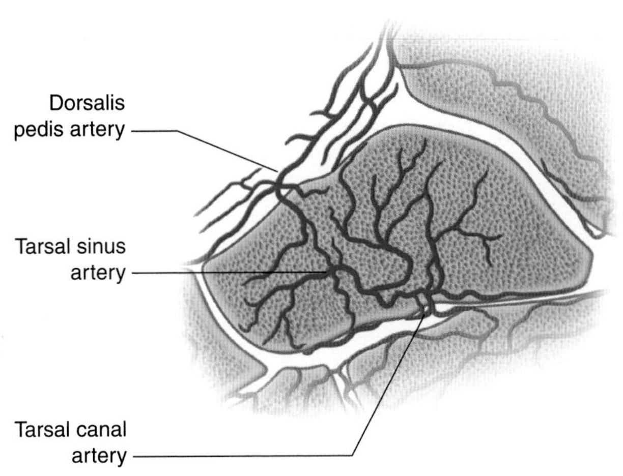

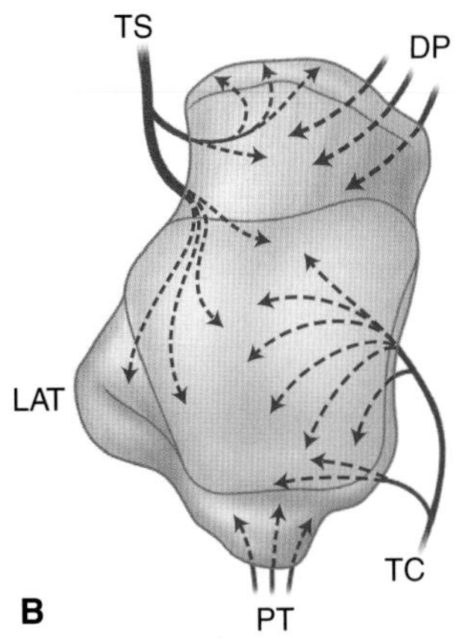

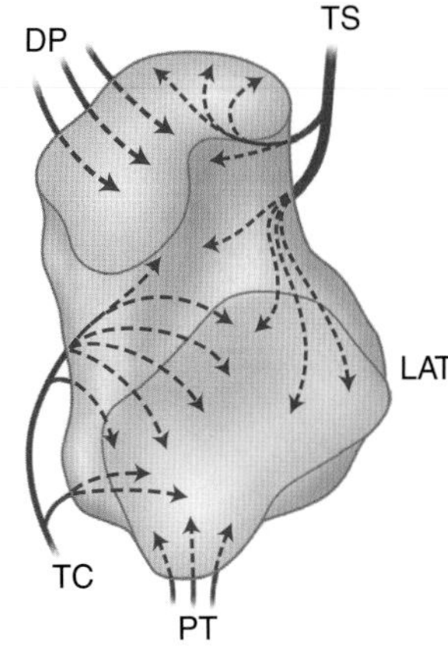

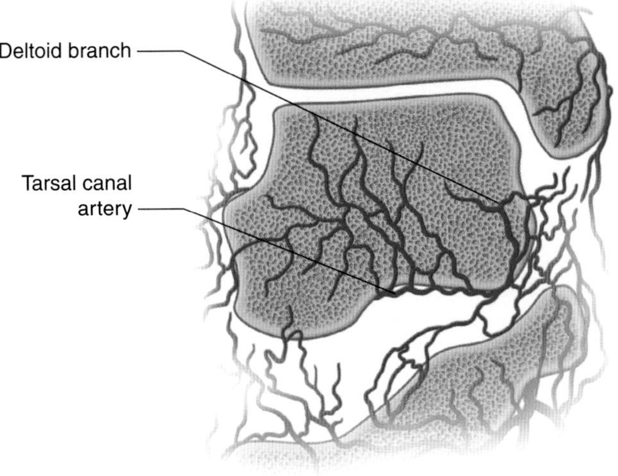

Figure 13.2. Photograph demonstrating the blood supply of the talus (**A**). Adapted from Sarrafian S. Anatomy of the Foot and Ankle: Descriptive, Topographic, Functional. 1st ed. Lippincott Williams & Wilkins: 1993:334. Schematic of the blood supply of the superior talus (*left*) and inferior surface (*right*) (**B**). TS, artery of the tarsal sinus; DP, dorsalis pedis; PT, posterior tibial artery; TC, artery of the tarsal canal. Redrawn from Browner, et al. *Skeletal Trauma: Fractures, Dislocations, Ligamentous Injuries.* 3rd ed. Saunders, 2003:2381.

thought to have an ischemic event of the subchondral bone. The increased appreciation of the spectrum of ankle instability in the last decade provides increased support for repetitive chondral microtrauma as the mechanism of injury for what was previously thought to be idiopathic.

A number of studies have found an association of greater than 80% of lateral lesions with a history of trauma. Lichtman found that 18% of 25 patients studied with medial lesions had no history of trauma. There remains a subset of patients, particularly those with posteromedial lesions, with no apparent mechanical risk factors or systemic disease to explain their lesions (10). It is postulated that these patients may have de novo subchondral bone ischemic necrosis. Woods reported on identical twins—presenting 2 months apart in the absence of trauma—with arthroscopically confirmed medial osteochondral lesions and pain with activity (11).

TRAUMA

Berndt and Harty developed their models for injury that seemed to correlate with their observations of location on the talus. Lateral lesions were simulated by inversion–dorsiflexion injuries that cause the talus to rotate in the mortise causing impact of the lateral dome with the fibula. Medial lesions are usually larger and were simulated by Berndt and Harty via a combination of inversion, external rotation, and plantarflexion. These lesions were entirely anterior and might not reflect in vivo conditions, as Raikin showed that 77% of 484 lateral lesions were centrally located on the dome (12,13).

Noguchi has used a three-dimensional ankle model to show increased stress distribution on the medial side of the ankle when lateral ligaments were released. Defects can be partial thickness, full thickness, or detached (Fig. 13.3) (14).

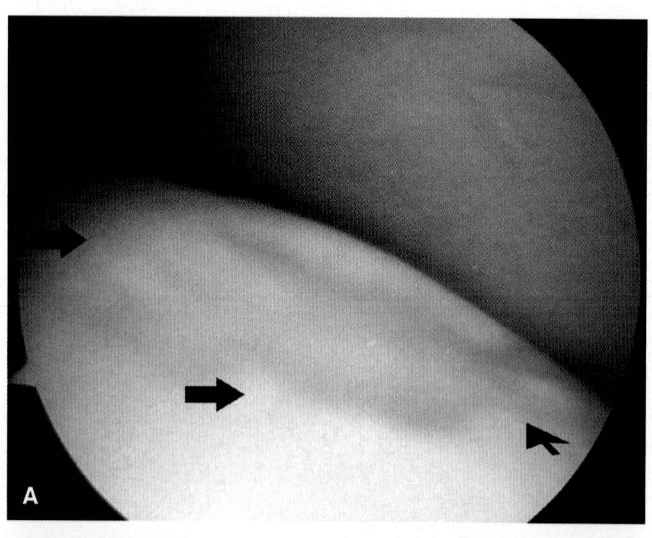

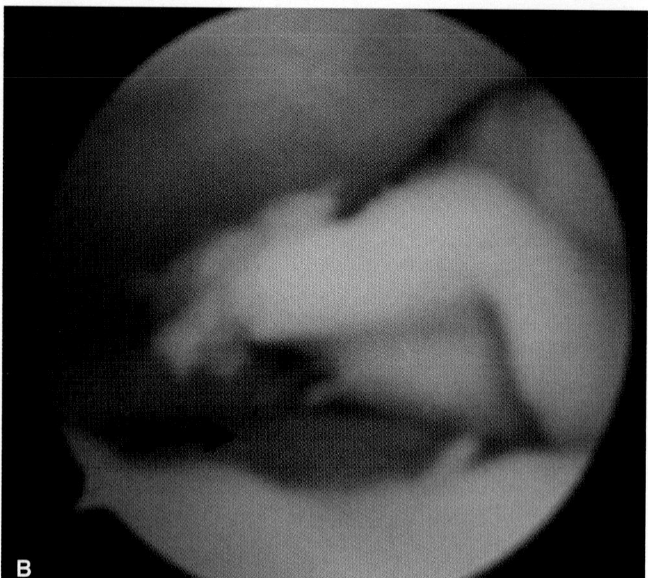

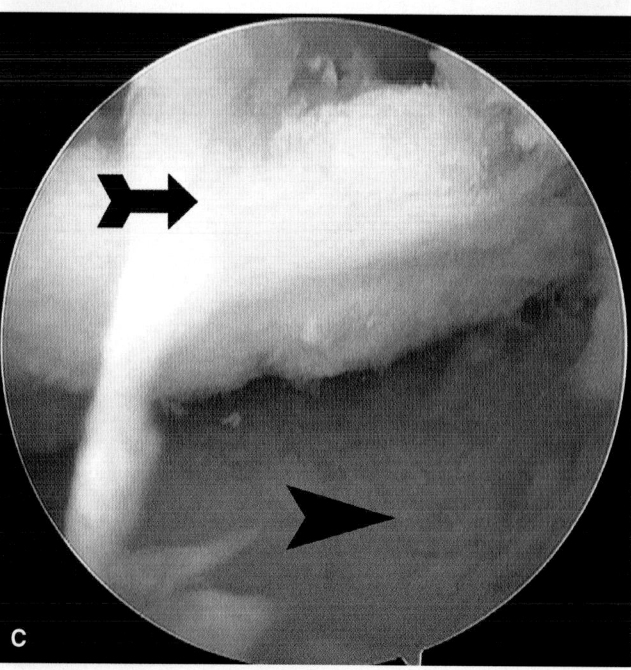

Figure 13.3. Arthroscopic photograph of a partial thickness lesion of the talus (*outlined by arrows*) **(A)**. Delamination injury of the lateral talus with intact subchondral bone **(B)**. Full thickness defect with attached bone (*arrow*) and exposed talus trabecular bone (*arrowhead*) **(C)**.

CHRONIC ANKLE INSTABILITY

Athletes with lateral ligament instability of the ankle have recurrent sprains with impaired dynamic stabilizers such as proprioception, peroneal coordination and peroneal strength. Attenuated or ruptured calcaneofibular and anterior talofibular ligaments along with reflex inhibition from mechanical instability allow pathologic articulation of the talus with respect to the tibia and fibula. Medial ligament instability is more difficult to evaluate, but when combined with lateral ligament insufficiency can allow even greater talar motion and rotational instability in the ankle mortise. Hintermann arthroscopically examined 523 ankles with chronic instability and described degrees of joint opening both laterally and medially. Cartilage lesions were found in 55% of unstable ankles while all ankles with complete deltoid ligament ruptures had damage to talar cartilage (5). There was no correlation between findings of cartilage lesions and degree of instability. Van Dijk evaluated patients with persistent medial pain after severe sprains and found that 66% have cartilage lesions. He concluded that every sprain has an additive effect and that ligament stabilization may slow the accrued damage over time and perhaps delay the onset of osteoarthrosis (15). Tochigi and McKinley found increased contact stresses with simulated instability in a stepped articular defect cadaver model; therefore, concomitant ligament stabilization should be addressed at the time of definitive osteochondral defect treatment (16).

EVALUATION OF TALUS INJURY

SYMPTOMS

Patients usually present with persistent pain after an ankle sprain. Time to presentation may be prolonged. In one study, the average time to presentation was 3 years for medial lesions and 1.5 years for lateral lesions (17). Pain is typically localized to the side of the lesion and may be accompanied by intermittent swelling, stiffness, and weakness. Mechanical symptoms such as locking and catching are variable. High-level athletes can usually tolerate the pain and may present after numerous injury events. A complete history pertaining to both medial and lateral ankle instability is paramount as findings on examination can be subtle. Alignment of the hindfoot should be noted as pes cavus deformity can contribute to inversion injuries. Stability should be tested with both anterior drawer testing and bilateral prone inversion challenge testing of the ankle and subtalar joints (Fig. 13.4).

Physical examination will show tenderness over the affected medial or lateral domes that can be localized as the ankle is moved from dorsiflexion into plantarflexion. Restricted range of motion with ankle weakness and a limp compared to the contralateral side is also common. The authors find that diagnostic injections of the ankle joint with marcaine/lidocaine can be helpful to determine if the pain is being generated by the intra-articular lesion or other factors. Other causes of pain should be considered and include mechanical ligament instability, talus bone contusions, loose bodies, lateral process fractures, injury to the peroneal tendons, accessory bones, neuropathic pain from stretch injury to the superficial peroneal nerve, and anterior/posterior impingement.

IMAGING

Plain weight-bearing AP, lateral, and oblique radiographs of the ankle are appropriate in the initial evaluation of the athlete with persistent pain after an ankle sprain. New images should be obtained if there have been recurrent instances of instability or more than 4 weeks have passed from initial radiographic evaluation. Radiographic images may reveal lucency in the dome but are limited for very proximal or distal lesions on the dome, for Stage 0 to II lesions, or early in the disease course. An imaging comparison study showed that routine radiographs failed to identify 50% of 92 lesions identified with other modalities (18).

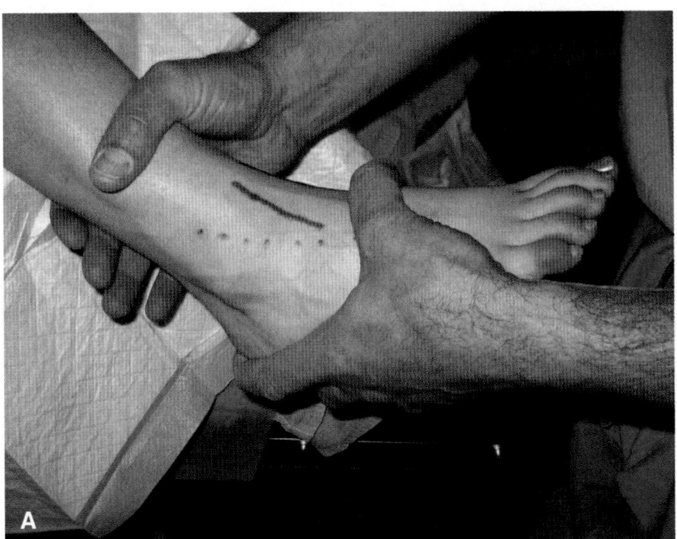

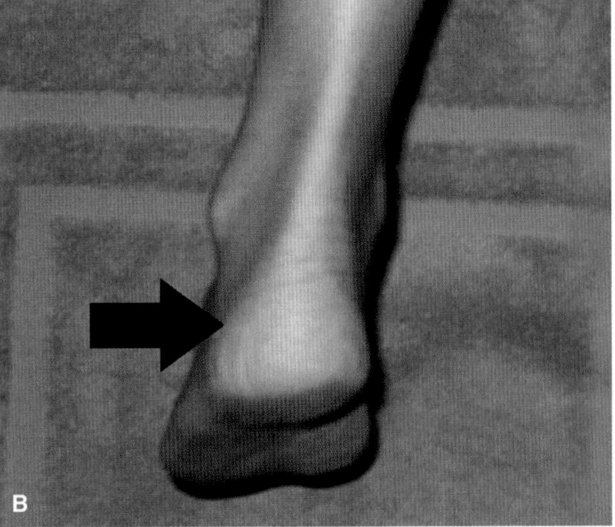

Figure 13.4. Photograph showing the anterior drawer examination of the ankle for ligamentous instability. The ankle is plantarflexed and a posterior to anterior force is applied with the ankle in slight internal rotation to test the anterior talofibular ligament **(A)**. Demonstration of prone ligament testing for lateral instability. A lateral to medial force in the direction of the arrow is placed on the hindfoot to test the calcaneofibular ligament **(B)**.

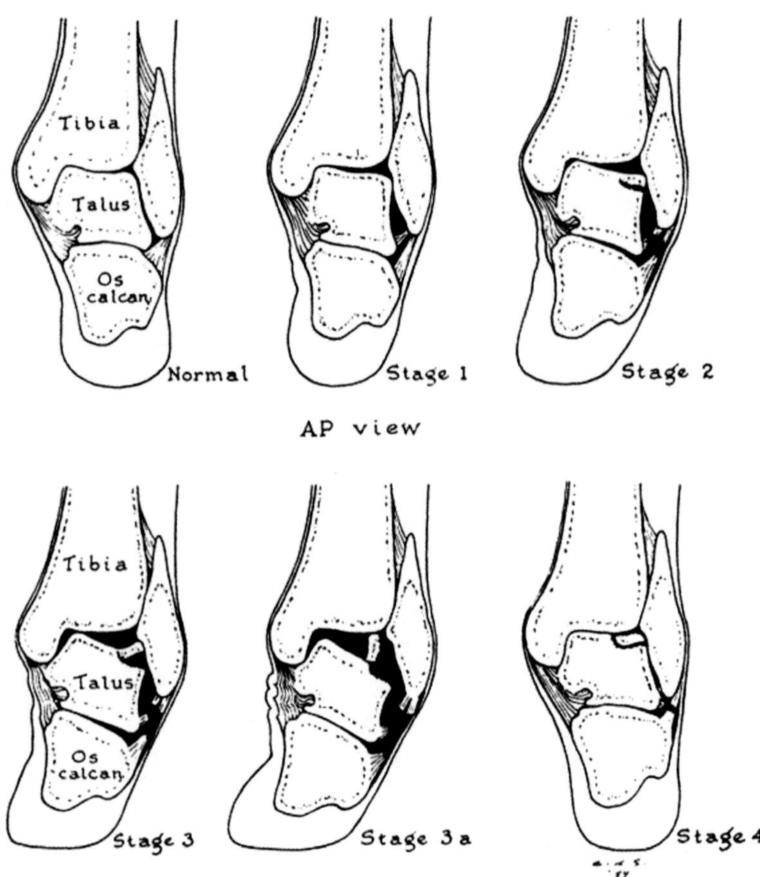

Figure 13.5. Drawing that shows the Berndt and Harty classification of transchondral fractures of the talus. Reprinted from Berndt AL, Harty M. Transchondral fractures (osteochondritis dissecans) of the talus. *J Bone Joint Surg Am* 1959;41-A:988–1020.

Pain after 8 weeks of conservative therapy warrants an MRI due to increased sensitivity for diagnosis and for characterizing the personality of lesions in preparation for possible surgical intervention. Stability of the lesion, delamination, location, and the presence of bone edema all aid in preoperative planning.

In 1959, Berndt and Harty investigated "transchondral fractures of the talus" with a literature review and attempted to elucidate mechanisms of injury with amputated specimens (Fig. 13.5). They simulated inversion injuries and developed a well-known four-stage system that is still used today. Although not originally specified whether their system was based on appearance or radiographs, it is used today for radiographic evaluation and extended by various authors to MRI and CT studies (12).

Other modalities have become routine for diagnosis and staging. High-resolution multiplanar CT was evaluated versus MRI and arthroscopy and found to be nearly equivalent (19). There is also a strong correlation with both MRI and arthroscopic findings (20,21). Bachmann questioned the sensitivity of plain radiographs and Mintz in 2003 showed MRI to be 95% sensitive for disease but with an inter-observer correlation Kappa score of 76% to 83% compared to findings at surgery (22,23).

Hepple and others have contributed to the classification and understanding of lesions by updating the classification schemes to include MRI findings and the addition of a fifth stage to denote the more severe lesions with subchondral cysts and impaired bone stock. MRI findings include lower signal on T1 images due to disruption of normal bone architecture and high signal on T2 images due to increased bone edema (Fig. 13.6) (24).

Higashiyama et al. studied two characteristic MRI findings following fixation of free fragments or drilling in a postoperative imaging study. A decrease in area of low signal intensity on T1-weighted sequences and disappearance of a fluid-filled signal rim between detached fragment and talar bed on T2-weighted images was observed. There was a trend of clinical improvement among those patients with these characteristic changes (25,26).

Various mechanisms have been suggested by authors to explain the location of lesions although there is no clear consensus. Raikin et al. examined 428 ankles by MRI and developed a 9-part grid to describe the location of injuries in the talar dome. They found that, both medial (62%) and lateral (34%) defects were most common at the equator or mid talar dome (13).

DISTAL TIBIAL OSTEOCHONDRAL DEFECTS

The incidence of lesions of the distal tibia account for 2% to 4% of osteochondral lesions in the ankle, and osteochondral defects (OCD) of the tibial plafond can be found in isolation or as a "kissing lesion" adjacent to a talus OCD. Kissing lesions can indicate a progression to osteoarthritis. Incongruity of the articular surface from a traumatic event, such as a pilon fracture, can make these injuries difficult to treat (Fig. 13.7) (27,28).

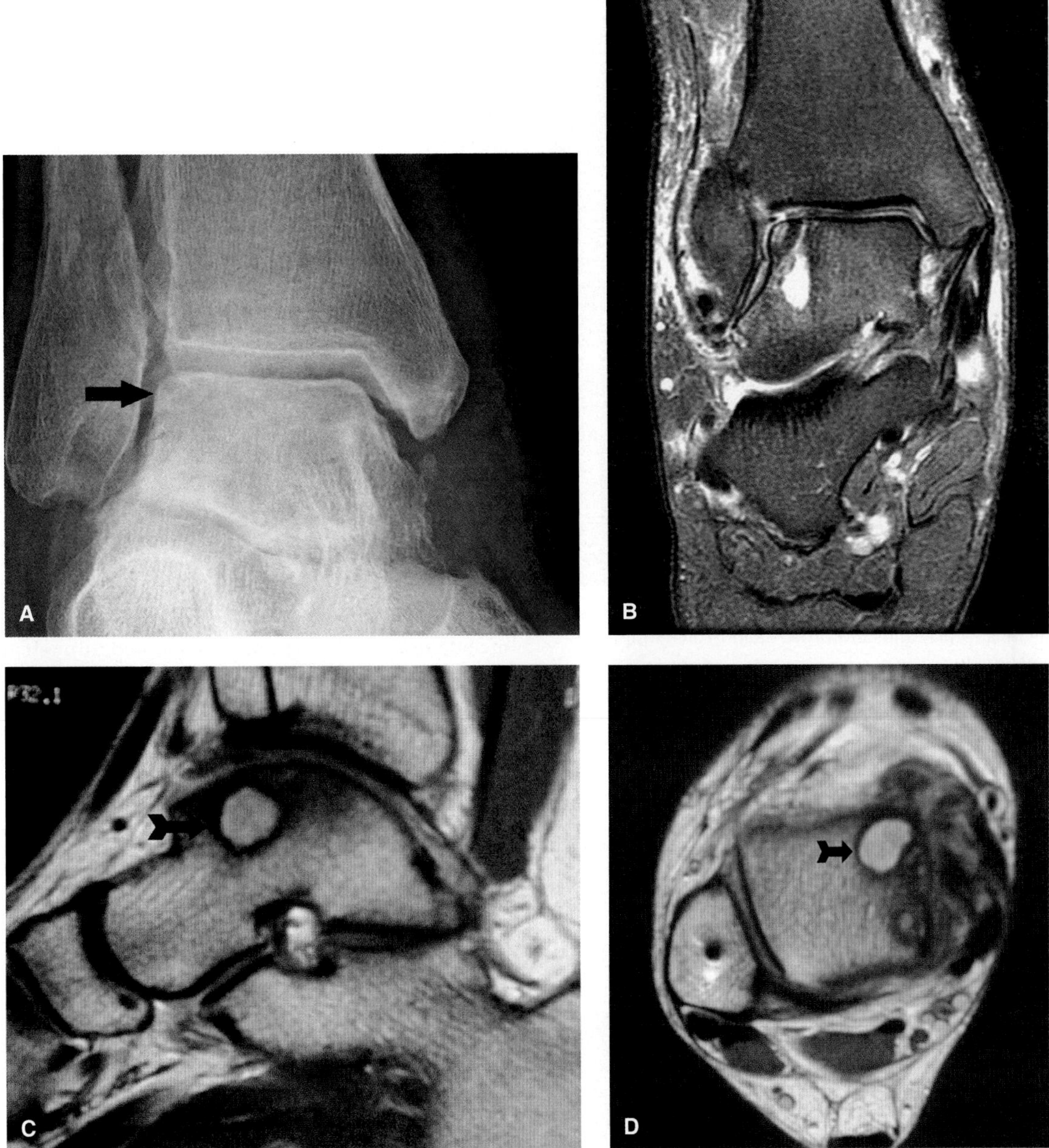

Figure 13.6. Plain radiograph showing a lateral talus OCD **(A)**. Note the loss of normal trabecular anatomy in the lateral talar dome with increased density in the adjacent subchondral bone (*arrow*). Corresponding T2-weighted MRI demonstrating the lesion with corresponding bone edema and cystic change **(B)**. Sagittal **(C)** and axial **(D)** T1 MRI of a large cystic lesion of the medial talar dome (*arrow*).

NON-SURGICAL TREATMENT

Conservative treatment is guided by the potential for a lesion to heal and patient preferences. Stage I and II lesions (stable) can be treated non-operatively with immobilization and protected weight bearing for 6 weeks followed by progressive weight bearing for another 6 weeks with a focus on range of motion and ankle-strengthening exercises (Fig. 13.8). Range of motion exercises are important for healing of cartilage by supporting the diffusion of nutrients in the synovial fluid though appropriate time for initial defect consolidation is a concern. Clinical effects of early fragment shear forces are a potential downfall of aggressive motion exercises (Algorithm 13.1).

A meta-analysis found an average 45% success rate with non-operative treatment. Time to heal and weight-bearing status varied widely in the study and no consensus exists on how long to keep an athlete from play (29). The authors suggest return to play on an individual basis after sport-specific drills and exercises are completed and pain has resolved to tolerable levels (30).

An MRI follow-up study of 29 lesions treated non-operatively at an average of 13.7 months showed that 45% had progressed, 24% improved, and 31% remained unchanged. Bone marrow edema and cysts, although featured prominently in revision staging systems, were not found to reliably predict progression of lesions (31). Clinical outcomes were not measured but MRI findings of cysts and bone marrow edema tended to improve

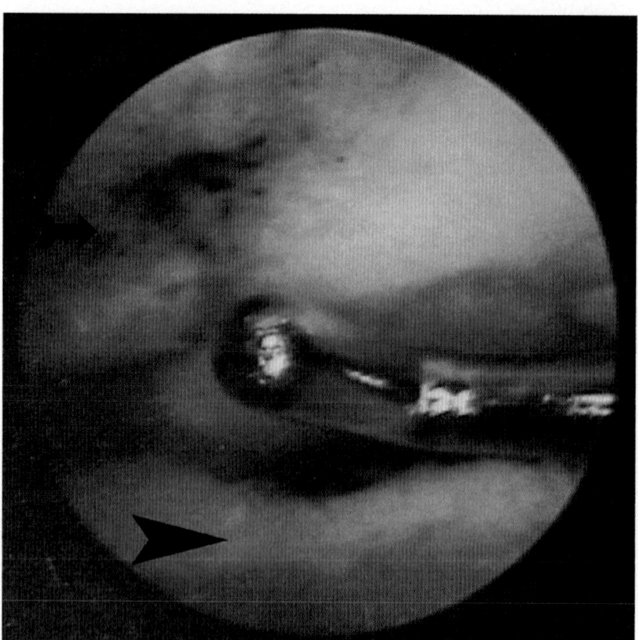

Figure 13.7. Intraoperative photograph of osteochondral "kissing lesions" of the tibia (*arrow*) and talus (*arrow head*) treated with microfracture of both lesions.

over time. Several studies have confirmed the lack of correlation between both MRI and CT with clinical outcomes (20,32).

SURGICAL TREATMENT AND OUTCOMES

For talus OCD, consistency in reporting of outcomes are inconsistent, and many studies have small sample sizes (33). O'Driscoll has posited that articular cartilage injury can be restored, replaced, relieved, or resected (the four r's) (34). Acute restoration is performed on the rare lesion with a bony defined fragment that is technically repairable. True osteochondritis dissecans lesions are possible candidates but overall relatively rare. Delamination must not be present and the best candidates are young athletes with good healing potential who are able to comply with weight-bearing restrictions. Techniques include open reduction and internal fixation with recessed transchondral screws, retrograde internal fixation and biodegradable fixation devices (Fig. 13.8). No large-scale studies are available to evaluate these techniques (35).

ARTHROSCOPY, CURETTAGE AND MICROFRACTURE/DRILLING

The initial surgical treatment for most lesions involves arthroscopy with curettage and microfracture. Arthroscopy is indicated for unstable lesions and those that have failed conservative treatment with stable lesions. Best results are seen in patients with small lesions (<1 cm^2) and having stable surrounding cartilage. Advanced osteoarthrosis and deformity are relative contraindications due to poor healing potential.

Several techniques are described to stimulate healing and include drilling (both transmalleolar and through an arthrotomy), retrograde talar drilling, curettage and microfracture. Lesions with intact cartilage can be retrograde drilled to stimulate medullary bleeding through subchondral bone (36). More advanced lesions with full thickness loss of surface cartilage necessitate antegrade drilling with 1.2 mm Kirschner wires or curettage and microfracture. Transmalleolar drilling allows access to posteromedial lesions that are troublesome to visualize from standard arthroscopic portals (25). A comparison of transmalleolar drilling and retrograde drilling of undetached fragments by Kono showed no significant difference between the two techniques at 2 years with similar outcomes

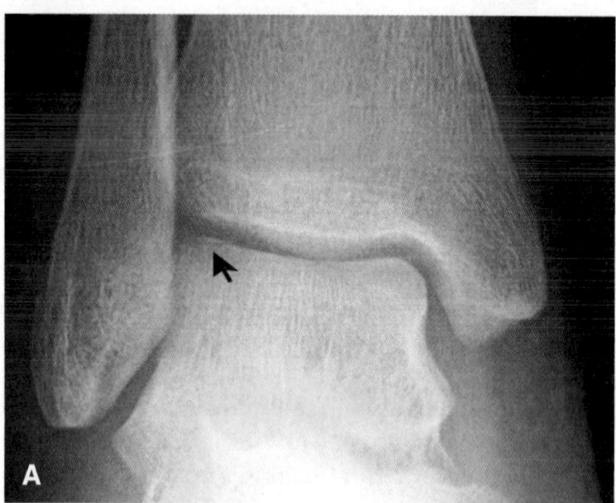

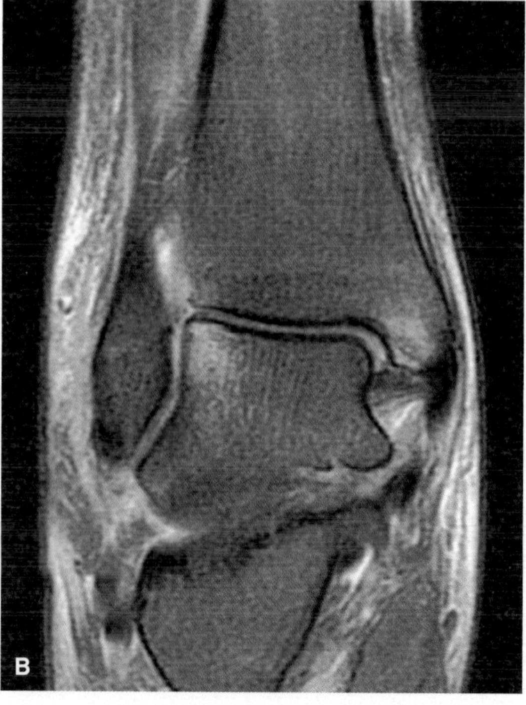

Figure 13.8. Plain radiograph of a 17-year-old female patient with an acute lateral talus injury with minimal displacement after a severe ankle sprain (*arrow*) **(A)**. T2-weighted MRI demonstrates edema in the lateral talus with minimal disruption of the chondral surface **(B)**. The patient responded well to 6 weeks of non–weight-bearing followed by a gradual progression of weight bearing and activity.

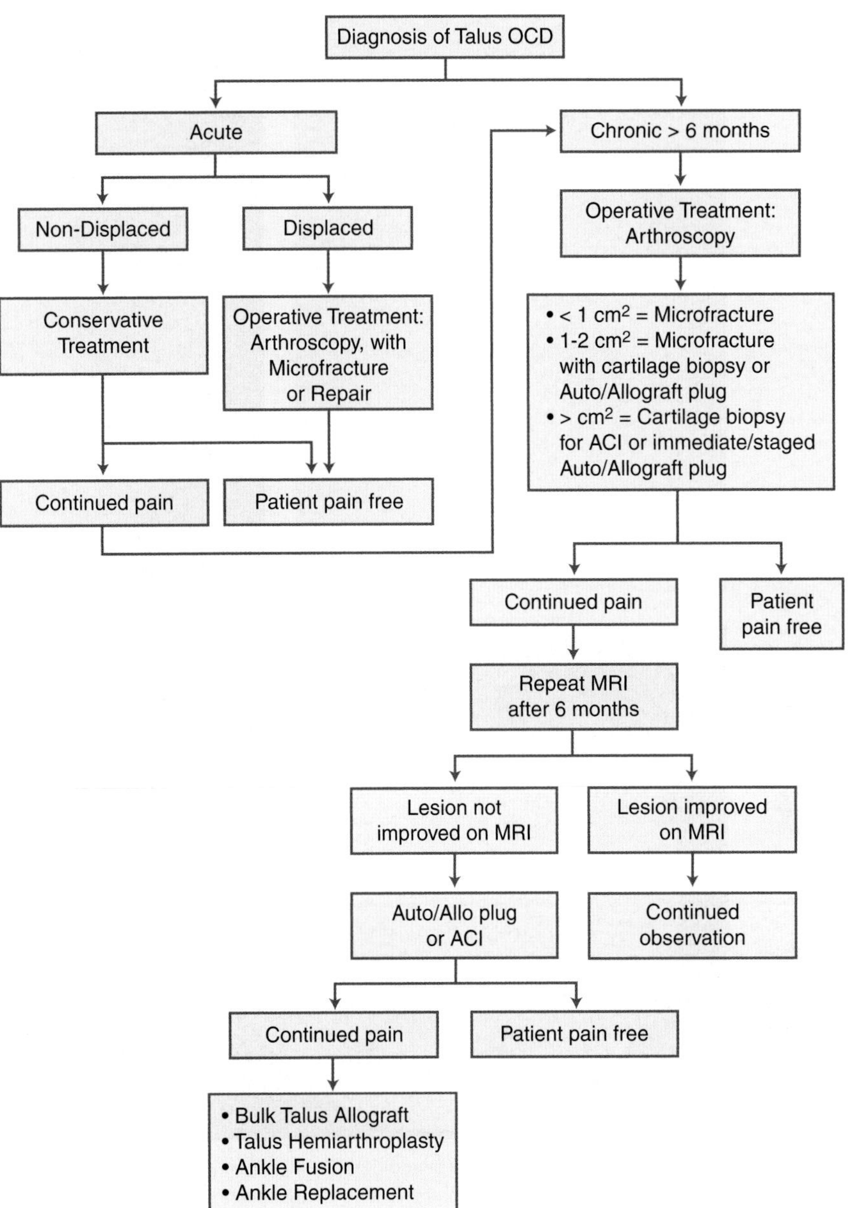

Algorithm 13.1. Treatment algorithm for the conservative and operative care of the talus osteochondral defect.

for clinical improvement of American Orthopaedic Foot and Ankle Society (AOFAS) score and MRI findings (37).

Clinical improvement in pain is seen in 85% of people in a number of studies with long-term follow-up (38–40). Schuman studied a combined group of 38 patients with 22 patients receiving microfracture as a primary procedure and 16 patients following a failed index procedure with a mean follow-up of 4.8 years. The revision group showed 75% good or excellent results and the primary group had 86% good or excellent results. The longest follow-up has been an average 71 months (24 to 152 months) with 72% excellent/good results, 20% fair and 8% poor. The average outcome AOFAS score was 84 but there was no preoperative baseline for comparison. The arthroscopic grade correlated with outcome and was best in patients with intact cartilage who received a drilling intervention to stimulate healing.

Repeat microfracture for continued pain after a primary procedure was efficacious at a mean of 5.9 years. Revision microfracture is indicated for patients with persistent pain who have imaging suggestive of incomplete healing and who are not candidates for more invasive procedures. Repeat microfracture or drilling appears to be a reasonable, low-complication procedure for patients who have failed primary attempts at healing if the lesion is one that clinically has a high expectation of healing (41).

Although the goal of drilling and microfracture is to stimulate healing and restoration of hyaline cartilage, defects usually heal with less organized fibrocartilage. Failed procedures after 4 months of healing and physical therapy should be scrutinized for concomitant pathology such as subtle instability or impingement of both bone and soft tissue. To ensure optimal outcome, alignment and stability should be restored along with the cartilage treatment. Recalcitrant lesions in active patients are candidates for grafting procedures. At this time, there are no long-term studies of treated defects which demonstrate the

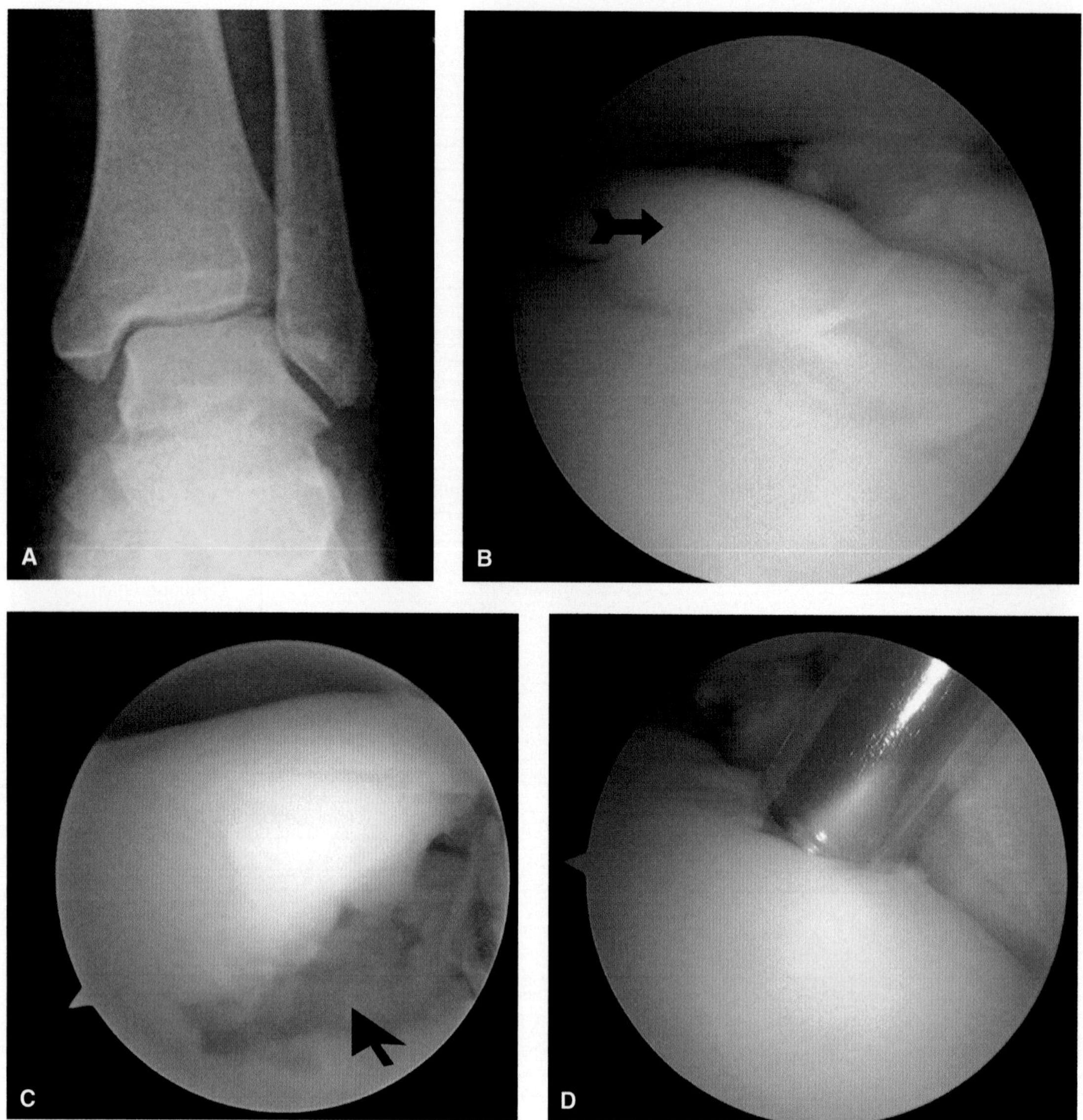

Figure 13.9. Preoperative radiographs showing a displaced lesion in a 13-year-old female **(A)**. Intra-operative photographs of the lesion (*arrow*) **(B)** with an attached subchondral fragment (*arrow*) **(C)**. Reduction and repair using bio-absorbable pins **(D)**.

time to secondary procedures for ankle arthritis, such as ankle fusion or arthroplasty.

KISSING LESIONS

Ferkel et al. reviewed 880 consecutive ankle arthroscopies and identified 23 patients (2.6%) with osteochondral lesions of the distal tibia (32). They reported on 17 patients with distal tibial OCD treated with microfracture. Six (35%) had osteochondral lesions of the tibia and talus; eleven had isolated lesions of the distal tibia. Treatment included excision, curettage, and abrasion arthroplasty in all patients. Five patients had transmalleolar drilling of the lesion, two had microfracture, and two had iliac bone grafting. Preoperatively, the median AOFAS ankle–hindfoot score was 52, and postoperatively, it was 87. The authors recommended arthroscopic treatment by means of debridement, curettage, abrasion arthroplasty, and, in some patients, transmalleolar drilling, microfracture, or iliac crest bone grafting. They found excellent and good results in 14 of 17 patients at 44 (24 to 99) months.

Carreira and Scranton have reported on the successful use of an autograft plug system to address osteochondral lesions of the distal tibia in two patients using a retrograde method. The osteochondral grafts were reversed and backed into the lesion, then secured in place with an interference screw (42).

AUTHORS' PREFERRED TECHNIQUE: ANKLE ARTHROSCOPY WITH CURETTAGE AND MICROFRACTURE

A standard arthroscopy setup including a well-padded leg holder is utilized (Fig. 13.10). A 30 degree 2.7 mm arthroscope is introduced via an anteromedial portal; however, it is

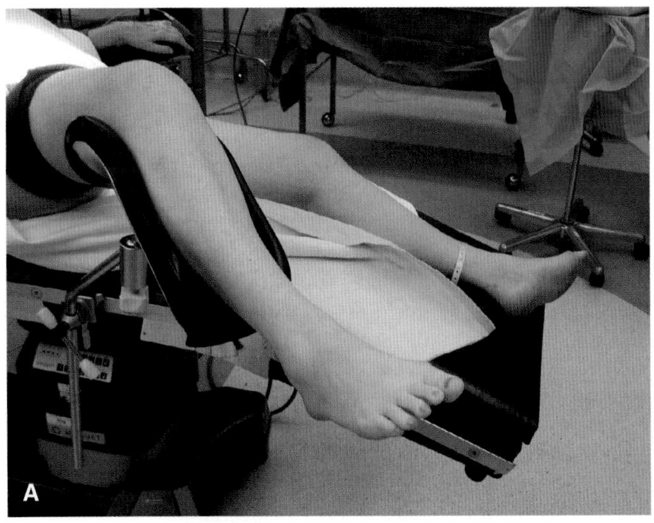

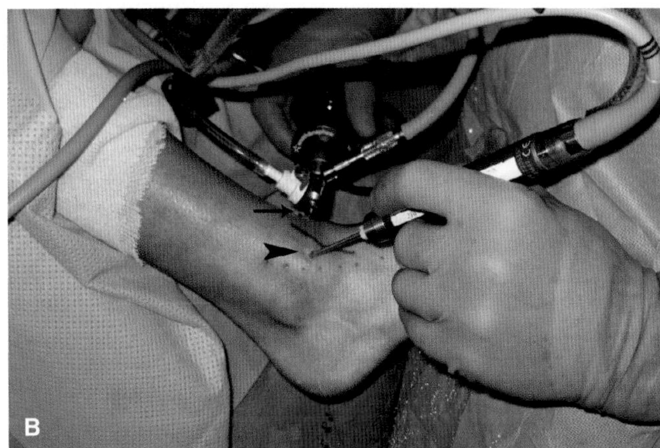

Figure 13.10. Operative-room setup for ankle arthroscopy **(A)**. The leg is placed in a well-padded holder and the foot of the bed is flexed. The leg holder is positioned so that distraction can be used if necessary. Photograph of ankle arthroscopy utilizing the anteromedial (*arrow*) and anterolateral (*arrowhead*) portals **(B)**. Note the *dotted line* lateral to the anterolateral portal marking the intermediate branch of the superficial peroneal nerve.

recommended to have a 70 degree 2.7 mm arthroscope and 1.9 mm arthroscope available. The anteromedial portal is established medial to the anterior tibial tendon at the level of the joint, and next an anterolateral portal is established under direct visualization just lateral to the peroneus tertius tendon. If possible, the branches of the superficial peroneal nerve should be palpated and marked prior to the procedure in order to decrease the possible complication of neuritis or nerve laceration. If necessary, a posterolateral portal can be used to access posterior lesions.

Access to the joint space is highly dependent on the ligamentous restraint and bony architecture. A joint distraction system is not always necessary, but should be available so that the entire articular surface of the tibia and talus can be inspected thoroughly. Removal of the anterior tibial and talar osteophytes should be performed to improve visualization and prevent anterior impingement. Anterior osteophyte removal should be performed without joint distraction to ensure that the anterior neurovascular structures are not tented over the anterior ankle joint.

Once it is identified, the size and extent of the lesion is carefully probed, and any loose or delaminated material is curetted or removed with a shaver (Fig. 13.11).

Soft or cystic bone is also removed and the cartilage is debrided to a stable border. The lesion is carefully measured and a microfracture procedure is performed with an awl through the subchondral bone (if intact). A tourniquet is used during the procedure and should be released to confirm a bleeding bed of bone. The technique can be performed entirely through standard arthroscopic portals for lesions at the equator of the dome and anterior. Any concomitant ligament stabilization

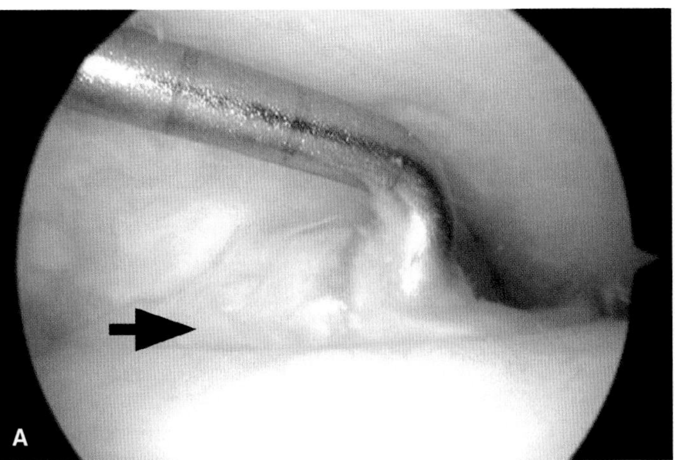

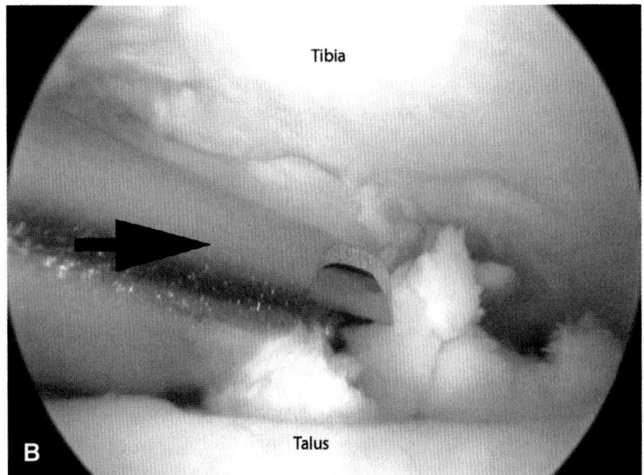

Figure 13.11. Microfracture of the talus OCD. The lesion (*arrow*) is probed to determine the depth and presence of delamination **(A)**. The loose cartilage is removed with a curette or shaver **(B)**.

should follow the arthroscopy procedure to avoid trauma to the repaired ligaments. Sample biopsy cartilage, including that from the lesion itself, can be harvested if subsequent chondrocyte implantation is foreseeable (28).

OSTEOCHONDRAL GRAFTS

Indications for osteochondral autografts include patients with focal talus lesions >1.5 cm^2, age less than 50 years and failure of either non-operative treatment or an index cartilage surgery. Kissing talo-tibial lesions and axial defects or deformity are contraindications (43). Autografts are harvested as full thickness cartilage with subchondral bone.

Multiple small-sized cylindrical plugs of varying small diameters (2 to 4 mm) are harvested to implant and cover a larger area in the mosaicplasty technique. The intervening spaces are filled with newly generated fibrocartilage, but hyaline-transplanted cartilage populates the bulk remainder.

A commercial system for larger single grafts is available (6 to 10 mm), and is called the osteochondral autograft transfer or "OATS." Concomitant donor site morbidity, usually from the ipsilateral knee femoral trochlea, is a concern although the technique can be used with fresh frozen allograft. Reddy examined changes in Lysholm score for 15 patients with asymptomatic knees undergoing talar osteochondral autograft mosaicplasty. At a mean follow-up of 47 months, the Lysholm score ranged from 49 to 100 with a mean of 81. Four patients were classified as "poor" by the Lysholm criteria (44).

Advantages for the OATS or mosaicplasty technique include the use of autograft tissue with robust fixation and a single-stage procedure that can be performed open or arthroscopically. Surgical exposure of the posterior talar dome, large defect size, and matching cartilage shape, curvature and depth of resection are all technically demanding skills that need to be practiced on a cadaver specimen with appropriate preoperative planning. Both techniques necessitate an orthogonal approach to the articular surface.

Osteochondral autograft of the talus was evaluated in a study of 19 patients with 16-month follow-up. 17 of 19 patients with an average postoperative AOFAS score of 88 indicated they would have the procedure again (45). Type V cystic lesions are thought to be the most difficult to treat with debridement, drilling or microfracture. Scranton showed 90% good to excellent results among 50 patients with Type V lesions. One of fifty patients experienced knee pain after the all arthroscopic harvest and 26 required a malleolar osteotomy for surgical exposure (28).

Mosaicplasty of the talus has been used extensively and was evaluated by Hangody with mean 4.2-year follow-up data showing 94% good to excellent results using the Hannover ankle score (46). Their basic science investigations of histologic retrieval in animal studies exhibit retainment of hyaline graft and fibrocartilage ingrowth in between plugs. Grafts are usually harvested from the periphery of the femoral trochlea because the cartilage thickness and curvature roughly matches that of the talus.

Controversy regarding the optimal open technique exists due to the paucity of strict surgical guidelines or level I evidence. The highest level of evidence for talar investigations is a trial of chondroplasty, microfracture and osteochondral autograft transplantation performed by Gobbi et al. (47). Statistically significant improvement as measured by the AOFAS hindfoot score was noted at 12 and 24 months for all techniques. Recommendations for surgical decision making among equivalent procedures are based on individual surgeon preferences, experience, and lesion location and character.

Muir et al. studied cadavers to evaluate the accessibility of the talar dome via various approaches about the ankle. The four arthrotomies and three osteotomies utilized and characterized the percentage of the talar dome that could be accessed in a perpendicular fashion with respect to the articular surface. They found that a medial malleolus osteotomy was needed for 17% of the dome, a lateral malleolus osteotomy was needed for 20% of the dome, and that 15% of the central dome could not be accessed in a perpendicular manner with any approach (48).

Cadaver allograft plugs can be used in place of an autograft and have the advantage of reducing donor site morbidity. The disadvantages include availability, the possibility of disease transmission, and increased cost.

Bulk fresh osteochondral allografts are replacement options for multifocal and large defects (>1 cm^2), particularly in the setting of avascular necrosis. Indications include subchondral and extensive diseases, possibly necessitating a bipolar graft and salvage procedures for failed autografting restoration attempts. Patients seeking to minimize the donor site morbidity of autograft procedures can be considered. Both fresh frozen and fresh osteochondral allografts are available; however, cryopreservation results in a loss of chondrocyte viability (49,50). Fresh grafts are preferred, but are less available due to tissue bank logistics and surgical timing (51–55). Early results of small studies have exhibited mixed outcomes (56,57). The technique is demanding and requires a large arthrotomy. Long-term graft survival and resorption is a concern although recent reports have been encouraging (50,58).

The use of a synthetic osteobiologic substitute have gained popularity recently and offer some attractive alternatives to autograft or allograft plugs which include ease of use, decreased cost, lack of donor site morbidity, and elimination of risk of transmittable diseases. The plugs create a porous scaffold that allows for ingrowth of bone and fibrocartilage. The construct includes a calcium sulfate core covered with a polylactide-co-glycolide cap which is press fit into the talus defect in the same fashion as an allograft or autograft osteochondral plug (Fig. 13.12). The copolymer resorbs in 6 to 9 months; however, radiographic fill of the defect can take up to 1 year (59).

AUTHORS' PREFERRED TECHNIQUE: MEDIAL MALLEOLUS OSTEOTOMY AND OATS AUTOGRAFT PLUG

In order to gain access to the medial talar dome, a medial malleolar osteotomy can be performed. Careful preoperative identification of the exact location of the lesion on CT or MRI is important to ensure that the osteotomy cut will allow access to the lesion.

The patient is positioned supine and a tourniquet is used (Fig. 13.13). The incision is centralized over the medial malleolus and careful dissection is performed to identify and protect the posterior tibial tendon.

Dissection proceeds anteriorly to identify the anteromedial aspect of the joint and a small arthrotomy is performed so that

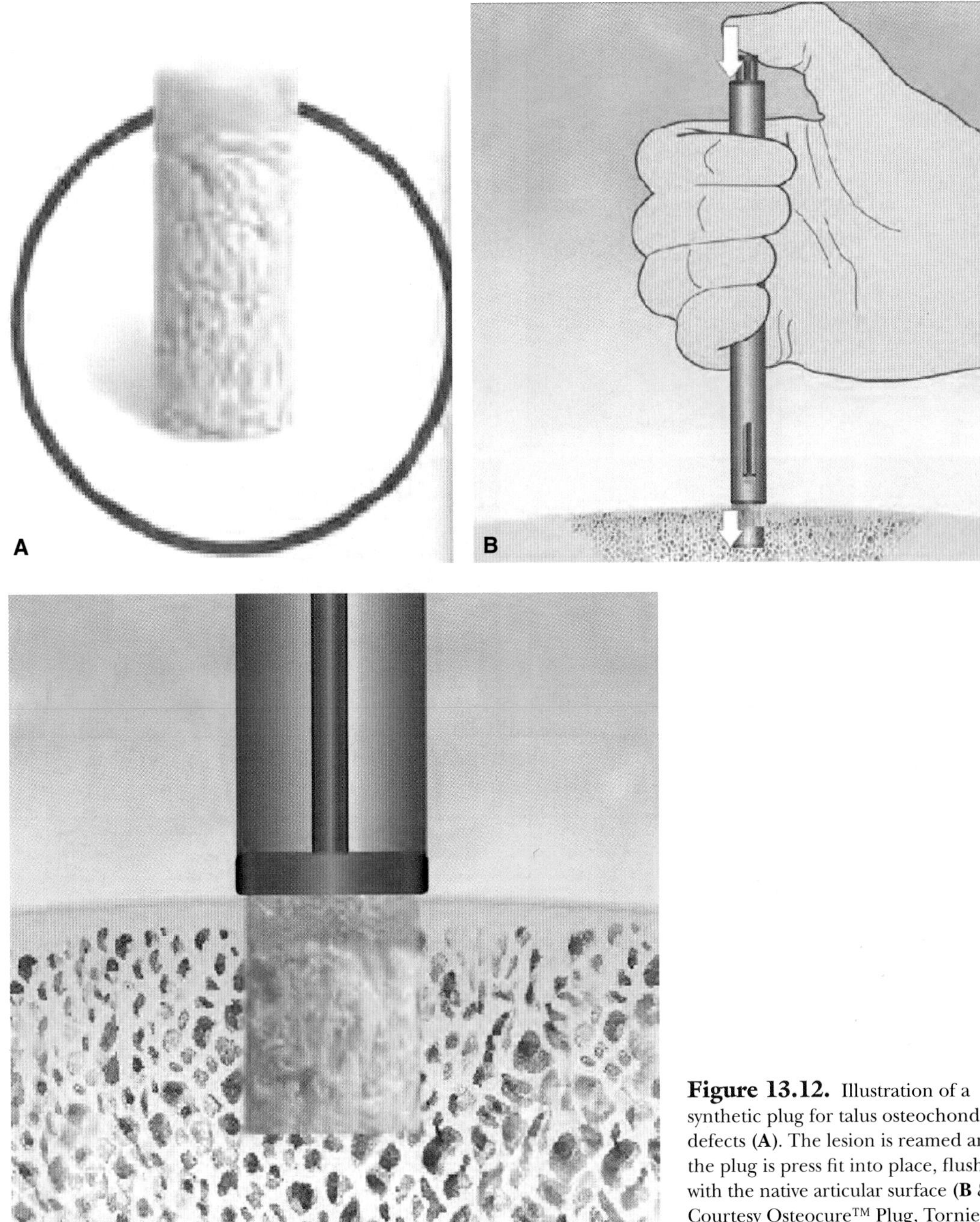

Figure 13.12. Illustration of a synthetic plug for talus osteochondral defects **(A)**. The lesion is reamed and the plug is press fit into place, flush with the native articular surface **(B & C)**. Courtesy Osteocure™ Plug, Tornier, Stafford, TX, USA.

the joint is properly identified, which aides in visualizing the angle of the osteotomy.

Drill holes for two 4.5 mm screws are placed across the planned osteotomy site. A chevron-type cut also ensures that the tibial plug will be reduced in a precise anatomic fashion. The cut is performed with an oscillating saw and osteotome. Care is taken to ensure that the talar cartilage is not disturbed. A suture can be passed through the drill holes to provide atraumatic retraction of the medial osteotomy.

The lesion is identified and carefully curetted to a stable border. It is then measured and templated for the donor plug. The guidewire is placed in the center of the lesion and reaming is performed to the desired depth. The contour of the talar dome is noted as careful harvest from the knee is needed to match the geometry of the lesion location on the talus. The harvest is performed from the ipsilateral knee and the authors prefer the superolateral surface of the lateral femoral condyle. The depth of the site on the talus is carefully measured and the harvested plug is trimmed to the appropriate size. Attention must be paid to the orientation of the plug as it is inserted. The insertion device is removed when the plug is still slightly prominent (1 to 2 mm), and then it is gently tamped into place. The osteotomy site is then reduced and secured with two 4.5 mm screws. Care is taken to ensure that the tibial articular surface is anatomically reduced and an ankle arthroscope can be introduced to verify the reduction (Fig. 13.14).

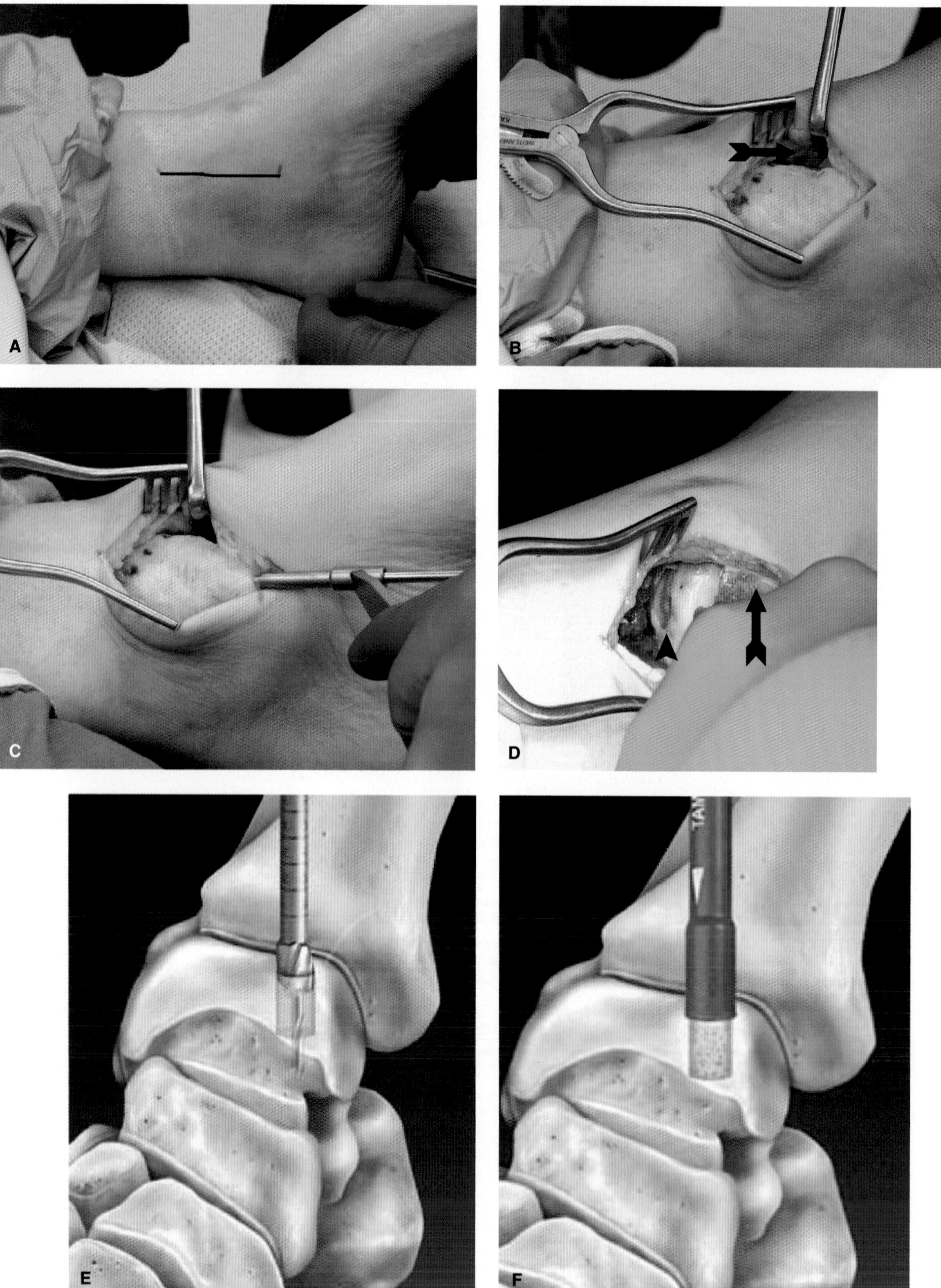

Figure 13.13. Medial malleolus osteotomy. The incision is centered over the medial malleolus **(A)**. An arthrotomy is made medial to the tibialis anterior tendon to visualize the joint (*arrow*) **(B)**. The medial malleolus is pre-drilled prior to the osteotomy **(C)**. The osteotomy cut is performed, and the lesion (*arrow head*) is visualized through the osteotomy site (*arrow*) **(D)**. The talus OCD lesion is reamed perpendicular to the surface of the talus **(E)**. After the auto or allograft plug is procured, it is implanted and then tamped gently into place flush with the native cartilage **(F)**. (*continued*)

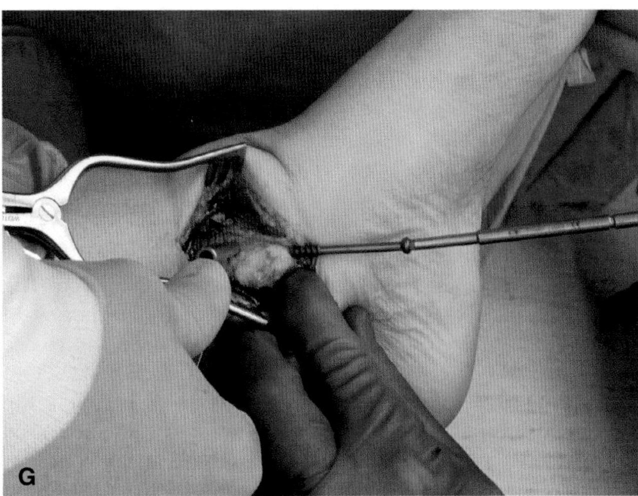

Figure 13.13. (*Continued*) The osteotomy is reduced and fixed using screws showing an anatomic reduction of the anterior limb of the osteotomy (*arrows*) (**G**). Courtesy of Arthrex Inc., Naples, FL, USA.

AUTOLOGOUS CHONDROCYTE IMPLANTATION (ACI)

Autologous chondrocyte implantation (ACI) uses cultured chondrocytes with a periosteal patch. Harvesting is first accomplished from either the knee or ankle, and can include the damaged area of chondral tissue (30). The biopsy typically yields 2 to 3 million cells and these cells can be stored for more than 1 year. Once the decision is made to transplant, the cells are cultured for 6 to 8 weeks and results in at least 12 million cells available for implantation. The process of growing the cells increases the number of viable cells for implantation by at least 10 fold. The ability to culture large numbers of cells for implantation is critical for the success of the procedure (60).

Whittaker et al. reported their results with ACI on 10 patients at 4-years follow-up (61). Eight of the ten patients had failed prior arthroscopic treatment. At a mean of 24 months, 90% were "pleased" or "extremely pleased" with the result of the surgery. Full thickness biopsies were obtained in five patients requiring repeat arthroscopy with two showing hyaline cartilage and three showing fibrocartilage. Results confirmed some donor site morbidity. The Lysholm knee score returned to normal in 3 patients at 1 year, but remained reduced by 15% in 7 patients.

Similar results have been found with other authors. Baums et al. reported on 12 patients with ACI at a mean follow-up of 63 months. There were six medial lesions and six

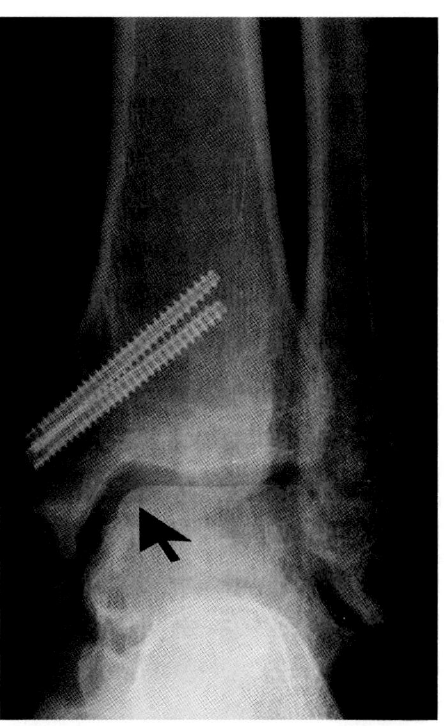

Figure 13.15. Radiograph of a 34-year-old female 6 months after a medial malleolus osteotomy and ACI for a medial talus defect that had failed microfracture. The patient was pain free 6 months after the operation.

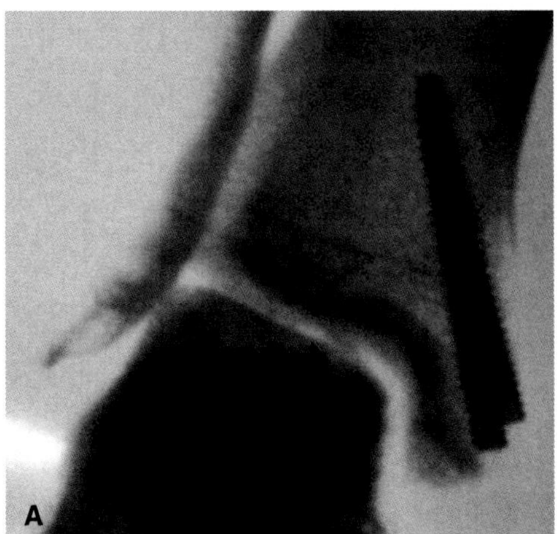

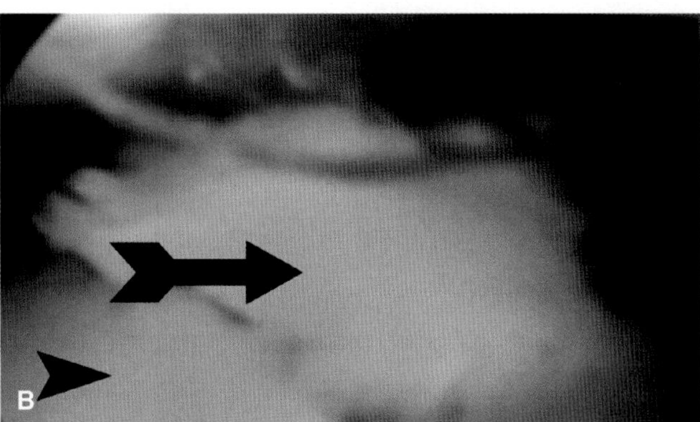

Figure 13.14. Talus osteochondral autograft intra-operative radiograph after the reduction showing the implanted osteochondral plug (*arrow*) (**A**). Arthroscopy photograph showing the implanted autograph plug (*large arrow*) and native cartilage (*arrowhead*) (**B**).

lateral lesions. The average size of the lesions was 2.3 cm^2. At 63-month follow-up, all patients were either very satisfied or satisfied with the result. Based on the Hannover score, there were seven excellent, four good and one satisfactory result. The preoperative AOFAS hindfoot score was 43.5 while the 63-month follow-up score was 88.4. MRI showed congruent graft incorporation in seven patients and four showed irregularity of the articular surface (62–64).

AUTHORS' PREFERRED TECHNIQUE: ACI

For traditional ACI, a medial or lateral malleolus osteotomy is performed as necessary. The tourniquet can be used for the osteotomy (Fig. 13.16). The lesion is curetted to a stable border and then a template is created using the foil sleeve from a suture packaging. Care is taken not to disturb the subchondral bone under the lesion as bleeding from the bone can disrupt the periosteal patch and injected chondrocytes. Epinephrine-soaked pledgets are placed on the lesion and the tourniquet is deflated. Next, the periosteal patch is harvested from the tibia. The optimal site is approximately 4 cm distal to the tibial tubercle. Careful dissection is carried out to remove the subcutaneous fat overlying the tibia without disturbing the periosteum. Next the template is centered on the tibia and the periosteum is cut with an extra 2 mm border around the template using a no. 15 scalpel.

The periosteum is carefully removed using a periosteal elevator and the cambium layer (closest to the bone) is noted as this will be placed facing the subchondral bone over the lesion. The tibial incision is closed in a standard fashion. The periosteal patch is then sutured to the lesion using 6-0 braided absorbable suture that has been lubricated with sterile mineral oil. Before placing the final suture at the distal portion of the lesion, the perimeter is sealed with fibrin glue and an angiocatheter is used to place some saline in the patch to ensure that the construct is sealed. Next, the cultured chondrocytes are injected into the lesion and the final suture is placed. The medial malleolus is reduced and then stabilized. A drain is placed in the anterior aspect of the joint and the incision is closed in a standard

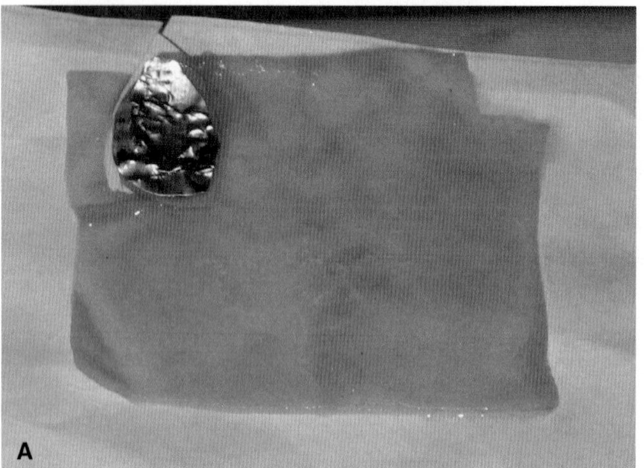

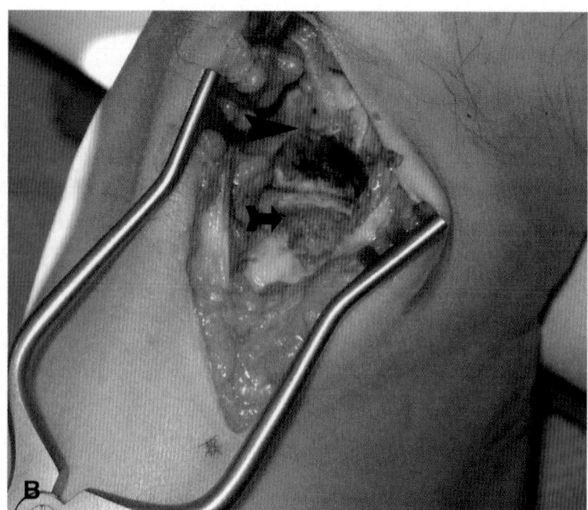

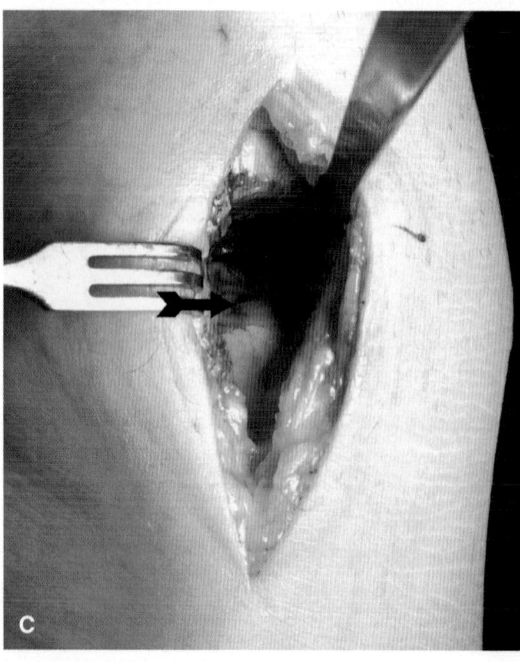

Figure 13.16. Photograph of a Matrix ACI (Genzyme, Cambridge, MA) membrane with template of talus OCD lesion **(A)**. Exposure of the medial talus lesion (*arrow*) through a medial incision utilizing a plafondoplasty of the tibia (*arrow head*) **(B)**. MACI membrane (*arrow*) in place after implantation and fixation with fibrin glue **(C)**.

fashion. The drain is removed after 24 hours and a splint is utilized until the incision has healed. The patient is encouraged to start gentle range of motion exercises 2 weeks postoperatively. Weight bearing is restricted until 6 weeks and then is gradually increased over the following 6 weeks in a cast boot. Full weight bearing without a boot is not permitted until 12 weeks postoperatively.

MATRIX-BASED CHONDROCYTE IMPLANTATION

Matrix-based chondrocyte implantation (MACI) is similar to ACI. Cells are first harvested from the ankle or knee. Next, chondrocyte cells are enzymatically separated from the matrix and cultured to produce 15 to 20 million cells. Instead of injecting the cultured chondrocytes under periosteum, the cells are imbedded in a type I/III collagen membrane bilayer. Similar to ACI, the MACI technique allows the surgeon to increase by at least ten fold the cells available for implantation into the defect. A second-stage operation is used to implant the membrane over the talar defect (60,65,66).

The advantages of MACI include that it is technically easier than ACI and no tibial/malleolar osteotomy is needed. Two operations are required and the cells can be stored for more than 1 year after initial harvest. Early results have been published in the literature (67).

Ronga and others have independently reported on series of patients with the MACI technique on six chondral defects in the ankle. The follow-up averaged 33.8 months, and the average age was 28.6 years. All defects were medial except for one "kissing" lesion. At 2-year follow-up, five ankles showed improvement in AOFAS scores. All ankles had a second-look arthroscopy, and the five with improved scores had hyaline-like cartilage that was stable to probing. The one ankle that did not improve had no detectable cartilage (68).

In a prospective study of 10 patients with full thickness defects who underwent MACI and followed for 2 years, Giza et al. showed a significant clinical improvement in both AOFAS and SF-36 scores. All patients felt they were subjectively improved by the surgery (69).

AUTHORS' PREFERRED TECHNIQUE: MACI

The size and location of the chondral defect are assessed by ankle arthroscopy, and harvesting of talar articular cartilage is performed (Fig. 13.16). The harvested chondrocytes are placed in a nutrient medium tube and sent to a cell laboratory (Genzyme Biosurgery, Boston, USA) along with 100 mL of autologous blood distributed in ten tubes. The cells are enzymatically separated from the matrix and cultured for 6 to 8 weeks in order to produce 15 to 20 million dedifferentiated cells. These cells are then imbedded in a type I/III collagen membrane bilayer and sent back to the surgeon for implantation (60).

The implant procedure is performed in a tourniquet-controlled bloodless field. The joint is exposed with a small anterolateral or anteromedial incision and the use of a malleolar osteotomy is generally not required. The use of a limited plafondoplasty, as described by Assenmacher et al., can improve access (70). The defect is prepared to stable margins using a curette and a template of the lesion is prepared. The graft is cut from the MACI membrane and placed into the defect on top of a layer of fibrin-tissue sealant. The graft stability is tested with range of motion of the ankle joint.

The postoperative protocol involved no weight bearing for 6 weeks. A splint was used until the incision was healed, and then gentle range of motion exercises were permitted. Partial weight bearing was allowed after 6 weeks, full weight bearing after 12 weeks, joint loading after 6 months, and return to sport was allowed after 12 months (Fig. 13.17).

AUTHORS' PREFERRED TECHNIQUE: FRESH HEMI-TALUS ALLOGRAFT

The patient is placed supine on the operating table. Perioperative antibiotics are given and a thigh tourniquet is placed. A small bump is placed under the ipsilateral hip. The operative lower extremity is prepped and draped in a sterile fashion. A unilateral external fixator is applied medially with half-pins in the talar neck, calcaneus, and two in the tibia. The external fixator

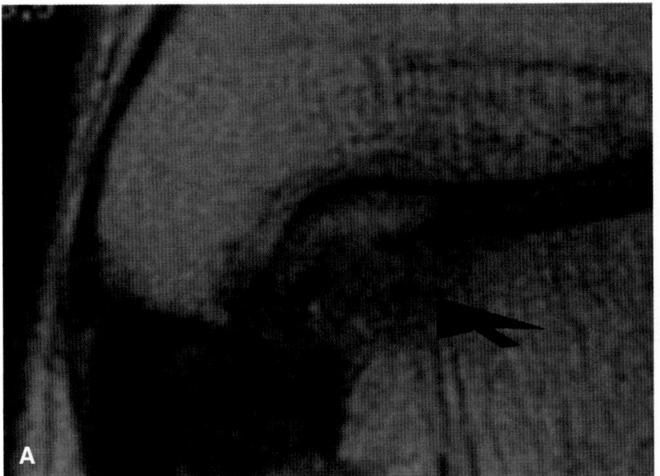

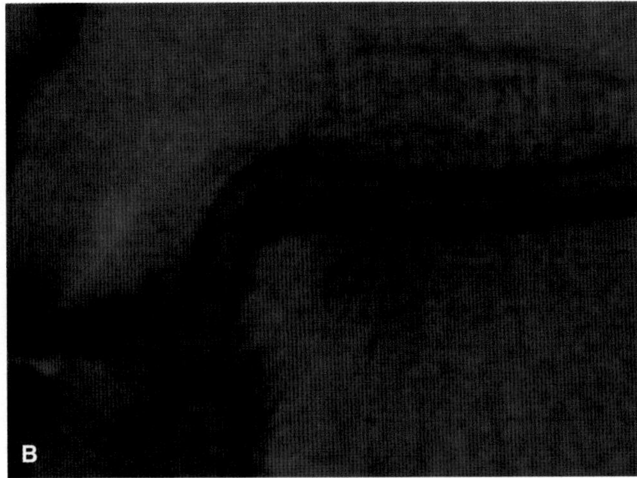

Figure 13.17. Preoperative coronal T1-weighted MRI showing a medial talus OCD which failed arthroscopy and microfracture *(arrow)* **(A)**. Postoperative T1 MRI 19 months after a MACI procedure showing restoration of the subchondral bone and cartilage **(B)**.

is locked into place to the patient's native alignment and then removed to be used later for joint distraction. The external fixator frame is removed and the pins left in place. The leg is exsanguinated and the tourniquet inflated to 275 mm Hg.

For medial-sided lesions, an anterior approach to the ankle is made between the interval of the extensor hallucis longus and tibialis anterior tendons. An anterolateral approach is made for lateral talar defects. Care is taken to avoid the branches of the superficial peroneal nerve and the deep bundle during the approach. The ankle joint is exposed by subperiostal dissection and debridement of osteophytes is performed with an osteotome and rongeurs. The external fixator is re-applied and is used to distract the ankle joint. Over-distraction is avoided to prevent disruption of the deltoid ligament (Fig. 13.18).

The medial or lateral osteochondral defect is clearly visualized at this point. The recipient site is first prepared with a scalpel to make a midline, full-length sagittal cut in the articular cartilage of the talar dome. A high-speed micro-oscillating saw with a long, 10 mm wide thin blade is used to make the midline sagittal and horizontal cuts in the talus to remove the lesion. The horizontal cut is started at the interface of the articular cartilage and talar neck, and directed posterior. The removed hemi-talus is used later as a template for the donor graft.

The fresh talar osteochondral allograft must be the same size, shape and match the same extremity (left/right) as the native talus. The allograft is prepared in a similar fashion to the recipient, and the thickness of the talar dome cut is approximately 7 mm. To minimize the potential for an immunologic response, wash the graft with high-pressure pulse lavage to remove marrow elements.

The donor graft is implanted into the recipient ankle carefully so as to not fracture the graft. The external fixator is removed and the ankle is brought through a range of motion. A graft that sits 1 to 2 mm proud is not problematic as the graft will likely settle over time as it incorporates. The image intensifier is used to confirm that the graft has complete apposition to bone and that the articular cartilage of the talus had been restored. The graft is fixed with cannulated, partially threaded,

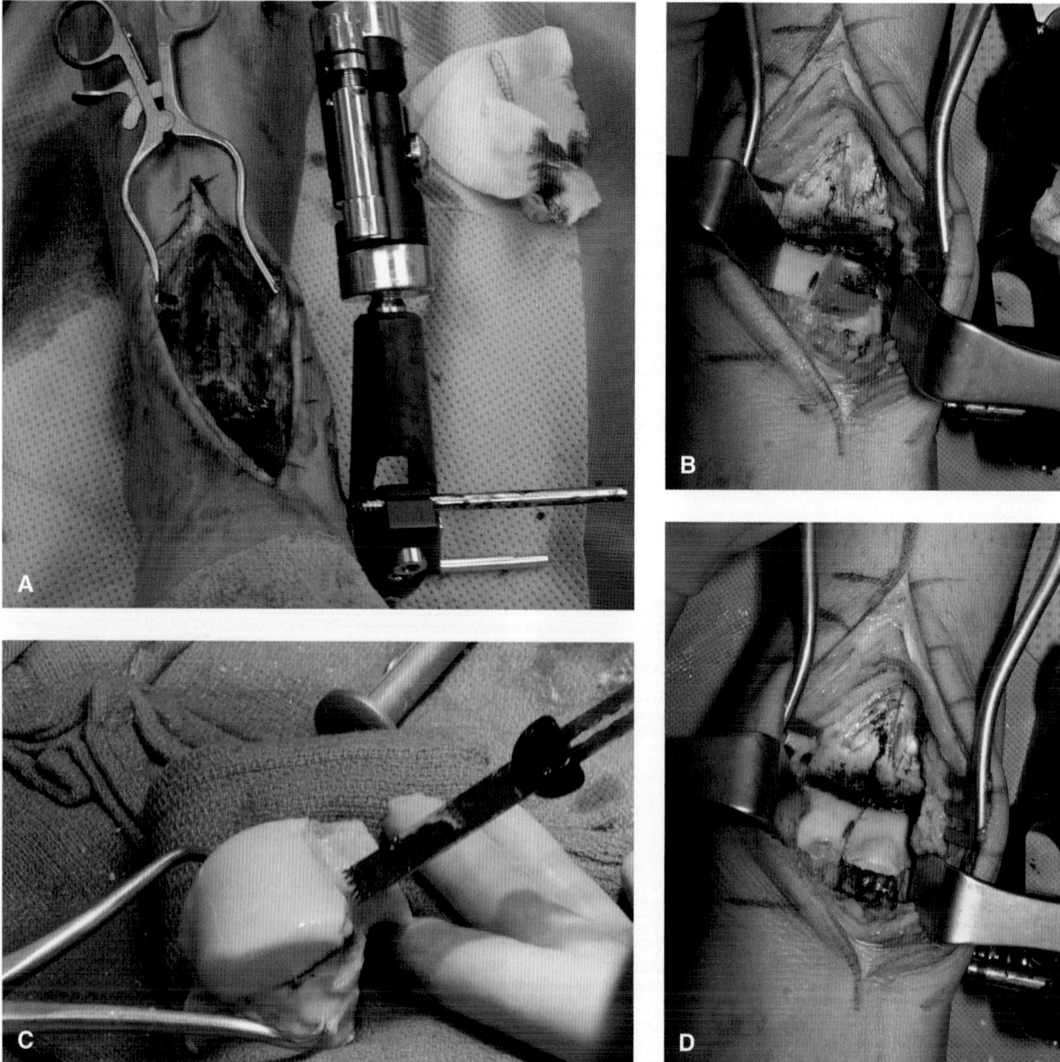

Figure 13.18. Intra-operative photograph of an ankle with a unilateral external fixator placed in preparation for a hemi-talus allograft (**A**). Photograph of the recipient talus prepared (**B**). Preparation of the allograft is performed on the back table (**C**). The allograft is then placed into the recipient (**D**).

countersunk screws to prevent subluxation. Testing for Achilles contracture is performed and treated tendoachilles lengthening as needed. The wounds are irrigated and the incision is closed in layers.

SUMMARY

Osteochondral defects of the talus in the athlete continue to be a challenging entity. The role of ankle instability as both an acute and chronic etiology is evident. Early attempts at stimulating healing, whether by curettage and/or drilling and microfracture have been shown to be equivalent. Patients with failed first-line treatments are candidates for cartilage replacement surgeries such as OATS, ACI and MACI. Larger, non-healing lesions are potential candidates for bulk osteochondral allografts. Development of precise indications, optimal rehabilitation, all-arthroscopic techniques, and advanced biomaterials to accelerate healing are current topics of ongoing investigation.

REFERENCES

1. Kannus P, Renström P. Treatment for acute tears of the lateral ligaments of the ankle. Operation, cast, or early controlled mobilization. *J Bone Joint Surg Am Vol* 1991;73(2):305–312.
2. Flick AB, Gould N. Osteochondritis dissecans of the talus (transchondral fractures of the talus): review of the literature and new surgical approach for medial dome lesions. *Foot Ankle* 1985;5(4):165–185.
3. Lindholm TS, Osterman K, Vankka E. Osteochondritis dissecans of elbow, ankle and hip: a comparison survey. *Clin Orthop Relat Res* 1980;(148):245–253.
4. Loren GJ, Ferkel RD. Arthroscopic assessment of occult intra-articular injury in acute ankle fractures. *Arthroscopy* 2002;18(4):412–421.
5. Hintermann B, Boss A, Schafer D. Arthroscopic findings in patients with chronic ankle instability. *Am J Sports Med* 2002;30(3):402–409.
6. Mulfinger GL, Trueta J. The blood supply of the talus. *J Bone Joint Surg Br* 1970;52(1):160–167.
7. Demirci S, Jubel A, Andermahr J, et al. Chondral thickness and radii of curvature of the femoral condyles and talar trochlea. *Int J Sports Med* 2008;29(4):327–330.
8. Athanasiou KA, Niederauer GG, Schenck RC Jr. Biomechanical topography of human ankle cartilage. *Ann Biomed Eng* 1995;23(5):697–704.
9. Sugimoto K, Takakura Y, Tohno Y, et al. Cartilage thickness of the talar dome. *Arthroscopy* 2005;21(4):401–404.
10. Alexander AH, Lichtman DM. Surgical treatment of transchondral talar-dome fractures (osteochondritis dissecans). Long-term follow-up. *J Bone Joint Surg Am* 1980;62(4):646–652.
11. Woods K, Harris I. Osteochondritis dissecans of the talus in identical twins. *J Bone Joint Surg Br* 1995;77(2):331.
12. Berndt AL, Harty M. Transchondral fractures (osteochondritis dissecans) of the talus. *J Bone Joint Surg Am* 1959;41-A:988–1020.
13. Elias I, Zoga AC, Morrison WB, et al. Osteochondral lesions of the talus: localization and morphologic data from 424 patients using a novel anatomical grid scheme. *Foot Ankle Int* 2007;28(2):154–161.
14. Noguchi K. Biomechanical analysis for osteoarthritis of the ankle. *Nippon Seikeigeka Gakkai Zasshi* 1985;59(2):215–222.
15. van Dijk CN, Bossuyt PM, Marti RK. Medial ankle pain after lateral ligament rupture. *J Bone Joint Surg Br* 1996;78(4):562–567.
16. Tochigi Y, Rudert MJ, McKinley TO, et al. Correlation of dynamic cartilage contact stress aberrations with severity of instability in ankle incongruity. *J Orthop Res* 2008;26(9):1186–1193.
17. Robinson DE, Winson IG, Harries WJ, et al. Arthroscopic treatment of osteochondral lesions of the talus. [see comment]. *J Bone Joint Surg Br* 2003;85(7):989–993.
18. Loomer R, Fisher C, Lloyd-Smith R, et al. Osteochondral lesions of the talus. *Am J Sports Med* 1993;21(1):13–19.
19. Verhagen RA, Maas M, Dijkgraaf MG, et al. Prospective study on diagnostic strategies in osteochondral lesions of the talus. Is MRI superior to helical CT? *J Bone Joint Surg Br* 2005;87(1):41–46.
20. Dipaola JD, Nelson DW, Colville MR. Characterizing osteochondral lesions by magnetic resonance imaging. *Arthroscopy* 1991;7(1):101–104.
21. Ferkel RD, Flannigan BD, Elkins BS. Magnetic resonance imaging of the foot and ankle: correlation of normal anatomy with pathologic conditions. *Foot Ankle* 1991;11(5):289–305.
22. Bachmann G, Jurgensen I, Siaplaouras J. The staging of osteochondritis dissecans in the knee and ankle joints with MR tomography. A comparison with conventional radiology and arthroscopy. *Rofo* 1995;163(1):38–44.
23. Mintz DN, Tashjian GS, Connell DA, et al. Osteochondral lesions of the talus: a new magnetic resonance grading system with arthroscopic correlation. *Arthroscopy* 2003;19(4):353–359.
24. Hepple S, Winson IG, Glew D. Osteochondral lesions of the talus: a revised classification. *Foot Ankle Int* 1999;20(12):789–793.
25. Kumai T, Takakura Y, Higashiyama I, et al. Arthroscopic drilling for the treatment of osteochondral lesions of the talus. *J Bone Joint Surg Am* 1999;81(9):1229–1235.
26. Anderson IF, Crichton KJ, Grattan-Smith T, et al. Osteochondral fractures of the dome of the talus. *J Bone Joint Surg Am* 1989;71(8):1143–1152.
27. Mologne TS, Ferkel RD. Arthroscopic treatment of osteochondral lesions of the distal tibia. *Foot Ankle Int* 2007;28(8):865–872.
28. Scranton PE Jr, Frey CC, Feder KS. Outcome of osteochondral autograft transplantation for type-V cystic osteochondral lesions of the talus. *J Bone Joint Surg Br* 2006;88(5):614–619.
29. Tol JL, et al. Treatment strategies in osteochondral defects of the talar dome: a systematic review. *Foot Ankle Int* 2000;21(2):119–126.
30. Mandelbaum BR, Gerhardt MB, Peterson L. Autologous chondrocyte implantation of the talus. *Arthroscopy* 2003;19 Suppl 1:129–137.
31. Elias I, Jung JW, Raikin SM, et al. Osteochondral lesions of the talus: change in MRI findings over time in talar lesions without operative intervention and implications for staging systems. *Foot Ankle Int* 2006;27(3):157–166.
32. Ferkel RD, Zanotti RM, Komenda GA, et al. Arthroscopic treatment of chronic osteochondral lesions of the talus: long-term results. *Am J Sports Med* 2008;36(9):1750–1762.
33. SooHoo NF, Vyas R, Samimi D. Responsiveness of the foot function index, AOFAS clinical rating systems, and SF-36 after foot and ankle surgery. *Foot Ankle Int* 2006;27(11):930–934.
34. O'Driscoll SW. The healing and regeneration of articular cartilage. *J Bone Joint Surg Am* 1998;80(12):1795–1812.
35. Kumai T, Takakura Y, Kitada C, et al. Fixation of osteochondral lesions of the talus using cortical bone pegs. *J Bone Joint Surg Br* 2002;84(3):369–374.
36. Taranow WS, Bisignani GA, Towers JD, et al. Retrograde drilling of osteochondral lesions of the medial talar dome. *Foot Ankle Int* 1999;20(8):474–480.
37. Kono M, Takao M, Naito K, et al. Retrograde drilling for osteochondral lesions of the talar dome. *Am J Sports Med* 2006;34(9):1450–1456.
38. Baker CL Jr, Morales RW. Arthroscopic treatment of transchondral talar dome fractures: a long-term follow-up study. *Arthroscopy* 1999;15(2):197–202.
39. Becher C, Thermann H. Results of microfracture in the treatment of articular cartilage defects of the talus. *Foot Ankle Int* 2005;26(8):583–589.
40. Schuman L, Struijs PA, van Dijk CN. Arthroscopic treatment for osteochondral defects of the talus. Results at follow-up at 2 to 11 years. *J Bone Joint Surg Br* 2002;84(3):364–368.
41. Savva N, Jabur M, Davies M, et al. Osteochondral lesions of the talus: results of repeat arthroscopic debridement. *Foot Ankle Int* 2007;28(6):669–673.
42. Carreira DS, Scranton PE Jr. Clinical tip: retrograde osteochondral autograft transfer system. *Foot Ankle Int* 2007;28(11):1200–1203.
43. Schäfer DB. Cartilage repair of the talus. *Foot Ankle Clin* 2003;8(4):739–749.
44. Reddy S, Pedowitz DI, Parekh SG, et al. The morbidity associated with osteochondral harvest from asymptomatic knees for the treatment of osteochondral lesions of the talus. *Am J Sports Med* 2007;35(1):80–85.
45. Al-Shaikh RA, Chou LB, Mann JA, et al. Autologous osteochondral grafting for talar cartilage defects. *Foot Ankle Int* 2002;23(5):381–389.
46. Hangody L. The mosaicplasty technique for osteochondral lesions of the talus. *Foot Ankle Clin* 2003;8(2):259–273.
47. Gobbi A, Kon E, Berruto M, et al. Patellofemoral full-thickness chondral defects treated with Hyalograft-C: a clinical, arthroscopic, and histologic review. *Am J Sports Med* 2006;34(11):1763–1773.
48. Muir D, Saltzman CL, Tochigi Y, et al. Talar dome access for osteochondral lesions. *Am J Sports Med* 2006;34(9):1457–1463.
49. Meehan R, McFarlin S, Bugbee W, et al. Fresh ankle osteochondral allograft transplantation for tibiotalar joint arthritis. *Foot Ankle Int* 2005;26(10):793–802.
50. Tasto JP, Ostrander R, Bugbee W, et al. The diagnosis and management of osteochondral lesions of the talus: osteochondral allograft update. *Arthroscopy* 2003;19 Suppl 1:138–141.
51. Ohlendorf C, Tomford WW, Mankin HJ. Chondrocyte survival in cryopreserved osteochondral articular cartilage. *J Orthop Res* 1996;14(3):413–416.
52. Rodrigo JJ, Thompson E, Travis C. Deep-freezing versus 4 degrees preservation of avascular osteocartilaginous shell allografts in rats. *Clin Orthop Relat Res* 1987;(218):268–275.
53. Stevenson S, Dannucci GA, Sharkey NA, et al. The fate of articular cartilage after transplantation of fresh and cryopreserved tissue-antigen-matched and mismatched osteochondral allografts in dogs. *J Bone Joint Surg Am* 1989;71(9):1297–1307.
54. Malinin T, Temple HT, Buck BE. Transplantation of osteochondral allografts after cold storage. *J Bone Joint Surg Am* 2006;88(4):762–770.
55. Williams SK, Amiel D, Ball ST, et al. Prolonged storage effects on the articular cartilage of fresh human osteochondral allografts. *J Bone Joint Surg Am* 2003;85-A(11):2111–2120.
56. Gross AE, Agnidis Z, Hutchison CR. Osteochondral defects of the talus treated with fresh osteochondral allograft transplantation. *Foot Ankle Int* 2001;22(5):385–391.
57. Kim CW, Jamali A, Tontz W Jr, et al. Treatment of post-traumatic ankle arthrosis with bipolar tibiotalar osteochondral shell allografts. *Foot Ankle Int* 2002;23(12):1091–1102.
58. Berlet GC, H.C., Philbin TM. *Successful use of fresh-frozen osteochondral allograft for the management of osteochondral lesions of the talus: A prospective study.* in *Presented at the American Orthopaedic Foot and Ankle Society 24th annual Summer Meeting, Denver.* 2008.
59. Myerson MS. *Synthetic (Nexa) plug.* in *American Orthopaedic Foot and Ankle Society, 23rd Annual Summer, Final Program.* 2007; Toronto.
60. Mandelbaum BR, Gerhardt MB, Peterson L. Autologous chondrocyte implantation of the talus. Arthroscopy: the journal of arthroscopic & related surgery: official publication of the Arthroscopy Association of North America and the International Arthroscopy Association. *Arthroscopy* 2003;19(Suppl 1):129–137.
61. Whittaker JP, Smith G, Makwana N, et al. Early results of autologous chondrocyte implantation in the talus. [erratum appears in J Bone Joint Surg Br. 2005 Jun;87(6):886]. *J Bone Joint Surg Br* 2005;87(2):179–183.

62. Koulalis D, Schultz W, Psychogios B, et al. Articular reconstruction of osteochondral defects of the talus through autologous chondrocyte transplantation. *Orthopedics* 2004; 27(6):559–561.
63. Giannini S, Buda R, Grigolo B, et al. Autologous chondrocyte transplantation in osteochondral lesions of the ankle joint. *Foot Ankle Int* 2001;22(6):513–517.
64. Baums MH, Heidrich G, Schultz W, et al. Autologous chondrocyte transplantation for treating cartilage defects of the talus. [reprint in J Bone Joint Surg Am. 2007 Sep;89 Suppl 2 Pt.2:170–182; PMID: 17768213]. *J Bone Joint Surg Am* 2006;88(2):303–308.
65. Zheng MH, Willers C, Kirilak L, et al. Matrix-induced autologous chondrocyte implantation (MACI): biological and histological assessment. *Tissue Eng* 2007;13(4):737–746.
66. Marlovits S, Striessnig G, Kutscha-Lissberg F, et al. Early postoperative adherence of matrix-induced autologous chondrocyte implantation for the treatment of full-thickness cartilage defects of the femoral condyle. *Knee Surg Sports Traumatol Arthrosc* 2005;13(6): 451–457.
67. Cherubino P, Grassi FA, Bulgheroni P, et al. Autologous chondrocyte implantation using a bilayer collagen membrane: a preliminary report. *J Orthop Surg (Hong Kong)* 2003;11(1):10–15.
68. Ronga M, Grassi FA, Montoli C, et al. Treatment of deep cartilage defects of the ankle with matrix-induced autologous chondrocyte implantation (MACI). *Foot Ankle Surg* 2005;11:29–33.
69. Giza E, Sullivan M, Ocel D, et al. Matrix induced Autologous chondrocyte implantation of talus articular defects. *Foot Ankle Int* 2010;31(9):747–753.
70. Assenmacher JA, Kelikian AS, Gottlob C, et al. Arthroscopically assisted autologous osteochondral transplantation for osteochondral lesions of the talar dome: an MRI and clinical follow-up study. *Foot Ankle Int* 2001;22(7):544–551.

CHAPTER

14

Clifford Jeng

Peroneal Tendon Disorders

ANATOMY

The lateral compartment of the calf contains the peroneus longus and peroneus brevis. The peroneus longus originates from the upper two-thirds of the fibula, the head of the fibula, the intermuscular septum, and the lateral condyle of the tibia. It inserts distally onto the plantar lateral margin of the base of the first metatarsal and the medial cuneiform. The peroneus brevis originates from the lower two-thirds of the fibula and the intermuscular septum. It inserts onto the styloid process of the base of the fifth metatarsal.

The peroneus longus and brevis are both innervated by the superficial peroneal nerve proximally in the calf. The blood supply to the tendons is derived from the posterior peroneal artery, which feeds the vinculae that attach posterolaterally on the peroneus longus and peroneus brevis tendons. A cadaver study demonstrated three hypovascular zones over the course of the peroneal tendons. Both tendons have an ischemic region at the tip of the fibula where they each make a sharp turn anteriorly. The third hypovascular zone occurs in the peroneus longus tendon as it passes sharply beneath the cuboid notch. Each of these areas represents a zone of high stress where "wringing out" of the vascularity to the tendon may occur. They also correspond to the most frequent locations where tears arise (1).

Proximal to the tip of the fibula, the two tendons share a common synovial sheath which extends 2.5 to 3.5 cm above the tip of the fibula. The peroneus brevis tendon has a flattened ovoid shape and lies directly against the posterior aspect of the lateral malleolus. The more round-shaped peroneus longus tendon lies posterior to the brevis and effectively compresses it up against the back of the fibula, causing significant mechanical pressure on the interposed tendon. This may lead to tears of the peroneus brevis over time.

Just distal to the tip of the fibula, both tendons make their first turn anteriorly toward the peroneal tubercle, a bony prominence on the lateral tuberosity of the calcaneus. The peroneus brevis passes superiorly over the peroneal tubercle, and the peroneus longus passes inferiorly beneath the tubercle. At the level of the peroneal tubercle, the tendons separate into their own individual tendon sheaths. The peroneus brevis continues distally to insert into the base of the fifth metatarsal. The peroneus longus makes a second turn inferomedially beneath the tubercle and then proceeds toward the cuboid notch where it makes its third turn running obliquely under the midfoot toward its insertion on the first metatarsal and medial cuneiform. As it passes anteromedially beneath the midfoot, it is covered by another synovial sheath, the plantar peroneal tunnel (2).

Two anatomical structures are primarily responsible for stabilizing the peroneal tendons within the retrofibular groove. A fibrocartilaginous ridge is present along the posterolateral border of the distal fibula. This prominent ridge deepens the retrofibular groove by 2 to 4 mm and blends with the periosteum laterally. It functions as a "bumper" to prevent the tendons from subluxing. The second stabilizing structure is the superior peroneal retinaculum (SPR) which is a strong fascial band that extends from the posterolateral surface of the fibula to the lateral wall of the calcaneus and Achilles sheath. This ligament, which begins approximately 2 cm above the tip of the fibula, confines the peroneal tendons within the retrofibular groove.

Both the peroneus longus and peroneus brevis muscles function to evert the foot and plantarflex the ankle. The peroneus longus provides 35% of the total hindfoot eversion power and the peroneus brevis provides 28%. In addition, the peroneus longus plantarflexes the first ray and is an antagonist to the anterior tibial tendon. The peroneus brevis is the primary abductor of the forefoot and is therefore an antagonist to the posterior tibial tendon. Both muscles are found to be active primarily during the stance phase of gait. The peroneals act as dynamic secondary stabilizers to ankle inversion injuries, and when trained appropriately can compensate for a torn or stretched lateral ligament complex (3).

PERONEUS BREVIS INJURY

MECHANISM OF INJURY

Pathology of the peroneus brevis can range from tendonitis to tenosynovitis to frank tearing of the tendon (Fig. 14.1). Mechanical factors, postural issues, and trauma are responsible for the acute inflammation of the tendon and tendon sheath which may lead to eventual thickening and rupture of the peroneus brevis tendon.

Anatomically, the peroneus brevis tendon lies wedged between the tendon of the peroneus longus and the posterior aspect of the fibula. As the two tendons turn sharply beneath the tip of the fibula to head toward their respective insertions, a significant amount of pressure is applied to the peroneus brevis

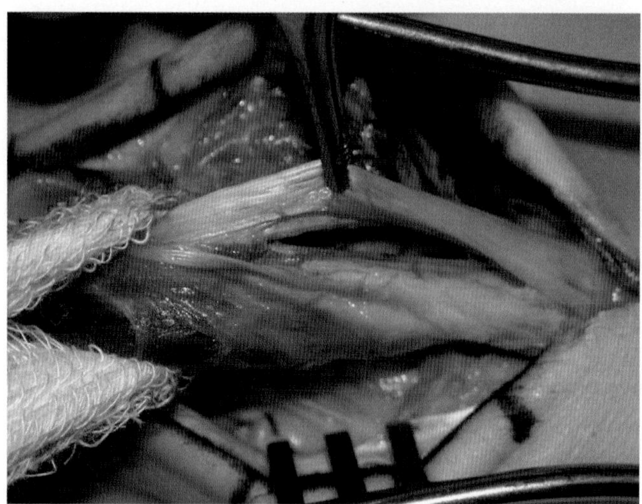

Figure 14.1. A central-splitting tear of the peroneus brevis is shown. Note the presence of a low-lying muscle belly which can overcrowd the peroneal tendon sheath and increase the risk for tears.

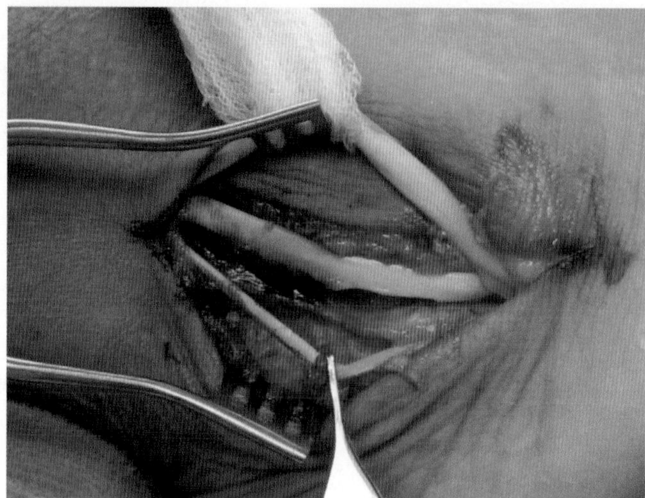

Figure 14.2. The third and smallest tendon shown at the bottom of the photograph is a peroneus quartus. This tendon originates from the peroneus brevis and inserts on the lateral wall of the calcaneus and can cause increased pressure within the peroneal sheath leading to tears.

potentially causing mechanical attrition of the tendon. Cadaver studies have consistently found peroneus brevis injuries to occur at this site, with a midsubstance longitudinal tear centered over the tip of the fibula within the retrofibular groove (4). This mechanical trauma can also result in inflammation and thickening of the tendon sheath which may impair free excursion of the tendon (5).

Additional anatomic factors may contribute to mechanical attrition of the peroneus brevis. The peroneus brevis has a very long musculotendinous junction which in some patients may extend inferior to the level of the ankle joint. Because the peroneal tendons are confined within the retrofibular groove by the peroneal retinaculum, the presence of a low-lying peroneus brevis muscle belly can result in a volume effect, over-stuffing the tendon sheath. Another contributing factor is the presence of an anomalous peroneus quartus muscle within the peroneal sheath. The peroneus quartus originates from the peroneus brevis muscle and inserts onto the peroneal tubercle on the lateral wall of the calcaneus. Its incidence has been quoted to be between 6.6% and 22%. It is yet another potential source of increased pressure within the peroneal tunnel, and its presence has been associated with stenosing tenosynovitis as well as with peroneal tubercle hypertrophy. The relative risk of a peroneus brevis tear in a patient with an anomalous peroneus quartus is doubled (4,6,7) (Fig. 14.2).

Postural problems such as significant hindfoot varus may be a source of peroneal pathology. Hindfoot varus dramatically increases the forces through both the peroneus longus and peroneus brevis. Trauma may also be responsible for peroneus brevis tears, particularly in patients with recurrent injuries such as frequent inversion sprains due to lateral ankle ligament instability. Up to 25% of patients with chronic lateral ankle ligament instability will have a peroneus brevis tear. 77% of these patients will have peroneal synovitis (8). Another mechanism of trauma is by subluxation or frank dislocation of the peroneal tendons out of the retromalleolar groove due to an incompetent SPR. The sharp posterolateral edge of the fibula can create a longitudinal split in an over-riding peroneus brevis. Intra-sheath subluxation of the tendons with an intact overlying retinaculum has also been described to cause longitudinal tears of the peroneus brevis (9).

Although acute inflammation is present in the earlier stages of peroneal pathology, the histology of brevis tears shows no inflammatory infiltrates within the tendon itself. Instead, there is splaying of the collagen bundles with proliferation of blood vessels and fibrovascular connective tissue. This may indicate that the primary causative factor for peroneus brevis tears is mechanical and not due to chronic inflammation leading to degeneration (10).

CLINICAL FINDINGS

The hallmark of peroneus brevis pathology is pain, swelling, and tenderness over the posterolateral ankle localized over the peroneal sheath. There may be either a history of acute injury or of repetitive overuse. Patients often report "snapping" or "popping" in the posterolateral ankle, and may even be able to voluntarily dislocate the tendons over the edge of the fibula. Muscle weakness or tendon subluxation may cause episodes of ankle instability. Long-standing peroneal tendon insufficiency can lead to a flexible or rigid hindfoot varus deformity.

On physical examination, peroneus brevis problems typically present with visible and palpable swelling and tenderness more proximally than peroneus longus injuries. The peroneus brevis is generally more symptomatic in the retrofibular groove region down to the tip of the fibula. Peroneus longus tenderness is most commonly found from the tip of the fibula down to the peroneal tubercle and extending to the cuboid notch.

Further findings on examination include pain with passive stretching of the tendons by plantarflexing and inverting the ankle. There may be weakness with resisted eversion strength testing of the ankle. However, normal eversion strength does not rule out peroneus brevis pathology, as the peroneus longus can compensate for a torn brevis. During resisted eversion testing, the examiner should also look for (1) pain elicited by the test, (2) palpable or visible snapping of the tendons within the sheath, and (3) subluxation or frank dislocation of the tendons over the posterolateral edge of the fibula.

It is important for the physician to have a clear understanding of the differential diagnoses that can cause lateral ankle pain so that he may rule out other sources for the patient's complaints. These include (1) syndesmotic injury, (2) fracture of the fibula, (3) osteochondral lesion of the talus, (4) lateral ankle ligament sprain, (5) lateral process of the talus fracture, (6) anterior process of the calcaneus fracture, (7) calcaneocuboid joint avulsion fracture, and (8) base of the fifth metatarsal fracture. During the examination, it is important that each of these sites is carefully palpated to identify possible concomitant injuries.

Injection of the peroneal tendon sheath with a bupivacaine solution may be both diagnostic and therapeutic. Temporary resolution of the pain may be helpful in determining the contribution of the peroneals to the patient's symptoms. However, in 15% of patients, there is a communication between the peroneal tendon sheath and the ankle joint or subtalar joint which may confound the results of the diagnostic injection. Forceful injection of the tendon sheath may also be effective in releasing adhesions which may limit tendon excursion (11).

Magnetic resonance imaging is the diagnostic test of choice for evaluating the peroneal tendons. MRI is capable of evaluating peroneal tenosynovitis, tendon tears, superior peroneal retinacular injuries, and the morphology of the retrofibular groove (12). Tenosynovitis appears as increased signal intensity on T2-weighted images surrounding the peroneal tendons. When there is circumferential fluid around the tendons of greater than 3 mm diameter, the sensitivity and specificity are 17% and 100% respectively for detecting peroneal tenosynovitis (13,14). Peroneus brevis tears appear on MRI as intermediate T2 signal changes within the tendon, enlargement of the tendon, or loss of continuity. Frank tears will make the brevis tendon look either c-shaped or bisected into two parts on the axial views (Fig. 14.3). The sensitivity of MRI to detect peroneus brevis tears compared to intra-operative findings has been quoted anywhere between 83% and 92%. The specificity has been cited between 75% and 80%. The accuracy of predicting a brevis tear by MRI is 80% (8,14–16). Conflicting reports in the literature state that MRI both overestimates as well as underestimates the presence of peroneal pathology (17).

Dynamic ultrasonography is another modality that has been described as a useful office tool in diagnosing peroneal tendon tears. It has been noted to be able to detect fluid within the tendon sheath, thickening of the tendon, as well as tears and frank ruptures with a sensitivity of 100%, specificity of 85%, and accuracy of 90%. As with all ultrasound diagnostic testing, the results have been shown to be user dependent (18).

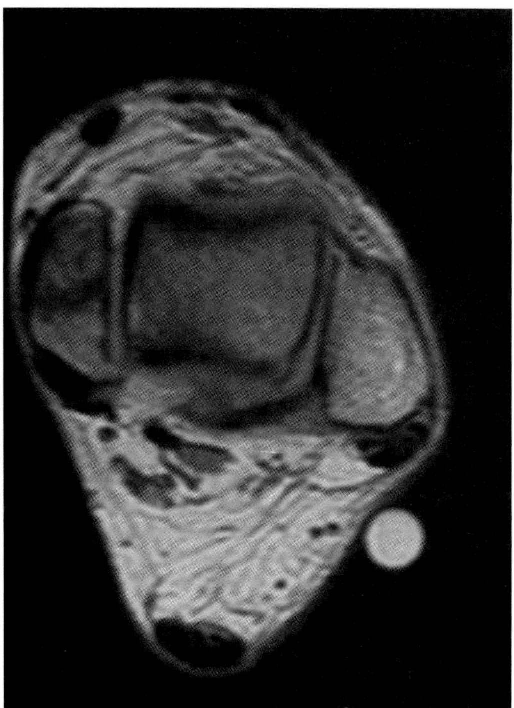

Figure 14.3. The axial T1-weighted image of the ankle shows a peroneus brevis tear. Note how the brevis which lies between the peroneus longus and the fibula appears to be bisected into two halves.

MANAGEMENT OF PERONEUS BREVIS INJURY

Conservative management for both peroneus brevis and peroneus longus pathology is similar. Because the tendons lie lateral to the subtalar joint axis, repetitive hindfoot inversion stretches the tendons and causes pain and inflammation. Immobilization with an ankle brace or cam walker can limit this motion providing symptomatic relief and allowing the tendons to recover. Perhaps even more effective is the use of a laterally posted shoe insert which forces the heel into valgus. This can further relax both peroneals within the tendon sheath.

Standard orthopedic modalities including non-steroidal anti-inflammatory drugs, cryotherapy, and rest may also be helpful for these conditions. Physical therapy may strengthen a weakened or injured peroneus brevis or longus. Brisement of the peroneal tendon sheath with bupivacaine may also release adhesions and permit more physiologic tendon excursion (11). Unfortunately, conservative management of peroneal pathology has been reported to fail in up to 83% of patients.

Surgical options for peroneus brevis problems range from simple tenosynovectomy to debridement of a low-lying muscle belly or accessory muscle, repair or debridement of a torn tendon, tenodesis to the longus, or tendon transfer. The surgical approach for each of these procedures is the same. Patients are positioned in the lateral decubitus position and a curvilinear skin incision is made over the course of the tendons just behind the fibula. The length of the incision is determined primarily by whether the patient's pain is located proximal or distal to the tip of the fibula. Subcutaneous dissection is carried out to expose the peroneal retinaculum, taking great care to avoid injuring the sural nerve. A critical step in all peroneal tendon surgery is correctly opening the SPR to expose the tendons. If the split in the SPR is made too anteriorly along the posterior edge of the fibula, there will be inadequate tissue to repair the posterior flap of the SPR at the end of the procedure. If the split in the SPR is made too far posterior to the fibular attachment, repair of the retinaculum may be impossible if a groove-deepening procedure is performed.

Once the tendons are exposed, there is usually a large amount of yellow proliferative synovitis surrounding the tendons. This is debrided off the tendons, being careful to avoid injury to the SPR which must be repaired later. If a low-lying muscle belly is found along the distal peroneus brevis tendon, this is excised as well to decompress the sheath. Similarly, if a peroneus quartus accessory muscle is identified, it should be excised. The tendons are then inspected individually for tears. It is important to carefully examine both the superficial and deep sides of each tendon looking for longitudinal splits along the length of the tendon or fusiform enlargement within the tendon.

If a peroneus brevis tear is identified, the decision must be made whether to repair or excise the tear. Krause recommended debridement of the damaged tendon and tubularization of the remaining intact peroneus brevis for Grade I tears which have greater than 50% of their cross-sectional area intact. Theoretically, there should be minimal functional deficit from this repair as demonstrated by the non-anatomic lateral ligament reconstructions (e.g., Chrisman–Snook) which routinely sacrifice half of the peroneus brevis. For Grade II tears in which greater than 50% of the cross-sectional area of the brevis is torn and not usable, Krause recommended resecting the diseased tendon and performing a tenodesis to the peroneus longus (19). The tenodesis should be done proximal to the tear in all cases so that the brevis muscle can contribute to eversion. Tenodesis distal to the tear should be done only if the distal tendon is healthy (20).

There are three other common scenarios which frequently occur while doing peroneal tendon surgery. The first is when the longitudinal tear is only on one side of the tendon and does not extend through to the other side. With a partial thickness tear, the interior of the tendon is debrided of any tendinosis or loose fibers and the edges are then repaired side-to-side with a running 4-0 suture. The second scenario is when the split in the tendon is directly down the middle with two reasonably healthy intact halves of the tendon available. When this occurs, it is up to the surgeon's judgment whether to sacrifice one limb of the torn tendon to avoid having to wait for tendon healing, or to repair the tear on both sides. Finally, in some cases, there is fusiform thickening and enlargement of the tendon seen with no tears visible on the surface of the tendon. If on pre-operative examination this area was felt to be the primary area of pain, the tendon should be incised longitudinally, the tendinosis debrided, and the cut edges of the tendon repaired with a running 4-0 suture.

Results following peroneus brevis repair show that although rehabilitation and return to maximum function may be prolonged, in general, a majority of patients report good to excellent results at final follow-up (19). In a recent series of patients following operative repair of the peroneal tendons, only 46% were able to successfully return to sports (16).

If a complete transverse rupture of the peroneus brevis is present, the distal end should be tenodesed to the peroneus longus so that the longus muscle can evert the hindfoot through a more biomechanically advantageous insertion into the base of the fifth metatarsal. If the rupture is recent and there is still good excursion of the peroneus brevis muscle, the proximal end should also be tenodesed to the longus to add additional hindfoot eversion power (21).

In the chronic situation where both the peroneus brevis and longus are ruptured and not usable, the tendons are excised and an allograft tendon can be interposed between the healthy muscle proximally and the tendon distally. However, if the proximal muscle belly is contracted and has poor excursion, a tendon transfer should be considered instead. Both the flexor digitorum longus (FDL) and the flexor hallucis longus (FHL) have been widely used for this purpose with good results (22,23). In patients with longstanding complete ruptures of both tendons, the peroneal sheath may become scarred or fibrotic (20). In this situation, a staged reconstruction is preferred with the temporary use of Hunter rods to re-establish the sheath and then secondary reconstruction with either an FDL or FHL transfer (20,23).

Associated pathology is common in patients with peroneal tendon tears, and these problems must also be addressed at the time of surgery to avoid failure or recurrence. In patients with peroneal tendon tears, 43% will have clinically significant lateral ankle ligament instability, 20% will have documented peroneal tendon subluxation, and anywhere from 32% to 82% will have some degree of hindfoot varus malalignment (17,20). Ankle instability can be corrected with either a Brostrom–Gould anatomic reconstruction or a non-anatomic repair using half of the peroneus brevis tendon if a tear is present. Peroneal tendon subluxation is addressed with either imbrication of the SPR or a groove-deepening procedure. A varus hindfoot must be re-aligned with a calcaneal osteotomy to relieve tension on the tendon repair (20).

Meticulous repair of the SPR is required after each of the above procedures to avoid subluxation of the tendons postoperatively. Early rehabilitation with passive mobilization of the tendons within the peroneal sheath is recommended to prevent painful scarring of the tendons.

PERONEUS LONGUS INJURY

MECHANISM OF INJURY

Tears of the peroneus longus are far less common than tears to the brevis (Fig. 14.4). They typically occur either at the tip of the fibula, at the peroneal tubercle, or at the cuboid notch. Each of these are areas of high stress and poor vascularity for

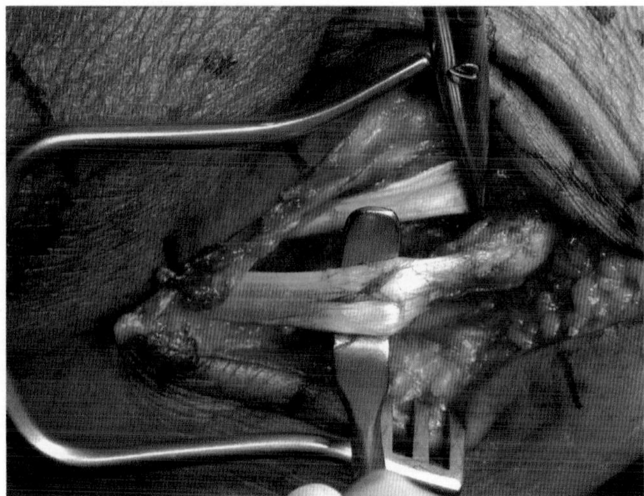

Figure 14.4. A longitudinal tear of the peroneus longus is shown overlying the retractor. Also note the enlargement of the peroneus longus tendon more distally due to the presence of an os peroneum.

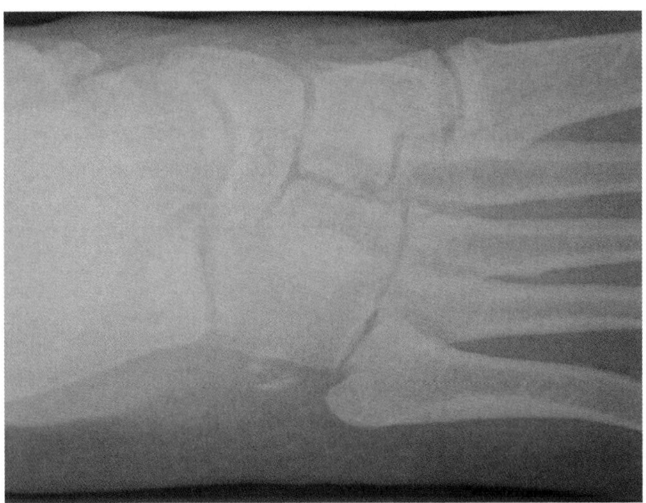

Figure 14.5. An os peroneum fracture is shown on this oblique radiograph of the foot. The fragmentation of the ossicle which can be seen here distinguishes it from a bipartite os peroneum.

the tendon (17). Because the peroneus longus and brevis are both secondary restraints to inversion stresses, they share similar risk factors for developing tears. Hindfoot varus was found to be present in 82% of patients with peroneus longus tendinopathy in one series. 33% of these patients also had associated peroneus brevis pathology (17). Peroneus longus tears are also frequently seen in patients with chronic lateral ankle ligament instability (24).

Painful os peroneum syndrome (POPS) is a term that was coined to indicate a spectrum of injuries related to the peroneus longus tendon. This syndrome includes the diagnoses of peroneus longus tenosynovitis, peroneus longus tears, enlarged peroneal tubercle, and os peroneum fracture (Figs. 14.4 and 14.5). These can all be sources of lateral hindfoot pain along the course of the peroneus longus from the tip of the fibula to the cuboid notch (25).

Tenosynovitis usually involves both peroneal tendons within their common sheath and may extend distally into their individual sheaths as well. A tear or a low-lying muscle belly may or may not be present. Peroneus longus tears can be either simple longitudinal tears or a complete rupture of the tendon proximal or distal to the os peroneum. An enlarged peroneal tubercle along the lateral wall of the calcaneal tuberosity can be the underlying cause for stenosing tenosynovitis or impingement of the peroneus longus. In an anatomic study, 29% of specimens had a prominent tubercle, whereas 70% had an either flat or concave peroneal tubercle (26).

An os peroneum fracture is the last diagnosis in the POPS spectrum. The os is a fibrocartilaginous sesamoid within the peroneus longus tendon that articulates with the cuboid notch as the tendon turns sharply to enter the plantar midfoot. It is uniformly present but is ossified in only 20% of patients (2). It is visible on plain radiographs of the foot in 10% to 20% of patients plantar to the cuboid near the calcaneocuboid joint. The os peroneum is anchored into the cuboid notch by two medial and two lateral ligamentous attachments resulting in minimal excursion of the tendon here. The os peroneum can be fractured either from a direct blow or from a forced eversion mechanism against a supinated foot (25).

CLINICAL FINDINGS

Patients with peroneus longus pathology often have a history of injury or ankle sprain. There may also be a history of an overuse injury or errors in training. They typically present with swelling and pain over the posterolateral ankle and hindfoot. A sensation of clicking, snapping or popping over the peroneals may be present. These patients often have a cavovarus foot alignment (17). Again, a useful generalization is that peroneus longus injuries are usually more symptomatic distal to the tip of the fibula, whereas brevis injuries have pain proximal to the tip of the fibula.

Plain x-rays are helpful in looking for a fractured os peroneum, as well as a proximally displaced os peroneum which would signify a peroneus longus complete rupture distal to the os. Radiographs can also identify signs of cavus foot deformity. Magnetic resonance imaging is useful in assessing for tenosynovitis along the length of the tendon. However, it can be difficult to evaluate peroneus longus tears due to the magic angle effect. Sometimes on the sagittal images, enlargement of the tendon or increased signal intensity within the tendon substance can be appreciated. MRI is also helpful in evaluating the size of the peroneal tubercle or edema within the os peroneum.

MANAGEMENT OF PERONEUS LONGUS INJURY

Non-operative treatment of peroneus longus injuries is similar to that of the brevis. Rest, immobilization, cryotherapy, and nonsteroidal anti-inflammatories are helpful in the acute stages of injury. Orthotic inserts with lateral heel posting to offload the peroneal tendons as well as early physical therapy to strengthen the muscles and promote smooth excursion of the tendons is critical in the later stages of rehabilitation. Conservative management will be successful in only 20% of patients, and the remaining 80% will usually require surgery (25).

Peroneus longus surgery often requires the skin incision to extend more distally along the course of the tendon to expose the os peroneum and the peroneal tubercle. The branches of the sural nerve are more prone to injury in this area and should be carefully identified and protected. Tenosynovitis should be debrided and accessory muscles or a low-lying muscle belly should be excised to decompress the tendons. The longus tendon is examined both on its deep and superficial aspects looking for tears or nodular thickening. Longitudinal tears are repaired with a running 4-0 suture. Tendinosis is incised and the degenerated portion of the tendon debrided, followed by repair of the split in the tendon. If there is a complete rupture of the tendon or if there is minimal salvageable tendon, then a tenodesis to the neighboring peroneus brevis is appropriate. Rarely, if a peroneus longus rupture distal to the os peroneum is diagnosed acutely, a direct end-to-end repair may be attempted (21).

A fractured os peroneum will usually be evident preoperatively. The fragments of the os peroneum should be excised sub-periosteally and the remaining shell of tendon reinforced with non-absorbable suture. Finally, if upon examination the peroneal tubercle is enlarged, both the peroneus longus and brevis sheaths are opened to decompress the tendons and the tubercle is exposed sub-periosteally (Fig. 14.6). An exostectomy is performed to relieve the abrasion and irritation on the peroneus longus. Bone wax is applied to the bleeding cancellous surface to prevent adhesions.

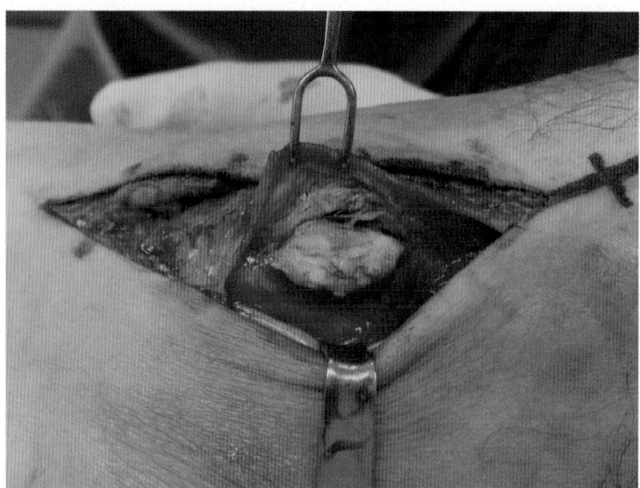

Figure 14.6. "Hypertrophic peroneal tubercle": A hypertrophic peroneal tubercle with the peroneus longus tendon retracted inferiorly. This enlarged tubercle can result in stenosing tenosynovitis and tears of the peroneus longus tendon.

PERONEAL TENDON DISLOCATION

MECHANISM OF INJURY

Subluxation or dislocation of the peroneal tendons can occur due to injury to the SPR, presence of a shallow or convex fibular groove, or generalized ligamentous laxity.

The SPR is the primary restraint to peroneal dislocation. The ligament arises from the posterior inferior edge of the fibula and has a variable insertion into either the calcaneus or the Achilles sheath or both. Five different patterns of SPR insertion have been described by Davis (27). Injury to the SPR can occur in four different patterns (Fig. 14.7). In Grade I injuries, the SPR remains attached but is lifted off the fibula sub-periosteally, creating a false pouch which the tendons can sublux into. This pattern occurs in 51% of cases. In a Grade II injury, the SPR remains attached but the fibrocartilaginous ridge is elevated. This occurs in 33% of patients. The SPR is avulsed off of the fibula in Grade III injuries along with a thin cortical fragment. Grade III injuries represent 16% of peroneal dislocation cases. Finally, Oden added a Grade IV to this classification system where the SPR is ruptured from its posterior attachments (28,29).

The shape of the posterior aspect of the fibula in the retromalleolar groove has been implicated as a potential cause for peroneal tendon dislocation. The fibular groove is concave in 82% of patients, flat in 11% of patients, and convex in 7% of patients (30). Flat or convex-shaped fibulas create a shallower groove which makes it easier for the tendons to dislocate. The groove is further deepened by the fibrocartilaginous cap on the posterolateral edge of the fibula. One histologic study showed that the groove depth was determined more by the fibrocartilaginous lip than by the posterior shape of the fibula (31).

Generalized ligamentous laxity can allow subtle subluxation of the peroneals over the posterolateral edge of the fibula bilaterally in normal asymptomatic patients. This repetitive slipping of the tendons may lead to tendon tears over time. Lateral ankle instability may predispose to SPR injury as well. Anatomic studies have demonstrated that the calcaneal band of the SPR runs parallel to the calcaneofibular component of the lateral

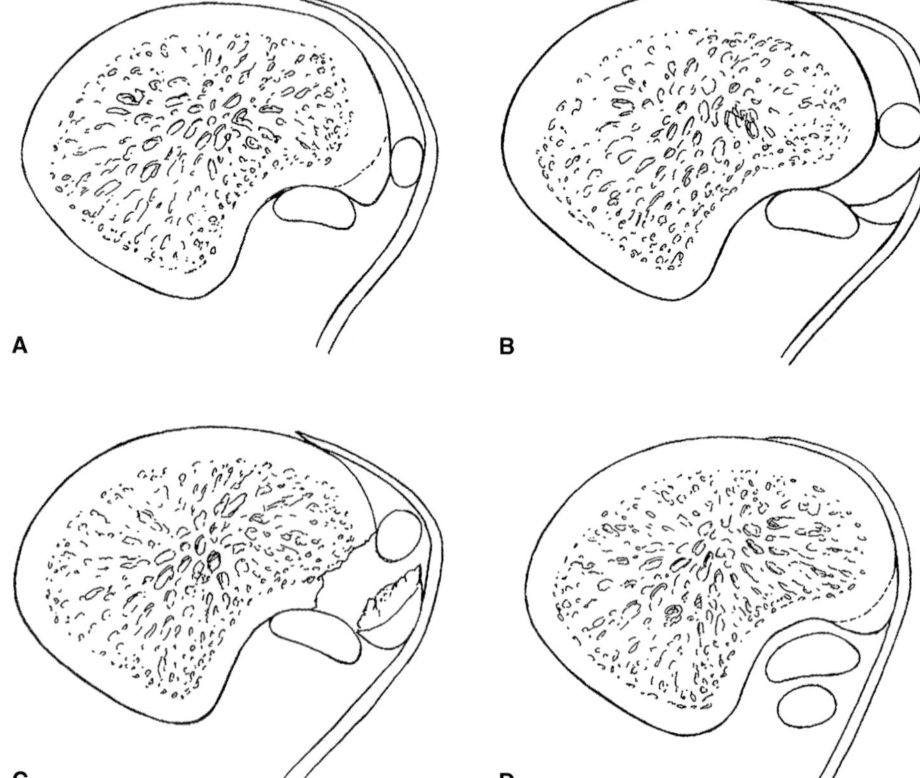

Figure 14.7. The classification for peroneal tendon dislocation injuries as described by Eckert and modified by Oden. **A:** In Grade I injuries, the SPR is lifted off the fibula sub-periosteally. **B:** In Grade II injuries, the fibrocartilaginous ridge is elevated off of the fibula. **C:** In Grade III injuries, the SPR is avulsed off of the fibula with a small cortical fragment attached. **D:** Oden added a Grade IV category to the classification system where the SPR ruptures from its posterior attachments on the calcaneus or Achilles sheath.

ankle ligament complex. Cutting studies confirm that dividing the lateral ankle ligaments places increased strain on the SPR, supporting the idea of the SPR being a secondary restraint to ankle inversion. Therefore in patients with chronic lateral ligament instability, the SPR can be injured or become attenuated leading to peroneal dislocation (32).

The most common mechanism of tendon dislocation is by a dorsiflexion and inversion type injury while the patient is forcefully contracting the peroneals. However, disruption of the SPR can also occur while the ankle is in plantarflexion, inversion, or eversion.

CLINICAL FINDINGS

Peroneal tendon dislocation often follows sporting injuries, particularly skiing. It is also commonly associated with ice skating, soccer, basketball, rugby, and gymnastics. 92% of cases are thought to be due to a traumatic incident (33). 42% of intra-articular calcaneus fractures have an associated dislocation of the peroneals (34).

Patients with peroneal dislocation complain of pain and swelling over the posterolateral ankle. They also report audible and visible "popping" or "snapping" of the tendons behind the malleolus which may cause buckling of the ankle secondary to pain. In many cases, the patient notices the tendon subluxing over the edge of the fibula or can voluntarily make the tendons dislocate. Unfortunately, delay in diagnosis is common, and more often than not the acute injury is misdiagnosed as a simple ankle sprain. What is clear is that, delay in diagnosis and treatment leads to poorer results and recurrence (35).

On physical examination, there is obvious tenderness and swelling over the peroneal sheath. There may be weakness with resisted eversion strength testing of the ankle. The subluxation and pain can be recreated with resisted dorsiflexion and eversion of the ankle from a plantarflexed and inverted position. Often the tendons may remain "locked out" over the edge of the fibula until manually reduced (Fig. 14.8). The apprehension test is done by performing the same provocative maneuver while manually stabilizing the tendons in the retrofibular groove. If the test is positive, holding the tendons in place relieves both the pain and apprehension of the tendons dislocating.

On plain radiographic examination, an avulsion fracture off of the lateral ridge of the fibula on the oblique ankle view is felt to be pathognomonic for a Grade III injury (28). MRI, however, is the study of choice to evaluate peroneal tendon dislocation. This can assess for disruption of the SPR, look for concurrent longus or brevis tendon tears, and evaluate the shape of the fibular groove (Fig. 14.9).

MANAGEMENT OF PERONEAL TENDON DISLOCATION

Conservative management of peroneal tendon dislocations consists of a short leg cast in plantarflexion and inversion for six weeks. Theoretically, this holds the tendons closely reduced within the retromalleolar groove allowing the SPR to heal and scar in as tightly as possible. Unfortunately, this treatment has been shown to have very high failure rates between 43% and 86% (28,35,36).

Due to these high failure rates, surgery may be indicated for acute SPR ruptures in younger patients or athletes. Surgical reconstruction should always be recommended for chronic dislocation. The various surgeries that have been described for the treatment of peroneal dislocations can be divided into five categories. These are (1) direct repair or imbrication of the SPR, (2) reconstruction of the SPR, (3) tendon rerouting procedures, (4) bone block procedures, and (5) groove-deepening procedures (Fig. 14.10).

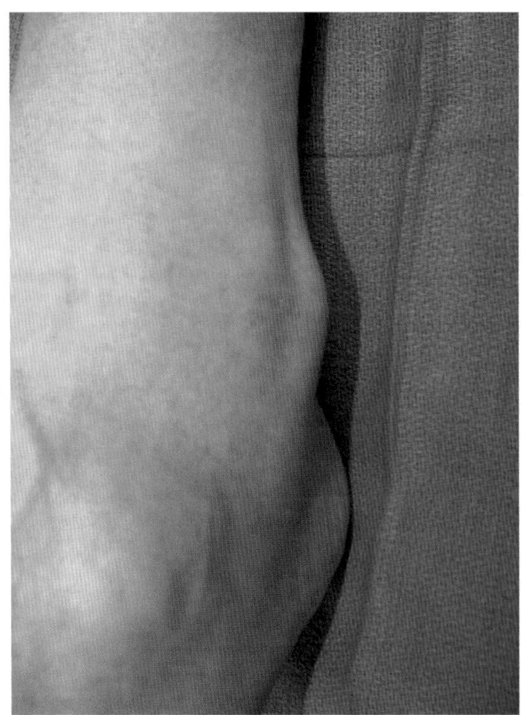

Figure 14.8. A patient with an SPR injury who could voluntarily dislocate his peroneal tendons.

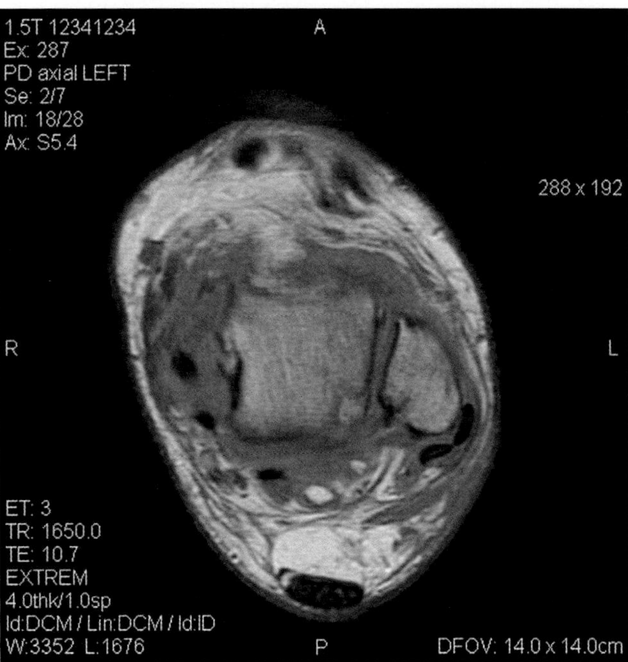

Figure 14.9. An axial T1-weighted MRI of a patient with peroneal tendon dislocation. Note the peroneal tendons sitting lateral to the fibula with the overlying avulsed SPR creating a false pouch.

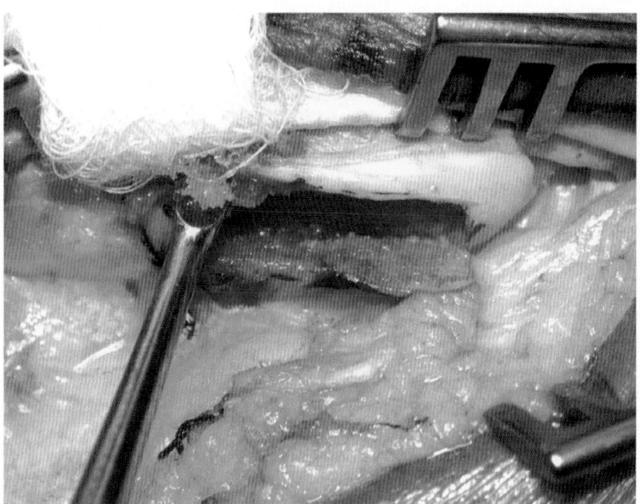

Figure 14.10. The fibular groove-deepening procedure for peroneal tendon dislocation. The osteoperiosteal hinge has been elevated and a curette is being used to remove the underlying cancellous bone to deepen the groove.

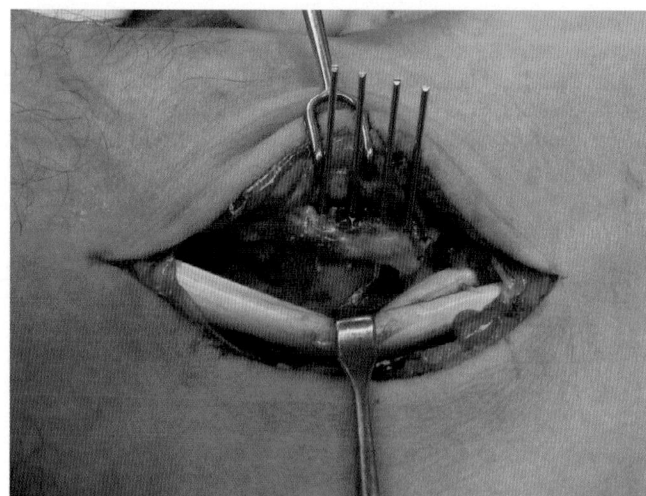

Figure 14.12. "Pins in fibula": Preparation for repair of the avulsed SPR begins with k-wire holes drilled into the posterolateral ridge of the fibula.

The surgical approach is the same as the preceding descriptions. Again, it is critical to correctly plan the location of the incision into the SPR so that the ligament can be properly repaired after the selected procedure. If a direct repair is planned, then an incision in the middle of the SPR with an adequate cuff of tissue left on the posterior edge of the fibula will allow ample ligament to imbricate the two edges. However, if a groove deepening is planned, then the incision in the SPR should be placed directly behind the fibula with no cuff of tissue remaining. This will provide a long posterior flap that can reach the deepened groove and cover the peroneal tendons adequately.

With direct repair, after a synovectomy is performed and any tears in the tendons addressed, the SPR is imbricated tightly in a pants-over-vest fashion to tighten the incompetent ligament. This has high reported success rates with anywhere from 85% to 100% good to excellent results at final 9.3-year follow-up (37). In Grade I and Grade II injuries where the SPR or fibrocartilaginous ridge has been avulsed off the posterolateral fibula, the ligament should be directly sutured back down onto the malleolus through K-wire holes drilled through the lateral ridge of bone (Figs. 14.11,14.12,14.13). This repair has 96% good to excellent results reported with only a 5% redislocation rate (28).

Reconstruction of an incompetent SPR can be performed in several ways. One approach is to mobilize the distal end of the CFL with an attached block of bone off the lateral wall of the calcaneus and then reattaching the bone block with the peroneal tendons contained underneath the ligament. This could similarly be done with a proximally based bone block

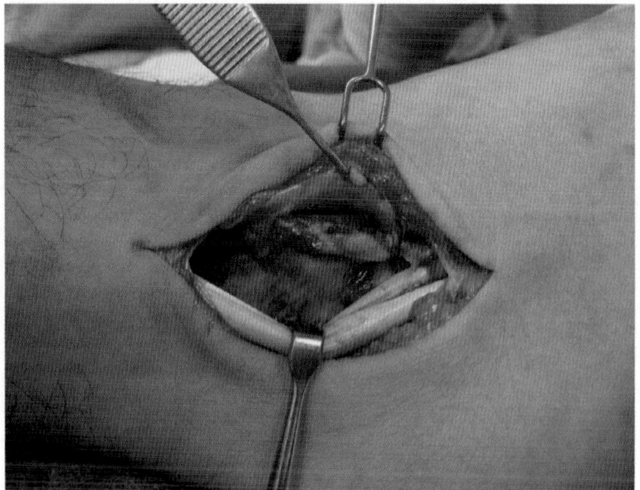

Figure 14.11. "Avulsion of the SPR": A patient with a 2-week-old injury who had a visible "fleck" sign on plain x-rays consistent with an Eckert Grade III injury. Surgical findings showed an avulsion of the SPR off of the fibula with slight thickening of the peroneus longus tendon.

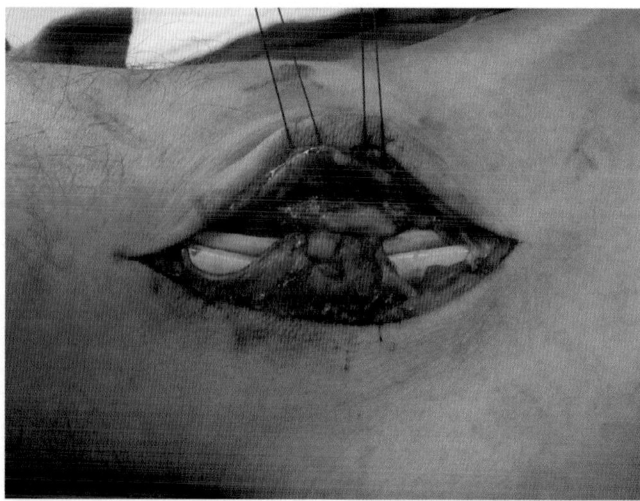

Figure 14.13. "SPR repair": SPR repair is completed by imbricating the posterior flap of the ligament into the retro-malleolar groove through the prepared k-wire holes in a pants-over-vest fashion and then tying down the avulsed anterior flap back onto the fibula.

off of the fibula (38). Another approach is to use a lateral slip of the Achilles tendon which can be re-routed anteriorly and attached to the back of the fibula to hold the peroneal tendons within the retromalleolar groove. This would simulate the calcaneal band of an intact SPR. This reconstruction has 96% good to excellent results at 6.8-year follow-up (35). Finally, Sarmiento described transversely dividing the peroneus brevis and longus tendons and rerouting them deep to the calcaneofibular ligament (CFL) to provide stability to the tendons. This technique was reported to have 100% good to excellent results at 30-month follow-up (39,40).

Bone block procedures have also been described in various ways. An osteotomy through the lateral wall of the fibula can be created and the resulting bone block translated posteriorly and fixed into position to restrain the tendons from subluxing. 92% to 100% good to excellent results have been reported with this procedure (41,42). Another option is to make a sagittal osteotomy through the distal end of the fibula and to rotate the lateral wall fragment posteriorly, thereby containing the tendons. This has been shown to have 82% good to excellent results (43). All bone block procedures carry with them risks of fibula fracture, nonunion, hardware complications, and redislocation.

The last category of surgeries involves deepening a flat or convex-shaped retro-malleolar groove to stabilize the tendons. The classic technique involves using a sagittal saw to elevate an osteoperiosteal flap along the posterior wall of the distal fibula, being careful to maintain a medial hinge. Once the flap is elevated, a portion of the cancellous bone within the fibula is removed with a burr or curettes to deepen the groove (Fig. 14.10). Then the osteoperiosteal flap is replaced into the deepened groove and a bone tamp is used to impact it into a more recessed position. The posterior edge of the SPR is sutured deeply within the groove through K-wire holes drilled into the lateral rim of the fibula. This helps both to maintain the reduction of the osteoperiosteal hinge deep within the groove, as well as to hold the tendons within the groove. In a series of 13 patients who underwent groove deepening, there were no recurrences at 3-year follow-up and 62% were able to return to their preinjury level of activity (44). In a biomechanical study, groove deepening resulted in significantly decreased pressures within the peroneal groove, primarily in the mid to distal region (45). A novel technique to deepen the groove has recently been popularized which drills a large hole longitudinally underneath the posterior cortex of the fibula. A bone tamp is then used to collapse the floor of the retro-malleolar groove into the created cavity. Early results show similar success rates (46).

REFERENCES

1. Petersen W, Bobka T, Stein V, et al. Blood supply of the peroneal tendons: injection and immunohistochemical studies of cadaver tendons. *Acta Orthop Scand* 2000;71:168–174.
2. Sarrafian SK. *Anatomy of the Foot and Ankle*. Philadelphia, PA: J.B. Lippincott; 1993.
3. Clarke HD, Kitaoka HB, Ehman RL. Peroneal tendon injuries. *Foot Ankle Int* 1998;19:280–288.
4. Sobel M, Bohne WH, Levy ME. Longitudinal attrition of the peroneus brevis tendon in the fibular groove: an anatomic study. *Foot Ankle* 1990;11:124–128.
5. Gray JM, Alpar EK. Peroneal tenosynovitis following ankle sprains. *Injury* 2001;32:487–489.
6. Zammit J, Singh D. The peroneus quartus muscle. Anatomy and clinical relevance. *J Bone Joint Surg Br* 2003;85:1134–1137.
7. Sobel M, Levy ME, Bohne WH. Congenital variations of the peroneus quartus muscle: an anatomic study. *Foot Ankle* 1990;11:81–89.
8. DiGiovanni BF, Fraga CJ, Cohen BE, et al. Associated injuries found in chronic lateral ankle instability. *Foot Ankle Int* 2000;21:809–815.
9. Raikin SM, Elias I, Nazarian LN. Intrasheath subluxation of the peroneal tendons. *J Bone Joint Surg Am* 2008;90:992–999.
10. Sobel M, DiCarlo EF, Bohne WH, et al. Longitudinal splitting of the peroneus brevis tendon: an anatomic and histologic study of cadaveric material. *Foot Ankle* 1991;12:165–170.
11. Mizel MS, Michelson JD, Newberg A. Peroneal tendon bupivacaine injection: utility of concomitant injection of contrast material. *Foot Ankle Int* 1996;17:566–568.
12. Rosenberg ZS, Bencardino J, Astion D, et al. MRI features of chronic injuries of the superior peroneal retinaculum. *AJR Am J Roentgenol* 2003;181:1551–1557.
13. Brodsky JW, Harms S, Negrine J. Surgical correlation of MRI characteristics of tendon tears about the ankle. AOFAS 11th Annual Summer Meeting. Vail, Colorado; 1995.
14. Kijowski R, De Smet A, Mukharjee R. Magnetic resonance imaging findings in patients with peroneal tendinopathy and peroneal tenosynovitis. *Skeletal Radiol* 2007;36:105–114.
15. Lamm BM, Myers DT, Dombek M, et al. Magnetic resonance imaging and surgical correlation of peroneus brevis tears. *J Foot Ankle Surg* 2004;43:30–36.
16. Steel MW, DeOrio JK. Peroneal tendon tears: return to sports after operative treatment. *Foot Ankle Int* 2007;28:49–54.
17. Brandes CB, Smith RW. Characterization of patients with primary peroneus longus tendinopathy: a review of twenty-two cases. *Foot Ankle Int* 2000;21:462–468.
18. Grant TH, Kelikian AS, Jereb SE, et al. Ultrasound diagnosis of peroneal tendon tears. A surgical correlation. *J Bone Joint Surg Am* 2005;87:1788–1794.
19. Krause JO, Brodsky JW. Peroneus brevis tendon tears: pathophysiology, surgical reconstruction, and clinical results. *Foot Ankle Int* 1998;19:271–279.
20. Redfern D, Myerson M. The management of concomitant tears of the peroneus longus and brevis tendons. *Foot Ankle Int* 2004;25:695–707.
21. Slater HK. Acute peroneal tendon tears. *Foot Ankle Clin* 2007;12:659–674, vii.
22. Borton DC, Lucas P, Jomha NM, et al. Operative reconstruction after transverse rupture of the tendons of both peroneus longus and brevis. Surgical reconstruction by transfer of the flexor digitorum longus tendon. *J Bone Joint Surg Br* 1998;80:781–784.
23. Wapner KL, Taras JS, Lin SS, et al. Staged reconstruction for chronic rupture of both peroneal tendons using Hunter rod and flexor hallucis longus tendon transfer: a long-term followup study. *Foot Ankle Int* 2006;27:591–597.
24. Sammarco GJ, DiRaimondo CV. Chronic peroneus brevis tendon lesions. *Foot Ankle* 1989; 9:163–170.
25. Sobel M, Pavlov H, Geppert MJ, et al. Painful os peroneum syndrome: a spectrum of conditions responsible for plantar lateral foot pain. *Foot Ankle Int* 1994;15:112–124.
26. Hyer CF, Dawson JM, Philbin TM, et al. The peroneal tubercle: description, classification, and relevance to peroneus longus tendon pathology. *Foot Ankle Int* 2005;26:947–950.
27. Davis WH, Sobel M, Deland J, et al. The superior peroneal retinaculum: an anatomic study. *Foot Ankle Int* 1994;15:271–275.
28. Eckert WR, Davis EA Jr. Acute rupture of the peroneal retinaculum. *J Bone Joint Surg Am* 1976;58:670–672.
29. Oden RR. Tendon injuries about the ankle resulting from skiing. *Clin Orthop Relat Res* 1987;(216):63–69.
30. Edwards ME. The relations of the peroneal tendons to the fibula, calcaneus, and cuboideum. *Am J Anat* 1928;42:213–253.
31. Kumai T, Benjamin M. The histological structure of the malleolar groove of the fibula in man: its direct bearing on the displacement of peroneal tendons and their surgical repair. *J Anat* 2003;203:257–262.
32. Geppert MJ, Sobel M, Bohne WH. Lateral ankle instability as a cause of superior peroneal retinacular laxity: an anatomic and biomechanical study of cadaveric feet. *Foot Ankle* 1993;14:330–334.
33. Clanton TO. *Surgery of the Foot and Ankle*. St Louis, MO: Mosby; 1999.
34. Ebraheim NA, Zeiss J, Skie MC, et al. Radiological evaluation of peroneal tendon pathology associated with calcaneal fractures. *J Orthop Trauma* 1991;5:365–369.
35. Escalas F, Figueras JM, Merino JA. Dislocation of the peroneal tendons. Long-term results of surgical treatment. *J Bone Joint Surg Am* 1980;62:451–453.
36. Stover CN, Bryan DR. Traumatic dislocation of the peroneal tendons. *Am J Surg* 1962; 103:180–186.
37. Hui JH, Das De S, Balasubramaniam P. The Singapore operation for recurrent dislocation of peroneal tendons: long-term results. *J Bone Joint Surg Br* 1998;80:325–327.
38. Pozo JL, Jackson AM. A rerouting operation for dislocation of peroneal tendons: operative technique and case report. *Foot Ankle* 1984;5:42–44.
39. Sarmiento A, Wolf M. Subluxation of peroneal tendons. Case treated by rerouting tendons under calcaneofibular ligament. *J Bone Joint Surg Am* 1975;57:115–116.
40. Martens MA, Noyez JF, Mulier JC. Recurrent dislocation of the peroneal tendons. Results of rerouting the tendons under the calcaneofibular ligament. *Am J Sports Med* 1986;14: 148–150.
41. Marti R. Dislocation of the peroneal tendons. *Am J Sports Med* 1977;5:19–22.
42. Micheli LJ, Waters PM, Sanders DP. Sliding fibular graft repair for chronic dislocation of the peroneal tendons. *Am J Sports Med* 1989;17:68–71.
43. Mason RB, Henderson JP. Traumatic peroneal tendon instability. *Am J Sports Med* 1996; 24:652–658.
44. Porter D, McCarroll J, Knapp E, et al. Peroneal tendon subluxation in athletes: fibular groove deepening and retinacular reconstruction. *Foot Ankle Int* 2005;26:436–441.
45. Title CI, Jung HG, Parks BG, et al. The peroneal groove deepening procedure: a biomechanical study of pressure reduction. *Foot Ankle Int* 2005;26:442–448.
46. Shawen SB, Anderson RB. Indirect groove deepening procedure: a biomechanical study of pressure reduction. *Tech Foot Ankle Surg* 2004;3:118–125.

CHAPTER

15

Kenneth S. Jung

Posterior Tibial Tendon Injuries in Sports

INTRODUCTION

Injuries to the posterior tibial tendon (PTT) in athletes are commonly due to overuse or acute trauma. Due to the position of the PTT at the foot and ankle joints, activities that involve pushing-off, lateral motion, and cutting utilize the tendon. Patients characteristically present with medial ankle pain and weakness. Tears, ruptures, and dislocations of the PTT exist in the literature as individual case reports or small series. Severe or long-standing injury to the PTT can result in collapse of the medial longitudinal arch, hindfoot valgus, forefoot abduction, and sinus tarsi pain. PTT pathology has been more commonly investigated with regards to PTT dysfunction and the adult-acquired flatfoot; thus, many of the diagnostic and treatment principles are applied to PTT injuries in a younger or athletic population.

ANATOMY

The PTT resides in the deep posterior muscle compartment of the lower leg, where it is innervated by the tibial nerve. It originates from the proximal third of the tibia, fibula, and interosseous membrane (Fig. 15.1). The musculotendinous junction is present in the distal third of the lower leg. The tendon courses posterior to the medial malleolus in the retromalleolar groove and then turns sharply within the tarsal tunnel toward the midfoot (1). At the level of the ankle, the PTT runs anterior and medial to the flexor hallucis longus tendon. These tendons are maintained in the retromalleolar groove by the flexor retinaculum, which spans the medial surface of the calcaneus to the medial malleolus (Fig. 15.2). The tendon inserts throughout the midfoot via anterior, middle, and posterior components. The anterior component inserts on the navicular, medial cuneiform, and inferior capsule of the naviculocuneiform joint. The middle component inserts on the middle cuneiform, lateral cuneiform, cuboid, second through fourth metatarsal bases, flexor hallucis brevis, and peroneus longus tendon near the first metatarsal base. The posterior component inserts on the anterior aspect of the sustentaculum tali. Of the total PTT width, the anterior band consists of 65%, the middle band consists of 15%, and the posterior band consists of 20% (2). Variable attachments have also been described to the abductor hallucis, spring ligament, and fifth metatarsal (3).

Proximally, the posterior tibial artery contributes muscular branches at the musculotendinous junction and branches via the paratenon. There is a longitudinal intratendinous network of vessels. Distally at the tendon–bone interface, branches in the epitenon are supplied by the periosteum via the medial plantar branch of the posterior tibial artery and medial tarsal artery (4–6). A zone of hypovascularity, spanning an average of

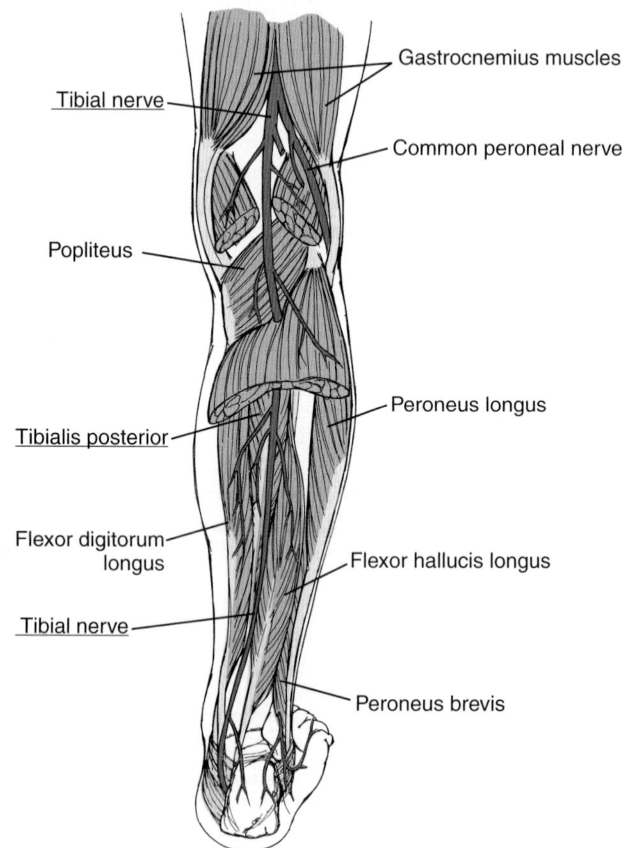

Figure 15.1. The PTT resides in the deep posterior muscle compartment of the lower leg, where it is innervated by the tibial nerve. It originates from the proximal third of the tibia, fibula, and the interosseous membrane.

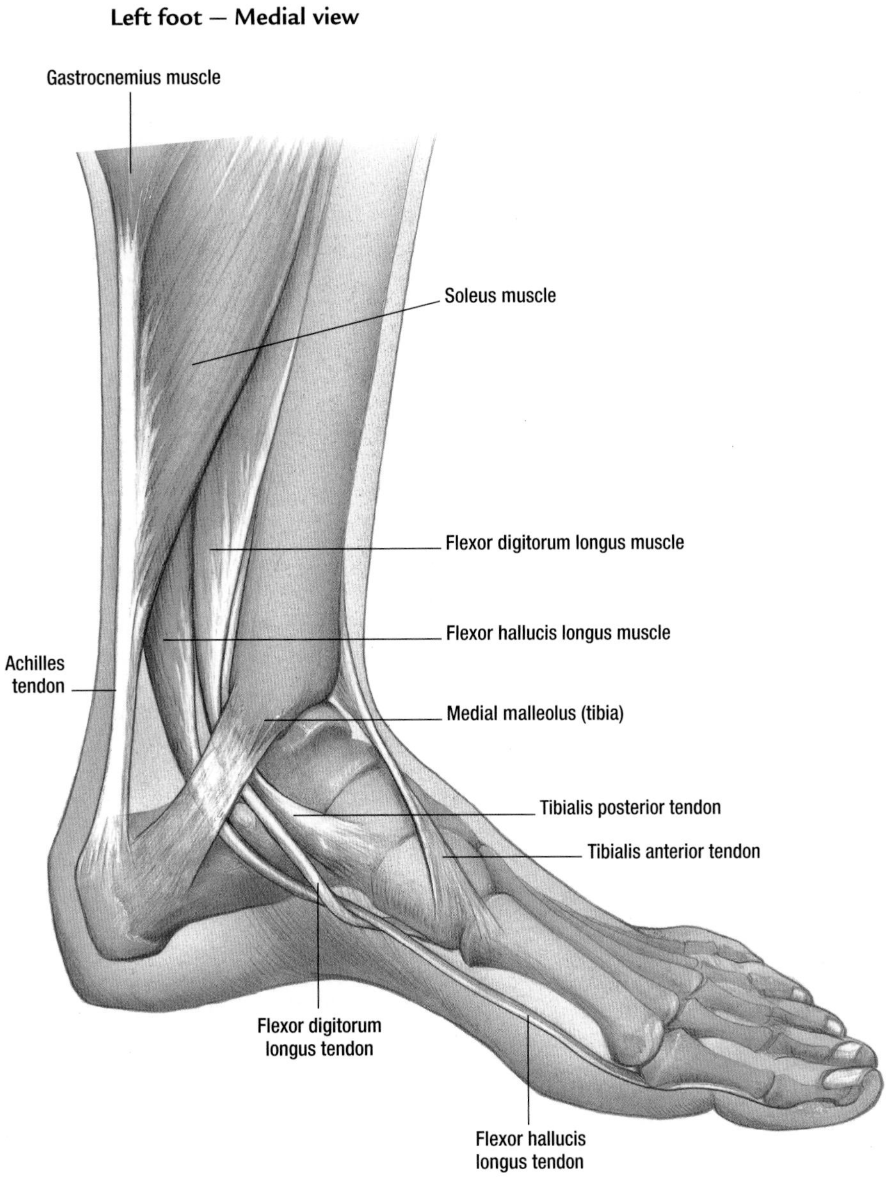

Figure 15.2. The PTT courses posterior to the medial malleolus deep to the flexor retinaculum.

14 mm, has been reported posterior and distal to the medial malleolus (4,5). This hypovascularity predisposes the tendon to degenerative changes and rupture. Prado et al. did not find an area of hypovascularity and proposed mechanical factors and age as possible causes of degeneration (6). Mechanical factors attributed to the PTT making a sharp turn around the medial malleolus have been proposed (7,8).

BIOMECHANICS

The PTT courses posterior to the ankle joint and medial to the subtalar joint, with insertions in the midfoot. Thus, the PTT plantarflexes the ankle, inverts the hindfoot, and adducts the midfoot. It functions as the primary inverter of the foot and provides dynamic stability to the medial longitudinal arch (9). Elongation of the PTT by 1 cm reduces its efficiency as the primary dynamic stabilizer (10). Static stability to the medial longitudinal arch is imparted by soft tissue structures, including the spring, deltoid, and talocalcaneal interosseous ligaments and the talonavicular capsule. The static restraints are weaker than the PTT and are prone to failure under repetitive biomechanical stress if the PTT is insufficient (1).

The PTT plays important roles in the stance phase of the gait cycle due to its actions at the ankle and transverse tarsal joints. At heel strike, the ground reactive force causes ankle dorsiflexion and hindfoot valgus. The PTT eccentrically contracts to resist these moments (11,12). From heel strike to foot flat, the PTT provides energy absorption by controlling the flexibility of the foot. The PTT insertion on the navicular provides it control of midfoot stability. In eversion, the axes of talonavicular and calcaneocuboid joints are parallel, which "unlocks" the midfoot. In this alignment the foot is flexible and absorbs force. PTT concentric contraction inverts and locks the midfoot by diverging the axes the talonavicular and calcaneocuboid joints, making the foot rigid. This action transitions the role of the foot from shock absorber to a lever arm. A locked midfoot provides a rigid lever arm for the gastrocnemius–soleus complex to act upon, producing more efficient push off. If the PTT is weak or dysfunctional, the primary dynamic stabilizer of the medial longitudinal arch is compromised, and forces act through the talonavicular joint. Eventually, the static structures of the medial longitudinal arch fail and flatfoot deformity results (7).

Individuals with increased hindfoot valgus have increased load on the PTT. In addition to the force vector in the sagittal plane, there is increased force in the coronal plane, resulting in subtalar eversion. Thus, the PTT absorbs the ground reactive force with eccentric contraction to resist dorsiflexion and eversion. Increased loads on the tendon make it more prone to injuries from overuse and failure. PTT in a flatfoot deformity have been shown to have increased gliding resistance, which places it at risk for micromechanical trauma and degeneration (13).

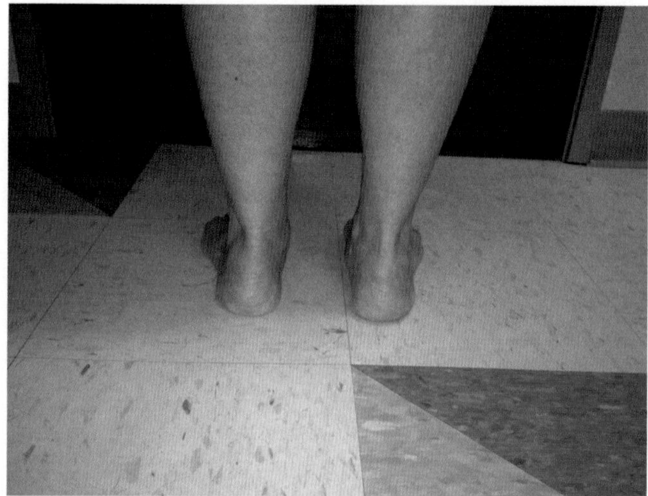

Figure 15.3. Demonstration of "too many toes" sign in the left foot. Swelling over the PTT is also noted.

PHYSICAL EXAMINATION

Early recognition, diagnosis, and treatment is important, in order to avoid foot deformity and prolonged disability (14). Clinical history regarding the nature of injury and onset of symptoms should be obtained. Mechanism of injury typically involves forced dorsiflexion of an everted ankle, although inversion has also been reported. Acute onset of pain or a sensation of a "pop" should alert the clinician to a tear or rupture. Acute onset or exacerbation of flatfoot deformity may indicate PTT rupture or insufficiency. An insidious onset of pain and deformity may indicate degeneration of the PTT. A history of corticosteroid injections should be noted. Questions regarding alterations in training intensity and frequency are posed to rule out overuse injuries. Injuries attributed to biomechanical causes may be due to alterations in equipment, such as shoe wear, bracing, or orthosis. The terrain or training surface the athlete utilizes is also important to ascertain. In addition, medical history regarding drug use and inflammatory disorders are noted.

Physical examination commences with an overall, comparative assessment of the subject's lower extremities in a standing position. The subject should be observed from front and behind. From the anterior perspective, midfoot pronation, prominence of the navicular, and forefoot abduction are assessed. Focal swelling at the medial aspect of the ankle as well as pitting edema of the entire extremity is noted. With increased medial swelling and fullness, the bony contour of the medial malleolus is obscured. From the posterior view, alignment of the hindfoot is compared. The "too many toes" sign can be appreciated, indicating increased forefoot abduction (15) (Fig. 15.3). The subject is asked to attempt a double-heel rise. Symmetric hindfoot inversion should be observed. This tests PTT strength and the flexibility of the subtalar joint. Inability to elevate and invert the hindfoot signifies PTT weakness or dysfunction (Fig. 15.4). A rigid or stiff subtalar joint can also lead to a failed trial. The subject then attempts a single-heel rise to assess hindfoot inversion, strength, and reproduction of pain. Failure to accomplish this feat may be attributed to pain or weakness of the PTT.

Physical examination continues with the patient in a seated position. The hallmark is tenderness to palpation along the course of the tendon. Palpation is performed from posterior to the medial malleolus to the navicular insertion, with the hindfoot in neutral, inversion, and eversion. Due to the paucity of subcutaneous fat in this region, the tendon should be palpable, especially with inversion. Swelling, thickening, and gaps may be detected. In the presence of pitting edema, the contour of the medial malleolus may be obscured. The posterior tibial edema sign has been described to aide in diagnosis of posterior tibial tendon dysfunction (PTTD). The spot tested is posterior and proximal to the medial malleolus along the PTT course. If pitting edema is greater in this area versus the anterior tibial region, the test is considered positive for PTTD (16). In addition, tendon stability is assessed with circumduction of the ankle while palpating the PTT. Apprehension may be caused by resisted inversion with the ankle plantarflexed or dorsiflexed.

Palpation of the osseous anatomy is also performed. Tenderness of the medial malleolus raises the awareness of stress

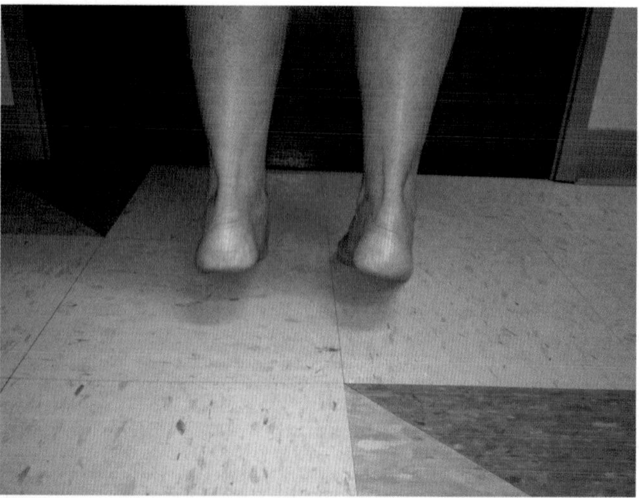

Figure 15.4. Double-heel rise demonstrating lack of hindfoot inversion of the left foot due to PTT weakness.

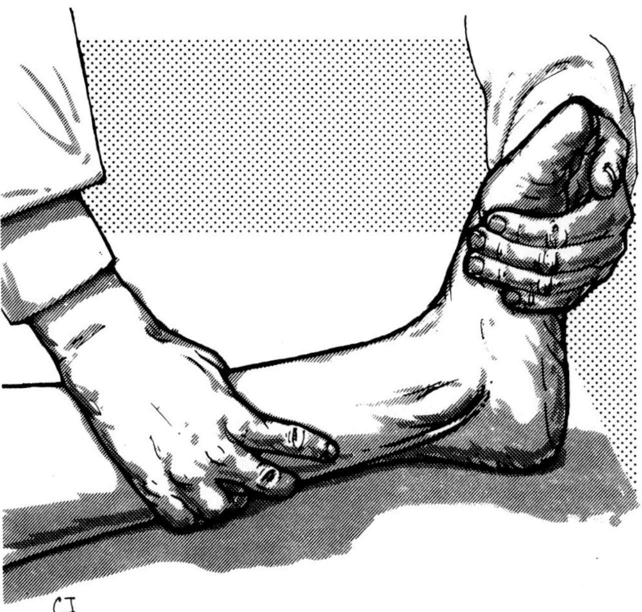

Figure 15.5. Examination of inversion of the foot. The patient attempts to invert the foot against resistance, from a starting position of plantarflexion, heel eversion and forefoot abduction. The PTT can be seen and palpated posterior to the medial malleolus.

reaction or fracture. The medial aspect of the navicular is palpated to elicit a symptomatic accessory navicular. Prominence of the navicular is noted as well as the presence of ulceration or callus. Medial prominence suggests an accessory navicular, and plantar prominence indicates collapse of the medial longitudinal arch. The calcaneus is also examined for tenderness, which may indicate a stress injury as well.

The mobility of the ankle, subtalar, and transverse tarsal joints are also assessed. If hindfoot valgus or forefoot abduction is present, the ability to passively correct to neutral is noted. Long-standing injuries may demonstrate decreased mobility or rigid deformities. Contracture of the Achilles tendon versus the gastrocnemius is assessed with the Silfverskiöld test. Passive ankle dorsiflexion is assessed with the knee extended and flexed. If ankle dorsiflexion is limited in knee extension, but not flexion, a gastrocnemius contracture is present. If dorsiflexion is limited in knee extension and flexion, an Achilles contracture is present (17).

Inversion against resistance can elicit pain and evaluate strength. A true assessment of PTT strength is evaluated from a starting position of plantarflexion, heel eversion, and forefoot abduction. This eliminates recruitment of the tibialis anterior tendon. Inversion against manual resistance is then attempted by the patient. Comparison to the contralateral side is noted (18) (Fig. 15.5).

IMAGING

Weight-bearing plain radiographs of the foot and ankle allow evaluation of bony alignment and alterations. The presence of an accessory navicular and bony changes should be noted. An external oblique view of the foot may be used to better visualize the medial navicular. Enthesopathy is suggested by hypertrophic changes at the insertion of the PTT on the navicular. A tibial spur adjacent to the PTT in the retromalleolar groove is a secondary sign of tendinopathy (19). Irregular periosteal reaction (20) on the medial malleolus or an avulsion fracture (21) has been reported in chronic PTT dislocation.

Chronic PTT injuries alter biomechanical stresses, which can lead to changes in the bony alignment of the foot and ankle. Lateral foot projection allows assessment of the longitudinal arch. The lateral talometatarsal angle or Meary's angle increases with loss of the medial longitudinal arch (22). The alignment of the talar head relative to the navicular is assessed for increased flexion of the talar head, which denotes weakness to supporting structures. Anteroposterior foot view allows assessment of forefoot abduction. As the forefoot abducts, there is decreased coverage of the talar head by the navicular. This is attributed to the increased pull of an unopposed peroneus brevis and attenuation of medial structures. The tibiotalar and subtalar joints are also assessed for alignment and degenerative changes. Particular attention to the calcaneus, medial malleolus, and navicular should be paid if considering stress fracture in the differential diagnosis.

MRI is considered the "gold standard" for assessing tendon disorders; however, ultrasound has been found to be comparable (23). Surrounding soft tissue structures, especially the deltoid ligament, spring ligament, flexor digitorum longus, and flexor hallucis longus, can also be assessed. Furthermore, the ability to detect edema aides in ruling out contusions and stress fractures in bony structures adjacent to the PTT, including the medial malleolus and calcaneus. The synchondrosis of an accessory navicular can be assessed for evidence of trauma and edema. Bone scan can further aide in the assessment of stress fractures and trauma to the accessory navicular synchondrosis. Ultrasound provides the added benefit dynamic assessment, which may aide in diagnosis of PTT subluxation or dislocation (19).

On MRI, the PTT normally is ovoid and twice the diameter of the flexor digitorum longus and flexor hallucis longus tendons distal to the level of the medial malleolus (19,24) (Fig. 15.6). PTT tears are classified into three types, based upon MRI and gross structural features (14). Type 1 tears demonstrate longitudinal splits without intrasubstance degeneration. MRI demonstrates homogenous black signal. Type 2 tears have wider longitudinal splits and intrasubstance degeneration. MRI demonstrates a narrow tendon due to degeneration and elongation. A grey signal within the tendon is seen. The examiner should be aware of the "magic angle" phenomena, which can affect intermediate or increased signal and mimic tendinopathy (25). Type 3 demonstrates complete tears of the tendon and possibly, an empty tendon sheath. Increased swelling and degeneration are seen.

DIFFERENTIAL DIAGNOSES

When considering PTT injuries in an athlete, it must be remembered that the incidence is low. Careful examination of surrounding structures must be performed in order to rule out other diagnoses, which can present with medial ankle pain.

Bone contusion and stress fractures of the medial malleolus, navicular, and calcaneus can be elicited with a history of alterations in training frequency and intensity. Diagnosis may be made with radiographs or MRI.

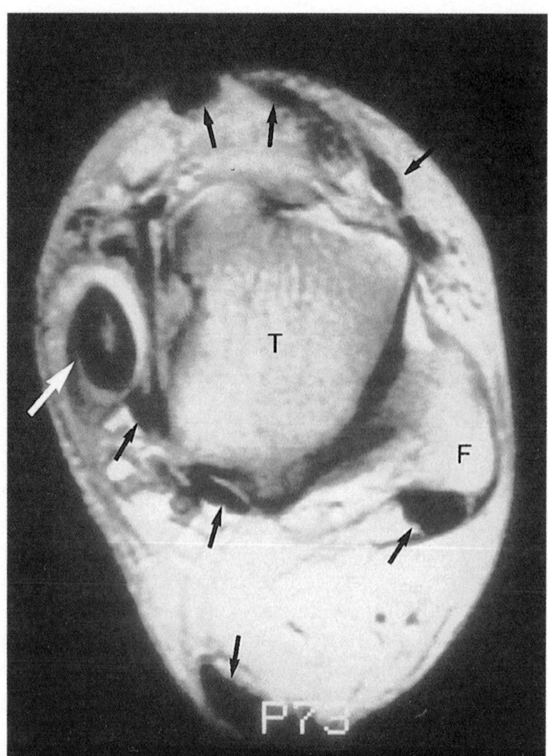

Figure 15.6. Magnetic resonance imaging of tendon pathology. Transverse T_2-weighted fast spin-echo image of the ankle of a patient with medial ankle pain and flatfoot deformity shows thickening and increased signal intensity of the PTT (*long arrow*) consistent with severe tendonitis. Compare this appearance with that of the normal tendons on the same image (*short arrows*). *T*, talus; *F*, fibula.

Adjacent soft tissues may also contribute to medial ankle symptoms. A portion of the deltoid ligament is palpated inferior to the medial malleolus and anterior to the PTT. Stress testing of the ankle in abduction or varus can also reproduce symptoms. Specifically in dancers, flexor hallucis longus tenosynovitis and posterior impingement are more common etiologies (26). The flexor hallucis longus tendon is plantar to the PTT and can be palpated while the hallux is brought through flexion and extension.

Patients may also present with inferior heel pain, as well as pain along the PTT. The heel pain triad of PTT dysfunction, plantar fasciitis, and tarsal tunnel syndrome has been described. It has been postulated that as a result of the failure of the static (plantar fascia) and dynamic (PTT) support of the medial longitudinal arch, a traction injury of the posterior tibial nerve results. Surgical treatment consisted of complete surgical release of the plantar fascia and tarsal tunnel, along with PTT reconstruction (27).

POSTERIOR TIBIAL TENDON INJURIES

Acute injuries in the athletic population tend to occur with forced dorsiflexion, combined dorsiflexion and eversion, or a neutral foot preparing to plant or push-off. Injuries have been reported to the tendon itself, as well as along the course of the PTT, from posterior to the medial malleolus to the navicular insertion.

When considering PTT injuries in athletes, they can be placed along a spectrum from tenosynovitis to rupture. This can be likened to the classification of PTTD, originally described by Johnson (28) and modified by Meyerson (29). Stage 1 demonstrates tenosynovitis. Stage 2 demonstrates partial tears with a flexible deformity. Stage 3 exhibits partial tears with a rigid hindfoot deformity. Stage 4 exhibits valgus alignment of the tibiotalar joint.

PTTD is the most common cause of adult-acquired flatfoot deformity. Clinical and histologic examinations of tendons from type 2 PTT patients have been examined. Clinically, findings of cloudy, thickened peritenon and increased synovial fluid were consistent with synovitis; however, histologic examination demonstrated findings consistent with degenerative tendonisis, rather than tendonitis (8). Progression of degeneration to insufficiency or rupture results in tendon dysfunction. Unlike PTTD, which commonly occurs in middle-aged women, PTT injuries in athletes are attributed to acute trauma or have insidious onset due to overuse. Nevertheless, the principles that guide the treatment of PTTD can be applied to PTT injuries in athletes. In addition to evaluating and treating PTT pathology, the alignment of the foot and ankle must be addressed. Bony realignment procedures may be performed in addition to soft-tissue procedures in order to protect the PTT reconstruction from recurrent, deforming forces.

TENOSYNOVITIS

Tenosynovitis was first described by Kulowski in 1936 (30). Patients present with tenderness and swelling over the PTT. PTT pain with resistance and single-heel rise may be present, rather than overt weakness and lack of inversion. Pes planus should be noted on examination, and if present, compared to the contralateral extremity. MRI is used to evaluate the PTT and fluid in the tendon sheath. Tendon sheath injections with local anesthetic have been shown to elucidate a diagnosis in patients with multiple pain generators as well as those with negative MRI findings and continued clinical suspicion. In a small series, patients with negative MRI findings and complete relief of symptoms with sheath injection had findings of inflammation at the time of surgery (31).

Initial management includes rest, activity modification, NSAID, physical therapy, and an orthosis. External support of the medial longitudinal arch is provided with an off-the-shelf or custom orthosis. Additional arch support can be provided with a motion-control shoe. Taping may also be utilized to help support the PTT, but this requires an individual trained with proper technique. If no improvement is made after 4 to 6 weeks, immobilization in a walking boot or cast is recommended (32).

Rehabilitation programs have been reported for treatment of PTT dysfunction stages 1 and 2 (33,34). Treatment included use of a short articulated ankle–foot orthosis or an orthosis with high medial and lateral trim lines. Rehabilitation included global strengthening of the posterior tibial, anterior tibial, peroneals, and gastrocnemius–soleus, as well as stretching of gastrocnemius–soleus complex. Over a median period of 4 months, patients had improvement in pain and function (34).

A 12-week rehabilitation program has been described. An initial 2-week period of gastrocnemius–soleus stretching and orthosis use was used to unload the tendon and diminish inflammatory symptoms. This was followed by a 10-week period of orthosis use, calf stretching, and eccentric PTT exercises. Symptomatic improvement and increase in function were reported 6 months after the program (33).

Surgical treatment, consisting of inspection and tenosynovectomy, is indicated if symptoms persist for 3 to 6 months (32,35). The tendon sheath is opened to allow exposure of the tendon from the posterior aspect of the medial malleolus to the navicular insertion. Thorough tenosynovectomy is performed. The entire tendon should be inspected circumferentially, as tears may be on the underside or lateral aspects. Palpation is also performed to appreciate thickening or thinning. A thinned tendon may indicate attenuation from intrasubstance tears. Any tears are debrided and repaired. McCormack et al. reported on a group of young athletes who underwent surgical debridement at an average of 8 weeks from initial evaluation. Tenosynovitis, stenosis of the tendon at the distal aspect of the sheath, and a repairable longitudinal tear were seen intraoperatively. Clearance to play was given 6 to 8 weeks after surgery. Successful return to sport was accomplished in all patients, with seven of eight reporting excellent results (36).

TEARS AND RUPTURES

Patients may initially be diagnosed and treated for an ankle sprain, which can delay definitive diagnosis and treatment for weeks to months (32,37–40). Persistent medial ankle pain and physical examination with specific attention to PTT pathology are vital to making a diagnosis. A symptomatic or weak PTT on single heel raise and resisted inversion raise clinical suspicion for PTT pathology. Flatfoot deformity may or not be present, depending on the degree and duration of the tear. MRI allows further evaluation and may demonstrate narrowing, thickening, intrasubstance changes, or tears. Tears may occur anywhere along the course of the tendon. Longitudinal tears appear as splits between tendon fibers. Intrasubstance tears with degeneration may be found in areas of thickening or attenuation. Intraoperative inspection reveals a continuous tendon and no longitudinal split; however, the tendon contains unorganized, fibrous tissue. Avulsion tears are found at the navicular insertion.

RUPTURE AND POSTERIOR TIBIAL TENDON DYSFUNCTION

PTTD is the most common cause of adult-acquired flatfoot deformity. Clinical and histologic examinations of tendons from type 2 PTT patients have been examined. Clinically, findings of cloudy, thickened peritenon and increased synovial fluid were consistent with synovitis; however, histologic examination demonstrated findings consistent with degenerative tendonisis, rather than tendonitis (8). Progression of degeneration to insufficiency or rupture results in tendon dysfunction.

In the athletic population acute ruptures are seen, rather than degeneration of the acquired adult flatfoot. Nevertheless, the principles of PTTD type 2 treatment can be applied to ruptures in the athlete. In addition to evaluating and treating PTT pathology, the alignment of the foot and ankle must be addressed. Bony realignment is performed in addition to soft-tissue procedures in order to protect the PTT reconstruction from deforming forces.

If a tear is diagnosed in a timely fashion, non-operative management consisting of boot or cast immobilization for 4 to 6 weeks may be initiated. Immobilization is followed by rehabilitation consisting of progressive stretching and resistance exercises (26). Use of an orthosis, depending on the athlete's activity, is considered upon return to participation.

Patients unresponsive to rehabilitation are indicated for surgical treatment. The tendon is visually inspected and palpated along its entire course. Circumferential inspection of the tendon must be performed, since tears may be present on the undersurface. Pathology is indicated by thickening, flattening, attenuation, or a palpable step-off. After synovectomy, debridement of the tear is performed. Split tears are repaired directly. Intrasubstance tears contain degenerated scar tissue which require debridement. Direct side-to-side repair is then performed. Attempts are also made to restore the ovoid morphology of the tendon. If the tendon is flattened, repair includes tubularization of the tendon. Avulsion tears are found near the navicular insertion. A step-off in the tendon may be appreciated in the case of partial tear with retraction (Fig. 15.7). Concomitant intrasubstance and longitudinal tears have been reported (32).

In order to achieve participation in upper-level sports, the goals of reconstruction and repair are restoration of normal length and tension in the tendon with maintenance of the anatomic arch (38). Avulsion and intrasubstance tears can lead to tendon elongation and insufficiency, which manifests as weakness and flatfoot deformity. Avulsion tears are directly repaired by advancing the tendon and re-securing it to the navicular with a suture anchor or bone tunnels. Prior to attachment, the site is decorticated to provide a bed of cancellous bone.

In cases of tendon elongation causing weakness or flatfoot deformity, the tension of the musculotendinous unit must be restored. After debridement, the PTT is advanced to the navicular insertion with the foot in plantarflexion and inversion. PTT advancement can be performed by longitudinally splitting the distal 1.5 cm to the navicular and elevating periosteal flaps dorsally and plantarly. The PTT is secured to the navicular with a suture anchor (38). A flexor digitorum longus tendon transfer is also recommended to supplement the repair and restore tension (Fig. 15.8). The flexor digitorum longus

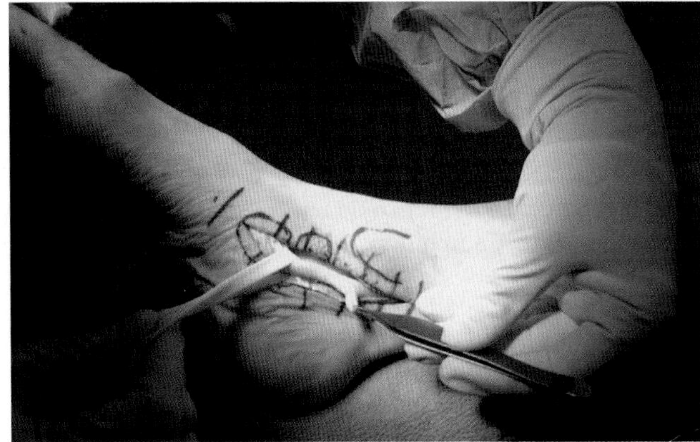

Figure 15.7. Intraoperative demonstration of a partial PTT tear with retraction. The tendon was debrided prior to transfer of the flexor digitorum longus tendon.

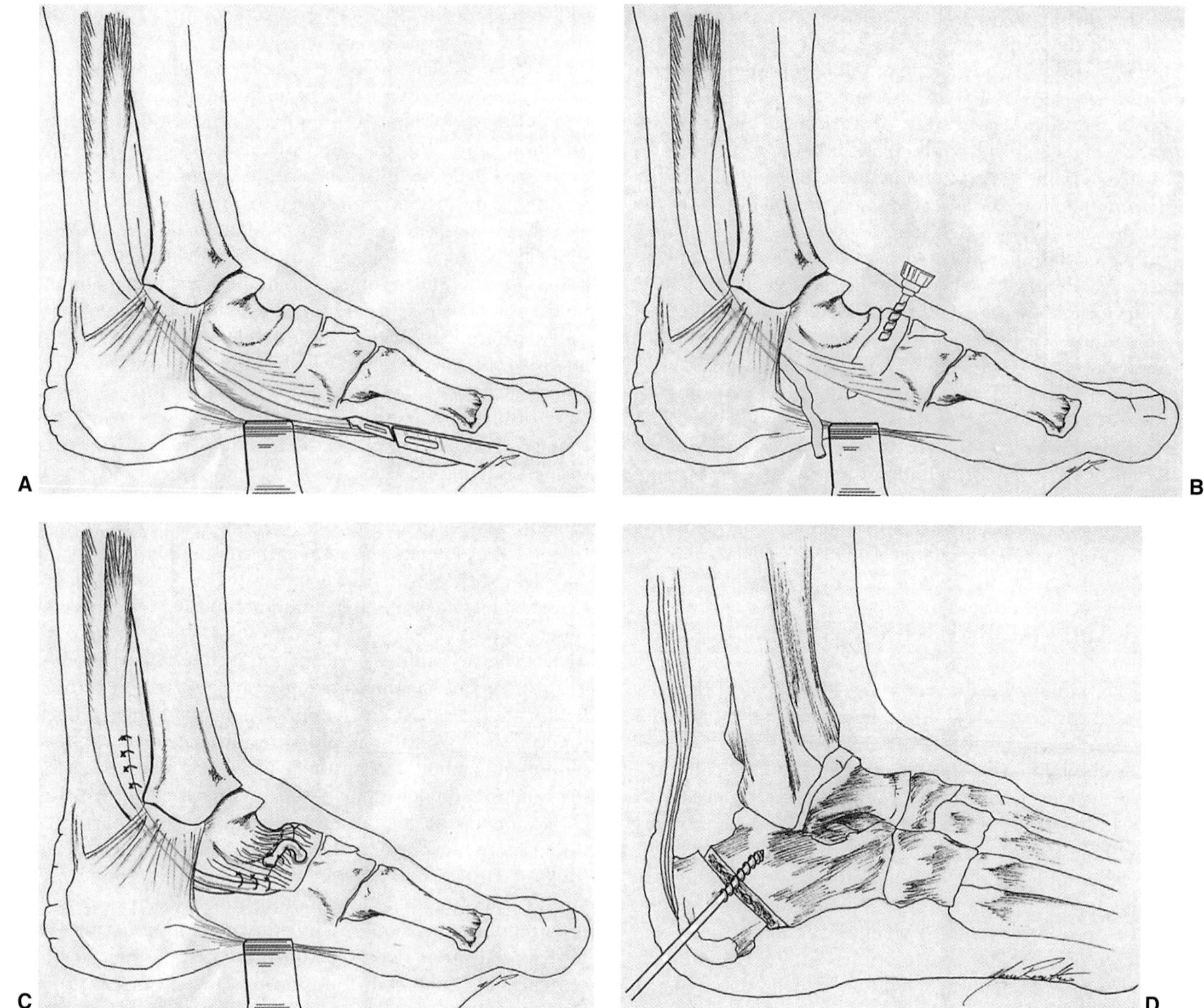

Figure 15.8. Demonstration of FDL transfer and medial displacing calcaneal osteotomy. **A:** FDL is traced to the Knot of Henry and released. **B:** FDL is transferred to the plantar surface of the navicular. A bone tunnel is prepared for passage of the tendon. **C:** FDL transfer is performed with the ankle in plantarflexion and inversion. FDL is secured with an interference screw or sewed onto itself through a bone tunnel. **D:** Calcaneal osteotomy is secured with screw fixation after medial displacement and correction of hindfoot valgus.

tendon is utilized due to its proximity and ability to balance the pull of the peroneus brevis. Furthermore, the flexor hallucis longus tendon is not used due to its roles in push-off and stabilizing the medial longitudinal arch (18). The FDL tendon is harvested plantar and medial to the PTT. It can be transferred to the plantar aspect of the navicular by means of a bone tunnel or interference screw fixation. The PTT repair and FDL transfer is performed with the ankle in plantarflexion and inversion. After the transfer is secured, mild resistance should be appreciated with the ankle and hindfoot in neutral alignment (38).

FDL transfer is also recommended when the proximal PTT stump does not have adequate length to reach the navicular (37). This may occur after debridement of scar tissue from a degenerated tendon or in chronic injuries with retraction. Full recovery of a collegiate hockey player has been reported with FDL transfer alone (40).

FDL transfer is recommended in highly competitive athletes to provide the best chance to return to competition (32); however, consideration of the athlete's specific activities and needs must be taken into account prior to performing an FDL transfer. Deland et al. reported successful outcomes in four dancers with PTT tears. Direct repair of the tendon without FDL transfer was performed in order to preserve toe function in dancers (26).

Evaluation must assess the PTT as well as any deformity that may have developed. If the PTT weakens or becomes dysfunctional, flatfoot deformity or hindfoot valgus may develop. In a series of six patients, Woods et al. noted excellent outcome in patients who had surgery relatively early after injury and maintained function of the PTT and an arch. Patients with a ruptured PTT, flattened longitudinal arch, and pronated foot noted improvement and returned to athletic activities. PTT debridement was felt to improve pain, but not correct flatfoot deformity, which can lead to problems with push-off in athletes (37). Operative treatment must address the PTT pathology as well as foot and ankle deformity. If hindfoot valgus is present, a medial displacing calcaneal osteotomy is performed (Fig. 15.8). With hindfoot valgus, Achilles' pull produces heel eversion. A medial displacing osteotomy alters the pull of the Achilles tendon to diminish this effect (Fig. 15.8). The osteotomy also addresses the valgus deformity that develops with PTT insufficiency. Equinus contracture is addressed by performing a gastrocnemius recession in Silfverskiöld positive subjects. In order to reinforce the static structures of the medial longitudinal arch, reconstructions of the spring (39) and deltoid ligaments have been advocated (32).

Post-operatively, patients are kept non–weight bearing, immobilized in slight inversion for 4 to 6 weeks. Non–weight bearing is stressed in order to permit wound healing. A boot is then used, which can be removed for range of motion. Dorsiflexion and plantarflexion are initiated, followed by inversion and eversion. Progressive weight bearing in a boot with an orthosis is initiated at 6 weeks for PTT repair and FDL transfer. If a calcaneal osteotomy is performed, progressive weight bearing begins at 6–8 weeks. Physical therapy is instituted upon initiation of range of motion and progressive weight bearing. Return to athletic participation is anticipated 6 to 8 months from surgery.

LACERATION

Lacerations occur in traumatic events. Diagnosis should be made upon exploration of the wound. However, if the wound is closed without recognition of the tendon laceration, diagnosis can be made on physical examination. A palpable defect in the PTT and lack of inversion are present. MRI or ultrasound can be used to assist with diagnosis.

Prompt primary repair of the tendon is recommended at the time of wound exploration (41,42). If tendon laceration is not recognized, chronic changes seen in PTT rupture may progressively develop. Injury to the PTT and alignment of the foot and ankle must be addressed.

Attempt at primary repair is recommended in a timely fashion in order to minimize retraction of the proximal stump and scarring of the tendon ends. The tendon is repaired end-to-end with a Krakow stitch using a nonabsorbable suture. The repair is supplemented with a peritendinous running suture using an absorbable suture. The tendon should be repaired under adequate tension with the foot inverted and plantarflexed. If the tendon ends are unable to be opposed or are attenuated, a FDL tendon transfer is performed. In the event of an undiagnosed rupture and the presence of hindfoot valgus, a medial displacing calcaneal osteotomy is performed to correct the deformity (35). Appropriate antibiotic coverage must also be provided in cases of laceration.

POSTERIOR TIBIAL TENDON DISLOCATION

The flexor retinaculum spans the medial surface of the calcaneus to the medial malleolus and helps to maintain the PTT in the retromalleolar groove. The occurrence of PTT dislocation is rare, as evidenced by case reports in the literature with small numbers. Due to its infrequent occurrence, PTT dislocations have been initially and mistakenly treated as simple ankle sprains (35). Lohrer et al. reported 58.5% of PTT dislocations were induced by sport and 53.1% were initially misdiagnosed (43). Complaints of medial ankle pain and swelling are noted. Weakness and inability to invert the foot may be present. If dislocated, the PTT is found medial or anterior to the medial malleolus. Subluxation of the tendon may be appreciated as well. The mechanism of injury typically is forced ankle dorsiflexion with the foot inverted and forceful contraction of the PTT (35,44,45). The PTT may initially appear reduced, but dislocation or apprehension can be reproduced with resisted plantarflexion and inversion.

Imaging studies, such as MRI or ultrasound, may aide in establishing a diagnosis. The clinician should also be aware of associated injuries, such as medial malleolus ankle fracture (46), flexor digitorum longus tendon dislocation (20), and Achilles rupture (47), which have been reported in combination with PTT dislocation. Radiographic examination should be performed with specific attention to the medial malleolus for irregular periosteal reaction (20) or an avulsion fracture (21).

Non-operative treatment is typically not successful in maintaining reduction of the PTT. Surgical intervention is performed with the goal of evaluating the PTT, flexor retinaculum, and retromalleolar groove. A hypoplastic or shallow flexor sulcus may predispose an individual to PTT dislocation (48). The PTT is also inspected, and any tears are debrided and repaired. At the time of surgical intervention, the flexor retinaculum may or may not be intact. If the flexor retinaculum is found intact, it will be lax or attenuated. Successful outcomes have been achieved with direct repair of the retinaculum (44,49) and reconstruction of the flexor retinaculum. Reconstruction consists of reattaching of the attenuated retinaculum to the anterior ridge of the PTT groove and imbricating the redundant tissue to supplement the repair (35,50). Suture anchors or bone tunnels can be employed to secure the flexor retinaculum to the tibia. Successful reconstruction of a chronic dislocation has also been achieved with an Achilles tendon flap (49,51). The retromalleolar sulcus is deepened if it is determined to be hypoplastic (46). The groove can be deepened by drilling the bone inferior to the sulcus and tamping the posterior aspect of the medial malleolus down with a mallet. Augmentation of the retromalleolar groove with a bone block has also been described (21,52).

ACCESSORY NAVICULAR

The first description of accessory navicular was by Bauhin in 1605 (53,54). Occurrence of accessory navicular ranges from 10% to 14% (55). It is more common in females (ratio 5:1) (56,57). Approximately 50% of patients have a pes planovalgus deformity, but an accessory navicular is not associated with the development of flexible flatfoot (58). Patients with symptomatic accessory naviculars present with medial pain and prominence.

Most cases are asymptomatic; however, symptomatic cases may be related to the type of accessory navicular. Type 1 demonstrates an ossicle within the PTT. Type 2 demonstrates a synchondrosis between the navicular and the ossicle (Fig. 15.9.) Type 3 demonstrates a fused synchondrosis that results in a prominent navicular tuberosity. Patients present with foot pain over the medial navicular. Type 2 are symptomatic due to chronic injury of the synchondrosis (56,59,60). Histologic

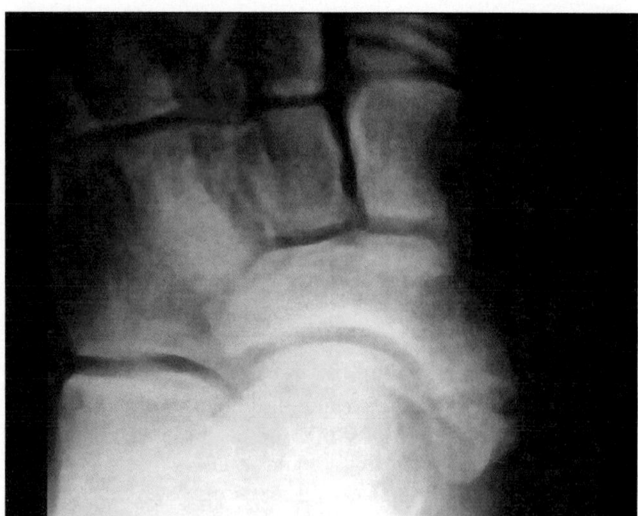

Figure 15.9. Anteroposterior radiograph demonstrating an accessory navicular.

examination of symptomatic ossicles exhibits a mixture of hyaline and fibrocartilage, as well as evidence of trauma hemorrhage, fibrous tissue, and callus-like reparative tissue (54). Type 3 are symptomatic due to the prominence of the medial navicular. Difficulty with shoe wear becomes more prevalent as the size of the prominence increases. Insertional pain of the PTT may also be present.

Radiographic examination should include an internal and external oblique views, which may allow better visualization of the accessory navicular. CT provides clearer definition of bony anatomy. Bone scan may show increased activity at the ossicle. MRI allows visualization of the ossicle, synchondrosis, and PTT. Physical examination of bilateral feet should be performed. Bony prominence of the medial navicular as well as tenderness should be noted. The PTT is also palpated to evaluate pathology of the tendon itself. The alignment of bilateral feet and ankles should be noted.

Symptoms often present in adolescence and with increased activity. For patients with activity-related symptoms, initial treatment includes rest and activity modification. Patients with pain during athletic participation are withheld from sport. NSAID and ice can also be used to provide relief of pain. An over-the-counter orthosis is used provide external arch support. Patients with tight heel cords are initiated in a stretching regimen. If no improvement is made, a period of immobilization in a walking cast or boot for 4 to 6 weeks is recommended. Patients who are symptomatic with ambulation, including activities of daily living, are placed in a boot initially.

In the event non-operative treatment is unsuccessful, surgical treatment is indicated. Several techniques have been described, including the Kidner procedure, ossicle excision, and arthrodesis.

Kidner described ossicle excision, leaving a sliver of bone within the tendon to be advanced and attached to the plantar aspect of the navicular. This technique attempts to change the line of pull of the PTT from medial to upward; thus, the mechanical advantage is increased (53).

Successful outcomes have also been achieved with ossicle excision and contouring the navicular tuberosity (61). Access to the ossicle is obtained via a longitudinal split between tendon fibers or elevating the PTT insertion off the navicular. A complete release of the PTT is not necessary. After ossicle excision, the PTT is reattached to the navicular with non-absorbable suture or suture anchors.

Achieving increased stability of the accessory navicular has also been described. A comparative study of arthrodesis with screw fixation versus the Kidner procedure yielded similar results. This technique is limited by the size of the accessory navicular and its ability maintain fixation by a 3.5 mm cannulated lag screw (62). Percutaneous drilling has also been described to achieve union between the ossicle and the navicular. Excellent results were reported in patients who achieved union. Fusion rates were higher in patients with an immature physis in the proximal phalanx of the hallux. Good to excellent results were achieved, even in patients with nonunion. Achieving increased stability at the synchondrosis was felt to contribute to symptomatic improvement (63). This method is more applicable to the skeletally immature patient. Due to the limited numbers of trials utilizing fusion techniques, the recommended treatment for symptomatic accessory naviculars is the Kidner procedure or ossicle excision.

Post-operatively, the patient is casted in inversion for 4 weeks. Progressive weight bearing in a boot with an orthosis is initiated. Physical therapy is instituted upon initiation of range of motion and progressive weight bearing. Return to athletic participation is anticipated 3 to 4 months from surgery.

CONCLUSION

PTT injuries in athletes are uncommon, but they demand a clinician's awareness due to the disability that may arise from a missed or delayed diagnosis. This is reinforced by the number of case reports found in the literature in which patients were initially treated for simple ankle sprains. In the course of history taking and physical examination, specific attention must be paid to medial ankle pain. The overall alignment of the athlete's foot and ankle must also be assessed. Recognizing hindfoot valgus or flatfoot deformity may clue the examiner to PTT injury or pathology. This recognition is also imperative in determining a course of treatment. Treatment focuses on correcting pathology and restoring PTT biomechanics, which maximizes the athlete's functional outcome.

REFERENCES

1. Mosier SM, Pomeroy G, Manili A. Pathoanatomy and etiology of posterior tibial tendon dysfunction. *Clin Ortho Rel Res* 1999;365:12–22.
2. Sarrafian SK. *Anatomy of the Foot and Ankle.* 2nd ed. Philadelphia, PA: J.B. Lippincott; 1993.
3. Bloome DM, Marymont JV, Varner KE. Variation on the insertion of the posterior tibialis tendon: A cadaveric study. *Foot Ankle Int* 2003;24(10):780–783.
4. Frey C, Shereff M, Greenidge N. Vascularity of the posterior tibial tendon. *J Bone Joint Surg Am* 1990;72:884–888.
5. Petersen W, Hohmann G, Stein V, et al. The blood supply of the posterior tibial tendon. *J Bone Joint Surg Br* 2002;84-B:141–144.
6. Prado MP, de Carvalho AE, Rodrigues CJ, et al. Vascular density of the posterior tibial tendon: A cadaver study. *Foot Ankle Int* 2006;27(8):628–631.
7. Funk DA, Cass JR, Johnson KA. Acquired adult flat foot secondary to posterior tibial-tendon pathology. *J Bone Joint Surg Am* 1986;68-A:95–102.
8. Mosier SM, Lucas DR, Pomeroy G, et al. Pathology of the posterior tibial tendon in posterior tibial tendon insufficiency. *Foot Ankle Int* 1998;19:520–524.
9. Basmajian JV, Stecko G. The role of muscles in arch support of the foot. *J Bone Joint Surg* 1963;45A:1184–1190.

10. Sutherland DH. An electromyographic study of the plantar flexors of the ankle in normal walking on the level. *J Bone Joint Surg* 1966;48A:66–71.
11. Sitler DF, Bell SJ. Soft tissue procedures: *Foot Ankle Clin N Am* 2003;8:503–520.
12. Reber L, Perry J, Pink M. Muscular control of the ankle in running. *Am J Sports Med* 1993;21(6):805–810.
13. Uchiyama E, Kitaoka HB, Fujii T, et al. Gliding resistance of the posterior tibial tendon. *Foot Ankle Int* 2006;27(9):723–727.
14. Conti SF. Posterior tibial tendon problems in athletes. *Orthop Clin North Am* 1994;25(1):109–121.
15. Augustin JF, Lin SS, Berberian WS, et al. Nonoperative treatment of adult acquired flat foot with the Arizona brace. *Foot Ankle Clin* 2003;8:491–502.
16. DeOrio JK, Shapiro SA, McNeil RB, et al. Validity of the posterior tibial edema sign in posterior tibial tendon dysfunction. *Foot Ankle Int* 2011;32(2):189–192.
17. Silfverskiöld N. Reduction of the uncrossed two-joints muscles of the leg to one-joint muscles in spastic conditions. *Acta Char Scand* 1924;56:315–328.
18. Mann RA, Thompson FM. Rupture of the posterior tibial tendon causing flat foot. Surgical treatment. *J Bone Joint Surg Am* 1985;67:556–561.
19. Kong A, Van der Vliet A. Imaging of tibialis posterior dysfunction. *Br J Radiol* 2008;81: 826–836.
20. Aguiar ROC, Cabral MVG, Moura BB, et al. Dislocation of the flexor digitorum longus and posterior tibial tendons without fracture dislocation of the ankle: A case report. *Foot Ankle Int* 2007;28(11):1187–1189.
21. Lee K, Byun WJ, Ha JK, et al. Dislocation of the tibialis posterior tendon treated with autogenous bone block: A case report. *Foot Ankle Int* 2010;31(3):254–257.
22. Gould N. Evaluation of hyperpronation and pes planus in adults. *Clin Orthop Relat Res* 1983;181:37–45.
23. Nallamshetty L, Nazarian L, Schweitzer M, et al. Evaluation of posterior tibial pathology: Comparison of sonography and MR imaging. *Skeletal Radiol* 2005;34:375–380.
24. Khoury NJ, El-Kjoury GY, Saltzman CL, et al. MR imaging of posterior tibial tendon dysfunction. *Am J Roentgenol* 1996;167:675–682.
25. Erickson SJ, Cox IH, Hyde JS, et al. Effect of tendon orientation of MR imaging signal intensity : a manifestation of the "magic angle" phenomenon. *Radiology* 1991;181:389–392.
26. Deland JT, Hamilton WG. Posterior tibial tendon tears in dancers. *Clin Sports Med* 2008; 27:289–294.
27. Labib SA, Gould JS, Rodriguez-del-Rio FA, et al. Heel pain triad: The combination of plantar fasciitis, posterior tibial tendon dysfunction and tarsal tunnel syndrome. *Foot Ankle Int* 2002;23(3):212–220.
28. Johnson KA, Strom DE. Tibialis posterior tendon dysfunction. *Clin Orthop Relat Res* 1989; 239:196–206.
29. Myerson M. Posterior tibial tendon insufficiency. In: Myerson M, ed. *Current Therapy in Foot and Ankle Surgery.* St. Louis, MO: Mosby-Year Book: 1993;123–135.
30. Williams R. Chronic non-specific tendovaginitis of the tibialis posterior. *J Bone Joint Surg Br* 1963;45B(3):542–545.
31. Cooper AJ, Mizel MS, Patel PD, et al. Comparison of MRI and local anesthetic tendon sheath injection in the diagnosis of posterior tibial tendon tenosynovitis. *Foot Ankle Int* 2007;28(11):1124–1127.
32. Porter DA, Baxter DE, Clanton TO, et al. Posterior tibial tendon tears in young competitive athletes: Two case reports. *Foot Ankle Int* 1998;19:627–630.
33. Kulig K, Lerhaus ES, Reischl S, et al. Effect of eccentric exercise program for early tibialis posterior tendinopathy. *Foot Ankle Int* 2009;30(9):877–885.
34. Alvarez RG, Marini A, Schmitt C, et al. Stage I and II posterior tibial tendon dysfunction treated by a structured nonoperative management protocol: An orthosis and exercise program. *Foot Ankle Int* 2006;27(1):2–8.
35. Gluck GS, Heckman DS, Parekh SG. Tendon disorders of the foot and ankle, Part 3: The posterior tibial tendon. *Am J Sports Med* 2010;38:2133–2144.
36. McCormack AP, Varner KE, Marymont JV. Surgical treatment for posterior tibial tendonitis in young competitive athletes. *Foot Ankle Int* 2003;34(7):535–538.
37. Woods L, Leach RE. Posterior tibial tendon rupture in athletic people. *Am J Sports Med* 1991;19(5):495–498.
38. Marks RM, Schon LC. Posttraumatic posterior tibialis tendon insertional elongation with functional incompetency: A case report. *Foot Ankle Int* 1998;19(3):180–183.
39. Brodsky JW, Baum BS, Pollo FE, et al. Surgical reconstruction of posterior tibial tendon tear in adolescents: Repair of two cases and review of literature. *Foot Ankle Int* 2005; 26(3):218–223.
40. Jacoby SM, Slauterbeck JR, Raikin SM. Acute posterior tibial tendon tear in an ice-hockey player: A case report. *Foot Ankle Int* 2008;29(10):1045–1048.
41. Bell W, Schon L. Tendon lacerations in the toes and foot. *Foot Ankle Clin* 1996;1:355–372.
42. Floyd DW, Heckman JD, Rockwood CA. Tendon lacerations in the foot. *Foot Ankle* 1983;4:8–14.
43. Lohrer H, Nauck T. Posterior tibial tendon dislocation. A systematic review of the literature and presentation of a case. *Br J Sports Med* 2010;44(6):398–406.
44. Nava BE. Traumatic dislocation of the tibialis posterior tendon at the ankle. *J Bone Joint Surg Am* 1968;50B(1):150–151.
45. Sharma R, Jomha NM, Otto DD. Recurrent dislocation of the tibialis posterior tendon. *Am J Sports Med* 2006;34:1852–1854.
46. Ouzounian TJ, Myerson MS. Dislocation of the posterior tibial tendon. *Foot Ankle* 1992; 13(4):215–219.
47. Boss AP, Hintermann B. Tibialis posterior tendon dislocation in combination with Achilles tendon rupture: A case report. *Foot Ankle Int* 2008;29(6):633–636.
48. Soler RR, Gallart Castany FJ, Riba Ferret J, et al. Traumatic dislocation of the tibialis posterior tendon at the ankle level. *J Trauma* 1986;26:1049–1052.
49. Rolf C, Guntner P, Ekenman I, et al. Dislocation of the tibialis posterior tendon: Diagnosis and treatment. *J Foot Ankle Surg* 1997;36(1):63–65.
50. Nuccion SL, Hunter DM, Difiori J. Dislocation of the posterior tibial tendon without disruption of the flexor retinaculum. *Am J Sports Med* 2001;29:656–659.
51. Ballesteros R, Chacon M, Cimarra A, et al. Traumatic dislocation of the tibialis posterior tendon: a new surgical procedure to obtain a strong reconstruction. *Trauma* 1995;39: 1198–1200.
52. Miki T, Kuzuoka K, Kotani H, et al. Recurrent dislocation of tibialis posterior tendon. A report of two cases. *Arch Orthop Trauma Surg* 1998;118:96–98.
53. Kidner FC. The pre-hallux (accessory scaphoid) in its relation to flat-foot. *J Bone Joint Surg Am* 1929;11:831–837.
54. Zadek I, Gold AM. The accessory tarsal scaphoid. *J Bone Joint Surg Am* 1948;30:957–968.
55. Geist E. The accessory scaphoid bone. *J Bone Joint Surg Am* 1925;7:570–574.
56. Lawson JP, Ogden JA, Sella E, et al. The painful accessory navicular. *Skeletal Radiol* 1984;12:250–262.
57. Mygind HB. The accessory tarsal scaphoid: clinical features and treatment. *Acta Orthop Scand* 1953;23:142–151.
58. Sullivan JA, Miller WA. The relationship of the accessory navicular to the development of the flat foot. *Clin Orthop Relat Res* 1979;144:233–237.
59. Chen YJ, Hsu RW, Liang SC. Degeneration of the accessory navicular synchondrosis presenting as rupture of the posterior tibial tendon. *J Bone Joint Surg Am* 1997;79: 1791–1798.
60. Grogan DP, Gasser SI, Ogden JA. The painful accessory navicular: A clinical and histopathological study. *Foot Ankle* 1989;10:164–169.
61. Macnicol MF, Voutsinas S. Surgical treatment of the symptomatic accessory navicular. *J Bone Joint Surg Br* 1984;66(2):218–226.
62. Scott AT, Sabesan VJ, Saluta JR, et al. Fusion versus excision of the symptomatic Type II accessory navicular: A prospective study. *Foot Ankle Int* 2009:30(1):10–15.
63. Nakayama S, Sugimoto K, Takakura Y, et al. Percutaneous drilling of symptomatic navicular in young athletes. *Am J Sports Med* 2005;33:531–535.

CHAPTER

16

Jonathan Kaplan
David B. Thordarson
Timothy P. Charlton

Achilles Pathology and Ruptures

ANATOMY

The Achilles tendon is the largest and strongest tendon in the body. It consists of the two heads of the gastrocnemius muscle and the soleus muscle to form the triceps surae tendon. In addition, there is a small contribution of the plantaris muscle, which is absent in 6% to 8% of the population. The course of the Achilles tendon is unique in that it spirals 90 degrees as it courses distally to its insertion, such that the medial proximal fibers insert posteriorly on the posterosuperior calcaneal tuberosity.

Unlike other tendons in the body, the Achilles tendon lacks a true synovial sheath. Instead, it is comprised of an outer paratenon layer consisting of both a visceral and parietal layer, followed by the mesotenon, epitenon, and finally the inner endotenon. The anterior surface of the paratenon is well vascularized with transverse arterioles penetrating the mesotenon while the posterior, medial, and lateral surfaces contain multiple thin layers rich in mucopolysaccharides that decrease friction during tendon excursion, allowing approximately 1.5 cm of tendon glide (1). The epitenon is a connective tissue layer rich in blood vessels as well.

It is important to have a good understanding of the blood supply to the Achilles tendon. Proximally, the tendon receives its vascularity via the musculotendinous junction from the recurrent branch of the posterior tibial artery. Distally, recurrent branches from the calcaneus via the fibular and posterior tibial arteries provide vascularity to the insertion site. There is a watershed area approximately 2 to 6 cm above the calcaneal insertion, in which the blood supply consists of vessels within the overlying paratenon as described above (2). Nuclear studies have showed that mesotenal arteries are fewest at this level as well as a decrease in intratendinous vessels 4 cm from the calcaneus. Additional studies have shown that with aging, the number of vessels decrease with age, which may contribute to increased injury rates with aging (3).

Many disorders of the Achilles are related to its surrounding structures. There are two main bursae surrounding the Achilles tendon. The retrocalcaneal bursa is located anterior to the Achilles tendon and posterior to the posterosuperior calcaneal tuberosity. Dorsiflexion of the foot increases pressure and plantarflexion decreases pressure on these bursae. The superficial bursa is located posterior to the Achilles tendon and anterior to the skin and subcutaneous tissue, and this superficial location predisposes it to chronic irritation due to external compression from shoe wear. In addition, patients should be evaluated for a Haglund deformity, which is a prominence on the posterosuperior lateral aspect of the calcaneus, which may predispose the patient to retrocalcaneal bursitis and mechanical irritation.

The Achilles tendon consists mostly of collagen, elastin, mucopolysaccharides, and glycoproteins. Mature fibroblasts within the Achilles produce both type 1 and type 3 collagen. The normal tendon is 95% type 1 collagen, however, when ruptured, there is an increase in production of type 3 collagen, which may alter the strength after healing. With aging, the tendon sustains a decrease in cell density, collagen fibril diameter and density, and a loss of fiber waviness, thereby resulting in higher injury susceptibility in older athletes (1).

BIOMECHANICS

The triceps surae crosses the knee, ankle, and subtalar joint, and therefore contributes to knee flexion, ankle plantarflexion for push-off gait, and foot supination. Studies have shown that the Achilles tendon is subjected to some of the highest loads in the body. It reaches peak forces 12.5 times body weight (9.0 kN) in response to running at full speed and 1.0 to 4.0 kN in activities such as jumping and cycling (4–7). The Achilles is very responsive to mechanical stimuli such that the diameter thickens in response to exercise while it atrophies in response to inactivity or immobilization. In addition, there is a decrease in stiffness seen with immobility and aging versus an increased stiffness with exercise. Multiple studies have shown that overstimulation leads to increased degenerative enzymes (8) while understimulation leads to extracellular matrix degradation and loss of tendon properties (9,10). Controlled training regimens have been shown to increase collagen turnover and thickening of collagen fibrils, resulting in increased tendon tensile strength and stiffness (1).

The stress–strain curve regarding the Achilles tendon is well documented (11) (Fig. 16.1). At rest, the tendon has a wavy configuration, which is lost with tensile stresses. Studies have shown a linear relationship to collagen fiber deformation with increasing tendon loads. Strains placed on the tendon less than 4% are within limits of most physiologic loads and therefore fibers return to original configuration. However, strain between 4% to 8% results in intermolecular cross-link failure and collagen fibers sliding past each other while strain beyond 8% cause tensile failure of collagen fibers and interfibrillar shear failure resulting in macroscopic rupture (12).

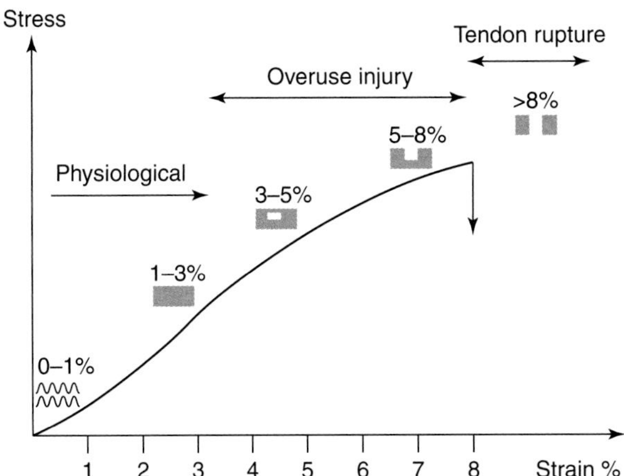

Figure 16.1. Stress–strain curve of Achilles tendon. Adapted from Maffulli N. Rupture of the Achilles tendon. *J Bone Joint Surg Am.* 1999 Jul;81(7):1019–1036.

EVALUATION

The evaluation of any suspected Achilles injury should involve a detailed history including mechanism of injury, previous injuries, as well as medical co-morbidities (such as diabetes or renal disease), medications (fluoroquinolones, corticosteroid injections), and social history (smoking, steroid use) which may contribute to diagnosing and treating these disorders. The examination should include a thorough lower extremity examination as well as specific maneuvers focused on diagnosing Achilles disorders. This includes inspection for ecchymosis and edema, palpation for any gaps or tenderness along the Achilles tendon, as well as a complete neurovascular examination including evaluation for peripheral vascular disease and peripheral neuropathy. The knee, ankle, and subtalar joints should all be examined.

In the presence of an Achilles rupture, contributions of the FHL and FDL tendons should be factored into the evaluation of the patient's ability to plantarflex the ankle as there are high rates of false negatives in the presence of a completely disrupted Achilles tendon. The Thompson test is one recommended test to diagnose Achilles tendon ruptures. The patient should be placed prone with the knee flexed to 90 degrees. The examiner should then squeeze the calf and observe for ankle plantarflexion. This test is considered positive if there is no plantarflexion when the calf is squeezed. The contralateral extremity should also be tested for comparing normal resting tension as well as plantarflexion in response to squeezing the calf. However, one must consider that false positives may exist with the Thompson test in patients with partially torn gastrocnemius muscle at or above the musculotendinous junction.

Imaging studies should be considered for almost all Achilles disorders. Radiographs are important to rule out fractures and may show a loss of the Kager triangle, which is a radiolucent triangle seen posteriorly on the lateral radiographs consisting of the area between the FHL and Achilles. Ultrasound has been shown to be valuable for diagnosis and treatment of Achilles tendinopathy as well as for evaluation of Achilles ruptures. MRI is useful for evaluation of tendinosis and paratenonitis as well as both acute and chronic Achilles tendon ruptures and it allows better estimation of tendon gap in chronic tears.

ACHILLES TENDINOPATHY

Achilles tendinopathy consists of a variety of disorders in which there is pain, swelling, and impaired performance of the Achilles tendon (11). There is an alteration in collagen structure in tendinopathy, which includes a loss in parallel orientation, separation of fibers, decrease in diameter and density of fibers, as well as an increase in type 3 collagen. A decrease in stiffness and force, decreased stress with a greater cross-sectional area, and increased strain and elongation result in a decreased Young's modulus, leading to a thicker tendon that is more elastic, that however produces less power.

The exact etiology of Achilles tendinopathy is unknown, however, it is frequently due to overuse and is multifactorial in nature. Tendinopathy may be related to host susceptibility and biomechanical malalignment. There is increased incidence of tendinopathy in patients with cavus feet, increased hindfoot inversion and decreased ankle dorsiflexion with the knee in extension, hyperpronation and limited mobility of the subtalar joint, and a varus forefoot (13,14). A leg-length discrepancy of 5 mm in elite athletes and 20 mm in non-elite athletes may predispose patients to tendinopathy. Muscle weakness or imbalances in strength, power, endurance, and flexibility also contribute to tendinopathy (4).

NONINSERTIONAL ACHILLES TENDINOPATHY

Noninsertional Achilles tendinopathy (NIAT) is considered a spectrum including tendinosis, paratenonitis, and paratenonitis with tendinosis. While it is important to understand the differences between these diagnoses, workup and treatment is often the same for all conditions that fall under NIAT (Table 16.1).

Pathogenesis

While exact pathogenesis is unknown, it is more commonly seen in athletes and is frequently due to overuse, altered training regimens including changes in frequency, duration and surface, poor training technique, poor environmental conditions, altered mechanics, and changes in shoe wear. Training errors have been reported to be involved in 60% to 80% of runners experiencing NIAT (4). The etiology has been referred to as the "Problem of Too—too much, too early, too fast."

TABLE 16.1 Spectrum of Noninsertional Achilles Tendinopathy

Tendinosis	Thickening of the tendon due to degeneration (aging, micro trauma, vascular compromise). Decreased cellularity with fatty degeneration and hypoxic degradation, no inflammatory cells seen on histopathology.
Paratenonitis	Inflammation and thickening isolated to the paratenon. Inflammatory infiltrate seen on histopathology.
Paratenonitis with tendinosis	Combination of inflammation within the paratenon as well as intratendinous degeneration. Histopathology shows findings consistent with both paratenonitis and tendinosis.

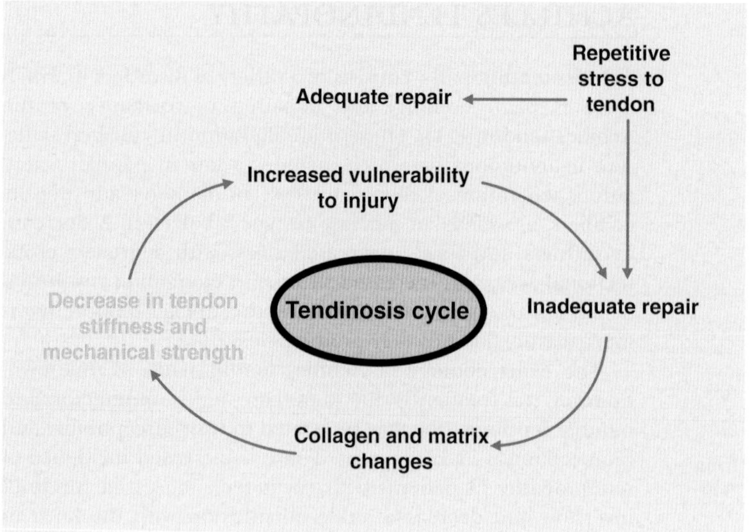

Figure 16.2. Tendinosis cycle.

The "tendinosis cycle" consists of a series of events leading to progressive worsening of NIAT (Fig. 16.2). Repetitive strain leads to inadequate repair and breakage of collage cross-linking. This results in tissue denaturation leading to inflammation and increased vulnerability to injury, thus restarting the cycle. It is believed that decreased arterial blood flow, local hypoxia, impaired metabolic activity, as well as free radical formation and exercise-induced hyperthermia leads to tendon degradation, however, this is controversial.

Presentation

Patients typically present with activity-related pain occurring within the substance of the tendon, approximately 2 to 6 cm above its insertion. Initially, patients experience pain, swelling, and warmth during exercise only as NIAT progresses; symptoms may become constant at rest and during activity, thus limiting ability to perform physical activities. Paratenonitis with tendinosis may have greater symptoms compared to those with either paratenonitis or tendinosis.

On exam, patients may have nodularity, warmth, swelling, and tenderness 2 to 6 cm above the insertion site. Patients with tendinosis will have a painless nodule that moves with tendon excursion while those with paratenonitis have a painful nodule that does not move with tendon excursion. Patients with NIAT may also have decreased push-off strength, increased dorsiflexion, and decreased plantarflexion. It is important to evaluate the patient for altered biomechanics including evaluation for leg-length discrepancy, ankle instability, malalignment, laxity, and stiffness or contractures that may predispose to NIAT (Fig. 16.3).

Diagnosis

Imaging studies may include plain radiographs, ultrasound (Fig. 16.4), and MRI. Radiographs are frequently normal, however, they may show intratendinous calcifications.

Ultrasound is considered beneficial because it is fast, inexpensive, more readily available, and may also be used for treatment modalities such as ultrasound-guided injections. Disadvantages include intra-user variability, limited soft tissue examination, and decreased sensitivity compared to MRI. Under ultrasound, the normal Achilles tendon is a homogenous fibrillar structure with well-defined borders and its adjacent paratenon typically measuring between 4 and 7 mm in thickness. With tendinosis, the tendon is found to be enlarged with a fusiform thickening, hypoechoic lesions within the tendon, and neovascularization seen with Doppler imaging. Studies have shown that 28% of normal individuals may have small microtears within the tendon while up to 82% of athletes have microtears (15). In paratenonitis, the tendon is normal appearing; however there is a circumferential hypoechogenic appearance around the tendon with hypervascularity seen within the paratenon (16).

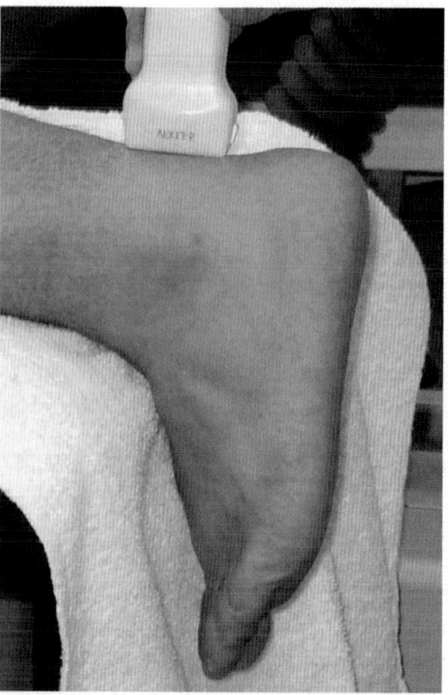

Figure 16.3. Achilles tendon examination.

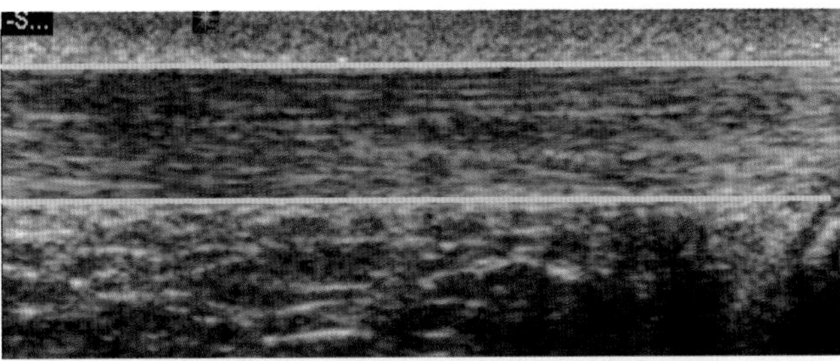

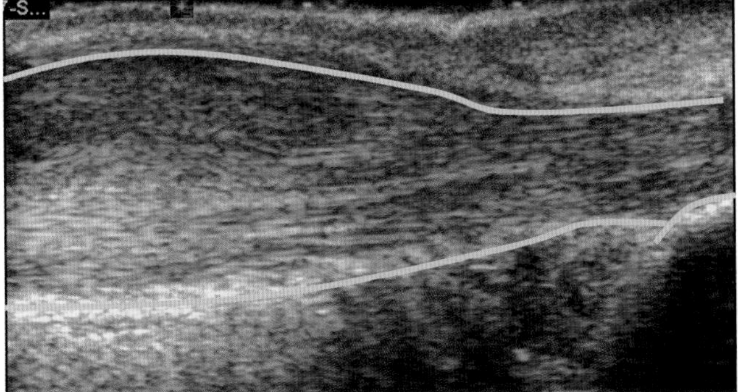

Figure 16.4. Normal and abnormal fusiform changes of the Achilles tendon on ultrasound.

While MRI is not necessary for the diagnosis of NIAT, it is frequently the preferred modality of imaging due to its increased sensitivity (Fig. 16.5). MRI provides better tissue contrast and higher spatial resolution allowing better identification of anatomic structures as well as evaluation of extent of pathology. Disadvantages include a higher cost, decreased availability, and it is more time consuming. In tendinosis, MRI shows a fusiform thickening (anterior to posterior diameter greater than normal limit of 6 mm) and intratendinous signal change. In paratenonitis, there is increased signal seen on T2 imaging within the paratenon and a normal-appearing tendon.

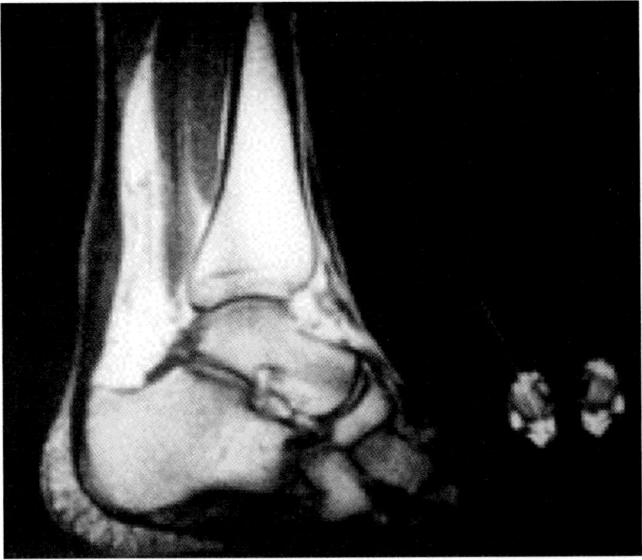

Figure 16.5. MRI shows fusiform elongation of the Achilles tendon consistent with a more advanced type 3 collagen change.

NONOPERATIVE TREATMENT

There is inconsistent data regarding treatment of NIAT; however, conservative treatment is typically the initial treatment of choice Table 16.2. This includes rest and activity modification, NSIADs, vasodilation cream, cryotherapy, immobilization, eccentric exercises, cross-training, stretching, shockwave therapy, and modification of risk factors such as the use of heel lifts and orthotics (Fig. 16.2). While there is no clear treatment algorithm, it is generally recommended that patients refrain from initiating activities for approximately 2 to 6 weeks prior to more invasive treatments and interventions. Up to 90% of patients with acute NIAT improve with nonoperative treatment, while chronic conditions are less consistent.

Eccentric exercises consist of elongation of the tendon while simultaneously contracting muscles. This creates tensile forces that decrease blood flow resulting in a decrease in neovascularization and associated pain receptors, leading to resolution of symptoms over a 12-week course (17,18). Shockwave therapy is believed to alleviate pain by stimulating soft tissue healing, regenerating tendon fibers, and inhibiting pain receptors (19). Shockwave transmits energy to the tendon producing intracellular damage, resulting in increased permeability of cell membranes as well as nerve depolarization to block transmission of pain signals (20). Results with this treatment are mixed, in addition to the treatment being costly.

Vasodilation cream consists of glyceryl trinitrate, which is a product of nitric oxide that may increase fibroblast collagen synthesis (21,22); however, it frequently results in painful headaches that limit patient compliance. This treatment is generally not recommended.

Other nonoperative treatment but more invasive treatments for NIAT include corticosteroid injections, PRP injections, and prolotherapy; however, data is insufficient for these modalities. Corticosteroid injections may provide short-term pain relief; however, intratendinous injections may have a catabolic effect on tendons. Steroid injections are strongly discouraged at our institution. PRP injections may cause delivery of cytokines to stimulate healing; however, there is insufficient evidence at this time. Prolotherapy consists of injecting a sclerosing agent, polidocanol, to target the vascular intima and cause thrombosis of vessels as well as to destroy local nerves; however, the results are inconsistent.

SURGICAL TREATMENT

Operative intervention is typically reserved for patients' refractory to conservative treatment, and noninvasive treatments should be attempted for at least 3 months prior to surgical intervention. Surgical treatment of paratendonitis includes injection brisement to breakup adhesions or paratenon excision with debridement. For tendinosis, options include debridement, micropuncture, and flexor hallucis longus (FHL) transfer. Despite surgical intervention, NIAT may be refractory in up to 25% to 50% of patients (4,23).

The goal of surgery is to resect degenerative tissue, stimulate healing, as well as augment tendon with vascularized graft if needed (19). It is generally recommended that FHL transfer to augment repair should be performed if greater than 30% to 50% of the tendon is involved. The FHL is preferred to other autographs because it is well vascularized and also functions as a strong plantarflexor within an axis similar to the Achilles tendon

(24,25). Topaz debridement can be done with a microcautery device through a 1.5 cm incision. Perforations of varying depths are placed into the degenerated tissue to theoretically promote a neovascularization into the diseased tissue.

Complications may exist in approximately 10% of patients undergoing surgical intervention; however, at 1 year most patients are satisfied with outcomes and return to the previous level of activity (4). Complications include skin necrosis, superficial and deep infections, seroma and hematoma formation, sural neuritis, new partial ruptures, deep vein thrombosis (DVT), and sensitive or hypertrophic scars. Maffulli showed females have worse outcomes, longer recovery time, more complications, and an increased incidence of reoperation (26).

INSERTIONAL ACHILLES TENDINOPATHY

Similar to NIAT, insertional tendinopathy is a spectrum of disorders which instead involves the insertion of the tendon at the superoposterior aspect of the calcaneus and adjacent areas. This includes retrocalcaneal bursitis, retrotendon Achilles bursitis, Haglund deformity, insertional paratenonitis, insertional tendinosis or tendonitis, and systemic enthesopathies.

Etiology

It is important to consider multiple concomitant disorders as they frequently are co-existent. A Haglund deformity is an enlarged posterior superolateral calcaneal projection that impinges on insertional fibers of the Achilles and the retrocalcaneal bursa. While it is not necessarily a pathologic condition alone, its predisposition to bursitis and Achilles impingement leading to paratenonitis and insertional tendinosis remains controversial. Kang et al. demonstrated that a Haglund prominence alone was not necessarily a factor in insertional Achilles tendonosis. Calcification may be seen within the Achilles tendon insertion, representing a degenerative area of the tendon.

Insertional tendinosis may be a biologic disorder due to constant intrinsic loading while insertional tendonitis is a true inflammatory process due to irritation from tendinosis, bursitis, or Haglund deformity. It is frequently found in obese patients and older recreational athletes (27). Retrocalcaneal bursitis is impingement of the bursa located between the Achilles and calcaneal process. Conversely, retrotendon Achilles bursitis is impingement of the bursa located between the Achilles tendon anteriorly and the skin posteriorly. It is frequently due to pressure of shoe wear against a prominent area.

While the majority of insertional Achilles tendinopathy disorders affect older recreational athletes, a separate subset of patients experience insertional Achilles tendinopathy due to enthesopathies. Conditions such as psoriasis, gout, and other spondyloarthropathies commonly affect young males. Symptoms are frequently bilateral. These conditions are beyond the scope of this chapter, however, warrant consideration and workup if indicated.

Presentation

Typically patients are older recreational athletes, commonly referred to as "weekend warriors". Symptoms typically consist of swelling, and slow onset, dull aching pain or startup pain located at the Achilles insertion. Pain is typically worse with activity and shoe wear. Symptoms may be exacerbated hill running, alterations in training regimen, and training errors. Dorsiflexion increases pain in retrocalcaneal bursitis by compressing the bursa between the Achilles and calcaneal process (27).

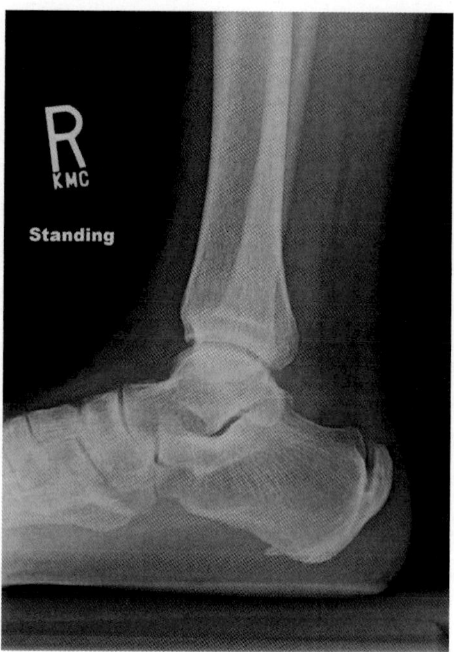

Figure 16.6. Calcification of the tendon is a poor prognostic sign for nonoperative treatment.

Examination frequently demonstrates swelling, warmth, and tenderness to palpation at the insertion site. It is important to evaluate the patient for contractures that may cause tension at the insertion site by performing the Silfverskiöld test.

Diagnosis

Similar to NIAT, imaging studies include radiographs, ultrasound, and MRI. Radiographs are beneficial for evaluating the anatomy of the calcaneus including the presence of Haglund deformity, tendon calcification, posterior calcaneal angle, and the parallel pitch line.

Ultrasound may show intratendinous calcifications, heterogeneity within the tendon, or thickening at its insertion site for insertional tendinosis or tendonitis (Fig. 16.6). In retrocalcaneal bursitis or retrotendon Achilles bursitis, ultrasound may show fluid with the bursa as well as peritendinous thickening (27).

MRI is valuable for visualizing the Achilles tendon, bursae, bony abnormalities, and the extent of the disease. Findings may be similar to that of NIAT however located at the Achilles insertion site. In addition, MRI may show increased fluid within the bursae with adjacent inflammation. It is more sensitive for demonstrating partial tears within the Achilles tendon.

Treatment

Initial treatment for insertional Achilles tendinopathy is similar to that of noninsertional tendinopathy. Nonoperative treatment is effective in approximately 90% of cases and consists of a period of rest Table 16.3, NSAIDs, physical therapy, shoe-wear modification,

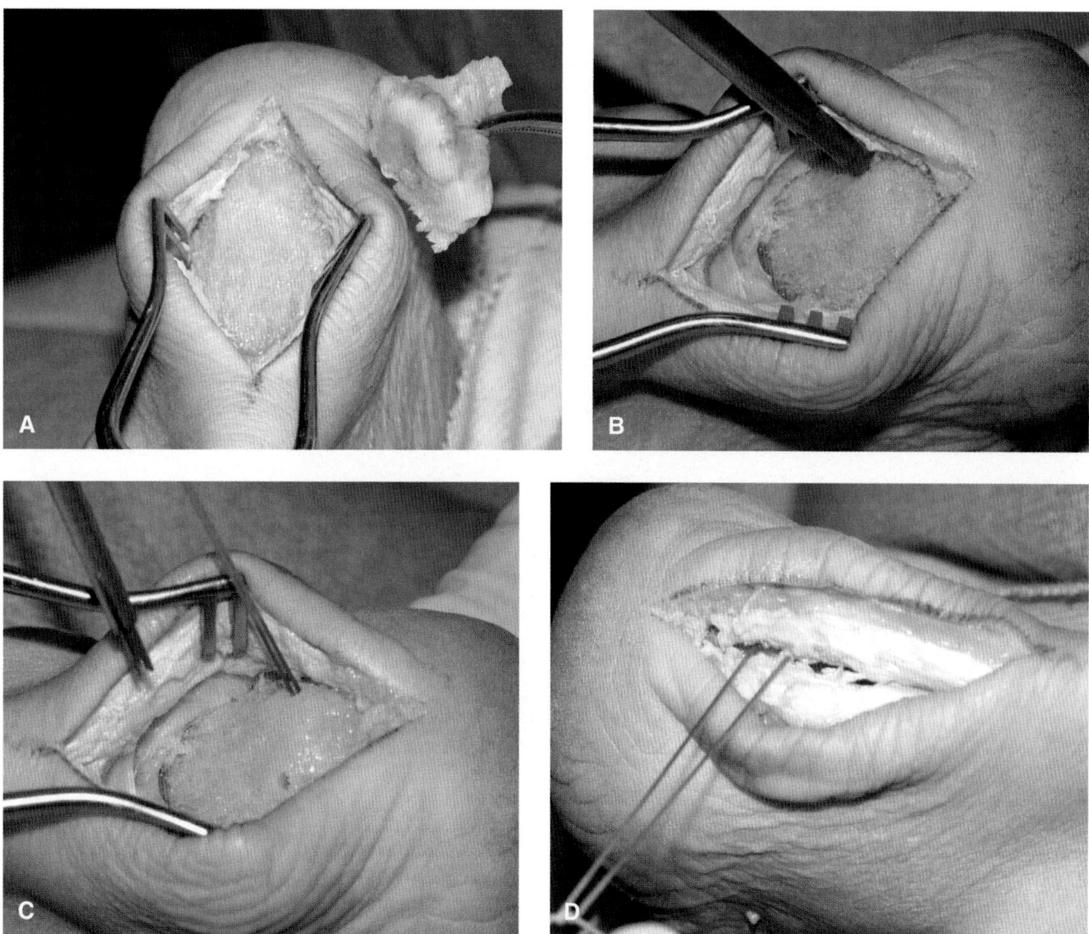

Figure 16.7. The Haglund deformity resection. **A:** Prominence is resected. **B–D:** Suture anchors in a single or double row construct are placed.

and alterations in training regimen or activity modifications. Corticosteroid injections should be avoided due to risk of tendon rupture.

Surgery is typically reserved for refractory cases of insertional Achilles tendinopathy. Operative interventions are typically directed at the underlying pathology and include open versus arthroscopic Haglund deformity resection (Fig. 16.7), bursa excision, debridement, and FHL transfer if greater than 50% of the tendon is involved. If calcifications are present on x-ray examination, then Haglund resection with reattachment using multiple suture anchor, double row construct is recommended.

ACUTE ACHILLES TENDON RUPTURES

The rate of Achilles tendon ruptures is increasing in industrialized countries due to a decrease in constant exercise and an increase in "weekend warriors" participating intermittently in physical activities (28). The typical age of patients with Achilles tendon ruptures is between 30- and 40-years old with a male to female ratio reported anywhere from 2:1 to 19:1. Seventy five percent of acute ruptures are sports related. It is more common for the left side to be ruptured than the right, which may be due to the possibility that more patients are right-side dominant and tend to push off with their left side. Of note, 80% of Achilles tendon ruptures occur in the watershed area located 2 to 6 cm above its calcaneal insertion. (29). Risk factors for Achilles tendon ruptures include sedentary lifestyle, corticosteroid injections due to collagen necrosis, anabolic steroid use due to collagen dysplasia and decreased tensile load, hyperthyroidism, renal insufficiency, gout, atherosclerosis, and fluoroquinolone use. In addition, systemic diseases may predispose the tendon to minor trauma.

Acute Achilles rupture is believed to be caused by a combination of mechanical overload as well as progressive degeneration of the tendon. Sedentary lifestyle leads to a decrease in vascularity, resulting in micro trauma and impaired healing until the tendon reaches macroscopic failure and rupture (30). This degenerative theory is supported by the fact that up to 15% of patients with Achilles tendon ruptures reported symptoms prior to rupture.

Presentation

Patients with acute Achilles tendon ruptures typically present with posterior ankle pain, difficulty with ambulation, decreased push-off strength, and may report an audible pop at the time of injury. The mechanism of injury may be due to (1) rapid dorsiflexion with a contracted gastrocsoleus complex, such as when a person steps onto a curb, (2) forced plantarflexion with

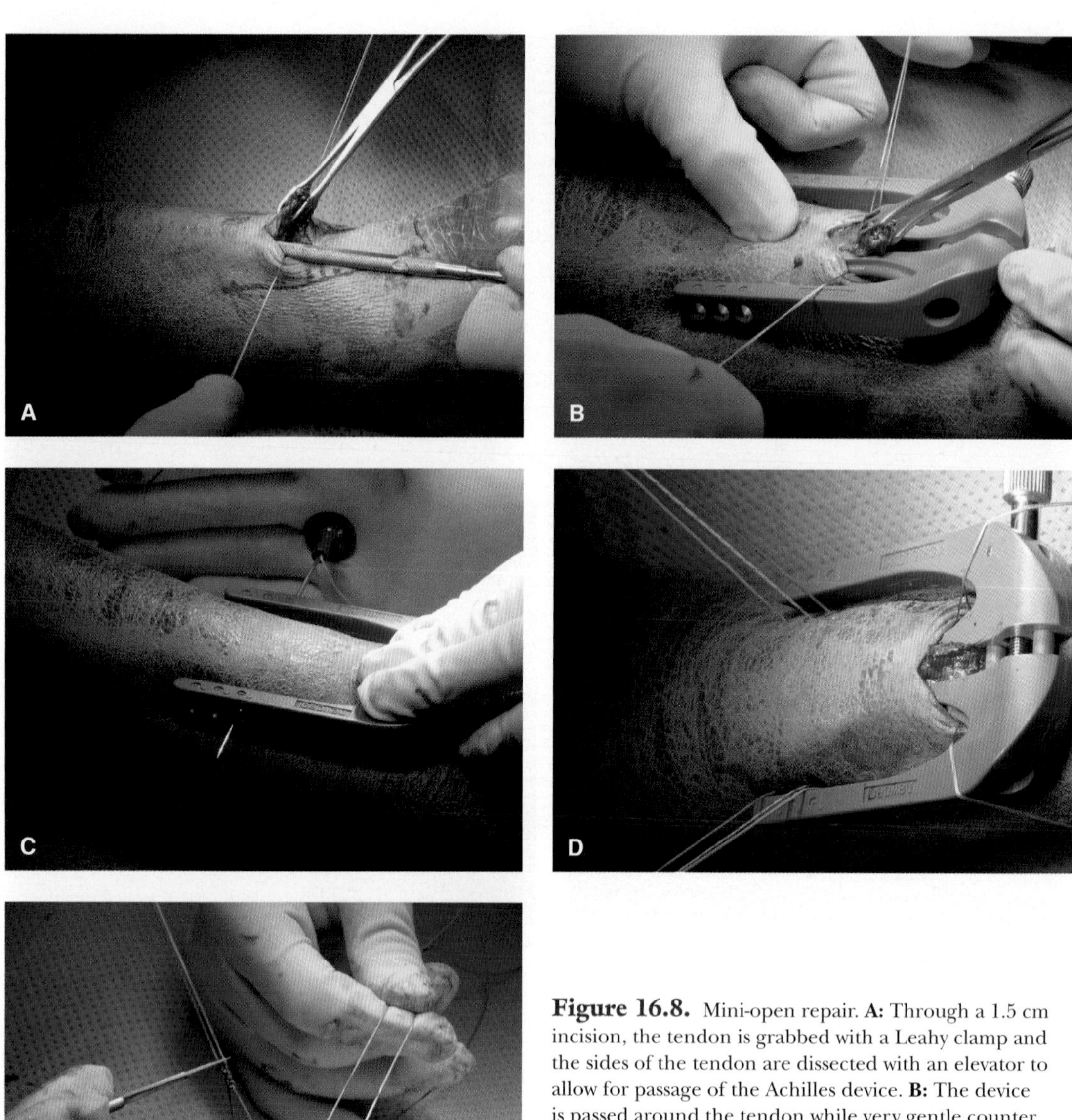

Figure 16.8. Mini-open repair. **A:** Through a 1.5 cm incision, the tendon is grabbed with a Leahy clamp and the sides of the tendon are dissected with an elevator to allow for passage of the Achilles device. **B:** The device is passed around the tendon while very gentle counter pressure is held with the Leahy clamp, such as to prevent the tendon from bunching while the device is passed. **C:** Needles with no. 2 suture are passed through the device. **D:** After three sutures are passed, the device is withdrawn and the suture will be within the paratenon. **E:** The sutures are tied on both ends and tension is established while the foot is held at 45 degrees knee flexion.

the knee extended, or (3) strong forced dorsiflexion on a fully plantarflexed foot, commonly seen in athletes with eccentric contraction during a jump or fall from height.

On examination, patients may have edema and ecchymosis, a palpable gap, point tenderness, and an increase in passive ankle dorsiflexion and decreased plantarflexion compared to the contralateral uninjured extremity (31). As described earlier, the examiner should perform the Thompson test to evaluate for an intact Achilles tendon as simply evaluating the ability of the patient to actively plantarflex may result in false negatives due to the ability of the flexor hallucis longus and flexor digitorum longus tendons to plantarflex the ankle. It is also important to compare the resting tension of the injured Achilles tendon to the contralateral side. Resting tensions of both extremities should be assessed in the prone position. An elongated resting tension should be considered highly suggestive of an Achilles tendon rupture.

Imaging

As diagnosis is generally based on presentation and examination, additional imaging may not be required unless there are equivocal history and examination findings (31). Radiographs may show a disruption of the Kager triangle, radiolucency proximal to the Achilles insertion, as well as a calcaneal avulsion.

Ultrasound has been shown to be reliable for diagnosing Achilles tendon ruptures and is more cost effective than MRI.

TABLE 16.2 Treatment

	Treatment	Results Expectation
Initial presentation	Heel lift (cowboy boot, high heels), NSAIDs, training modification	Mixed results due to compliance issues in activity
3–6 mos	Physical therapy with attention to eccentric rehabilitation	Reasonable in the absence of a large palpable nodule
Surgical	Open debridement or Topaz debridement	Extended recovery up to 9 mos

Patients with an Achilles tendon rupture will have a hypoechogenic area over the rupture tendon. Kotnis showed that dynamic ultrasound may be valuable for selecting appropriate nonoperative patients as patients with a gap less than 5 mm showed no difference in operative versus nonoperative treatment in regards to the re-rupture rate (32). However, while it is possible to measure the gap using ultrasound, this is operator dependent and therefore may not be as reliable as MRI. While MRI is more expensive and time consuming, it allows better evaluation of the extent of rupture as well as adjacent soft tissue injury. On MRI, there will be a disruption of signal on T1 and T2 images.

Treatment

There is no consensus for optimal treatment of acute Achilles tendon ruptures; however, there is a trend toward operative intervention for younger, more active individuals (28) Table 16.4.

NONOPERATIVE TREATMENT

Nonoperative treatment is generally reserved for elderly, more sedentary patients or patients with medical co-morbidities. Patients with diabetes, heavy tobacco use, venous stasis, morbid obesity, renal failure, and chronic steroid use are typically treated nonoperatively due to the high risk of complications with surgical intervention. Conservative treatment involves immobilization in plantarflexion to approximate the tendon edges. Patients are placed in a plantarflexed short leg cast or brace for 4 weeks followed by an additional 4 weeks of immobilization in neutral. Data shows that there are lower rates of re-rupture with functional bracing (2.4%) than with casting (12.4%) (28).

TABLE 16.3 Treatment of Insertional Achilles Tendinopathy

	Treatment	Results Expectation
Initial presentation	Heel lift (cowboy boot, high heels), NSAIDs, training modification	Mixed results due to compliance issues in activity
3–6 mos	Physical therapy (eccentric rehabilitation less effective)	Mixed results particularly in patients with visualized calcification on x-ray
Surgical	Open debridement, Haglund resection and reattachment	Extended recovery up to 9 mos. Good results

TABLE 16.4 Acute Achilles Tendon Ruptures: Treatment Results

	Strength	Infection	Re-rupture	Nerve Injury
Open	High	High	Low	Medium
Percutaneous	High	Low	Low	High
Mini-open	High	Low	Low	Low
Closed	Low	Zero	High	Zero

With nonoperative treatment, there is a higher risk of re-rupture (12.7%) compared to open Achilles repair (3.5%); however, there are no risks of surgical complications such as sural nerve injury, wound healing, and scar sensitivity, which are present in up to 34% of open Achilles repairs. There is a 0% risk of infection with nonoperative treatment compared to a 4.0% risk of infection with open Achilles repair (28). Still, patients treated nonoperatively have been found to have decreased plantarflexion strength (78% nonoperative compared to 87% operative), worse return to athletic activities (63% nonoperative compared to 71% operative), and decreased ankle motion (33,34). Therefore, despite higher risks of complications with surgery, it is generally recommended that younger, more athletic patients undergo surgical intervention to return them to a more normal pre-injury functional level.

Surgical interventions include percutaneous repair, mini-open repair, and open Achilles tendon repair. The goals for surgery are to restore normal resting length and tension, approximate tendon edges, and minimize complications. Benefits to surgical intervention compared to nonoperative treatment include lower re-rupture rates, earlier return to function, increased strength, and greater ankle range of motion. Surgical repair restores greater strength due to organization of the collagen fibrils during the remodeling phase to resist tensile stress as well as providing intrinsic tendon healing with collagen cross-linking during the maturation phase of healing. Risks of surgical intervention include sural nerve injury, wound complications, superficial and deep infections, and scar sensitivity with shoe wear.

DVT is a very controversial topic in Achilles tendon rupture. The risk of wound infections is offset with the catastrophic complication of a pulmonary embolism. When factoring in the fact that this complication happens to an otherwise healthy patient population, the issue becomes particularly sensitive to the surgeon. While DVTs have been well documented with Achilles repair, Patel et al. demonstrated that there is a lower risk of DVT than previously believed, and is slightly less than 0.5%. Use of chemoprophylaxis is not routinely used at our institution for prevention of DVT, but is a reasonable consideration. The limited incision size of a mini-open repair may also be more amenable to chemoprophylaxis versus the standard open incision.

Percutaneous repair of Achilles tendon ruptures has been shown to have decreased operative times, lower wound complications (8.3% compared to 26.1% in open repair), decreased

TABLE 16.5 Postoperative Rehabilitation for Achilles Tendon Rupture

Time	Accelerated Treatment	Non-accelerated Treatment
0–2 wks	Non–weight bearing in cast/splint	Non–weight bearing in cast/splint
2–4 wks	Gentle ROM in articulated CAM Walker	Non–weight bearing in cast
4–6 wks	Partial weight bearing in articulated CAM Walker	Gentle ROM in articulated CAM Walker
6–8 wks	Heel to neutral in CAM walker	Partial weight bearing in articulated CAM Walker
8–12 wks	Heel lift in a shoe with gradual reduction in heel lift	Heel to neutral in CAM walker
12–16 wks	Gentle physical therapy	Heel lift in a shoe with gradual reduction in heel lift
4–6 mos	Sports specific physical therapy	Gentle physical therapy
Anticipated return to sports	6–9 mos	1 yr

infections (0% compared to 19.6% in open repair), and a more cosmetic wound (11,35). Soubeyrand showed that the use of ultrasound improved correct positioning of all needles and tendon approximation (36). Also, according to a meta-analysis performed by Khan in 2005 showed lower rates of re-rupture compared to open Achilles repair (2.1% vs. 4.3%) (28). Conversely, percutaneous Achilles repair is associated with higher rates of sural nerve injury (4.5% to 2.8% in open repair) (11,35).

Open Achilles tendon repair consists of performing an end-to-end repair with the Krackow-, Bunnell-, or Kessler-type sutures. It has been shown that the modified Krakow stitch provides a stronger repair which is associated with higher rates of wound complications. Adjuncts include gastrocnemius turndown flap, overlapping repair with the plantaris, or using a graft jacket to improve strength; however, these procedures are generally reserved for treatment of re-rupture or delayed presentations (27). In addition, the plantaris can be released and fanned over the repair site to decrease adhesions and improve healing. As described above, open Achilles repair is associated with lower rates of sural nerve injury which are also associated with greater wound complications and rates of infections as well as greater rates of re-rupture.

The mini-open repair involves the use of a smaller incision combined with percutaneous fixation (Fig. 16.9). This allows direct visualization and precise control of tendon ends while avoiding excessive dissection, thereby decreasing risk of infection (37,38). It has been shown that the use of the mini-open technique provides a higher load to failure than the standard open 4-strand Krackow repair (39).

Postoperative rehabilitation for Achilles tendon ruptures includes a short period of immobilization followed by early range of motion exercises. Athletes may benefit from an accelerated rehabilitation program Table 16.5 including range of motion at 72 hours postop, ambulation in CAM walker 2 weeks postop, and full weight bearing at 6 weeks postop. This has been shown to allow 93% of athletes to return to sports by 6 months with only 2% to 3% deficit of pre-injury power and strength (40). In addition, postoperative casting followed by bracing has been shown to provide lower rates of adhesions, changes in sensation, hypertrophic scar formation, infection, and overall complications compared to casting alone (28).

REFERENCES

1. Saltzman CL, Tearse DS. Achilles tendon injuries. *J Am Acad Orthop Surg* 1998;6:316–325.
2. O'Brien M. The anatomy of the Achilles tendon. *Foot Ankle Clin* 2005;10:225–238.
3. Strocchi R, De Pasquale V, Guizzardi S, et al. Human Achilles tendon: morphological and morphometric variations as a function of age. *Foot Ankle* 1991;12:100–104.
4. Paavola M, Kannus P, Järvenin TA, et al. Achilles tendinopathy. *J Bone Joint Surg Am* 2002;84:2062–2076.
5. Komi PV. Biomechanics and neuromuscular performance. *Med Sci Sports Exerc* 1984;16: 26–28.
6. Komi PV, Salonen M, Järvenin M, et al. In vivo registration of Achilles tendon forces in man. I. Methodological development. *Int J Sports Med* 1987;8(Suppl 1):3–8.
7. Komi PV, Fukashiro S, Järvenin M. Biomechanical loading of Achilles tendon during normal locomotion. *Clin Sports Med* 1992;11:521–531.
8. Archambault JM, Hart DA, Herzog W. Response of rabbit Achilles tendon to chronic repetitive loading. *Connect Tiss Res* 2001;42:13–23.

8a. Archambault JM, Effervig-Wall MK, Tsuzaki M, et al. Rabbit tendon cells produce MMP-3 in response to fluid flow without significant calcium transients. *J Biomech* 2002;35:303–309.

9. Lavagnino M, Arnoczky SP, Tian T, et al. Effect of amplitude and frequency of cyclic tensile strain on the inhibition of MMP-1 mRNA expression in tendon cells: an in vitro study. *Connect Tiss Res* 2003;44:181–187.
10. Arnoczky SP, Lavagnino M, Egerbacher M. The mechanobiological aetiopathogenesis of tendinopathy: is it the over-stimulation or the under-stimulation of tendon cells? *Int J Exp Pathol* 2007;88:217–226.
11. Maffulli N. Rupture of the Achilles tendon. *J Bone Joint Surg Am* 1999;81:1019–1036.
12. O'Brien M. Functional anatomy and physiology of tendons. *Clin Sports Med* 1992;11: 505–520.
13. Kvist M. Achilles tendon injuries in athletes. *Ann Chir Gynaecol* 1991;80:188–201.
14. Kaufman KR, Brodine SK, Shaffer RA, et al. The effect of foot structure and range of motion on musculoskeletal overuse injuries. *Am J Sports Med* 1999;27:585–593.
15. Gibbon WW, Cooper JR, Radcliffe GS. Sonographic incidence of tendon microtears in athletes with chronic Achilles tendinosis. *Br J Sports Med* 1999;33:129–130.
16. Mitchell *JBJS* 2009;11:1405–1409.
17. Knobloch K. Eccentric rehabilitation exercise increases peritendinous type I collagen synthesis in humans with Achilles tendinosis. *Scand J Med Sci Sports* 2007;17:298–299.
18. Ohberg L, Alfredson H. Effects on neovascularization behind the good results with eccentric training in chronic mid-portion Achilles tendinosis? *Knee Surg Sports Traumatol Arthrosc* 2004;12:465–470.
19. Courville XF, Coe MP, Hecht PJ. Current concepts review: noninsertional Achilles tendinopathy. *Foot Ankle Int* 2009;30:1132–1142.
20. Ogden JA, Alvarez R, Levitt R, et al. Shock wave therapy for chronic proximal plantar fasciitis. *Clin Orthop Relat Res* 2001;387:47–59.
21. Rompe JD, Nafe B, Furia JP, et al. Eccentric loading, shock-wave treatment, or a wait-and-see policy for tendinopathy of the main body of tendo Achilles: a randomized controlled trial. *Am J Sports Med* 2007;35:374–383. [Erratum in *Am J Sports Med.* 2007;35:1216.]
22. Roos EM, Engström M, Lagerquist A, et al. Clinical improvement after 6 weeks of eccentric exercise in patients with mid-portion Achilles tendinopathy – a randomized controlled trial with 1-year follow-up. *Scan J Med Sci Sports* 2004;14:286–295.
23. Johnston E, Scranton P Jr, Pfeffer GB. Chronic disorders of the Achilles tendon: results of conservative and surgical treatments. *Foot Ankle Int* 1997;18:570–574.
24. Wapner KL, Pavlock GS, Hecht PJ, et al. Repair of chronic Achilles tendon rupture with flexor halluces longus tendon transfer. *Foot Ankle* 1993;14:443–449.
25. Wilcox FAI 2000;12(12):1004–1010.
26. Maffulli N, Testa V, Capasso G, et al. Surgery for Chronic Achilles tendinopathy produces worse results in women. *Disabil Rehabil* 2008;30:1714–1720.
27. Heckman DS, Gluck GS, Parekh SG. Tendon disorders of the foot and ankle, part 2: Achilles tendon disorders. *Am J Sports Med* 2009;37:1223–1234.

28. Khan RJ, Fick D, Keogh A, et al. Treatment of acute Achilles tendon ruptures. A meta-analysis of randomized, controlled trials. *J Bone Joint Surg Am* 2005;87:2202–2210.
29. Hattrup SJ, Johnson KA. A review of ruptures on the Achilles tendon. *Foot Ankle* 1985;6:34–38.
30. Kannus P, Józsa L. Histopathological changes preceding spontaneous rupture of a tendon. A controlled study of 891 patients. *J Bone Joint Surg* 1991;73:1507–1525.
31. Schepsis AA, Jones H, Haas AL. Achilles tendon disorders in athletes. *Am J Sports Med* 2002;30:287–305.
32. Kotnis R, David S, Handley R, et al. Dynamic ultrasound as a selection tool for reducing Achilles tendon ruptures. *Am J Sports Med* 2006;34:1395–1400.
33. Bhandari M, Guyatt GH, Siddiqui F, et al. Treatment of acute Achilles tendon ruptures: a systematic overview and metaanalysis. *Clin Orthop Relat Res* 2002;400:190–200.
34. Cetti R, Christensen SE, Ejsted R, et al. Operative versus nonoperative treatment of Achilles tendon rupture. A prospective randomized study and review of the literature. *Am J Sports Med* 1993;21:791–799.
35. Cretnik A, Kosanovic M, Smrkolj V. Percutaneous versus open repair of the ruptured Achilles tendon: a comparative study. *Am J Sports Med* 2005;33:1369–1379.
36. Nadaud JP, Parks BG, Schon LC. Plantar and calcaneocuboid joint pressure after isolated medial column fusion: a biomechanical study. *Foot Ankle Int* 2011;32:1069–1074.
37. Assal M, Jung M, Stern R, et al. Limited open repair of Achilles tendon ruptures: a technique with a new instrument and findings of a prospective multicenter study. *J Bone Joint Surg Am* 2002;84:161–170.
38. Kakiuchi M. A combined open and percutaneous technique for repair of tendo Achilles. Comparison with open repair. *J Bone Joint Surg Br* 1995;77:60–63.
39. Huffard, et al. *Knee Surg Sports Traumatol Arthrosc* 2003;11:409–414.
40. Mandelbaum BR, Myerson MS, Forster R. Achilles tendon ruptures. A new method of repair, early range of motion, and functional rehabilitation. *Am J Sports Med* 1995;23:392–395.

CHAPTER

17

Mark L. Prasarn
Clément ML. Werner
Dean G. Lorich
David L. Helfet

Ankle Fractures and Disruptions of the Syndesmosis

INTRODUCTION

Ankle fractures are among the most common injuries seen by the orthopedic surgeon (1). Although many regard them as "simple" fractures, it is our contention that these injuries are far from "simple". Malleolar fractures and soft-tissue injuries about the ankle have not received the attention they truly deserve secondary to the presence of the higher-energy pilon fracture. In our minds, both entities truly represent a clinical problem that even in the most experienced hands can ultimately lead to a poor outcome.

It has been shown by Ramsey and Hamilton that even a 1 mm shift of the talus within the mortise produces a decrease of 42% of joint contact area (2). This inevitably leads to increased joint contact pressures and alterations in peak-pressure distributions, resulting in articular cartilage degeneration. Long-term clinical studies have demonstrated that residual articular displacement and a malaligned mortise predisposes to an unsatisfactory result (3,4). It is generally agreed that restoration of an anatomic ankle mortise and normal tibiotalar contact area will result in the optimum clinical outcome.

It is therefore the goal of the treating surgeon to achieve a stably fixed anatomic reduction with a perfectly aligned ankle mortise. In order to do so, all aspects of the injury pattern must be recognized and addressed. Following the attainment of a stable ankle, early and aggressive rehabilitation must be undertaken.

ANATOMY

The ankle joint is a synovial joint surrounded by a thin hyaline capsule. It has several contributing osseous and ligamentous components:

OSSEOUS

The ankle joint is a complex joint consisting of three bones. The tibial contribution consists of the tibial plafond (including the posterior malleolus) and the medial malleolus. The most distal part of the fibula, or lateral malleolus, lies on the lateral side of the ankle joint. The most inferior osseous portion is the talus.

The distal tibial plafond is a concave surface from anterior to posterior. The posterior border is lower than the anterior border. The medial malleolus is continuous with the plafond on the medial side. It consists of an anterior and posterior colliculi. A posterior lip on the back of the plafond, or posterior malleolus, articulates with the talus and is a mechanical block to posterior subluxation.

The lateral malleolus is a bony prominence on the lateral aspect of the distal fibula. It is more posterior and projects further distally than the medial malleolus. Medially, the triangular surface covered by cartilage articulates with the talus. It lies slightly more proximally in a groove on the posterolateral surface of the distal tibia known as the incisura.

The talus is almost entirely covered by articular cartilage, and has no musculotendinous attachments. It transfers body weight from the tibia to the calcaneus. The superior surface is convex and articulates with the tibial plafond superiorly and the malleoli laterally and medially.

Inman demonstrated that the talus is not a perfect hinge joint with the body of the talus closely resembling a section of a frustum (a shape cut from a cone with the apex oriented medially) (5). The dome of the talus is wider anteriorly than posteriorly. As the ankle dorsiflexes, the fibula externally rotates to accommodate the widened anterior surface of the talar dome.

LIGAMENTOUS

In addition to the osseous restraints, several periarticular ligaments enhance ankle stability.

On the medial aspect of the ankle is a double-laminar ligament known as the deltoid ligament. The superficial portion originates from the anterior colliculus and inserts distally onto the talus, calcaneus and navicular. The synovial covered deep portion arises from the posterior colliculus and goes to the talus. The deep deltoid is the primary medial stabilizing soft-tissue structure.

On the posterior aspect of the ankle, there is a complex consisting of two main ligaments: The posterior tibiotalar and the posterior talofibular. This complex is strengthened by the posterior tibiofibular ligament.

The lateral (fibular) collateral ligaments are divided into three groups: The posterior talofibular, the calcaneofibular and the anterior talofibular ligaments.

The most significant ligamentous structure that maintains ankle stability is the syndesmotic complex. It consists of the anterior tibiofibular, posterior tibiofibular, transverse tibiofibular, and interosseous ligaments. The interosseous membrane provides some stability between the tibia and fibula as well.

PHYSICAL EXAMINATION

Ankle fractures in the athlete are usually the result of low-energy torsional forces and typically present with swelling, pain, deformity, and an inability to bear weight. A complete history of the event should be recorded. Age, previous injuries, past medical history, medications, and activity level are all important factors involved in making a definitive treatment decision.

Gross visual inspection should first be performed to rule out an open fracture or ankle dislocation. Unless rapid radiographic evaluation is available, any ankle dislocation should be immediately close reduced and immobilized in a well-padded splint. Open fractures should be irrigated and debrided in the operating suite in an emergent fashion. Any fracture blisters and the amount of initial swelling should be noted to plan how expediently surgery can be performed if necessary.

All bony and ligamentous landmarks of the leg, ankle, and midfoot should be meticulously palpated to localize pain or crepitus. The joints of the ankle should then be stressed to rule out ligamentous rupture with instability. The presence or absence of medial injury/tenderness, is a very important finding and can help to determine whether or not operative versus conservative treatment is indicated. The compartments of the leg and foot should be examined to rule out compartment syndrome. A thorough neurovascular evaluation is performed in all cases.

The anterior drawer maneuver evaluates the integrity of the anterior talofibular ligament. The knee is flexed to 90 degrees and the ankle in neutral. The foot is held in place and a posterior force is applied to the distal tibia. Posterior translation of the tibia with respect to the talus as compared to the contralateral side implies ankle instability. Inversion stress to the foot tests the lateral calcaneofibular ligament. Eversion stress in the neutral position tests the competency of the deltoid ligament. A positive “squeeze test”, performed by compressing the tibia and fibula proximally and eliciting pain at the syndesmosis, may be indicative of syndesmotic disruption.

RADIOLOGY

The Ottawa ankle rules are a set of guidelines to help determine when radiographs are indicated following injury to ankle. The criteria evaluated involve tenderness of the malleoli and the ability/inability to bear weight (6). Three views of the ankle (AP, lateral, mortise) are routinely obtained and evaluated for fracture and talar subluxation. Evaluation of the medial clear space, talocrural angle, and tibiofibular clear space are utilized to determine the alignment of the ankle. The medial clear space is the distance from the lateral border of the medial malleolus and the medial border of the talus, and should equal the space between the tibial plafond and the superior talus. The talocrural angle is the angle subtended by a line drawn parallel to the plafond and another connecting the tips of the malleoli. This averages 83 ± 4 degrees and is a reliable indicator of the relationship of the malleoli to the plafond. Abnormalities in either of these two measurements are representative of an abnormal ankle mortise. The distance from the medial cortex of the fibula to the incisura surface on the tibia is the tibiofibular clear space. This measurement should be less than 6 mm on either view, and greater values may represent syndesmotic disruption (Fig. 17.1).

CLASSIFICATION

The two main classifications in use today are that of Lauge-Hansen and Danis–Weber:

LAUGE-HANSEN CLASSIFICATION

The experimental, clinical and radiographic studies conducted by Lauge-Hansen resulted in the classification system that bears his name. More than 95% of ankle fractures can be classified into four groups in this system. An additional group, pronation–dorsiflexion, was later added for fractures caused by an axial load. In this system, the first word is the position of the foot at the time of injury, and the second word is the direction of the force. Each group is divided into several of the stages based on a sequence of injured structures observed in cadaver specimens (Fig. 17.2) (7). Each group is further described below.

Supination–Adduction (SA)

1. Transverse fracture of the fibula below the level of the joint, or rupture of the lateral collateral ligaments
2. Vertical fracture of the medial malleolus

Supination–Eversion (External Rotation) (SER)

1. Rupture of the anterior tibiofibular ligament
2. Spiral or oblique fracture of the distal fibula
3. Rupture of the posterior tibiofibular ligament or fracture of posterior malleolus
4. Rupture of deltoid ligament or fracture of the medial malleolus

Pronation–Abduction (PA)

1. Fracture of the medial malleolus or rupture of deltoid ligament
2. Rupture of the syndesmotic (anterior and posterior tibiofibular) ligaments or avulsion fracture of their osseous attachments
3. Short, oblique fracture of the fibula above the level of the joint

Pronation–Eversion (External Rotation) (PER)

1. Rupture of the deltoid ligament or avulsion fracture of the medial malleolus
2. Rupture of the anterior tibiofibular and interosseous ligament
3. Short spiral fracture of the fibula above the level of the joint
4. Rupture of the posterior tibiofibular ligaments or avulsion fracture of posterior tibial margin

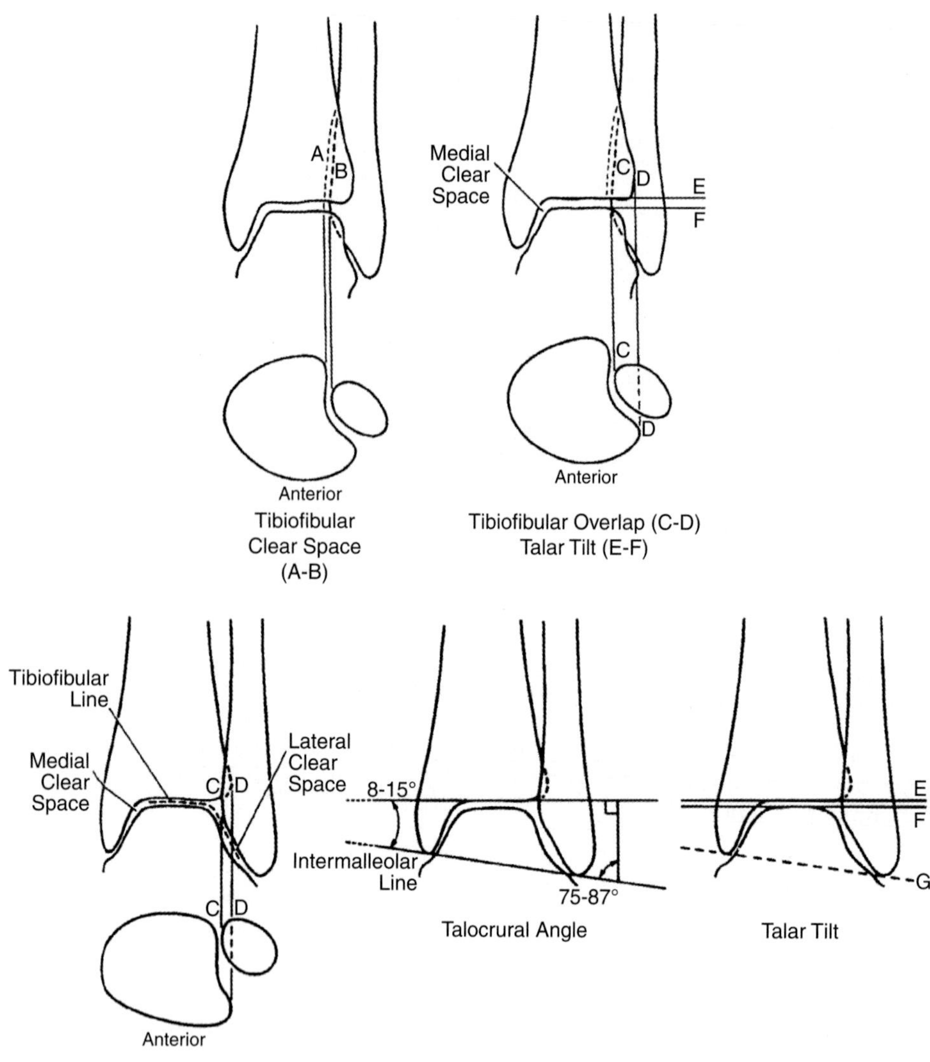

Figure 17.1. Radiographic measurements of the ankle. Adapted from Müller ME, Allgöwer M, Schneider R, et al. Manual of Internal Fixation. 3rd ed. New York, NY: Springer-Verlag; 1990. With permission.

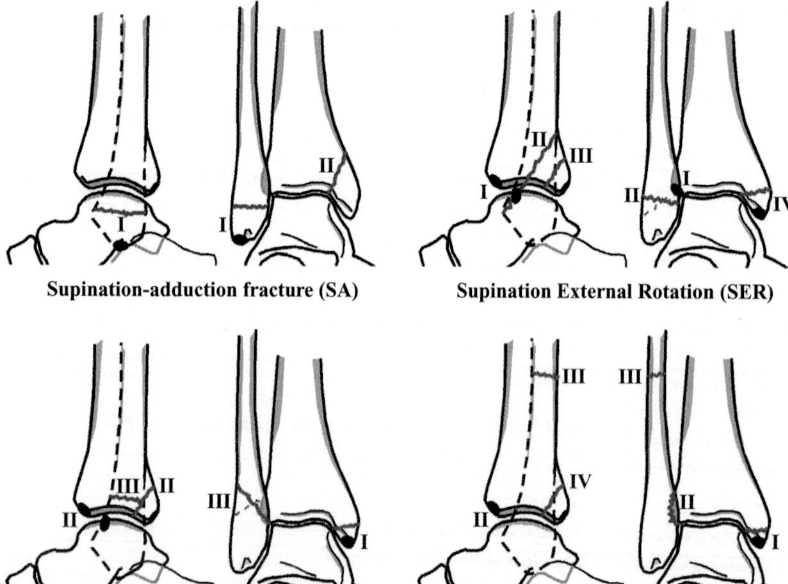

Figure 17.2. Lauge-Hansen classification system.

Pronation–Dorsiflexion (PD)

1. Fracture of the medial malleolus
2. Fracture of the anterior margin of the tibia
3. Supramalleolar fracture of the fibula
4. Transverse fracture of the posterior tibial surface

DANIS–WEBER CLASSIFICATION

In 1949, Danis described an anatomic classification which was later modified by Weber and now known as the Danis–Weber, or AO/ASIF group classification. In this system, the ankle fracture is divided into three classes (A, B, or C) according to the relationship of the fibular fracture to the syndesmosis and interosseous ligaments: Type A fractures are infrasyndesmotic, Type B are transsyndesmotic, and Type C are suprasyndesmotic.

These three types have been further classified into groups and subgroups, by Maurice Müller in the "Comprehensive Classification of Fractures" in order to qualify the spectrum of the injury according to the morphologic complexity of the fracture (Fig. 17.3) (8).

AO/ASIF CLASSIFICATION

Type A fractures are distal to both the interosseous ligament and syndesmosis (infrasyndesmoidal):

A1—isolated.
A2—with fracture of the medial malleolus.
A3—with a posteromedial fracture.

Type B fractures, which occur obliquely through the fibula, involve part or all of the syndesmosis and have an unstable syndesmosis approximately 50% of the time. They are typically at the level of the syndesmosis (transsyndesmotic).

B1—isolated.
B2—medial lesion (ligament or malleolus).
B3—with medial lesion and fracture of the posterolateral margin.

Type C fractures include fractures of the fibula proximal to the distal tibiofibular ligament and syndesmosis. These high fractures above the level of the syndesmosis (suprasyndesmotic) are considered unstable.

C1—simple diaphyseal fracture.
C2—complex fracture of the diaphysis.
C3—proximal fracture of the fibula.

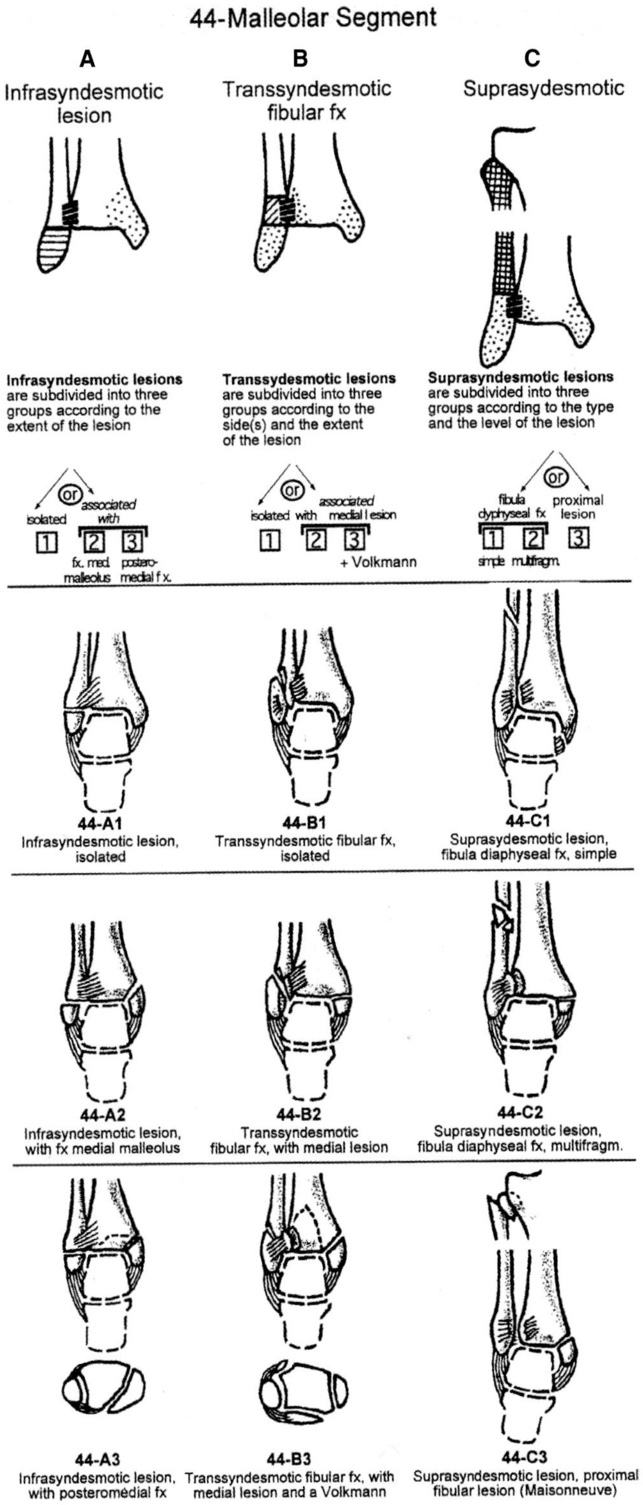

Figure 17.3. AO/ASIF classification system. Adapted from Maurice E. Müller. Comprehensive Classification of Fractures of the Ankle. In: Müller ME, Nazzarin S, Koch P, eds. Classification AO des fractures. 1: Les os longs; New York, NY: Springer Verlag Berlin-Heidelberg; 1987. Reprinted with permission.

ANKLE STABILITY FOLLOWING INJURY

Any injury pattern that does not compromise ankle stability may be considered for conservative management. An ankle is deemed unstable when loss of normal constraints results in the talus moving in a non-physiologic manner (9). There has been much clinical and basic science investigation into defining the relationship between injury pattern and ankle stability (3,4,7,8,10–16).

Isolated injuries to the lateral malleolus do not represent unstable fractures and do not require operative intervention. It has been shown that stability is not compromised unless there is also injury to the medial side of the ankle through either a complete tear of the deltoid or medial malleolus fracture (9,17). Therefore, bimalleolar fractures and lateral malleolus fractures with complete tears of the deltoid ligament, or bimalleolar equivalents, require open reduction and internal fixation to obtain the best possible outcome (14,15). We assume that the deltoid is incompetent if the patient has ecchymoses, swelling or tenderness just distal to the medial malleolus as well as an incongruent mortise on radiographic evaluation.

Weber B ankle fractures with an intact mortise pose a dilemma to the treating surgeon.

There has been considerable debate regarding the specificity of stress views and clinical signs of medial injury for predicting combined injury patterns. McConnell et al. demonstrated that soft-tissue indicators alone were not predictive of medial instability and recommended stress views (18). A recent paper by Koval et al. failed to demonstrate a correlation between positive stress views and complete deltoid rupture as seen on MRI (19). We do not rely solely on soft-tissue indicators alone, and do not perform stress radiographs. If the competency of the deltoid ligament is in question, we recommend evaluation by MRI.

FRACTURES OF THE LATERAL MALLEOLUS

Isolated fractures of the lateral malleolus may be treated conservatively if an adequate reduction can be maintained with a well-padded cast or splint. Patients should be monitored closely with regular radiographic follow-up to ensure maintenance of reduction. Good results have been demonstrated in clinical studies evaluating non-surgical management of such injuries (13,16).

If medial injury (medial malleolus fracture or complete deltoid tear) is diagnosed in conjunction with a lateral malleolus fracture, then surgical intervention is indicated.

Anatomical reduction of the fibula is crucial if high contact forces and subsequent osteoarthritis of the lateral aspect of the ankle joint are to be prevented. Malreduction of the fibula in terms of malleolar widening can be well controlled by assessment of the tibiofibular clear space (should be less than 6 mm). Longitudinal or rotational malreductions of the fibula, on the other hand, are more difficult to detect (20). Should there be a Maisonneuve fracture, we tend to open reduce the fracture to avoid any malrotation distally.

Several constructs have been proposed for fibula fracture fixation, including lateral plates with lag screws, lag screws alone, and posterior antiglide plates. While lateral plating might be more easily performed, it is often subject to symptomatic hardware, and leaves the hardware subcutaneously under the incision (21). Lag screws alone might obviate the need for hardware removal, but the technique might not be applicable in certain fracture configurations as well as osteopenic patients (22). The posterior antiglide plates have been shown to have the best resistance to torsional forces, but have been associated with peroneus brevis tendon irritations.

FRACTURES OF THE MEDIAL MALLEOLUS

The fracture pattern of the medial malleolus can greatly vary and has been described to be more vertical in Danis–Weber A (adduction) fractures, and more horizontal in Danis–Weber B and C (abduction and external rotation) fractures. Although both the Danis–Weber and the Lauge-Hansen classification give us an idea on certain injury mechanisms, they are not universally applicable. Also, the mechanical stress pattern encountered in the ankle after ORIF is not necessarily identical to the injury mechanism. It is advisable for more vertically oriented fracture patterns to provide maximal stress resistance against the two most commonly encountered mechanical forces on the medial side (varus stress and axial compression), regardless of the initial injury mechanism.

This is especially the case for the relatively vertical medial fracture patterns, which tend to migrate proximally if only fixed by two oblique lag screws. These vertically oriented medial malleolar fractures are occasionally associated with marginal impaction of the medial articular surface. Disimpaction and restoration of the articular surface leaves a metaphyseal defect which may further compromise the stability of medial-to-lateral lag screws. Therefore, we tend to apply an additional antiglide plate on the medial side (Fig. 17.4), with the lag screws inserted through the plate. Care must be taken not to extend the plate too distally to avoid prominence especially with shoe wear.

For horizontal fracture patterns at the level of the plafond, we advocate using mini-fragment plates and screws for fixation. The fragment is typically small in these cases and in many instances does not accommodate the 4.0 mm malleolar screws recommended by the AO manual. We contour a 2.4 mm plate around the medial malleolus and insert the corresponding screws through the plate that then serves as a washer as well as an antiglide plate. This fixation is often enhanced with 2.7 mm or 3.5 mm screws placed bicortically into the lateral distal tibial cortex from the tip of the medial malleolus (Fig. 17.5).

INJURIES OF THE SYNDESMOTIC COMPLEX

Syndesmotic injuries have classically been addressed surgically, although there are few reports in the literature regarding non-operative management of these injuries (23). The diagnosis of syndesmotic injuries based on plain radiographs is problematic, and even stress radiographs cannot be absolutely reliable (24). CT and MRI have been proposed as diagnostic tools, but are unlikely to become routine methods of assessment for these injuries. External rotation stress radiographs are the most frequently used method for assessing syndesmotic integrity (18). These should always be compared to the contralateral uninjured side.

Intra-operatively, we assess syndesmotic complex integrity through direct visualization and by placing a Hohmann retractor in the interosseous space and inducing an external rotation stress. Since it has been shown that the accuracy of reduction based on intraoperative image intensifier views alone is unreliable, (25) it may be advisable to directly reduce all syndesmotic disruptions. This allows direct assessment of the reduction by visualization and palpation of the anterior edge of the fibula at the anterior border of the incisura.

A multitude of techniques have been described to stabilize the syndesmosis: One versus two screws, screws of different diameters, tricortical versus quadricortical screws, bioresorbable devices, wires, etc. The use of locking screws in conjunction with 1/3 tubular locking plates allows for fixed angle stabilization, which may be advantageous biomechanically, and may

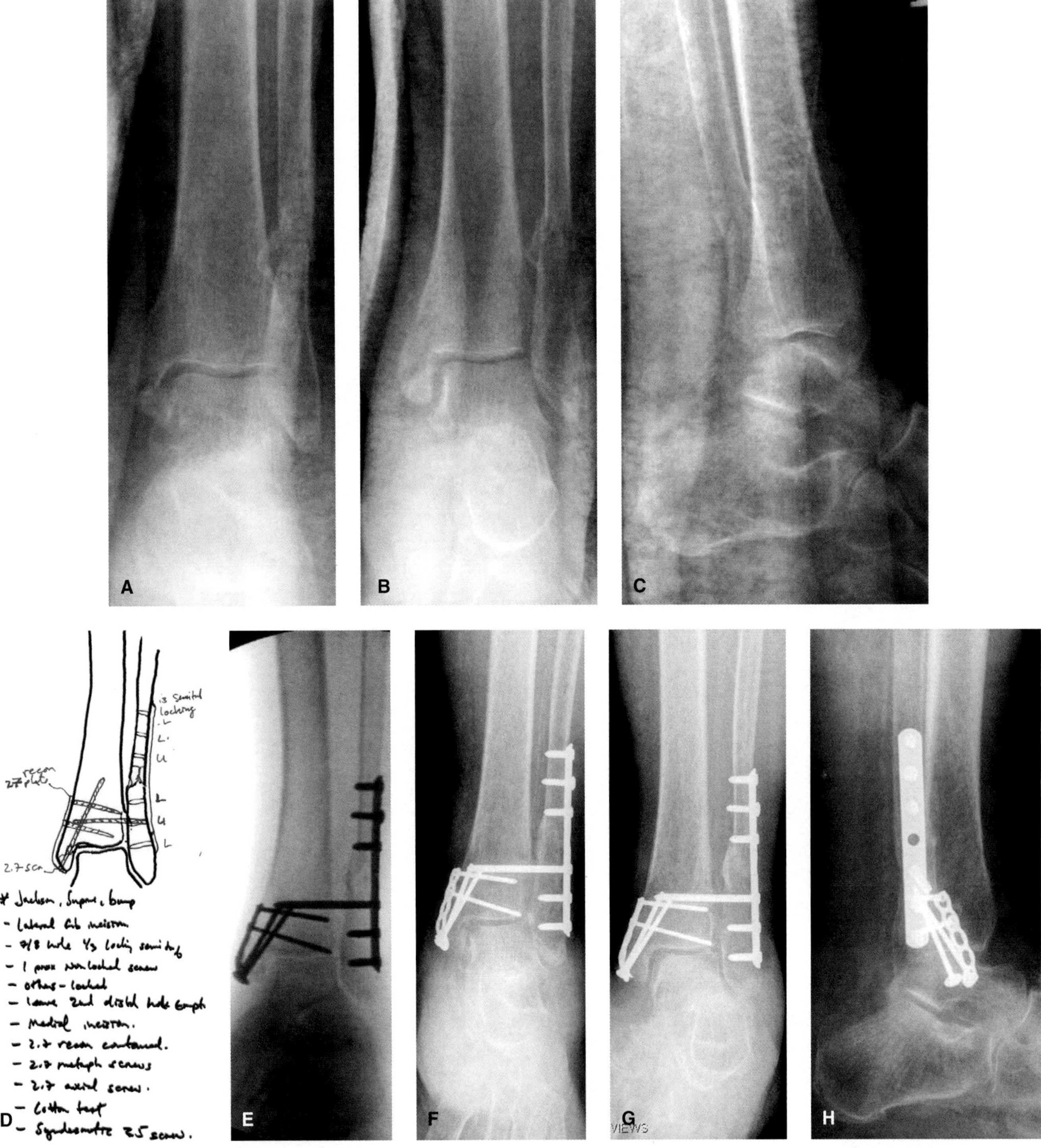

Figure 17.4. A 59-year-old female presented with left ankle pain and swelling after a fall while walking to the bathroom. Radiographs revealed a Lauge-Hansen-type SER IV displaced left-sided bimalleolar ankle fracture. Open reduction and internal fixation was performed with placement of a 7-hole 1/3 semitubular plate across the fibular fracture and a syndesmotic screw. A 5-hole mini-fragment plate was contoured across the medial malleolus as a medial malleolus antishear plate. The patient returned for follow-up 6 months following fracture surgery with excellent clinical and radiographic results including fracture union, full pain-free range of motion and a return to her previous activities of daily living. **A, B, C:** Anteroposterior (AP), mortise, and lateral radiographic views. **D, E:** Preoperative plan for open reduction and internal fixation and intraoperative fluoroscopic image illustrating acceptable reduction and fixation. **F, G, H:** AP, mortise, and lateral radiographic views 6 months following fracture surgery.

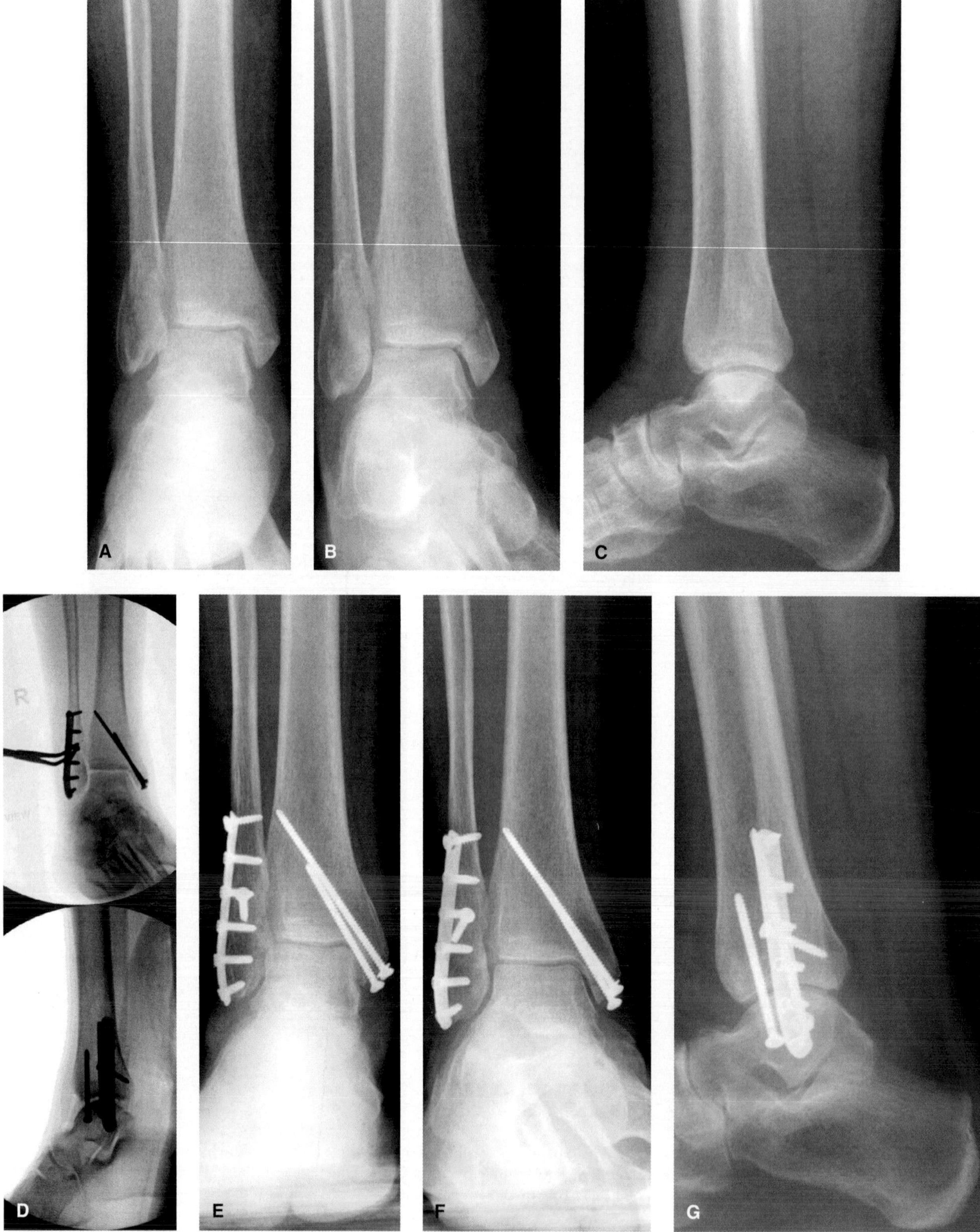

Figure 17.5. A 63-year-old female insulin-dependent diabetic fell while walking and sustained a Lauge-Hansen type SER IV displaced right bimalleolar ankle fracture. Open reduction and internal fixation was performed with placement of a 6-hole 1/3 tubular locked plate and screws and additional lag screw across the fibular fracture. A syndesmotic screw was not used as the syndesmosis appeared stable upon intraoperative examination. Two bicortical medial malleolar screws were placed across the medial malleolus fracture for additional purchase. The patient returned for follow-up 7 months following fracture surgery with excellent clinical and radiographic results including fracture union, full pain-free range of motion and a return to her previous activities of daily living. **A, B, C:** AP, mortise, and lateral radiographic views. **D:** Intraoperative fluoroscopic images demonstrating examination of the stability of the ankle syndesmosis and acceptable reduction and fixation. **E, F, G:** AP, mortise, and lateral radiographic views 7 months following fracture surgery.

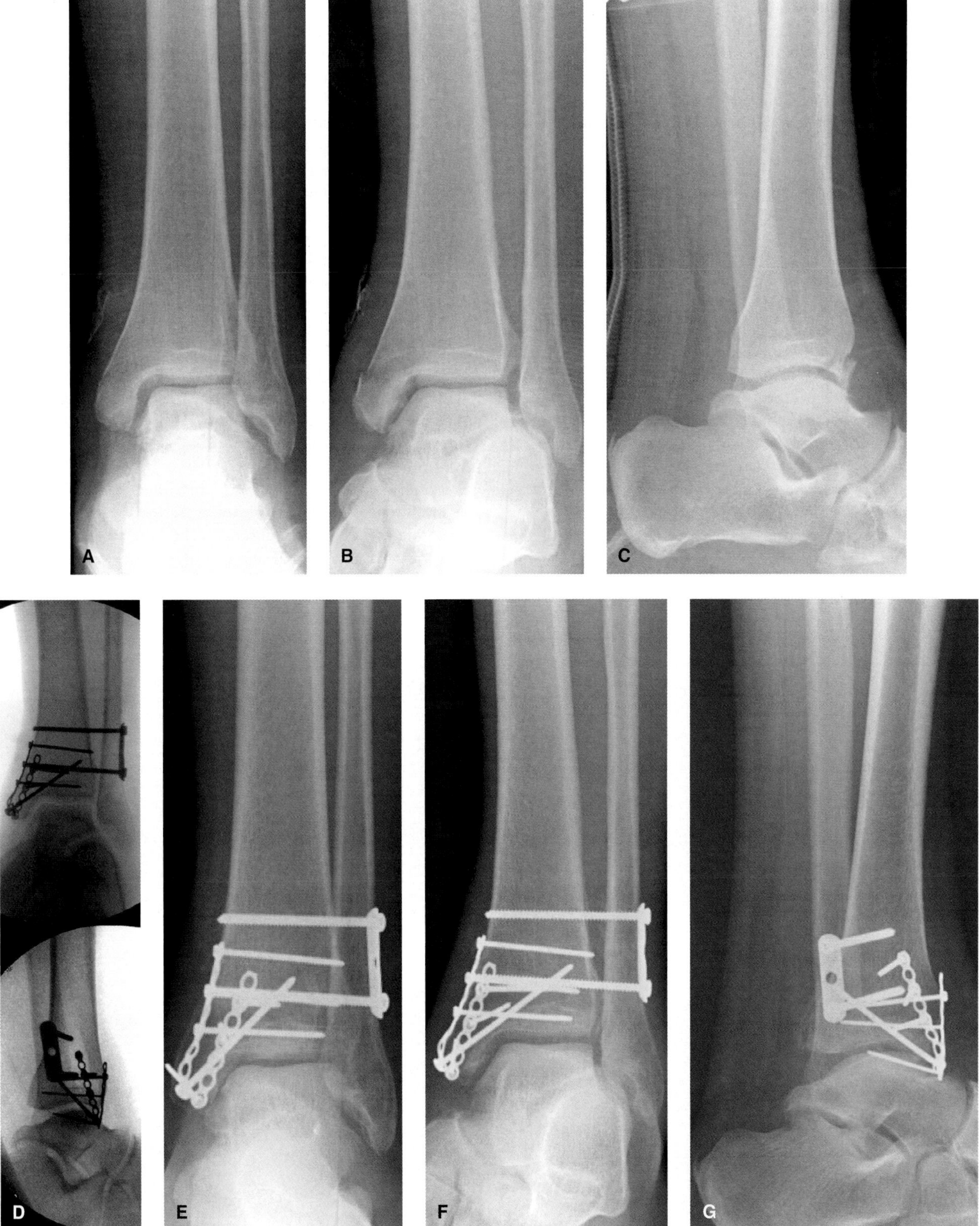

Figure 17.6. A 72-year-old male fell while walking and presented with right ankle pain and swelling. Radiographs revealed a right-sided Lauge-Hansen type SER IV variant medial malleolus ankle fracture and widening of the ankle mortise. Open reduction and internal fixation was performed with placement of 7- and 8-hole locked mini-fragment plates and screws across the medial malleolus fracture and a 1/3 tubular locking plate with two bicortical locking screws across the syndesmosis. The patient returned for follow-up 6 months following fracture surgery with excellent clinical and radiographic results including fracture union, pain-free range of motion and a return to his previous activities of daily living. **A, B, C:** AP, mortise, and lateral radiographic views. **D:** Intraoperative fluoroscopic images demonstrating acceptable reduction and fixation. **E, F, G:** AP, mortise, and lateral radiographic views 6 months following fracture surgery.

help avoid over-compression of the ankle mortise. Although biomechanical and clinical data regarding this technique is not yet available, this is our preferred method of fixation (Fig. 17.6). This plate gives additional rotational control and leads to a more even buttress force for stabilization of rotational forces as the syndesmosis heals. Additionally, restoration of syndesmotic stability may be achieved by fixation of the posterior malleolus in lieu of syndesmotic screws. Although further investigation is warranted, this may obviate the need for syndesmotic screw fixation in select patients.

FRACTURES OF THE POSTERIOR MALLEOLUS

Involvement of the posterior malleolus, also referred to as Volkmann's fragment, is seen in up to 25% of all ankle fractures. If stability of this posterior fragment is not restored, talar subluxation or articular incongruity may result, both leading to posttraumatic arthritis. The prognosis to develop such posttraumatic arthritis has been correlated to the size of the posterior malleolar fragment, with larger fragments involving more than 25% of the articular surface, doing poorer (26–28).

While much controversy exists about the treatment of this type of fracture, small avulsion fragments may be effectively treated nonoperatively (29), especially since the weight-bearing area involved is minimal in fractures of less than 25% of the total articular surface. However, when a small avulsion fragment exists, the posterior syndesmotic ligaments are invariably attached to this fragment (30), and even if gross tibiotalar stability is present, the posterior restraining buttress of the ankle is disrupted. In our anecdotal experience, this can lead to micro-instability of the tibiotalar joint and subsequent early posttraumatic articular degeneration. Although this is a topic which demands further study, perhaps more attention should be paid to reconstruction of these posterior structures.

Whether or not anatomical reduction and fixation is essential for larger fragments greater than 25% of the joint surface, is also a matter of debate (23,29,31) and is often dictated by intraoperative clinical or radiographic signs of posterior tibiotalar instability. Most authors would recommend internal fixation for posterior fragments comprising >25% to 30% of the articular surface (29). Unfortunately, assessment of the size of the posterior malleolar fragment is not very accurate through the use of plain radiographs and might be underestimated or even missed.

Posterior malleolar fractures can either be fixed percutaneously by applying anteroposterior lag screws, or through an open posterolateral Harmon approach. The latter has the advantage of allowing direct visualization of the posterior malleolus, an

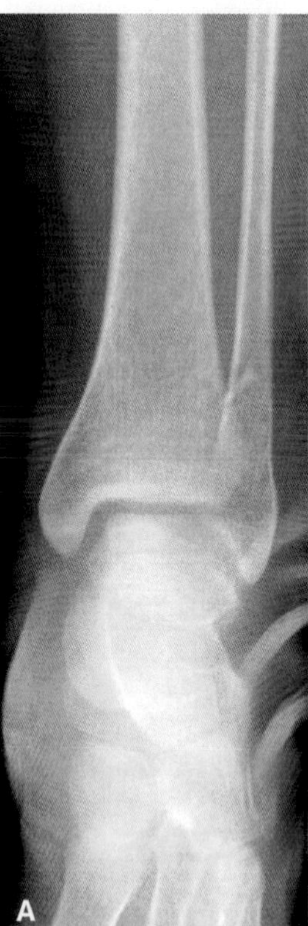

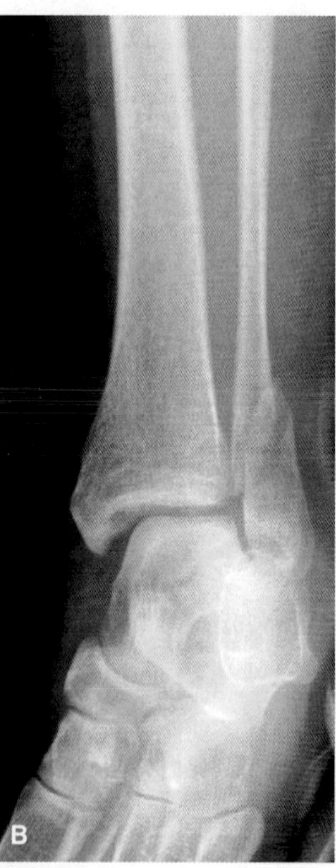

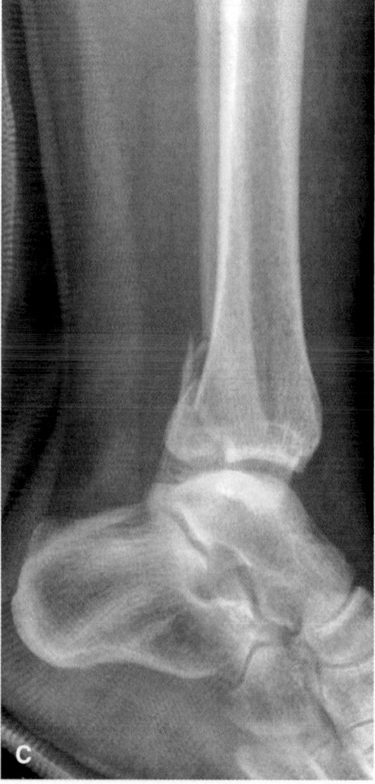

Figure 17.7. A 41-year-old female fell 10 feet from a fire escape and presented with left-sided ankle pain and swelling. Radiographs revealed a Lauge-Hansen type PA variant displaced left-sided ankle fracture with a lateral malleolus fracture and posterior malleolus fracture. Open reduction and internal fixation was performed with placement of a 6-hole 1/3 semitubular plate across the fibular fracture. A syndesmotic screw was not used as the syndesmosis appeared stable upon intraoperative examination. A 4-hole mini-fragment plate and screws were placed across the posterior malleolus fracture. The patient returned for follow-up 8 months following fracture surgery with excellent clinical and radiographic results including fracture union, full pain-free range of motion and a return to her previous activities of daily living. **A, B, C:** AP, mortise, and lateral radiographic views. (*continued*)

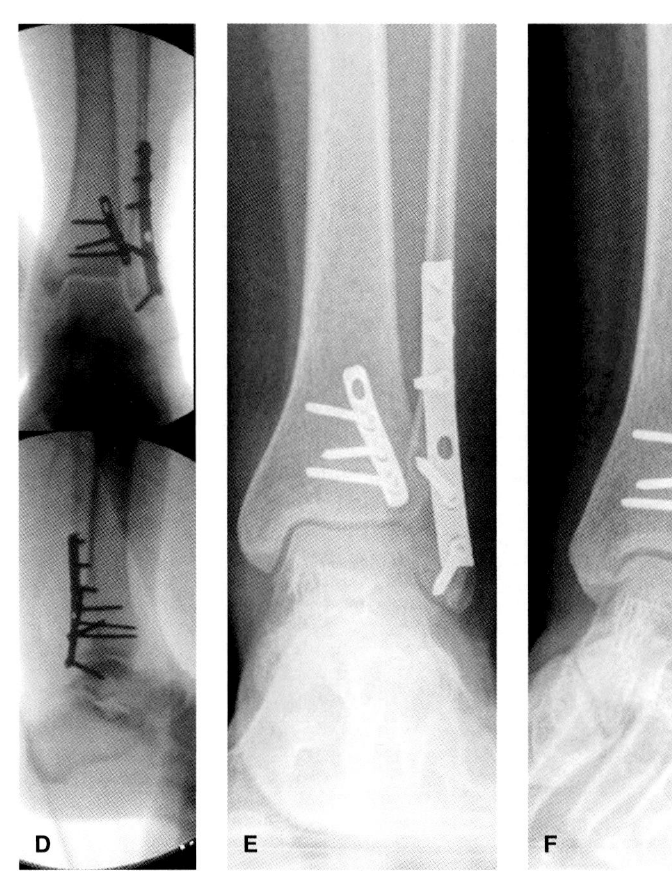
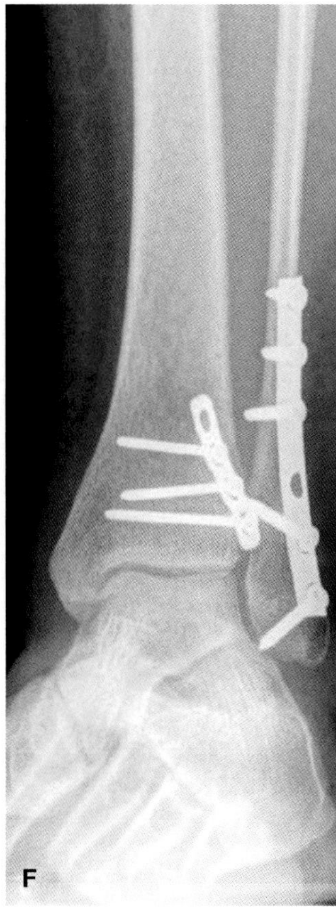
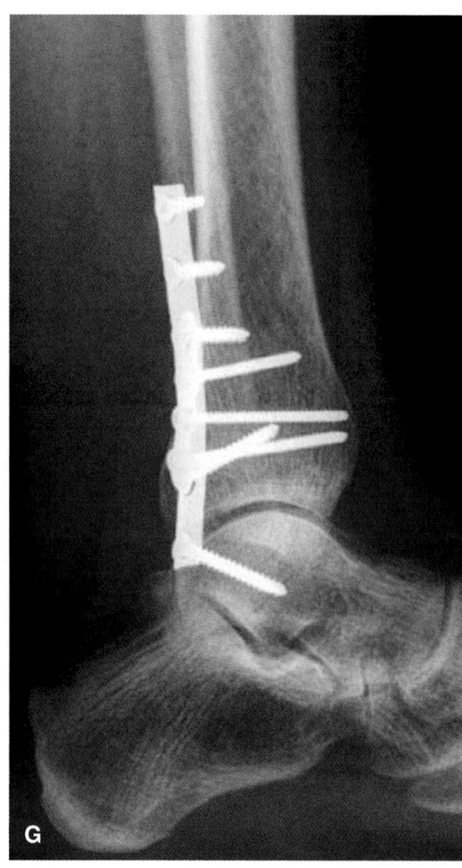

Figure 17.7. (*Continued*) **D:** Intraoperative fluoroscopic images demonstrating acceptable reduction and fixation. **E, F, G:** AP, mortise, and lateral radiographic views 8 months following fracture surgery.

antiglide plate can be applied at the fracture apex, and the fibula can be plated posterolaterally through the same incision.

A recent study showed that fixation of the posterior malleolar fragment might restore the ligamentous PITFL and might obviate the need for syndesmotic screws (30). An earlier investigation, on the other hand, demonstrated that the posterior malleolus could be stabilized adequately if stable fixation of the fibular fragments can be achieved (32). Based on our experience, we tend to stabilize the posterior malleolar fragment even if it is smaller than 25% of the articular surface to restore the posterior buttress and minimize talar instability (Fig. 17.7).

POSTOPERATIVE MANAGEMENT

Controversy exists on how to treat these injuries postoperatively and this obviously depends upon a multitude of factors: Age of the patient, strength of the construct achieved intraoperatively, compliance of the patient with non–weight-bearing, time elapsed between index operation and discharge of the patient, and associated injuries. The postoperative protocol may range from full weight bearing in a boot, to non–weight-bearing in a cast. Immediate weight bearing has been shown to be of some benefit in terms of shorter time to full weight bearing and time until return to work (33). This protocol might be restricted, however, to compliant and motivated patients with a stable osteosynthesis.

The majority of patients will be placed in a splint immediately postoperatively, which can be replaced by a walking boot after regression of the initial swelling, but before discharge. The patient remains toe-touch weight bearing until the first postoperative visit. If the wound is healing, the sutures can be removed and the ankle is then put in a boot for an additional 5 to 6 weeks. During this phase, the patient is allowed to be toe-touch weight bearing and is encouraged to start ROM exercises with physical therapy.

Regular follow-up x-rays are necessary for all patients, especially in the first several weeks after surgery. Within this timeframe, the bone has not healed yet and an eventual loss of reduction which needs to be addressed operatively can still be carried out before bone healing.

REFERENCES

1. Carr JB. Malleolar fractures and soft tissue injuries of the ankle. In: Browner BD, Jupiter JB, Levine AM, Trafton PG, eds. *Skeletal Trauma*. Philadelphia, PA: Saunders; 2003: 2307–2374.
2. Hamilton WC. *Disorders of the Ankle*. New York, NY: Springer-Verlag; 1984.
3. Hughes JL, Weber H, Willenegger H, et al. Evaluation of ankle fractures: Non-operative and operative management. *Clin Orthop* 1979;(138):111–119.
4. Yde J. Ankle fractures: Primary and late results of operative and non-operative treatment. *Acta Orthop Scand* 1980;51:981–990.
5. Inman VT. *The Joints of the Ankle*. Baltimore, MD: Williams & Wilkins; 1976.
6. Stiell IG, Greenberg GH, McKnight RD, et al. A study to develop clinical decision rules for the use of radiography in acute ankle injuries. *Ann Emerg Med* 1992;21:384–390.
7. Lauge-Hansen N. Fractures of the ankle: II. Combined experimental-surgical and experimental-roentgenologic investigations. *Arch Surg* 1950;60:957–985.
8. Muller ME, Allgower M, Schneider R, Willenegger H. *Manual of Internal Fixation*. New York, Springer-Verlag, 1979.
9. Michelson JD, Ahn UM, Helgemo SL. Motion of the ankle in a simulated supination-external rotation fracture model. *J Bone Joint Surg* 1996;78:1024–1031.

10. Bauer M, Bergstrom B, Hemborg A, et al. Malleolar fractures: Non-operative versus operative management. A controlled study. *Clin Orthop* 1985;199:17–27.
11. Bauer M, Johsson K, Nilsson B. Thirty-year follow-up of ankle fractures. *Acta Orthop Scand* 1985;56:103–106.
12. DeSouza LJ, Gustilo RB, Meyer TJ. Results of operative treatment of displaced external rotation-abduction fractures of the ankle. *J Bone Joint Surg* 1985;67:1066–1074.
13. Kristensen KD, Hansen T. Closed treatment of ankle fractures: Stage II supination-eversion fractures followed for 20 years. *Acta Orthop Scand* 1985;56:107–109.
14. Phillips WA, Schwartz HS, Keller CS, et al. A prospective, randomized study of the management of severe ankle fractures. *J Bone Joint Surg* 1985;67:67–85.
15. Yde J, Kristensen KD. Ankle fractures: Supination-eversion fractures of stage IV. Primary and late results of operative and non-operative treatment. *Acta Orthop Scand* 1980;51: 981–990.
16. Yde J, Kristensen KD. Ankle fractures: Supination-eversion fractures stage II. Primary and late results of operative and non-operative treatment. *Acta Orthop Scand* 1980;51: 695–702.
17. Earll M, Wayne J, Brodrick C, et al. Contribution of the deltoid ligament to ankle joint contact characteristics: A cadaveric study. *Foot Ankle Int* 1996;17:317–324.
18. McConnell T, Creevy WR, Tornetta P. Stress examination of supination external rotation-type fibular fractures. *J Bone Joint Surg Am* 2004;86:2171–2178.
19. Koval KJ, Egol KA, Cheung Y, et al. Does a positive ankle stress test indicate the need for operative treatment after lateral malleolus fracture? A preliminary report. *J Orthop Trauma* 2007;21:449–455.
20. Gardner MJ, Demetrakopoulos D, Briggs SM, et al. Malreduction of the tibiofibular syndesmosis in ankle fractures. *Foot Ankle Int* 2006;27:788–792.
21. Brown OL, Dirschl DR, Obremskey WT. Incidence of hardware-related pain and its effect on functional outcomes after open reduction and internal fixation of ankle fractures. *J Orthop Trauma* 2001;15:271–274.
22. Tornetta P, Creevy W. Lag screw only fixation of the lateral malleolus. *J Orthop Trauma* 2001;15:119–121.
23. Yamaguchi K, Martin CH, Boden SD, et al. Operative treatment of syndesmotic disruptions without use of a syndesmotic screw: a prospective clinical study. *Foot Ankle Int* 1994;15:407–414.
24. Nielson JH, Gardner MJ, Peterson MG, et al. Radiographic measurements do not predict syndesmotic injury in ankle fractures: an MRI study. *Clin Orthop Relat Res* 2005;436: 216–221.
25. Gardner MJ, Demetrakopoulos D, Briggs SM, et al. The ability of the Lauge-Hansen classification to predict ligament injury and mechanism in ankle fractures: an MRI study. *J Orthop Trauma* 2006;20:267–272.
26. Broos PL, Bisschop AP. Operative treatment of ankle fractures in adults: correlation between types of fracture and final results. *Injury* 1991;22:403–406.
27. Jaskulka RA, Ittner G, Schedl R. Fractures of the posterior tibial margin: their role in the prognosis of malleolar fractures. *J Trauma* 1989;29:1565–1570.
28. McDaniel WJ, Wilson FC. Trimalleolar fractures of the ankle. An end result study. *Clin Orthop Relat Res* 1977;122:37–45.
29. Haraguchi N, Haruyama H, Toga H, et al. Pathoanatomy of posterior malleolar fractures of the ankle. *J Bone Joint Surg* 2006;99:1085–1092.
30. Gardner MJ, Brodsky A, Briggs SM, et al. Fixation of posterior malleolar fractures provides greater syndesmotic stability. *Clin Orthop Relat Res* 2006;447:165–171.
31. Harper MC, Hardin G. Posterior malleolar fractures of the ankle associated with external rotation-abduction injuries. Results with and without internal fixation. *J Bone Joint Surg* 1988;70:1348–1356.
32. Raasch WG, Larkin JJ, Daraganich LF. Assessment of the posterior malleolus as a restraint to posterior subluxation of the ankle. *J Bone Joint Surg* 1992;74:1201–1206.
33. Simanski CJ, Maegele MG, Lefering R, et al. Functional treatment and early weightbearing after an ankle fracture: a prospective study. *J Orthop Trauma* 2006;20:108–114.

Basil J. Alwattar
Michael J. Gardner

CHAPTER 18

Syndesmosis Injuries

INTRODUCTION

The ankle syndesmosis is the articulation of the distal tibia and fibula. Four main ligaments stabilize this articulation, which represent secondary stabilizers of the ankle joint. Although isolated injuries of the ankle syndesmosis do occur, most occur in conjunction with ankle fractures or other fractures of the distal tibia or fibula. Physical examination and traditional radiographic markers have been shown to be less reliable than previously thought, as both the diagnosis and treatment of syndesmotic injuries remain a challenging aspect of ankle injuries. Reduction of the syndesmosis and the stability of the tibiofibular joint is necessary to avoid a decreased tibiotalar contact area, early articular degeneration, and a potentially poor clinical outcome (1,2).

ANATOMY

The ankle syndesmosis is comprised of the anterior-inferior tibiofibular ligament (AITFL), the posterior-inferior tibiofibular ligament (PITFL), the transverse ligament and the interosseous ligament (IOL) (Fig. 18.1). The AITFL runs obliquely from the anterolateral tibial tubercle (Chaput tubercle) and proceeds distally and laterally to the anteromedial aspect of the distal fibula at approximately a 45 degree angle. The PITFL runs from the posteromedial tubercle of the distal tibia (Volkmann's tubercle) to the posteromedial aspect of the distal tibia. The transverse ligament represents a thickened aspect of the deep, distal-most portion of the PITFL and functions like a labrum, deepening and stabilizing the tibiotalar joint. The IOL is the thickened, distal portion of the tibiofibular interosseous membrane and connects the fibula to the tibia 0.5 to 2 cm above the tibial plafond (3,4).

The bony architecture of the syndesmosis is unique, as the medial aspect of the distal fibula is convex and lies within the fibular notch (incisura fibularis tibiae) of the distal tibia, a concave area between the distal tibial tubercles (Chaput and Volkmann). Great variety of this bony architecture can exist, which contributes to the difficulty in diagnosing syndesmotic injuries (4).

BIOMECHANICS—NORMAL MOVEMENT OF THE DISTAL TIBIOFIBULAR JOINT

The uninjured syndesmosis allows for motion in the coronal, sagittal and rotational (axial) planes (3,4,5). This movement is important when considering treatment options for syndesmotic injuries. Injury to the syndesmosis alters the normal motion between the fibula and tibia, and consequently the tibia and talus. In cadaveric sectioning studies, the AITFL was found to provide 35% of the syndesmotic strength with the PITFL providing 9%, the transverse ligament providing 33%, and the IOL providing 22% of the total syndesmotic strength (6). The amount of displacement and altered mechanics that occur with sequential sectioning of the syndesmotic ligaments significantly affect the widening and rotation about the syndesmosis, confirming the importance of a well-reduced, functional syndesmosis (6,7).

DIAGNOSIS OF SYNDESMOTIC INJURY

Patients with syndesmotic injury most often relay a history of an external rotation moment of the foot with respect to the tibia (8,9). A hyperdorsiflexion moment has also been described, but is a less frequent mechanism (9). Patients present with ankle pain and variable ability to bear weight. Greater force is necessary to cause a syndesmotic injury compared to a standard rotational ankle fracture or sprain (9). Syndesmotic injuries should be considered in all patients with ankle injuries, but especially in patients who have sustained higher-energy injuries.

Physical examination of the ankle should include a standard evaluation of the neurovascular status of the foot and lower leg. Ecchymosis, swelling and tenderness to palpation about the anterior and posterior syndesmotic ligaments are consistently present with syndesmotic injuries (10). Hopkinson et al. described a squeeze test to evaluate injured ankles for involvement of the syndesmosis (Fig. 18.2) (11). With the squeeze test, the examiner compresses the fibula to the tibia together above the mid portion of the lower leg, causing a separation at the syndesmosis and pain (11,12). The squeeze test is sensitive but not very specific for syndesmotic injuries, as it is positive in many painful conditions of the ankle joint including fracture and infection (11). An external rotation stress test (Fig. 18.3), recreating the mechanism of injury by applying an external rotation force on the foot while stabilizing the tibia, and a dorsiflexion/compression test have also been described (9,10). Beumer et al. evaluated the reliability of physical examination findings to diagnose syndesmotic injuries, and found that the test with the most accuracy and fewest false positives was the external rotation test (13). Although physical examination findings may

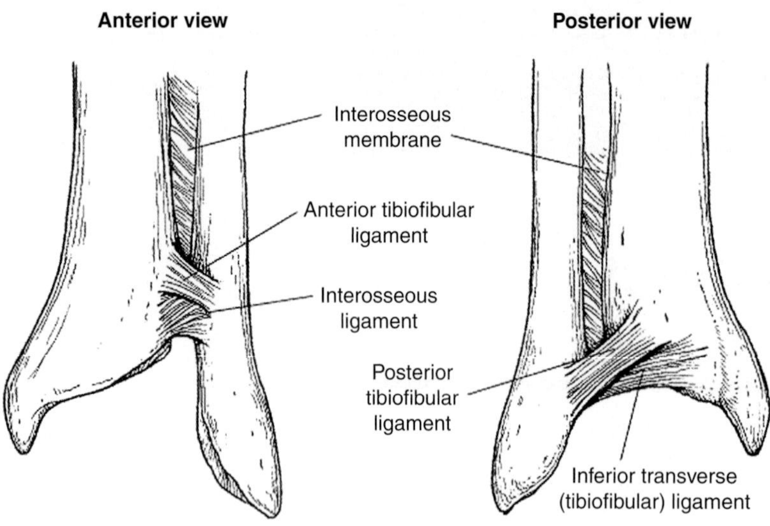

Figure 18.1. Ligaments of the distal syndesmosis. Adapted from Wuest TK. Injuries to the distal lower extremity syndesmosis. *J Am Acad Ortho Surg* 1997;5: 172–181. With permission.

be helpful, they are not reliable and should be combined with radiologic imaging when considering a syndesmotic injury (13).

With any suspected syndesmotic injury, three standard radiographic views of the ankle should be obtained (AP, lateral, and mortise views). Traditional markers of syndesmotic injury include increased tibiofibular clear space and decreased tibiofibular overlap measured on both the AP and mortise views (Fig. 18.4). These values are measured 1 cm proximal to the tibial plafond, opposite the highest point of the lateral talus. The overlap of the fibula on the anterior tibial tubercle, the tibiofibular overlap, should be greater than 1 mm on the mortise view and greater than 6 mm on the AP view, or 42% of the width of the fibula. The tibiofibular clear space is the distance between the medial fibula and the incisura fibularis

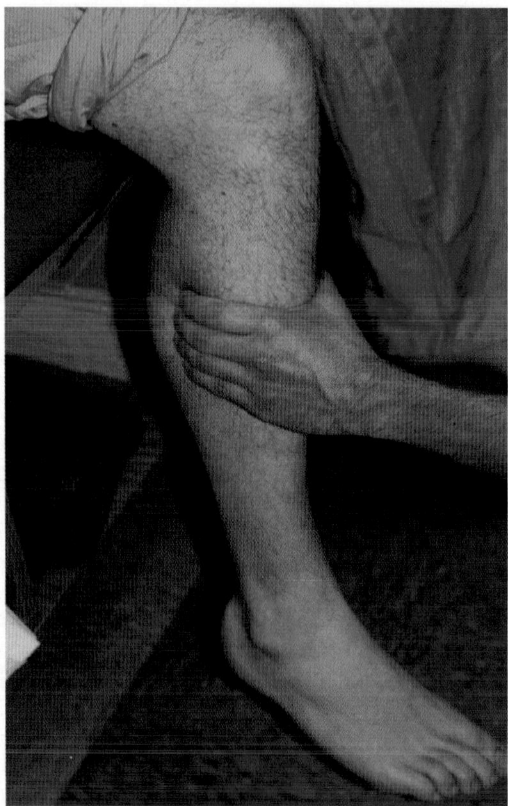

Figure 18.2. The squeeze test for syndesmotic injury. Adapted from Casillas MM. Operative treatment of acute syndesmotic injuries with screw fixation and without direct exposure or repair of the syndesmotic ligaments. *Tech Foot Ankle Surg* 2006;5:27–33. With permission.

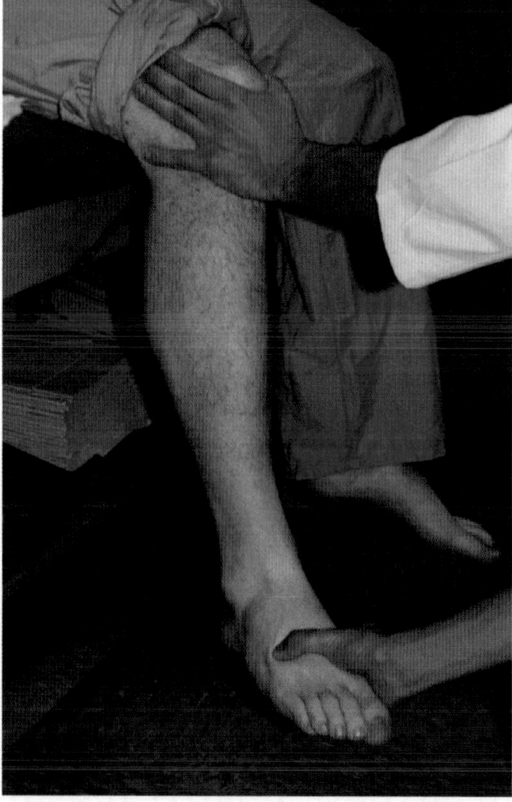

Figure 18.3. The external rotation test for syndesmotic injury. Adapted from Casillas MM. Operative treatment of acute syndesmotic injuries with screw fixation and without direct exposure or repair of the syndesmotic ligaments. *Tech Foot Ankle Surg* 2006;5:27–33. With permission.

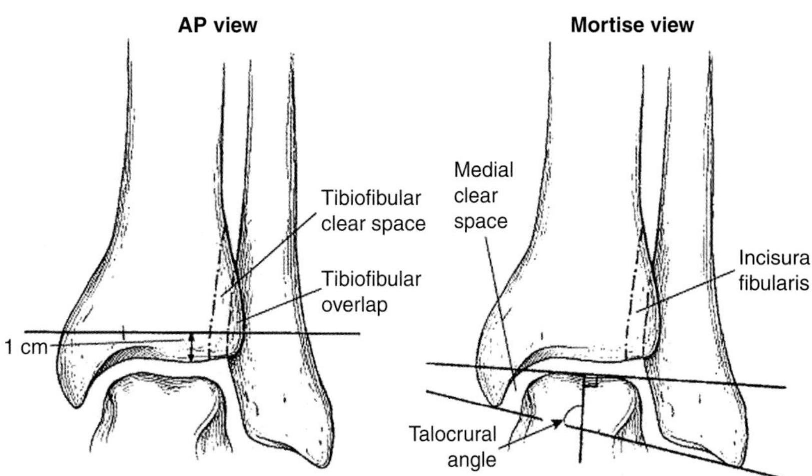

Figure 18.4. Radiographic measurements of the ankle syndesmosis. Adapted from Wuest TK. Injuries to the distal lower extremity syndesmosis. *J Am Acad Ortho Surg* 1997;5:172–181. With permission.

and should be approximately 6 mm on the AP or mortise view (14). More recent studies have shown that plain radiographs have a limited role in the evaluation of syndesmotic injuries (15,16,17), because the relationship between the distal tibia and fibula change with rotation of the limb, affecting both the tibiofibular overlap and clear space (16). Overall, tibiofibular overlap is more constant and should never be less than 1 mm on the mortise view, regardless of radiograph rotation or anatomic variation (17). Obtaining contralateral radiographs for comparison may be beneficial to account for anatomic variations.

The presence of a high fibula fracture on radiographs has traditionally been considered predictive for syndesmotic injury, but this has recently been called into question. Nielson et al. demonstrated that the level of the fibula fracture does not consistently correlate to the level of the syndesmotic ligament injury (15). Similarly, proximal third fibula fractures, the so-called Maisonneuve fractures, which were thought to indicate medial ankle injury with complete syndesmotic/interosseous membrane injury, may not always have a complete syndesmotic disruption(18–20). MRI and arthroscopic studies have shown that more often the posterior syndesmotic ligaments remain intact and act like a hinge (19,20). Therefore high fibula fractures may have an intact or partially injured syndesmosis that may be treated non-operatively (18,21).

CT evaluation of the syndesmosis is much more sensitive than plain radiographs and can detect syndesmotic incongruities within several millimeters (22). But CT scans are static images, and syndesmotic injuries may only be apparent with stress (23). Stress radiographs can be used preoperatively and intraoperatively to determine the extent of syndesmotic injury (7). Classically, the mortise stress radiograph has been performed by placing an external rotation stress on the foot in neutral dorsiflexion while stabilizing the tibia. A change in tibiofibular overlap or clear space is noted to be significant for a syndesmotic injury. Lateral radiographs that evaluate posterior displacement of the fibula with stress have been shown to demonstrate a more pronounced movement of the fibula and a better radiographic assessment of the syndesmosis than the mortise view (24).

Cotton described a test for syndesmotic injury which is performed by placing a bone hook around the fibula with a lateral force after fracture fixation (25). Mortise radiographs are obtained and considered positive with increased widening of the syndesmosis or talar shift with stress (Fig. 18.5). Recent study has confirmed that, as with preoperative stress radiographs, posteriorly directed forces examined with lateral

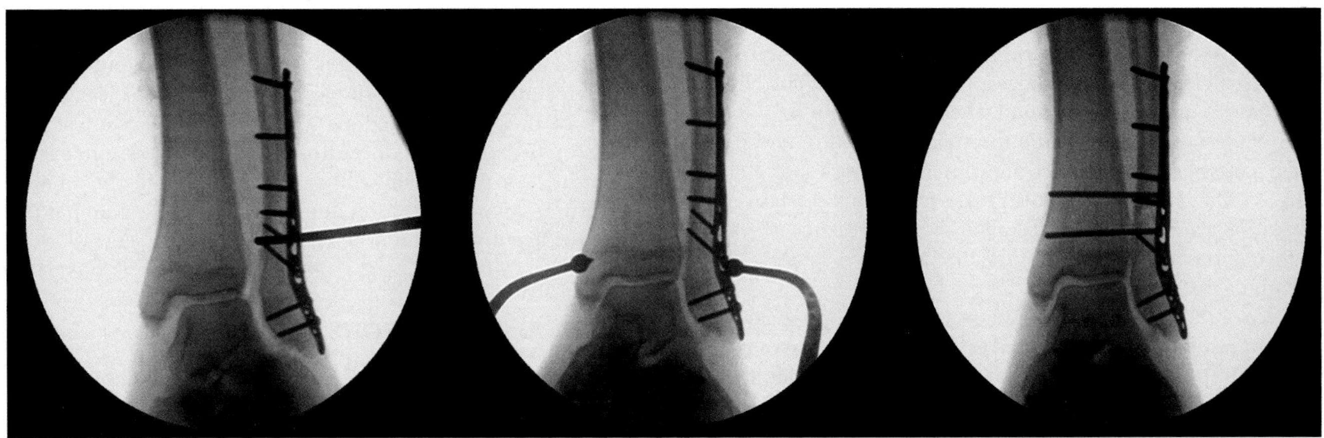

Figure 18.5. After fixation of the fibula, the Cotton test is performed and demonstrates talar shift and syndesmotic widening. This is treated with syndesmotic clamp reduction and screw fixation.

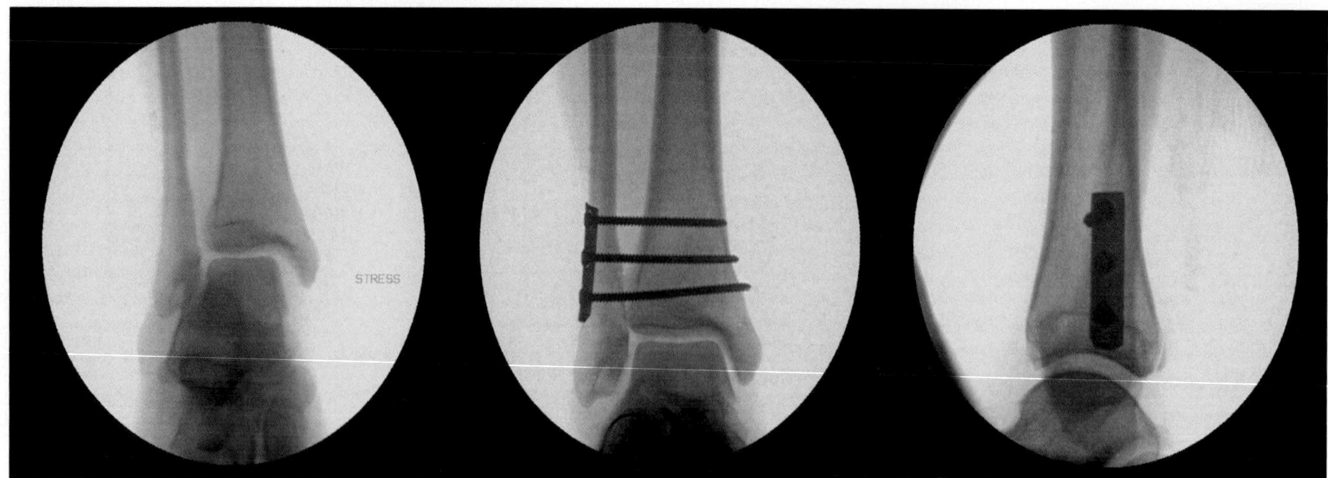

Figure 18.6. In patients with frank syndesmotic diastasis that is unable to be maintained reduced with closed treatment; surgical intervention should be strongly considered.

radiographs demonstrate larger excursion and higher sensitivity for injury (24).

MRI is a highly accurate imaging modality for assessing the syndesmosis (15,26–28). MRI has high specificity and sensitivity, and has a high interobserver reliability (27). As MRI becomes more accessible, it may become a more common component of preoperative evaluation of ankle injuries with suspected syndesmotic injuries and equivocal radiographic studies.

SYNDESMOTIC INJURY WITHOUT ASSOCIATED FRACTURE

The "high ankle sprain" represents a more significant injury with longer recovery time and a possible need for surgical intervention when compared to the typical common lateral ankle sprain (9,11,23). Syndesmotic sprains complicate between 1% and 18% of all ankle sprains and are generally associated with a higher-energy mechanism (9,11,29). Boytim et al. reported that 18% of ankle sprains sustained by professional football players had an associated syndesmotic injury. Isolated syndesmotic injuries have also been described in professional athletes, and Army cadets due to high-energy external rotation mechanisms (11,30).

The squeeze test and external rotation tests are helpful when considering these injuries, as are stress radiographs and MRI, particularly when radiographs are negative but clinical suspicion is high. Edwards and DeLee reported on six patients with syndesmotic injury without associated fracture and developed a classification for these injuries (23). Injuries were classified as either having latent or frank syndesmotic diastasis, with the latter group being subclassified by the presence of plastic deformation of the fibula and the direction of displacement of the fibula or talus.

In general, syndesmotic sprains take longer to heal than uncomplicated ankle sprains, and will keep athletes out of participation in sports for a significantly longer period of time (9,11). Surgery is considered in patients with frank diastases whose syndesmosis cannot be anatomically reduced closed (Fig. 18.6). Surgical intervention also avoids prolonged casting and the discomfort and morbidities associated with it.

TREATMENT OF SYNDESMOTIC INJURIES

Syndesmosis is a secondary ankle stabilizer, yet plays an integral role in the overall ankle function. Combined with the deltoid ligament, the syndesmosis maintains ankle congruency. Restoration of this anatomy is the goal of treatment of the syndesmotic injuries. Ramsey and Hamilton, in their classic article on tibiotalar contact forces, demonstrated that a lateral talar shift by 1 mm decreases the contact area of the ankle joint by 42%, increasing the point loading on the ankle and predisposing to subsequent arthritis (1). These results have been both confirmed and refuted in the literature, but persist as a justification for the surgical stabilization of syndesmotic injuries (31–34). More recent clinical studies have confirmed that reduction of the syndesmosis is important in the functional outcome of ankle fractures (35). A retrospective review evaluated 51 ankle fractures with associated syndesmotic injuries that were treated surgically, and found that the only significant factor related to improved functional outcome was the radiographic reduction of the syndesmosis (35). In contrast, Gardner et al. examined 25 patients who had ankle fractures with syndesmotic injuries, both of which underwent surgical stabilization and were evaluated by postoperative CT scan. In this series, over 50% were reduced asymmetrically in the fibular incisura on CT scan. More than half of these were not detectable on plain radiographs (36). The clinical significance of these malreductions was not studied. Syndesmotic malreduction detected on radiographs may represent a gross malreduction that is clinically significant, while the smaller magnitudes of malreduction detected only on CT scan has not been studied and may not be clinically relevant (Fig. 18.7).

SURGICAL INDICATIONS

The intact medial malleolus and deltoid ligament complex have been identified as the primary stabilizers of the ankle and as such the stability of the medial side is critical to overall ankle kinematics (37,38). In an attempt to quantify surgical indications, Boden et al. tested two groups of cadaveric specimens

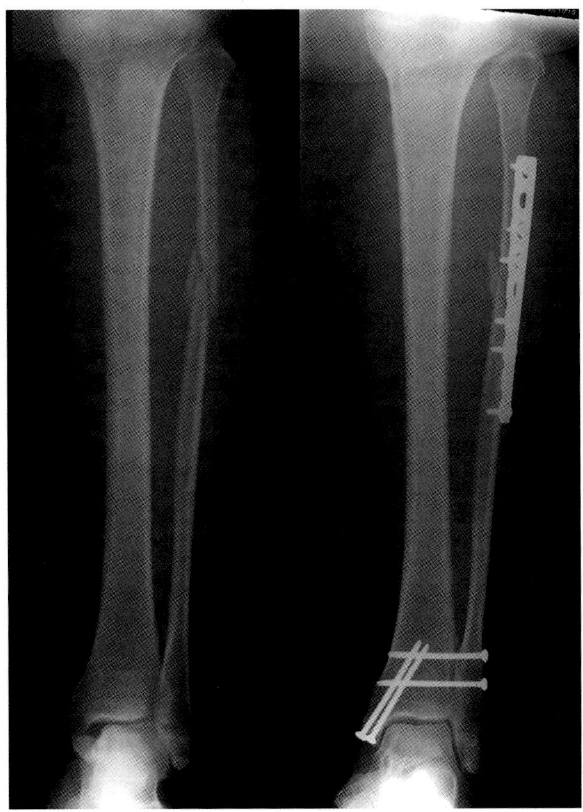

Figure 18.7. Anatomic reduction of the syndesmosis requires anatomic reduction of the fibular fracture. Often the only way to ensure fibular reduction is open reduction and internal fixation, even in more proximal fractures.

with simulated pronation-external rotation injuries. They reported that with a rigidly fixed medial malleolar fracture, sectioning of the syndesmosis provided minimal widening of the syndesmosis. With a deltoid ligament injury and sectioning of the syndesmosis, significant ankle diastases occurred with sectioning of the interosseous membrane at a level 3 to 4.5 cm above the tibial plafond. The author thus recommended that fibular fractures/syndesmotic injuries that extended 3 to 4.5 cm above the tibial plafond with associated deltoid injuries should be treated surgically (38). Other cadaver studies confirmed the finding that an intact or rigidly fixed medial complex of the ankle can provide adequate stability to the ankle (37,39). In a clinical study by Yamaguchi et al., 21 high fibular fractures sustained from rotational ankle injuries were reviewed. Three patients were found to have a medial-sided deltoid ligament injury. The syndesmosis in these 3 cases was fixed surgically. The syndesmosis injuries of the other 18 patients were treated non-operatively and showed no signs of ankle mortise widening at 1 year (40). The authors concluded that only those injuries with a concomitant deltoid injury needed surgery.

These recommendations should be interpreted with caution. First, this treatment algorithm assumes that the fibula fracture correlates to the level of a syndesmotic injury, which, as previously stated, is not necessarily universal. Second, Tornetta et al. demonstrated that a deltoid injury can occur concomitantly with a medial malleolar fracture and that rigid fixation of a medial malleolus fracture may not provide stability to the medial side of the ankle (41). The diagnosis of a deltoid injury with associated medial malleolar fracture is important and can be difficult to determine preoperatively prior to fixation of bony injuries (42). External rotation stress radiographs are useful in determining deltoid injury when no fracture of the medial malleolus exists. However, stress examination of an ankle with associated bimalleolar fracture cannot be performed until fixation of the lateral and medial malleolar fractures has been performed.

OPTIONS FOR SURGICAL FIXATION

A wide variety of methods have been described for the surgical fixation of syndesmotic injuries. These have included screws, ligament repairs, syndesmotic staples, K-wires, ring external fixators, syndesmotic hooks, and cerclage wires (43,44). AO technique describes screw fixation of the syndesmosis with a 3.5 mm stainless steel screw (Fig. 18.8). Debate persists as to the optimum screw size, position, material, and number (45). In addition, no consensus exists regarding postoperative timing of weight-bearing status or removal of implants. More recently, bioabsorbable and flexible implants have been introduced with early reports showing variable but promising results.

The syndesmosis should be stabilized 2 to 4 cm above the tibial plafond with a posterior to anterior angulation of 30 degrees to account for the posterolateral position of the fibula (46,47). Traditionally, 3.5 or 4.5 mm fully threaded, stainless steel screws have been used. Cadaver studies showed no difference between the two different screw sizes as well as no difference between stainless steel and titanium screws (48,49). 4.5 mm screws can provide greater resistance to shear stress, but the clinical significance of this is unclear (50). Two screws

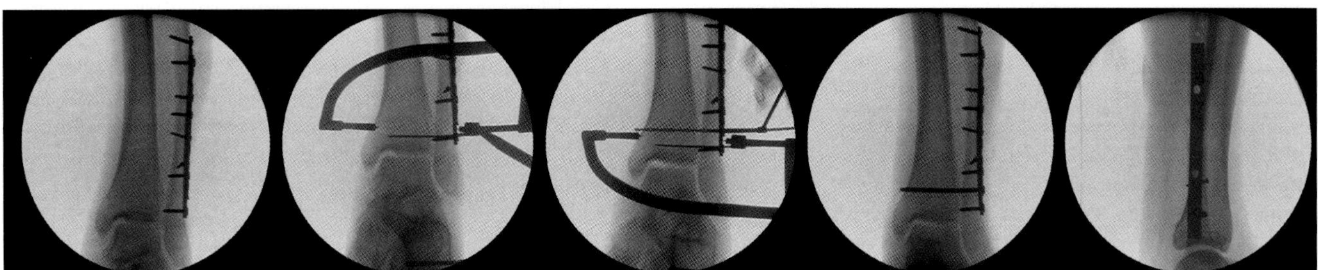

Figure 18.8. Surgical sequence of typical syndesmotic reduction and fixation, including clamp reduction, K-wire stabilization, and screw fixation. If any doubt exists as to the reduction, an open reduction with direct syndesmotic visualization should be considered.

are stronger than one, although again this may be clinically insignificant (7). Hoiness and Stromsoe compared one quadricortical 4.5 mm screw and two tricortical 3.5 mm screws in a prospective, randomized clinical trial and found no functional or clinical difference between the two groups at 1-year follow-up (51). Expert opinions have suggested that 4.5 mm screws should be considered in highly unstable fracture patterns, obese patients, patients with large fibulas and in non-compliant patients (26,43,44).

Controversy exists as to whether syndesmotic screws should engage three or four cortices (two of the fibula and one or two of the tibia). While four cortical purchase is biomechanically more stable, three cortical fixation theoretically allows some motion at the syndesmosis, which may be beneficial. Little clinical difference exists between 3 and 4 cortices of screw purchase (49,52). Moore et al. followed 127 patients with syndesmotic injuries treated surgically with 3.5 mm screws that were either tri-cortical or quadricortical in a prospective randomized trial. They quantified hardware failure, loss of reduction, and need for hardware removal, and found no significant difference between the two groups. Some suggest that four cortical fixation facilitates easier removal of hardware if necessary, but the overall difference between three and four cortical fixation does not appear to be clinically significant.

Normally, a substantial amount of movement occurs about the ankle syndesmosis (8,53). Rigid screw fixation across the syndesmosis does not allow for this movement, suggesting that perhaps all syndesmotic screws should be removed, possibly before allowing the patient to bear weight on the extremity. Recommendations have ranged from allowing patients to bear weight at 4 weeks with retained hardware to planned removal of all screws at 12 weeks without weight bearing until after screw removal (45,52,54–56). Retaining the syndesmotic screw may lead to a higher screw breakage rate, and has been related to an increased rate of osteolysis, although this has not been shown to affect clinical outcomes (55). Screw removal may be performed in an office setting under local anesthesia, but is associated with all the risks of an additional incision and surgical procedure. At least one reported case of septic arthritis leading to eventual tibiotalar fusion related to a removal of a syndesmosis screw has been reported in the literature (57). Retaining hardware often causes fatigue failure of a metal screw and osteolysis, but the clinical significance of this has not been determined either. At this time, no Level 1 evidence exists supporting empiric syndesmotic screw removal.

POSITION OF ANKLE DURING REDUCTION

The talar dome is trapezoidal in shape, on average 2.5 mm wider anteriorly than posteriorly (58). Because of this anatomic feature, the intramalleolar distance increases with dorsiflexion of the ankle, and decreases with plantarflexion (53). Earlier studies and texts recommended stabilizing the syndesmosis with the ankle in maximal dorsiflexion to avoid overtightening the syndesmosis (59). A cadaver study tested the limitation of dorsiflexion when the syndesmosis was fixed in plantarflexion. He reported that there was a loss of 0.1 degrees of dorsiflexion for every 1 degree of plantarflexion in which the syndesmosis was stabilized (59). Recent reports have refuted this recommendation (60,61). Tornetta et al. performed a cadaveric study of 17 ankles which were fixed with 4.5 mm lag screws in plantarflexion and found no difference in pre- versus post-fixation dorsiflexion. The recommendation to fix the syndesmosis while holding the ankle in dorsiflexion appears unnecessary. Tornetta suggested that a dorsiflexion force, which has been suggested as a possible mechanism of syndesmotic injury, may in fact cause displacement of the syndesmosis and lead to a malreduction (61). An accurately reduced syndesmosis is unlikely to be over compressed. This may not apply for a malreduced syndesmosis.

BIOABSORBABLE AND TIGHTROPE FIXATION

Bioabsorbable implants, made of poly-L-lactic acid/poly-glycolic acid (PLLA/PGA), do not need to be removed, avoiding secondary procedures; they theoretically lead to a gradual transfer of stresses to adjacent tissues and do not interfere with imaging modalities, such as MRIs and CT scans, as metal implants do (62). Reports of syndesmotic fixation using bioabsorbable implants have demonstrated equivalent clinically relevant biomechanical results as well as good clinical results when compared to metal implants (57,62–66). In a clinical study, Hovis et al. fixed 33 ankle fractures with lateral plates and one, four cortical 4.5 PLLA absorbable syndesmotic screw. All patients were reported to have excellent (83%) or good (17%) outcomes at the latest follow-up (65). Other clinical studies have confirmed these results (57,64,67).

A new technique for syndesmotic fixation with a suture endobutton has recently been described with early results. Fixation with a non-absorbable suture allows for motion at the syndesmosis while maintaining the fibula within the incisura fibularis. A cadaver model showed comparable mechanical properties to a 4.5 mm stainless steel screw, but these specimens were not loaded to failure (68). The first report of the use of the suture Tightrope™ (Arthrex™) to treat syndesmotic injuries reviewed 25 patients who were treated with syndesmosis fixation with one or two Tightrope™ suture buttons. The authors reported excellent or good results in all but two patients (69). Additional study of endobutton fixation of syndesmotic injuries is needed to evaluate the future of this fixation for this ligamentous injury.

REHABILITATION AND RETURN TO SPORTS

Recovery from ankle injuries with syndesmotic injury is significantly longer than those without syndesmotic involvement (9,11,70). Syndesmosis injuries with associated fractures or diastasis, that are treated operatively, are managed with a period of 6 to 12 weeks of non–weight-bearing, with variable opinions as to the need for syndesmotic fixation removal. Range of motion of the ankle and subtalar joint can start within a few days of operative fixation with a possible delay occurring for concerns of wound breakdown. Physical therapy then focuses on range of motion, proprioception and strengthening as described below for syndesmotic sprains. Return to play is often delayed for 4 to 6 months.

In syndesmotic sprains without associated fracture or diastasis (high ankle sprains), recovery is significantly longer than uncomplicated lateral ankle sprains (9,11,70). No clinical trials have been performed examining post-injury rehabilitation protocols, but multiple approaches have been described. Early reports recommended 4 to 6 weeks of non–weight-bearing and immobilization (11). More current reports emphasize the individualization of treatment protocols based on patient symptoms and injury severity (71). Three- and four-phase rehabilitation protocols for the management of syndesmotic ankle sprains have recently been described (71–74). Williams et al. recently reported a three-phase program: Phase one is the acute phase, focusing on pain control and management of edema. Rest, immobilization, elevation, icing, and non–weight-bearing proceed based on the patient's tolerance of pain and the persistence of swelling and usually last for a period of 1 to 4 days. Range of motion exercises of the ankle and subtalar joint are started during this phase and continue during the second phase of rehabilitation. During the second phase, or subacute phase, weight bearing progresses to full although assistive ambulatory devices should be used until walking is pain free. Strengthening, stretching and proprioceptive therapy begin during phase two which lasts from a few days to a few weeks. Progression to phase three proceeds when patients are able to jog and hop on the injured leg multiple times pain free. Phase three, or the advanced training phase, concentrates on sport-specific activities. Return to sport is based on the ability to perform highly functional tasks such as running, single-leg hops, vertical hops, cutting, figure-8 drills and back pedaling. Return to sport can be recommended when these activities are pain free. Taping and use of stirrup braces has been recommended but no brace has been shown to prevent or alter the treatment of these injuries and continued strengthening and proprioceptive exercises are recommended even after symptoms have resolved to prevent future, repeat injuries.

Return to sporting activity is quite variable and should be individualized to each patient. Boytim et al. found an average return at 14 days in professional football players while Wright et al. reported an average return at 42 days in professional hockey players with syndesmotic sprains. Wright though noted that these players reported continued discomfort for months after return to sport, that did not fully resolve until the following season with a prolonged period of rest (9,70). On average, the length of time until full return to sport of an ankle syndesmotic sprain is typically 6 to 8 weeks.

OUTCOMES

Reduction and stability of the syndesmosis is an important determinant in patient outcome after ankle injuries (2,35,36,75–77). Pettrone et al. retrospectively reviewed 146 ankle fractures with at least 1-year follow-up, and scored outcomes based on a scale that placed more emphasis on clinical outcome versus anatomic reduction (2,75). Overall outcomes were worse for patients with disruption of the syndesmosis. Leeds and Ehrlich retrospectively evaluated 34 patients with supination-external rotation and pronation-external rotation bimalleolar and trimalleolar fractures (76). They found significant associations between the syndesmotic malreduction with late syndesmotic instability, poor clinical outcome, and the development of late arthritis. Chissell and Jones reviewed 43 high fibula fractures associated with rotational ankle injuries (Weber C) and found that syndesmotic malreduction was present in 44% of patients who had clinically poor results (77). These studies confirm that syndesmotic malreduction leads to clinically worse results.

CONCLUSION

The ankle syndesmosis is an integral part of ankle stability and crucial to normal ankle biomechanics. Diagnosis of syndesmotic injury is difficult, as history, physical examination, and radiographic measurements may be variable and difficult to interpret. The presence of a syndesmotic injury with or without fracture denotes a significant injury, and diligence should be paid to anatomic reduction, as malreduction is associated with poor outcomes. A high index of suspicion should exist with all ankle injuries for the presence of a syndesmotic injury, and surgical fixation is pursued when indicated. The optimal surgical fixation of the syndesmosis has not been determined. New fixation methods continue to be developed and may provide solutions to the current questions that pertain to surgical treatment of syndesmosis disruptions.

REFERENCES

1. Ramsey PL, Hamilton W. Changes in tibiotalar area of contact caused by lateral talar shift. *J Bone Joint Surg Am* 1976;58-A:356–357.
2. Pettrone FA, Gail M, Pee D, et al. Quantitative criteria for prediction of the results after displaced fracture of the ankle. *J Bone Joint Surg Am* 1983;65:667–677.
3. Rasmussen O. Stability of the ankle joint: Analysis of the function and traumatology of the ankle ligaments. *Acta Orthop Scand* 1985;211:1–75.
4. Clanton TO, Paul P. Syndesmosis injuries in athletes. *Foot Ankle Clin N Am* 2002;7:529–549.
5. McCullough CJ, Burge PD. Rotatory stability of the load-bearing ankle: an experimental study. *J Bone Joint Surg Am* 1980;62(A):460–464.
6. Ogilvie-Harris DJ, Reed SC, Hedman TP. Disruption of the ankle syndesmosis: biomechanical study of the ligamentous restraints. *Arthroscopy* 1994;10:558–560.
7. Xenos JS, Hopkinson WJ, Mulligan ME, et al. The tibiofibular syndesmosis: Evaluation of the ligamentous structures, methods of fixation, and radiographic assessment. *J Bone Joint Surg Am* 1995;77(6):847–856.
8. Rasmussen O, Tovborg-Jensen I, Boe S. Distal tibiofibular ligaments: Analysis of function. *Acta Orthopaedica* 1982;53:681–686.
9. Boytim MJ, Fischer DA, Neumann L. Syndesmotic ankle sprains. *Am J Sports Med* 1991; 19:294–298.
10. Alonso A, Khoury L, Adams R. Clinical tests for ankle syndesmosis injury: Reliability and prediction of return to function. *J Orthop Sports Phys Ther* 1998;27:276–284.
11. Hopkinson WJ, St Pierre P, Ryan JB, et al. Syndesmosis sprains of the ankle. *Foot Ankle* 1990;10:325–330.
12. Tietz CC, Harrington RM. A biomechanical analysis of the squeeze test for sprains of the syndesmotic ligaments of the ankle. *Foot Ankle Int* 1998;19:489–492.
13. Beumer A, Swierstra BA, Mulder PGH. Clinical diagnosis of syndesmotic ankle instability: Evaluation of stress tests behind the curtains. *Acta Orthop Scand* 2002;73:667–669.
14. Harper MC, Keller TS. A radiographic evaluation of the tibiofibular syndesmosis. *Foot Ankle* 1989;10:156–160.
15. Nielson JH, Gardner MJ, Peterson MG, et al. Radiographic measurements do not predict syndesmotic injury in ankle fractures, an MRI study. *Clin Orthop Relat Res* 2005;436: 216–221.
16. Pneumaticos SG, Noble PC, Chatziioannou SN, et al. The effects of rotation on radiographic evaluation of the tibiofibular syndesmosis. *Foot Ankle* 2002;23:107–111.
17. Beumer A, van Hemert WL, Niesing R, et al. Radiographic measurement of the distal tibiofibular syndesmosis has limited use. *Clin Orthop Relat Res* 2004;423:227–234.
18. Merrill KD. The Maisonneuve fracture of the fibula. *Clin Orthop Relat Res* 1993;287: 218–223.
19. Yoshimura I, Naito M, Kanazawa K, et al. Arthroscopic findings in Maisonneuve fractures. *J Orthop Sci* 2008;13(1):3–6.
20. Morris J, Lee J, Thordarson D, et al. Magnetic resonance imaging of acute Maisonneuve fractures. *Foot Ankle Int* 1996;17:259–263.
21. Gardner MJ, Demetrakopoulos D, Briggs SM, et al. The ability of the Lauge-Hansen classification to predict ligament injury and mechanism in ankle fractures: An MRI study. *J Orthop Trauma* 2006;20:267–272.
22. Ebraheim N, Lu J, Yang H, et al. Radiographic and CT evaluation of tibiofibular syndesmotic diastasis: A cadaver study. *Foot Ankle Int* 1997;18:693–698.
23. Edwards GS, DeLee JC. Ankle diastasis without fracture. *Foot Ankle* 1984;4:305–312.
24. Candal-Cuoto JJ, Burrow D, Bromage S, et al. Instability of the tibio-fibular syndesmosis: Have we been pulling in the wrong direction? *Injury* 2004;35:814–818.
25. Cotton F. *Dislocations and Joint Fractures*. Philadelphia, PA: WB Saunders Co; 1911:535–588.
26. Oae K, Takao M, Naito K, et al. Injury of the tibiofibular syndesmosis: Value of MR imaging for diagnosis. *Radiology* 2003;227:155–161.
27. Vogl TJ, Hochmuth K, Diebold T, et al. Magnetic resonance imaging in the diagnosis of acute injured distal tibiofibular syndesmosis. *Invest Radiol* 1997;32:401–409.
28. Takao M, Ochi M, Oae K, et al. Diagnosis of a tear of the tibiofibular syndesmosis. *J Bone Joint Surg Br* 2003;85-B:324–329.

29. Fallat L, Grimm DJ, Saracco JA. Sprained ankle syndrome: Prevalence and analysis of 639 acute injuries. *J Foot Ankle Surg* 1998;37:280–285.
30. Fritschy D. An unusual ankle injury in top skiers. *Am J Sports Med* 1989;17:282–286.
31. Pereira DS, Koval K, Resnick R, et al. Tibiotalar contact area and pressure distribution: The effect of mortise widening and syndesmosis fixation. *Foot Ankle Int* 1996;17:269–274.
32. Brown TD, Hurlbut PT, Hale JE, et al. Effects of imposed hindfoot constraint on ankle contact mechanics for displaced lateral malleolar fractures. *J Orthop Trauma* 1994;8:511–519.
33. Clarke MH, Michelson JD, Cox QG, et al. Tibio-talar stability in bimalleolar ankle fractures: A dynamic in vitro contact area study. *Foot Ankle* 1991;11:222–227.
34. Yablon I, Heller F, Shouse L. The key role of the lateral malleolus in displaced fractures of the ankle. *J Bone Joint Surg Am* 1977;59A:169–173.
35. Weening B, Bhandari M. Predictors of functional outcome following transsyndesmotic screw fixation of ankle fractures. *J Orthop Trauma* 2005;19:102–108.
36. Gardner MJ, Demetrakopoulos D, Briggs SM, et al. Malreduction of the tibiofibular syndesmosis in ankle fractures. *Foot Ankle Int* 2006;27(10):788–792.
37. Michelson JD, Waldman B. An axially loaded model of the ankle after pronation external rotation injury. *Clin Orthop Relat Res* 1996;328:285–293.
38. Boden SD, Labropoulos PA, McCowin P, et al. Mechanical considerations for the syndesmosis screw. A cadaver study. *J Bone Joint Surg Am* 1989;71:1548–1555.
39. Burns WC, Prakash D, Adelaar R, et al. Tibiotalar joint dynamics: Indications for the syndesmotic screw- a cadaveric study. *Foot Ankle* 1993;143:153–158.
40. Yamaguchi K, Martin CH, Boden SD, et al. Operative treatment of syndesmotic disruptions without use of a syndesmotic screw: A prospective clinical study. *Foot Ankle Int* 1994;15:407–414.
41. Tornetta P. Competence of the deltoid ligament in bimalleolar ankle fractures after medial malleolar fixation. *J Bone Joint Surg Am* 2000;82:843–848.
42. McConell T, Creevy W, Tornetta P. Stress examination of supination external rotation-type fibular fractures. *J Bone Joint Surg Am* 2004;86:2171–2178.
43. Van den Bekerom MP, Lamme B, Hogervorst M, et al. Review of operative techniques for stabilising the distal tibiofibular syndesmosis. *Foot Ankle Int* 2007;28(12):1302–1308.
44. van den Bekerom MP, Hogervost M, Bolhuis HW, et al. Operative aspects of the syndesmotic screw: Review of current concepts. *Injury* 2008;39:491–498.
45. Mueller ME, Allgower M, Schneider R, et al. Malleolar fractures. In: *Manual of Internal Fixation.* 3rd ed., New York, Berlin, Heidelberg: Springer-Verlag; 1991:595–612.
46. Kukreti S, Faraj A, Miles JN. Does position of the syndesmotic screw affect functional outcome in ankle fractures? *Injury* 2005;36:1121–1124.
47. McBryde A, Chiasson B, Wilhelm A, et al. Syndesmotic screw placement: A biomechanical analysis. *Foot Ankle Int* 1997;18:262–266.
48. Thompson MC, Gesnik D. Biomechanical comparison of syndesmosis fixation with 3.5- and 4.5 millimeter stainless steel screws. *Foot Ankle Int* 2000;21:737–741.
49. Beumer A, Campo MM, Niesing R, et al. Screw fixation of the syndesmosis: a cadaver model comparing stainless steel and titanium screws and three and four cortical fixation. *Injury* 2005;36:60–64.
50. Hansen M, Le L, Werthheimer S, et al. Syndesmosis Fixation: Analysis of Shear Stress via Axial Load on 3.5-mm and 4.5-mm quadricortical syndesmotic screws. *J Foot Ankle Surg* 2006;45:65–69.
51. Hoiness P, Stromsoe K. Tricortical versus quadricortical syndesmosis fixation in ankle fractures. *J Orthop Trauma* 2004;18:331–337.
52. Moore JA, Shank JR, Morgan SJ, et al. Syndesmosis fixation: A comparison of three and four cortices of screw fixation without hardware removal. *Foot Ankle Int* 2006;27:567–572.
53. Scranton PE, McMaster JG, Kelly E. Dynamic fibular function: A new concept. *Clin Orthop Relat Res* 1976;118:76–81.
54. de Souza LJ, Gustilo RB, Meyer TJ. Results of operative treatment of displace external rotation-abduction fractures of the ankle. *J Bone Joint Surg Am* 1985;67:1066–1074.
55. Bell DP, Wong MK. Syndesmotic screw fixation in Weber C ankle injuries–should the screw be removed before weight bearing? *Injury* 2006;37:891–898.
56. Needleman RL, Skrade DA, Stiehl JB. Effect of the syndesmosis screw on ankle motion. *Foot Ankle* 1989;10:17–24.
57. Kaukonen JP, Lamberg T, Korkala O, et al. Fixation of syndesmotic ruptures in 38 patients with malleolar fracture: A randomized study comparing a metallic and a bioabsorbable screw. *J Orthop Trauma* 2005;19:392–395.
58. Close JR. Some applications of the functional anatomy of the ankle joint. *J Bone Joint Surg Am* 1956;38:761–781.
59. Olerud C. The effects of the syndesmotic screw on the extension capacity of the ankle joint. *Arch Orthop Trauma Surg* 1985;104:299–304.
60. Bragonzoni L, Russo A, Girolami M, et al. The distal tibiofibular syndesmosis during passive foot flexion. RSA-based study on intact, ligament injured and screw fixed cadaver specimens. *Arch Orthop Trauma Surg* 2006;126:304–308.
61. Tornetta P, Spoo JE, Reynolds FA, et al. Overtightening of the ankle syndesmosis: Is it really possible? *J Bone Joint Surg Am* 2001;83:489–492.
62. Thoradson DB, Hedman TP, Gross D, et al. Biomechanical evaluation of polylactide absorbable screws used for syndesmosis injury repair. *Foot Ankle Int* 1997;18:622–627.
63. Thoradson DB, Samuelson M, Shepard L, et al. Bioabsorbable versus stainless steel screw fixation of the syndesmosis in pronation-lateral rotation ankle fractures: A prospective randomized trial. *Foot Ankle Int* 2001;22:335–338.
64. Sinisaari IP, Luthje PM, Mikkonen RH. Ruptured tibio-fibular syndesmosis: Comparison study of metallic to bioabsorbable fixation. *Foot Ankle Int* 2002;22:744–748.
65. Hovis WD, Kaiser BW, Watson JT, et al. Treatment of syndesmotic disruptions of the ankle with bioabsorbable screw fixation. *J Bone Joint Surg Am* 2002;84:26–31.
66. Cox S, Mukherjee DP, Ogden AL, et al. Distal tibiofibular syndesmosis fixation: A cadaveric, simulated fracture stabilization study comparing bioabsorbable and metallic single screw fixation. *J Foot Ankle Surg* 2005;44:144–151.
67. Miller SD, Carls RJ. The bioresorbable syndesmotic screw: Application of polymer technology in ankle fractures. *Am J Orthop* 2002;31:18–21.
68. Thornes B, Walsh A, Hislop M, et al. Suture-endobutton fixation of ankle tibio-fibular diastasis: A cadaver study. *Foot Ankle Int* 2003;24:142–146.
69. Cottom JM, Hyer CF, Philbin TM, et al. Treatment of syndesmotic disruptions with the arthrex tightrope: a report of 25 cases. *Foot Ankle Int* 2008;29:773–779.
70. Wright RW, Barile RJ, Surprenant DA, et al. Ankle syndesmosis sprains in national hockey league players. *Am J Sports Med* 2004;32(8):1941–1945.
71. Williams GN, Jones MH, Amendola A. Syndesmotic ankle sprains in athletes. *Am J Sports Med* 2007;35(7):1197–1207.
72. Nussbaum ED, Hosea TM, Sieler SD. Prospective evaluation of syndesmotic ankle sprains without diastasis. *Am J Sports Med* 2001;29(1):31–35.
73. Gerber JP, Williams GN. Persistent disability associated with ankle sprains: A prospective examination of an athletic population. *Foot Ankle Int* 1998;19(10):653–660.
74. Brosky T, Nyland J, Nitz A, et al. The ankle ligaments: Consideration of syndesmotic injury and implications for rehabilitation. *J Orthop Sports Phys Ther* 1995;21(4):197–205.
75. Joy G, Patzakis MJ, Harvey JP. Precise evaluation of the reduction of severe ankle fractures: Technique and correlation with end results. *J Bone Joint Surg Am* 1974;56:979–993.
76. Leeds HC, Ehrlich MG. Instability of the distal tibiofibular syndesmosis after bimalleolar and trimalleolar ankle fractures. *J Bone Joint Surg Am* 1984;66:490–503.
77. Chissell HR, Jones J. The influence of a diastasis screw on the outcome of Weber type-C ankle fractures. *J Bone Joint Surg Br* 1995;77:435–438.

Kirstina Olson
Robert Anderson

CHAPTER 19

Lisfranc Injury in the Elite Athlete

INTRODUCTION

Injuries to the foot and ankle are one of the most common occurrences in athletic events, and have been reported to comprise almost 16% of all athletic injuries (1). Injuries to the midfoot that disrupt the tarsometatarsal joints, commonly referred to as the Lisfranc complex, are less frequent but can be devastating injuries to athletes. Sports-related Lisfranc injuries are often subtle and can be overlooked if a high index of suspicion is not present. Some studies have reported that up to 20% of Lisfranc injuries are missed on initial evaluation, due to discrete radiographic findings (2). However, this injury was found to occur in nearly 4% of all football players per year, with 29% of those occurring in offensive linemen (3). Subtle Lisfranc injuries in athletes have become concerning due to inferior long-term outcomes when initial diagnosis and treatment is delayed. Even partial capsular tears in elite athletes, which may present with minimal clinical symptoms or radiographic diastasis, can result in suboptimal performance.

STRUCTURAL ANATOMY

The structural anatomy of the midfoot is comprised of bony articulations and ligamentous attachments involved in intricate relationships that provide inherent static stability (4,5). The midfoot includes the navicular, cuboid, and the three cuneiform bones with their respective tarsometatarsal linkages. The innate osseous architecture of the five metatarsal bases forms a "Roman arch" configuration in the axial plane, acting as a buttress for the midfoot. The trapezoidal shape and configuration of the metatarsal bases creates a scaffolding which prevents plantar subluxation and acts as a foundation for the transverse arch. In addition, in the coronal plane, the second metatarsal base is recessed proximally and wedged between the three cuneiforms forming a "keystone." This mortise alignment provides added stability. Peicha et al. demonstrated the importance of this anatomic relationship through radiographic analysis of patients with Lisfranc injury. A shallow mortise was found in a significantly greater number of injured patients as compared to their controlled counterparts (6).

Dorsal, plantar, and interosseous ligaments run in longitudinal, oblique, and transverse planes adding to static midfoot stability (5,7). Transverse fibers connect the dorsal and plantar bases of the second through the fifth metatarsals. The plantar fibers are stronger and larger, which may account for the more commonly seen dorsal dislocations. Similarly, intercuneiform ligaments exist that are more defined and robust plantarly. Numerous authors have shown that disruption of the plantar ligament extending from the medial cuneiform to the second and third metatarsal bases is the greatest predictor of instability of the tarsometatarsal joints (8,9). The interosseous group of ligaments which lie between the dorsal and plantar ligaments is the strongest. These fibers run between and attach to the base of each of the five metatarsals; however, there is an absence of the expected interosseous ligament between the first and second metatarsals. Instead, a ligament is present that extends from the base of the second metatarsal to the medial cuneiform, termed Lisfranc ligament. This well-defined oblique structure provides additional plantar reinforcement for the medial column. It is the largest and the sturdiest of the interosseous ligaments. The Lisfranc joint "complex" additionally incorporates all of the neighboring tarsometatarsal joints, as well as the intercuneiform joint, representing the bridge between the midfoot and forefoot.

The soft-tissue structures surrounding the midfoot also aid in dynamically supporting the midfoot. The tibialis posterior tendon and the peroneus longus tendon both act to preserve the longitudinal and transverse arches, respectively (10). The anterior tibial tendon inserts into the dorsomedial aspect of the first metatarsal base and the medial cuneiform, adding medial column support. However, this tendon has additionally been documented as one of the possible underlying causes preventing the reduction of a Lisfranc dislocation (11). When a portion of the lateral slip becomes interposed between the two bones, the Lisfranc joint becomes irreducible. These tendons work in conjunction with the intrinsic muscles and the plantar fascia to further support the arches of the midfoot.

Adjacent structures of relevance in this area include the dorsalis pedis artery and the deep peroneal nerve. The perforating branch of the dorsalis pedis artery dives plantarly between the bases of the first and second metatarsals, approximately 1 to 2 cm after it crosses the Lisfranc joint. The deep peroneal nerve is intimately associated with the dorsalis pedis artery and provides sensation to the first dorsal webspace. These structures are at risk at the initial time of injury as well as during surgical exposures. The integrity of the two structures must be assessed and documented in every patient, both clinically and at the time of surgery (12).

BIOMECHANICS

The midfoot and forefoot have often been described as three columns. The medial column incorporates the medial cuneiform and the first metatarsal, which functions as a rigid level to allow propulsion of the foot during the push-off stage of gait. The middle column includes the middle and lateral cuneiforms with their respective distal articulations to the second and third metatarsals. The cuboid junction with the fourth and fifth metatarsals forms the lateral column. The middle column is the most rigid with the medial column additionally imparting stability to maintain the arch. The lateral column has been found to have the most motion of the three columns; this flexibility of the lateral column allows accommodation of the forefoot on uneven ground (13). These tenants are important to remember when reconstructing a Lisfranc injury involving all the three columns, which often necessitates varying the types of fixation used.

MECHANISM

Lisfranc injuries result in patterns of tarsometatarsal instability that may include primarily the Lisfranc ligament, fractures of the associated bones, dislocations of the surrounding joints, or a spectrum of all of the above. They are commonly seen after a motor vehicle accident or a fall from a height (2). This high-energy injury tends to produce a more obvious deformity from the subsequent force transmitted through the foot. Conversely, there exists a more subtle mechanism seen in the athletic population that is becoming increasingly recognized as an equally devastating injury, and possibly more common than that from trauma. The force and rotation which takes place at the initial insult determines the degree and direction of the instability and/or displacement. Injury patterns usually result from twisting of the forefoot, axial loading with the foot fixed in equinus, or a direct compression mechanism. Lisfranc disruptions have been further divided into direct and indirect types, referencing where the force is applied. Direct Lisfranc injuries involve a plantarward force that is delivered immediately over the Lisfranc complex, as seen when a weight is dropped onto the midfoot. These direct injuries are often associated with severe crush injuries, soft-tissue destruction and a variable degree of bony comminution. More commonly, indirect injuries occur when the foot is in plantarflexion and axially loaded or twisted. The transmitted force indirectly causes a midfoot disruption that may go unnoticed or unrecognized. This low-energy mechanism is what accounts for the "athletic" variety and produces more predictable injury patterns (14).

The athletic variety tends to present with more subtle and discreet signs because of the low-energy mechanism which often results in primarily ligamentous injuries. Historically, these are thought to occur by an axial load transmitted through a plantarflexed foot, most commonly seen when a football player falls back onto the heel of another player whose forefoot is planted in the ground. With the forefoot fixed to the ground, the metatarsophalangeal joints may hyperextend which in turn forces the midfoot into hyperplantarflexion. This maneuver ruptures the weak dorsal ligaments, followed by either a disruption of the plantar capsule or a fracture of the plantar metatarsal base. After the metatarsal bones have lost their check reins, they are allowed to displace dorsally; when a rotational force is present, they may also shift laterally and/or medially.

Recent analysis of these injuries finds that a non-contact mechanism may actually be more common; a twisting abduction force which disrupts the Lisfranc complex. When the forefoot is forcefully abducted while the hindfoot is fixed, a fracture at the second metatarsal base is often noted. This mechanism is manifested in equestrian players or jockeys when the foot becomes caught in the stirrup and the body sustains a powerful twisting force against the fixed foot. Similarly, Lisfranc injuries have been described when surfboarders fall backward and the foot becomes caught in the strap. Any severe rotational force transmitted through the midfoot may produce a tarsometatarsal injury.

Subtle Lisfranc injury variants can extend proximal to the tarsometatarsal joints; the force from the injury enters the intercuneiform joints between the medial and middle cuneiforms and exits out of the medial navicular–cuneiform joint (Fig. 19.1A, B). Myerson describes this more extensive injury as the Lisfranc joint "complex" when proximal tarsal involvement is present (2). In addition, with excessive metatarsal abduction and lateral displacement, a compression fracture of the cuboid is occasionally visualized. When this "nutcracker" fracture is identified, it should raise one's suspicion for a Lisfranc injury. The same holds true for the metatarsophalangeal joints; the initial hyperextension maneuver at that level of the foot may cause a subluxation or dislocation of the joint or fracture of the head/neck of the metatarsal. There is a possibility that the subluxed joints may spontaneously reduce, making the diagnosis even more challenging. There has been an increasing incidence of subtle Lisfranc injuries in all field sports, particularly football, and a keen appreciation of this injury is necessary.

DIAGNOSIS

Subtle Lisfranc variants that go unrecognized can lead to long-term dysfunction of the medial column of the midfoot (Fig. 19.2). Lisfranc injuries among competitive football players appear to be escalating in number and identification of the injury is crucial (15). The most vital part of diagnosing these inconspicuous injuries is to keep a high index level of suspicion and to beware of the diagnosis of "midfoot sprain" in any athlete, elite, or otherwise. It is imperative to examine the midfoot and tarsometatarsal joint complex in any athlete who complains of foot or ankle pain, even amidst distracting injuries such as ankle sprain. Clanton and McGarvey state that midfoot sprains in athletes rarely occur as isolated injuries, but rather in association with fractures or ankle sprains (14). Poor functional results have been repeatedly documented in athletes for whom the diagnosis was delayed (10,14,15).

HISTORY

A thorough history and physical examination is paramount in diagnosing subtle Lisfranc injuries. When a specific injury is recalled, it is best to have the patient describe the exact details, attempt to reproduce the mechanism, and localize the pain to

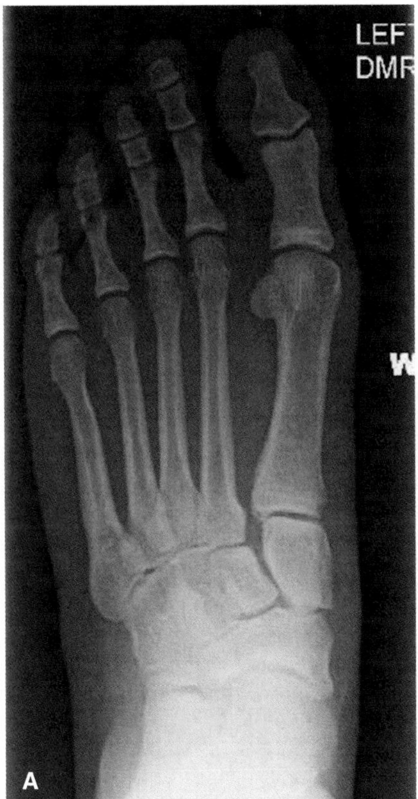

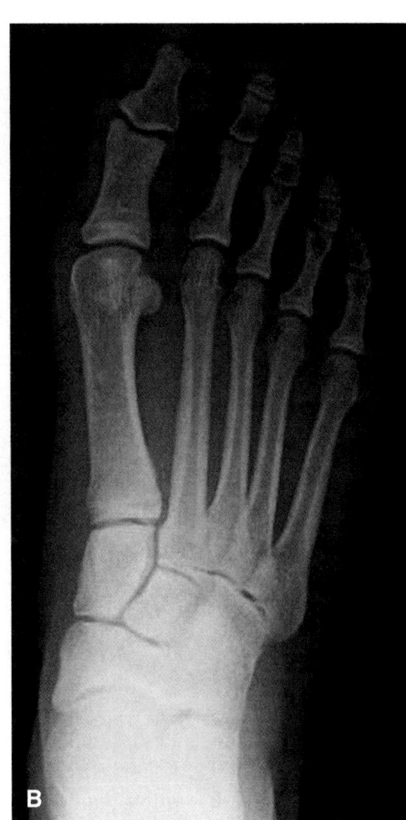

Figure 19.1. **A:** AP standing radiograph illustrating subtle diastasis of the intercuneiform joint with medial subluxation of the cuneiform at the naviculo-cuneiform joint. **B:** Comparison AP standing radiograph of the contralateral uninjured foot.

a specific area of the foot. A specific event that led to the condition may not always be recollected; however, in a series of 15 athletes, 12 of the 15 were able to remember a specific event that led to their pain and subsequent decrease in performance (16). Subtle proximal variants with an unstable first ray cause athletes to report difficulty with push-off strength or decreased ability to come out of a stance (15). The athlete may initially be unable to bear weight on the involved foot and may complain of either foot or ankle pain. When reviewing Lisfranc disruptions in collegiate football players, Meyer and colleagues noted that the inability of a player to perform a one-legged toe raise and cutting or jumping maneuvers in the setting of midfoot pain implies a significant injury to the tarsometatarsal joint complex (3).

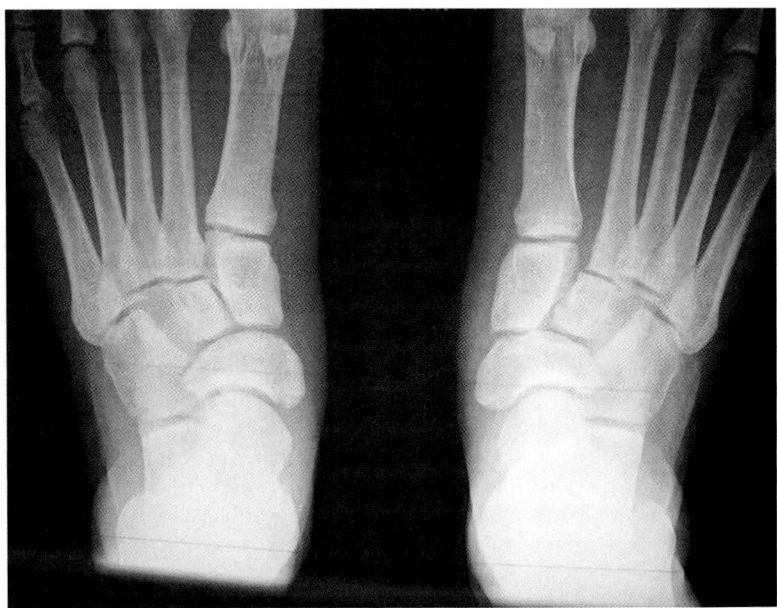

Figure 19.2. AP standing radiographs of the feet in a 21-year-old football player with chronic midfoot pain following a subtle Lisfranc injury 7 months prior. Note the advanced degeneration of the intercuneiform and naviculo-cuneiform joints with chronic subluxation.

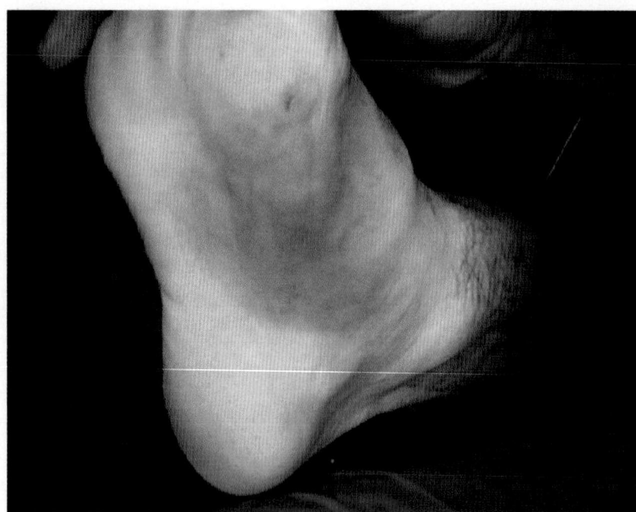

Figure 19.3. Clinical photo demonstrating the plantar ecchymosis of the midfoot that can occur in association with a Lisfranc injury.

PHYSICAL EXAMINATION

When examining for a subtle Lisfranc injury, inspection of the plantar surface of the foot should be performed routinely. Plantar ecchymosis has been described as a pathognomonic sign in a Lisfranc complex disruption (Fig. 19.3), although it may appear late or not at all in subtle injuries (17). Swelling of the midfoot may be observed and should be compared to the contralateral foot. It may be less obvious in a low-energy injury. Bony deformity is variable as well and there may or may not be a "gap sign" where a diastasis is noted between the hallux and the second toe (18). Tenderness to palpation over the tarsometatarsal joints is often present even in occult Lisfranc injuries. With more proximal variants, the tenderness may lie over the medial naviculo-cuneiform joint. Pain may be elicited with manipulation and provocative maneuvers. When reviewing ruptures of Lisfranc ligaments in athletes, Shapiro found that compression of the midfoot from side to side and moving the first metatarsal head in the sagittal plane while stabilizing the second metatarsal reproduced pain in the interval between the bases of the first and second metatarsals (19). Reproduction of pain by passive pronation and abduction of the midfoot were found to be the most reliable indicators of minor sprains in collegiate football players by some authors (3). Examination of the forefoot may confirm tenderness, swelling, or instability of the metatarsophalangeal joints. As above, the inability of the athlete to perform a single limb heel raise may heighten one's suspicions for this subtle injury.

IMAGING

Three standard views of the affected foot, including anteroposterior, 30-degree internal oblique and lateral are the mandatory initial radiographs which should be taken. Some authors also advocate performing 30-degree external oblique radiographs to better evaluate the medial column (2). The x-rays should be weight bearing, in an attempt to accentuate a subtle diastasis or subluxation that may not have been revealed otherwise. Even better may be a single limb weight-bearing radiograph, which will create significant stresses through the medial column of the foot. The longitudinal arch height should also be evaluated and compared to the contralateral side. The use of comparison weight-bearing radiographs of the unaffected foot has been emphasized by numerous authors in order to appreciate normal variants (14,16,19).

When evaluating either standing or stress radiographs, there have been certain parameters found to predict tarsometatarsal midfoot instability. On an anteroposterior (AP) film, the most sensitive indicator of Lisfranc injury is the line that connects the medial border of the second metatarsal and the medial edge of the middle cuneiform. These two (perimeters) should align and form a continuous parallel line. Similarly, the lateral base of the first metatarsal should line up with the lateral border of the medial cuneiform. In an oblique radiograph, the medial border of the fourth metatarsal should form a continuous line with the medial edge of the cuboid. The superior aspect of the first and second metatarsals should be congruent with the superior border of the cuneiforms on the lateral view. Faciszewski et al. postulated that the position of the medial cuneiform in relation to the base of the fifth metatarsal on a lateral weight-bearing x-ray helps to determine the prognosis of a Lisfranc injury. This relationship represents a measure of the longitudinal arch and when maintained, was found to be associated with a better functional outcome (20). Some authors report that if the actual distance between the first and second metatarsals is greater than 2 mm, a diastasis is present. However, a more reliable measure is a comparison view of the opposite side or stress views with a 1 to 2 mm variation in either study implying instability (10,14,16,21).

Other specific radiographic findings should also raise the physician's suspicion to a higher level. A fracture in the base of the second metatarsal warrants evaluation for a Lisfranc injury. This "fleck sign" represents a small avulsion fracture of the medial base of the second metatarsal at the attachment site of the Lisfranc ligament (Fig. 19.4). As mentioned previously, a compression fracture of the cuboid has been associated with

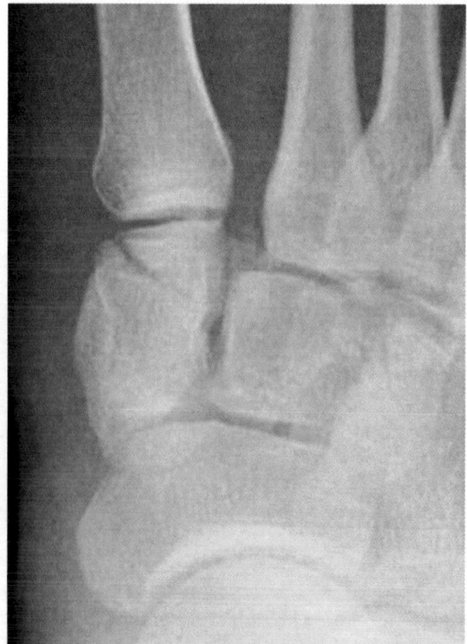

Figure 19.4. Radiograph highlighting the "fleck sign," representative of an avulsion of the Lisfranc ligament from the base of the second metatarsal.

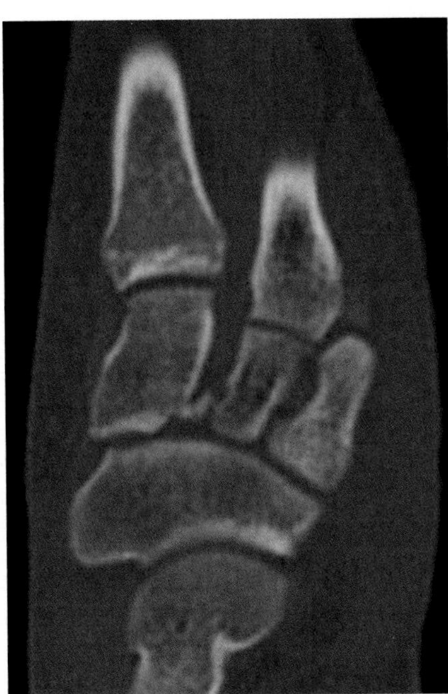

Figure 19.5. CT image confirming intercuneiform diastasis as well as intraarticular debris.

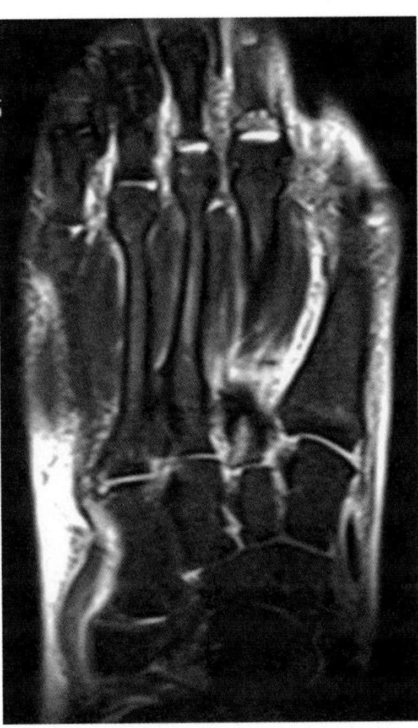

Figure 19.6. Axial MRI imaging used to confirm a complete disruption of the plantar Lisfranc ligament; a finding typically associated with an unstable midfoot pattern.

Lisfranc injuries. This related injury has been coined a "nutcracker" fracture from the force the cuboid sustains between the abducted fourth and fifth metatarsals and the anterior portion of the calcaneus. As mentioned above, metatarsal neck fractures or metatarsophalangeal dislocations have been associated with subtle Lisfranc variants as well.

A computed tomography (CT) scan is an additional radiographic tool that may provide more detailed information of the Lisfranc complex. This helps to define fracture patterns, assess for plantar comminution, and identify subtle injuries (Fig. 19.5). Lu et al. demonstrated that 1 to 2 mm of subluxation of the tarsometatarsal joint that was not appreciated by standard radiographs was able to be detected by CT scan (22). A specific technique that has been described in the literature is the "splay view," which is a coronal view of the midfoot, transformed from a mortise configuration to a flattened plane. It provides additional detail of the associated tarsometatarsal joints (23,24). This view remains more of a historical technique rather than one of common use, since most current CT scans can be performed in greater detail through thin cuts with three-dimensional reconstruction. However, the inherent problem of CT images is that they are not weight bearing.

Magnetic resonance imaging (MRI) may be helpful when radiographs and CT scans are equivocal and there remains a high index of suspicion for a Lisfranc "sprain." The continuity of the Lisfranc ligament and the presence of an occult injury may be able to be discerned with a MRI (Fig. 19.6). Recently Raikin et al. evaluated the reliability of MRI in attempting to determine the stability of subtle Lisfranc injuries (8). MR image evaluations were compared to intraoperative findings using manual stress radiographs under anesthesia and surgical intervention as reference points to further delineate the Lisfranc joint complex stability. They concluded that MRI may be used as an accurate tool to reliably predict midfoot stability when the plantar ligament bundle between the medial cuneiform and the bases of the second and third metatarsals is intact. However, it is unclear how easily detectable this ligament is on routine MR images. There may also be inconsistency depending not only on the quality of the MRI scan itself but regarding the caliber of the person reading it as well. For both CT and MRI scans, since neither are performed while the patient is weight bearing, there still exists the potential for an inconclusive study.

Other authors have concluded that the detection of subtle Lisfranc injuries may be best detected through the use of bone scintigrams. They concluded that the combined use of weight-bearing radiographs and bone scans provide a sensitive, reproducible, and inexpensive means of detecting subtle injuries (16). In addition, bone scans remain positive for nearly a year after the injury.

With the increasing availability and ease of office fluoroscopy, many authors have noted that this is the most reliable effective tool to stress the tarsometatarsal joint complex and determine stability (9,15,16). This has become the mainstay for detection of a suspected Lisfranc injury. Stress radiographs can be performed by applying an abduction and pronation force to the midfoot, followed by adduction and supination (Fig. 19.7). A regional ankle block can be used to facilitate the necessary radiographs or stress views.

CLASSIFICATION

Lisfranc injuries were historically classified by Quénu and Küss (1909) into three categories: homolateral, divergent, and isolated, with respect to the number of the metatarsals and the direction of displacement (25). This was further modified by Hardcastle in 1982 with the goal of attempting to guide treatment management by incorporating a greater variety of displacement (26). He divided the injuries into three patterns

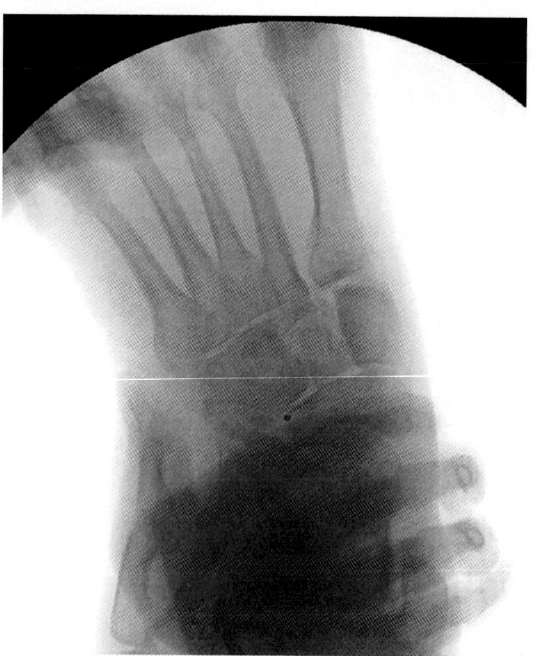

Figure 19.7. Stress radiograph maneuver used to confirm instability. Note the subluxation at the first tarsometatarsal joint.

of instability (A, B, and C). Type A (Total) represents a complete displacement of all of the tarsometatarsal joints with incongruity of the entire joint complex in one direction. Type B (Partial) describes a displacement of one or more metatarsals and involves only a part or section of the five tarsometatarsal joints. Type C (Divergent) comprises a diverging instability pattern, with the first metatarsal displaced medially and any number of the remaining metatarsals shifted laterally. Although the current treatment guidelines differ today than originally described by Hardcastle, the classification system is still widely used and accepted. Myerson has added subdivisions to the original classification; however, this modified classification system more appropriately describes high energy or direct types of Lisfranc injuries. His subclassification does highlight the potential for variant patterns with more proximal joint involvement (2).

Nunley has recently introduced a new classification system specifically directed toward athletic midfoot injuries and management (16). Grade I represents a Lisfranc ligament sprain with no diastasis or loss of arch height on weight-bearing radiographs. These injuries typically exhibit increased uptake on bone scintigram. They represent a dorsal capsular tear without elongation of the Lisfranc ligament. Stage II denotes a 1 to 5 mm diastasis between the first and second metatarsal as compared with the unaffected foot, with no loss of arch height. Type III injuries demonstrate a diastasis in addition to flattening of the arch as previously described (20). They noted that patients with midfoot tarsometatarsal sprains who maintained their arch showed a favorable outcome as compared with those who did not.

TREATMENT

The overall long-term goal of treatment is to preserve a painless, stable, plantigrade foot. This objective is best accomplished by obtaining a precise anatomic reduction to restore stability and alignment while maintaining motion. Treatment is generally guided by the degree of displacement and instability, which is determined using the above-mentioned radiographic assessment tools. Each athlete must also be evaluated on an individual basis with regard to their sport, position, time point during the season, and recovery period. Short- and long-term goals should always be discussed with the player, their family, agent, and coaches to provide everyone with a realistic anticipated return to play estimate and long-term prognosis.

Current recommendations incorporate the need for inherent stability through the medial column while maintaining the normal motion present in the lateral column. Stable anatomic reduction has been repeatedly found to provide the best long-term outcomes and minimize posttraumatic arthritis (2,10,14,16,21,26,27). Isolated ligamentous injuries, most often seen with the subtle athletic variant, have been documented to have worse outcomes when compared to high-energy displaced bony fractures (27,28). Surgical indications should be based largely on instability rather than on the specific measured degree of displacement. All of the surrounding joint complexes should be evaluated, including the tarsometatarsal, intercuneiform, and navicular–cuneiform articulations.

NON-OPERATIVE TREATMENT

Non-operative treatment has been documented to provide good results with successful return to activity when the injury pattern is stable (Nunley Stage I). This scenario must be documented radiographically and the athlete should be followed closely. Repeated stress views after 10 to 14 days are strongly suggested to ensure that stability is maintained. A period of immobilization in a cast with limited weight bearing for 4 to 6 weeks has been shown to provide excellent results (16,19). In a series by Meyer, only 50% of the athletes with "more severe" injuries were casted or splinted, and only 33% of those remained non–weight bearing (3). Although he did report favorable results with minimal long-term problems, four recurrences were noted.

If the athlete continues to feel pain after the initial 6-week time period, a controlled ankle motion boot or walking cast may be considered. In addition, the topic of surgical intervention may be readdressed, and repeated imaging can be useful. Nunley and Vertullo treated their Stage I Lisfranc ligament sprains with a non–weight-bearing cast for 6 weeks and then transitioned the athletes into custom-molded orthotics with excellent outcomes. Even with non-operative treatment, the athlete must be educated about the lengthy recovery process and the prognosis must be accurately portrayed.

OPERATIVE TREATMENT

INDICATIONS

Absolute indications for open reduction and internal fixation include open fractures and/or dislocations, vascular compromise, and compartment syndrome. These associated conditions are extremely rare in the low-energy athletic type of Lisfranc injuries. Current recommendations continue to emphasize the importance of maintaining stability and alignment. Most experts agree that a diastasis greater than 2 mm when compared

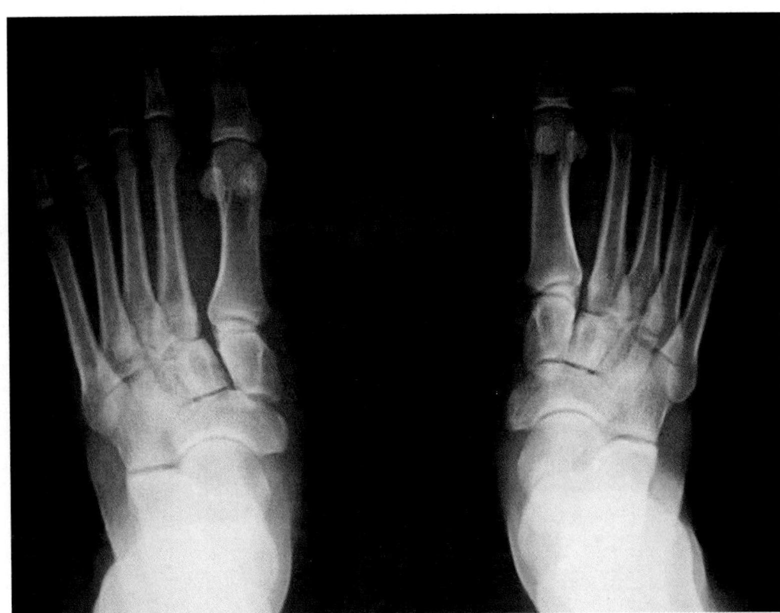

Figure 19.8. AP standing radiograph of the feet illustrating classic Lisfranc injury pattern on the left. Note the subluxation of the second metatarsal base occurring in association with proximal extension of injury to the naviculo-cuneiform joint (proximal variant pattern).

with the unaffected side on weight-bearing films or stress radiographs (Stage II) represents an unstable injury requiring operative intervention (10,14,16,28). There have been documented successful results with athletes treated non-operatively with 2 to 5 mm distance between the metatarsal bases on weight-bearing radiographs; however, this data was collected retrospectively in a limited number of patients (19). The physician also needs to consider the "acute-on-chronic" injury where the diastasis present may be longstanding. Therefore, a specific amount of diastasis on a single radiograph is not as useful as identifying true instability patterns on standing or stress imaging, or recognizing progressive diastasis on serial radiographs. Athletes sustaining a proximal variant injury pattern where the force of the injury extends through the intercuneiform joint to exit out the naviculo-cuneiform joint demonstrate instability of the first ray and difficulty with push-off and nearly always require surgical stabilization (Fig. 19.8) (15).

TECHNIQUE

The timing of midfoot surgery is dictated by the status of the soft tissues surrounding the foot. Incisions are performed only after the swelling and edema has subsided, which may delay the definitive procedure for up to 2 weeks after the injury. Skin wrinkling is a reliable indicator that the foot is able to tolerate an operative intervention. Closed treatment with percutaneous pin reduction and fixation does not allow for adequate reduction in the majority of cases. Results from the literature have shown less than promising results with this method. Although absolute indications are still relatively controversial in subtle athletic Lisfranc injuries, most authors agree that if instability is present which requires surgical intervention, open reduction is usually warranted (2,14,16,27,29). An attempt at a closed reduction may precede an open approach, as one may consider for an isolated subluxation of the second metatarsal base, but the surgeon should be prepared to proceed with open incisions should closed reduction fail. Nunley advocates an initial attempt at reduction with fluoroscopy under anesthesia for Type II injuries (displacement of 2 to 5 mm) (16). If the joint is not able to be reduced with percutaneous clamps or reduction maneuvers, then an open incision should be performed. This allows for debridement of all interposed bone and cartilage fragments, assessment of the articular surfaces, and anatomic reduction. While it is important to remove interposed debris that may block reduction, soft tissues that comprise ruptured ligaments are left in place to scar in. Subtle ligamentous injuries that extend to the proximal midfoot should always be anticipated and evaluated in the operating room using stress fluoroscopy or direct open exploration (Fig. 19.9A, B). The disrupted joint complex is most often approached through one or more dorsal longitudinal incisions. Whether it is centered over the first tarsometatarsal joint or the first interspace, the dorsalis pedis artery and the deep peroneal nerve must be identified and protected (16). If more than one incision is needed, the distance between incisions must allow for an adequately sized skin bridge. Failure to do so may result in vascular compromise and subsequent skin necrosis.

The role of primary arthrodesis remains controversial, but has become a popular subject of debate. Ly and Coetzee randomized 41 patients with ligamentous Lisfranc injuries to treatment with primary arthrodesis versus open reduction with internal fixation (28). Five patients from the traditional open reduction internal fixation group developed deformity and/or osteoarthritis, necessitating eventual arthrodesis. After 2 years, the American Orthopedic Foot and Ankle Society (AOFAS) scores and postoperative activity levels of the primary arthrodesis group (68.6, 92%, respectively) were significantly better than those from the open reduction internal fixation group (88, 65%, respectively). Henning et al. also performed a randomized controlled prospective study comparing these two cohorts and found no significant differences with regards to the Short Form-36 (SF-36) and Short Musculoskeletal Function Assessment (SMFA) questionnaires (30). Sangeorzan et al. also supported primary arthrodesis as a better option for ligamentous

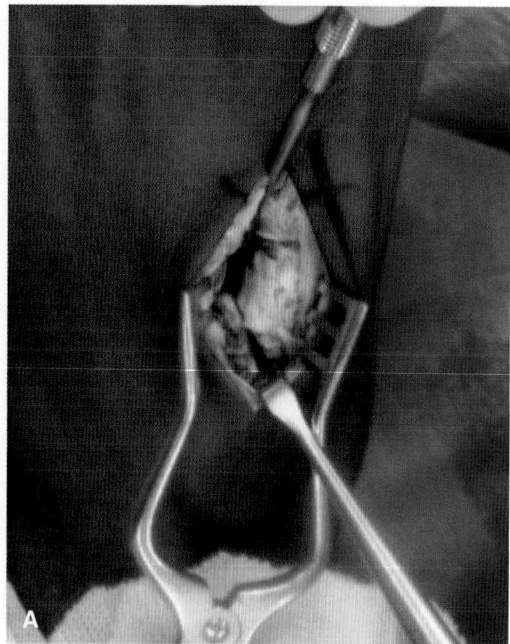

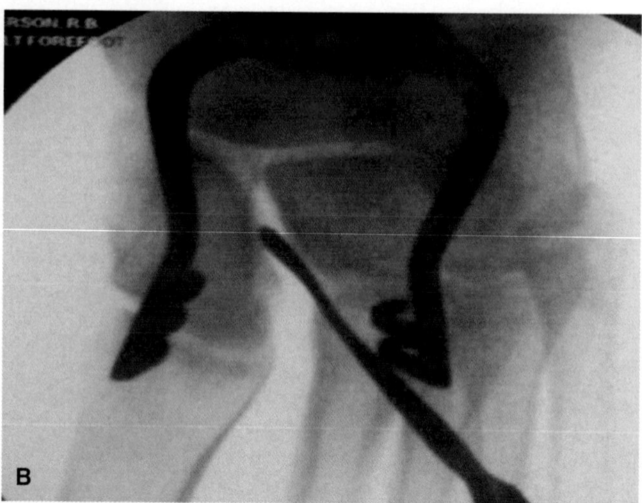

Figure 19.9. **A:** Intraoperative photo depicting the dorsal longitudinal incision used to explore the injured joints. Note the diastasis that extends between the first and second cuneiform bones. **B:** Intraoperative fluoroscopic imaging confirming the gross instability consistent with a proximal variant injury.

injuries in their study (31). This idea was refuted by Mulier who found that there was more pain, stiffness of the forefoot, loss of the metatarsal arch, and sympathetic dystrophy in the arthrodesis group (32). In conclusion, it is reasonable to perform a primary fusion in the setting of significant joint and cartilage comminution, as one may see with higher-energy injuries, but how to best manage ligamentous injuries is still being disputed. Furthermore, there has been no true documentation regarding how an elite athlete would perform with a midfoot fusion. With arthrodesis there exists the potential risk of a symptomatic nonunion or a dorsiflexion malunion with secondary lesser metatarsal overload, leading to further complications and dysfunction. Each individual must be considered on a case-by-case basis and the risks and benefits weighed accordingly.

Anatomic reduction remains the most important factor when treating a Lisfranc injury and may be achieved through differing operative techniques, as described by Easley et al. (33). Some surgeons prefer to reduce the base of the second metatarsal into the keystone of the surrounding cuneiforms. The joint is reduced and held with a large clamp extending from the base of the second metatarsal into the medial cuneiform. Once this is reduced and stabilized, the surrounding joints are then further evaluated in sequential order. An alternative method is to provisionally pin all of the unstable articulations with Kirschner wires (K-wires) before placing the definitive internal fixation across the joints. It is found helpful to start with the medial column (first tarsometatarsal joint) first and then work laterally. Both are acceptable treatment methods.

FIXATION

After the reduction is obtained, fixation must be implemented. K-wires, screws, plates, and external fixation devices have been described in the past. K-wires may be used for definitive fixation only when a significant bony component to the injury is present, often one with comminution. They are easily inserted and may be removed in the office, but have an increased risk of pin tract infection and subsequent loss of correction (34). They are most commonly reserved for holding the fourth and fifth tarsometatarsal joints reduced or buttressing the lateral column.

Current treatment regimens support solid internal fixation of the medial and middle columns, with optional pin fixation of the lateral column. Screws provide superior stability of the medial and middle columns when compared with K-wire pin fixation in biomechanical studies (35). Cannulated and solid screws have been described for fixation of the medial column joints, with 3.5 mm cortical screws being adequate in most patients. Consideration should be taken for placing larger screws in larger athletes, particular the "home run" screw placed from the medial cuneiform to the second metatarsal base. Compression across joints should be avoided and lag techniques are unnecessary if an adequate reduction is performed, as noted by Kuo et al. (27). The specific number of screws and pattern should be determined by the involved unstable joints.

An alternative type of fixation involves dorsal plating of the Lisfranc articulations. The theory behind this mode of treatment is to maintain stability while avoiding iatrogenic articular cartilage injury when drilling and placing screws across the tarsometatarsal joints. Alberta et al. performed a biomechanical comparison of dorsal plating and transarticular screw fixation in ten matched pairs of cadavers (36). No difference was found between the matched pairs of differing implants in resisting tarsometatarsal joint displacement. Dorsal plating can be used to span comminuted fractures; with the advent of low profile plates, soft-tissue irritation may be avoided. Although dorsal plating on the compression side has been found to be inferior to that of plantar tension plating, it provides results comparable to transarticular screw fixation (34).

Recently, there have been comparisons using screw fixation with suture-button fixation in 14 cadaveric specimens (37). After loading the feet with sectioned Lisfranc ligaments, no significant difference in displacement was noted between the two differing types of implants.

Thordarson et al. described using polylactide (PLA) absorbable screw fixation in Lisfranc injuries to circumvent the need for screw removal (29). There were no incidences of reaction to the screws, hardware osteolysis, or loosening. The reduction was maintained in all patients.

AUTHORS' PREFERRED APPROACH

The authors' treatment philosophy rests on the caveat that anatomic reduction is mandatory to provide optimal results for elite athletes with Lisfranc injuries. Any instability documented by CT images, stress fluoroscopy, or weight-bearing comparison radiographs in an acute injury warrants operative intervention. In the authors' opinion, when an unstable Lisfranc injury is recognized in an athlete, the need for an absolute accurate reduction outweighs the potential risks of a skin incision; therefore, an extremely low threshold to perform an open reduction is utilized. Open exploration is also the most assured way to assess for proximal variant instability patterns, those that involve the intercuneiform and naviculo-cuneiform joints.

The athlete is positioned supine on the operating table with a bump fashioned under the ipsilateral hip. The heel of the foot is situated at the very end of the table, allowing for easy access to intraoperative fluoroscopy. A dorsal longitudinal incision is performed in the interval between the first and second tarsometatarsal joints, allowing direct visualization and anatomic reduction of the diastasis. The incision is carried down in the interval between the extensor hallucis longus (EHL) and the extensor hallucis brevis (EHB). The dorsalis pedis artery and the deep peroneal nerve are identified laterally and protected throughout the case. The dorsal capsular ligaments are invariably torn upon initial presentation. If the navicular–cuneiform joints are also disrupted, the incision may be extended proximally to assess the area under direct visualization. All bony and cartilaginous fragments are debrided and removed, with care taken to preserve the plantar and interosseous ligaments. If the first tarsometatarsal joint is found to be unstable, we find it helpful to provisionally fix it with a K-wire first, confirming the reduction and alignment with fluoroscopy. The second metatarsal is then reduced with a large clamp extending from the lateral metatarsal base to the medial border of the medial cuneiform. The reduction is verified under direct visualization as well as fluoroscopy. A guide pin or K-wire is advanced following the trajectory of the native Lisfranc ligament. Cannulated drilling is performed in a standard, non-lag technique. The guide pin and drill are removed, and a 3.5 mm or larger, fully threaded, solid, cortical screw is advanced across the Lisfranc joint, recreating the ligament. This "home run" screw avoids the articular surfaces of both the first and the second tarsometatarsal joint. Attention is then returned to the first tarsometatarsal joint where, if unstable, is definitively fixed with either a screw or a dorsal plate. When screws are placed across the tarsometatarsal joints from distal to proximal, dorsal notching must be performed to avoid cortical fractures. To provide maximum fixation, the screws should be aimed and positioned generally parallel to the sole of the foot, exiting through the plantar cortex just distal to the naviculo-cuneiform joint. Over the past 3 years we have preferred the use of dorsally applied "bridge" plates, used with locked or non-locked screws. It is our preference to use non-locked screws for plate holes in closest proximity to the joint so as to direct the screw away from the joint itself, thus preventing articular injury (Fig. 19.10). At this point, the surrounding tarsometatarsal joints, as well as the proximal intercuneiform and navicular–cuneiform joints, are assessed for instability. If needed, a second longitudinal incision may be placed overlying the axis of the fourth metatarsal that allows visualization of the third tarsometatarsal joint. With an anatomic reduction of the Lisfranc ligament performed, the fourth and fifth articulations will often reduce spontaneously. K-wires can be placed from the fifth metatarsal proximally into the cuboid or lateral cuneiform in order to temporarily maintain this reduction. K-wires are preferred over screws at this location as they avoid the potential for arthrofibrosis that may limit the important compensatory motion which occurs along this lateral column. They are also easily removed in the office setting. Intercuneiform instability is managed with a single cortical screw inserted from the medial cuneiform into the second. This screw, along with the "home run" screw to the second metatarsal, is usually adequate to stabilize the naviculo-cuneiform joint and therefore we rarely pass fixation across this more proximal joint (Fig. 19.11A, B, C).

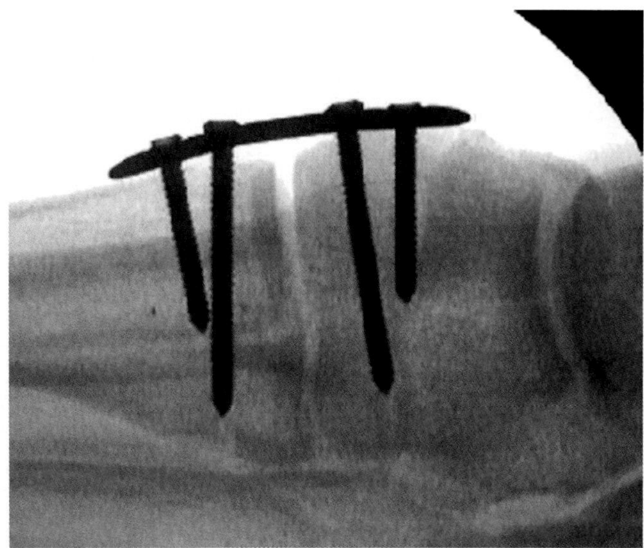

Figure 19.10. Example of dorsal bridge plating of an unstable first tarsometatarsal joint. Note the use of non-locked screws which are directed away from the articular surface.

When an athlete presents with a chronic, partially treated, or recurrent diastasis, the surrounding athletic situation should be taken into consideration and a treatment plan should be made on an individual basis. Less reliable and less favorable results have been documented in a chronic scenario; therefore, alternative treatments may be attempted. Currently, there are professional football players performing at a high level with chronic Lisfranc injuries; however, this is not the ideal situation or the standard of care, so caution should be taken when making such

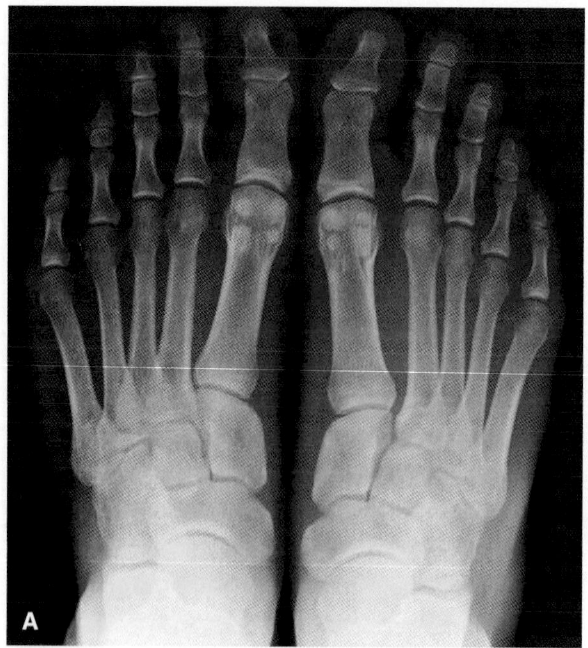

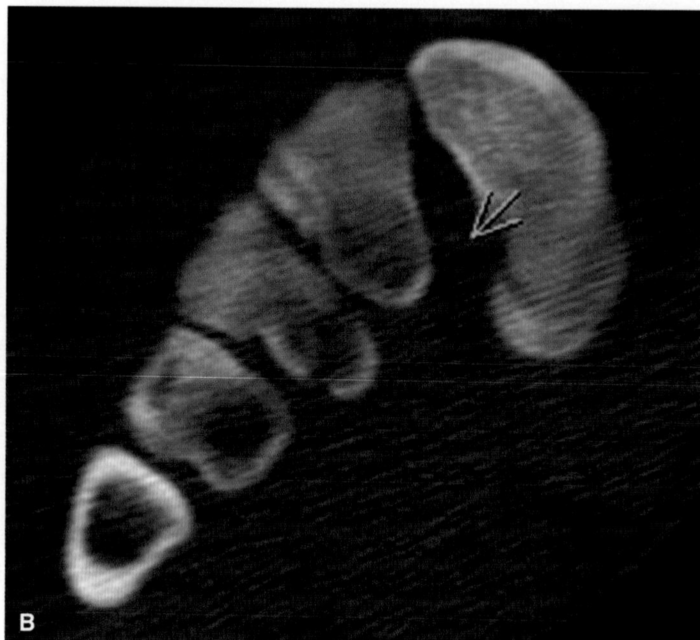

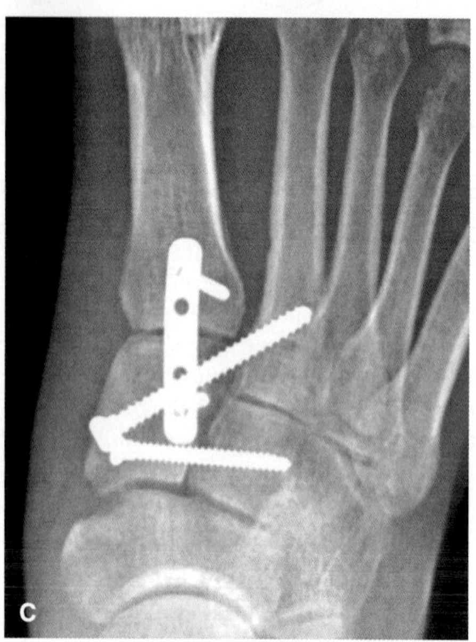

Figure 19.11. **A:** AP standing radiograph in a professional football player suffering a subtle Lisfranc injury on the right. **B:** Coronal CT image highlights the diastasis between the cuneiforms (green *arrow*). **C:** AP standing radiograph 6 weeks postoperative which illustrates the combined use of screws and bridge plating. A 4.5 mm solid screw was used for the "home run" position, while a 3.7 mm screw was place across the cuneiforms.

recommendations. For these difficult circumstances, it is best to refer to an athletic foot specialist for definitive treatment recommendations, which may include limited arthrodeses.

POSTOPERATIVE MANAGEMENT

Postoperatively, the patient should be placed into a well-padded splint in neutral dorsiflexion to allow for further swelling. Non–weight-bearing status should be initiated for 10 to 14 days and elevation of the lower extremity should be emphasized to minimize wound complications. After the incisions are healed and the sutures are removed, a short leg, non–weight-bearing cast or boot should be placed onto the leg for an additional 4 to 6 weeks. The athlete is transitioned into a controlled ankle motion boot for 4 to 6 more weeks, allowing for full weight bearing and rehabilitation. The boot is removed to allow for non-impact activities such as pool therapy and stationary bike. Shoewear modified with an orthotic device with pronounced arch support and midsole rigidity should be worn for 3 to 6 months afterward.

Hardware removal remains controversial. Most authors agree that pins, when used, should be removed from the lateral column joints at 6 weeks after the initial surgery. Screw or plate removal should be delayed for a minimum of 4 months to allow for adequate ligament healing. It is recommended that hardware crossing the tarsometatarsal joints be removed. Unless symptomatic, one may consider leaving an isolated "home run" Lisfranc ligament screw in place indefinitely. It is also advisable to maintain intercuneiform screw fixation permanently, in order to provide a "spot weld" that may assist in preventing recurrent diastasis. Another option to consider is to exchange the "home run" screw with a suture-button device at 3 to 4 months, providing ongoing protection without the ongoing risk of hardware failure. This alternative method and its results have yet to be reported in the literature.

COMPLICATIONS

Hardware failure always remains a potential complication when internal fixation is not removed. This can become a challenging problem when retained broken screws are present in the face of an athlete with recurrent symptomatic diastasis. This is one of the reasons that dorsal bridge plating has become attractive.

Another common complication of a Lisfranc disruption is posttraumatic arthritis. When specific joints are symptomatic, they can be managed with selective joint injections under fluoroscopic imaging. Anti-inflammatories and accommodative bracing may also play a role, but to a lesser extent. Since adequate immobilization of the midfoot requires a brace that encompasses a significant portion of the foot and ankle, an elite athlete may not be able to adequately perform while wearing such a brace. When all conservative measures fail, posttraumatic arthritis can be managed with an arthrodesis of the symptomatic joints. In the largest series of Lisfranc injuries documented by Myerson, over 44% of the 52 patients required further surgery, with 17 of the 27 procedures encompassing arthrodeses (2). However, these injuries were not of the subtle athletic variety. The incidence of symptomatic lateral column arthritis is significantly less than the medial side. If operative intervention does become necessary, interpositional arthroplasty may be an alternative to arthrodesis in an effort to preserve the inherent motion of the lateral column.

Other complications including infection, neuritis, neuroma, compartment syndrome, deep venous thrombosis, nonunion, malunion, residual deformity, and reflex sympathetic dystrophy have all been described as related to Lisfranc injuries. These present very rarely but can be difficult to cope with in an athlete who is already facing a prolonged recovery period.

RECOVERY

When reviewing college football players, although many returned to play within a few weeks, the average time to maximal performance was prolonged (mean: 40.5 days; range: 2 to 215 days) (3). However, others have found that time to return to competition averaged nearly 4 months (19,39). Symptoms following injury to the Lisfranc complex have been reported to improve until an average of 1.3 years after the injury (39).

PROGNOSIS

Although Ly and Coetzee found that patients with primary medial arthrodesis fared better in the short and the medium term than those patients treated with open reduction with internal fixation, it has not been documented how a high-level athlete would perform with a midfoot fusion (28). Anderson and others similarly found no significant differences in SF-36 and SMFA between those patients treated with a primary fusion as compared with those who underwent an open reduction with internal fixation (30,32). This holds true in the average patient population excluding the elite athlete.

In the largest series, Myerson and colleagues found that excellent functional results were closely correlated to the quality of the initial reduction (2). This remains a point of emphasis throughout the literature. In addition, poor functional results were noted in those athletes for whom diagnosis was delayed (38). Despite an often benign radiographic appearance, the delay in return to sport often signified the severity of the injury. Purely ligamentous Lisfranc injuries have been found to have a worse prognosis as compared with fracture dislocations by various authors (27,40). Sangeorzan documented a trend toward poorer outcomes despite anatomical reduction and screw fixation in purely ligamentous injuries. In regards to the outcome, there exists no significant difference when comparing age, gender, and mechanism of injury (40,41).

Functional results were quantitatively investigated by Teng et al., who reported on 11 patients at 41 months postoperatively (42). Using an in-shoe pressure monitoring system, F-scan gait analyses were performed and did not reveal any significant difference between the affected foot and normal controls.

CONCLUSION

Lisfranc injuries are rare, but can be devastating to the elite athlete. The "athletic" variant is typically a purely ligamentous injury and may present with subtle findings and more proximal joint involvement than the classically described injury pattern. Long-term function is best achieved through early recognition and appropriate treatment; therefore, a high index of suspicion is mandatory. Stability should be the guiding force regarding the treatment path and anatomic reduction must be maintained for optimal results. Non-operative treatment is accepted in Stage I sprains; however, careful observation and documentation of maintained stability should be instituted. In situations where acute instability is present, anatomic reduction and rigid fixation is recommended for the medial column while preserving motion in the lateral column. The role of primary arthrodesis in the setting of ligamentous injuries in the elite athlete has yet to be determined and should be exercised with caution. Immobilization is often prolonged and the long-term prognosis is guarded. The athlete, agent, coach, and family must be educated about the recovery period and serious nature of these injuries.

REFERENCES

1. Latterman C, Goldstein JL, Wukich DK, et al. Practical Management of Lisfranc Injuries in Athletes. *Clin J Sports Med* 2007;17(4):311–315.
2. Myerson MS, Fisher RT, Burgess AR, et al. Fracture dislocations of the tarsometatarsal joints: end results correlated with pathology and treatment. *Foot Ankle* 1986;6:225–242.
3. Meyer SA, Callaghan JJ, Albright JP, et al. Midfoot sprains in collegiate football players. *Am J Sports Med* 1994;22(3):392–401.
4. Kura H, Zuo ZP, Kitaoka HB, et al. Mechanical behavior of the Lisfranc and dorsal cuneometatarsal ligaments: In vitro biomechanical study. *J Orthop Trauma* 2001;15(2):107–110.
5. Anderson RB. Injuries to the midfoot and forefoot. *Orthopaedic knowledge update: foot and ankle.* 2nd ed. Rosemont: AAOS; 1994.
6. Peicha G, Labovitz J, Seibert FJ, et al. The anatomy of the joint as a risk factor for Lisfranc dislocation and fracture-dislocation: An anatomical and radiological case control study. *J Bone Joint Surg Br* 2002;84-B(7):981–985.
7. Solan M, Moorman CT 3rd, Miyamoto RG, et al. Ligamentous restraints of the second tarsometatarsal joint: a biomechanical evaluation. *Foot Ankle Int* 2001;22(8):637–641.

8. Raikin SM, Elias I, Dheer S, et al. Prediction of midfoot instability in the subtle Lisfranc injury. *J Bone Joint Surg Am* 2009;91:892–899.
9. Karr S, Femino J, Morag Y. Lisfranc joint displacement following sequential ligament sectioning. *J Bone Joint Surg Am* 2007;89-A(10):2225–2232.
10. Mantas JP, Burks RT. LisFranc injuries in the athlete. *Clin Sports Med* 1994;13(4):719–731.
11. Ashworth MJ, Davies MB, Williamson DM. Irreducible Lisfranc's injury: the 'toe up' sign. *Injury* 1997;28(4):321–322.
12. Gissane W. A dangerous type of fracture of the foot. *J Bone Joint Surg Br* 1951;33:535–538.
13. Ouzounian T, Shereff MJ. In vitro determination of midfoot motion. *Foot Ankle* 1989;10:140–146.
14. Clanton TO, McGarvey W. Athletic injuries to the soft tissues of the foot and ankle. In: Coughlin MJ, Mann RA, Saltzman CL, eds. *Surgery of the foot and ankle.* 8th ed. Philadelphia, PA: Mosby, Elsevier Inc.; 2007:1425–1563.
15. Anderson RB, Hammit N. Recognizing and treating the subtle Lisfranc injury. Presented to the NFL Physicians Society/ NFL Combine. *Indianapolis* 2005.
16. Nunley JA, Vertullo CJ. Classification, investigation, and management of midfoot sprains: Lisfranc injuries in the athlete. *Am J Sports Med* 2002;30(6):871–878.
17. Ross G, Cronin R, Hauzenblas J, et al. Plantar ecchymosis sign: a clinical aid to diagnosis of occult Lisfranc tarsometatarsal injuries. *J Orthop Trauma* 1996.
18. Davies MS, Saxby TS. Intercuneiform instability and the "gap" sign. *Foot Ankle Int* 1999;20:606–629.
19. Shapiro MS, Wascher DC, Finerman GA. Rupture of Lisfranc's ligament in athletes. *Am J Sports Med* 1994;22(5):687–691.
20. Faciszewski T, Burks RT, Manaster BJ. Subtle Injuries of the Lisfranc Joint. *J Bone Joint Surg Am* 1990;72-A(10):1519–1522.
21. Anderson RB. *Lisfranc fracture-dislocation. Current Practice in Foot and Ankle Surgery.* New York, NY: McGraw Hill; 1993:129–159.
22. Lu J, Ebraheim NA, Skie M. Radiographic and computed tomographic evaluation of Lisfranc dislocation: A cadaver study. *Foot Ankle Int* 1997;18:351–355.
23. Goiney RC, Connell DG, Nichols DM. CT evaluation of tarsometatarsal fracture-dislocation injuries. *AJR Am J Roentgenol* 1985;144:985–990.
24. Leenan LP, Van der Werken C. Fracture-dislocations of the tarsometatarsal joint, a combined anatomical and computed tomographic study. *Injury* 1992;23:51–55.
25. Quénu E, Küss G. Étude sur les luxations du metatarse (luxations métatarsotarsiennes) du diastasis entre le 1er et le 2e metatarsien. *Rev Chir* 1909;39:281–336,720–791,1093–1134.
26. Hardcastle PH, Reschauer R, Kutscha-Lissberg E, et al. Injuries to the Tarsometatarsal joint: incidence, classification and treatment. *J Bone Joint Surg Br* 1982;64-B(3):349–356.
27. Kuo R, Tejwani NC, Digiovanni CW, et al. Outcome after open reduction and internal fixation of Lisfranc joint injuries. *J Bone Joint Surg Am* 2000;82A:1609–1618.
28. Ly TV, Coetzee JC. Treatment of primary ligamentous Lisfranc joint injuries: primary arthrodesis compared with open reduction and internal fixation. *J Bone Joint Surg Am* 2006;88-A:514–520.
29. Thordarson DB, Hurvitz G. PLA screw fixation of Lisfranc injuries. *Foot Ankle Int* 2002;23(11):1003–1007.
30. Henning JA, Jones CB, Sietsema DL, et al. Open reduction internal fixation versus primary arthrodesis for Lisfranc injuries: a prospective randomized study. *Foot Ankle Int* 2009;30(10):913–922.
31. Sangeorzan BJ, Veith RG, Hansen ST. Salvage of Lisfranc's tarsometatarsal joint by arthrodesis. *Foot Ankle* 1990;10(4):193–200.
32. Mulier T, Reynders P, Dereymaeker G, et al. Severe Lisfrancs injuries: primary arthrodesis or ORIF?*Foot Ankle Int* 2002;23(10):902–905.
33. DeOrio M, Erickson M, Usuelli FG, et al. Lisfranc injuries in sport. *Foot Ankle Clin N Am* 2009;14(2):169–186.
34. Sangeorzan BJ, Hansen ST. Early and late posttraumatic foot reconstruction. *Clin Orthop Relat Res* 1989;243:86–91.
35. Lee CA, Birkedal JP, Dickerson EA, et al. Stabilization of Lisfranc joint injuries: a biomechanical study. *Foot Ankle Int* 2004;25:365–370.
36. Alberta FG, Aronow MS, Barrero M, et al. Ligamentous Lisfranc joint injuries: a biomechanical comparison of dorsal plate and transarticular screw fixation. *Foot Ankle Int* 2006;26(6):462–473.
37. Panchbhavi VK, Vallurupalli S, Yang J, et al. Screw fixation compared with suture-button fixation of isolated Lisfranc ligament injuries. *J Bone Joint Surg Am* 2009;91:1143–1148.
38. Curtis MJ, Myerson M, Szura B. Tarsometatarsal joint injuries in the athlete. *Am J Sports Med* 1993;21(4):497–502.
39. Brunet JA, Wiley JJ. The late results of tarsometatarsal joint injuries. *J Bone Joint Surg* 1987;69B:437–440.
40. Richter M, Wippermann B, Krettek C. Fractures and fracture dislocations of the midfoot: occurrence, causes and long-term results. *Foot Ankle Int* 2001;22:392–398.
41. Calder JD, Whitehouse SL, Saxby TS. Results of isolated Lisfranc injuries and the effect of compensation claims. *J Bone Joint Surg Am* 2004;86-B:527–530.
42. Teng AL, Pinzur MS, Lomasney L, et al. Functional outcome following anatomic restoration of tarsal-metatarsal fracture dislocation. *Foot Ankle Int* 2002;23:922–926.

CHAPTER

20

Daryl C. Osbahr
Answorth A. Allen

Stress Fractures of the Foot and Ankle

INTRODUCTION

Stress fractures are overuse injuries most commonly seen in athletes and military recruits. In his assessment of "Olympic Victors", Aristotle (384 to 322 BC) described the deleterious effects of overuse injuries by stating that successful athletes are "those who do not squander their powers by early and over-training." Although the effects of overtraining had been known for centuries, stress fractures were first described in 1855 by Breithaupt, a Prussian military physician (1). Based on his clinical observations of an overuse injury to the metatarsal in military recruits after long marches, the "march fracture" became synonymous with this impairment (2). In 1958, Devas associated stress fractures of the tibia with "shin soreness" and subsequently became the first to describe these injuries in the athletic population (3).

Stress fractures are now known to occur in a diverse patient population, ranging from military recruits and athletes to patients with chronic medical conditions. Considering the diversity in affected patient populations, stress fractures are routinely encountered in the office as well as the training room and require a complex and unique management algorithm to decrease morbidity and negate potential catastrophic consequences. Despite the potential for varying presentations, stress fractures are still typically considered a pathologic occurrence of physically active patients as repetitive stress during endurance training is mostly commonly associated with the athletic population.

Stress fractures have been encountered throughout the entire body; nevertheless, they are more common in the lower extremity as the weight-bearing bones encounter excessive loads, particularly the foot and ankle. Stress fractures may occur in any bone of the foot and ankle, and individual sports are commonly associated with injury to specific anatomical locations as repetitive stresses result in an insult to a particular bone. This chapter will review the science behind stress fractures and provide critical information concerning the diagnosis and management of these injuries according to specific anatomic locations in the foot and ankle.

EPIDEMIOLOGY

With a growing focus on improved fitness in the general population as well as more sophisticated diagnostic technology, stress fractures are now more frequently identified resulting in enhanced management of these injuries. Stress fractures have a reported incidence of less than 1% in the general athletic population (4); however, they account for approximately 10% of all injuries in athletes (4,5). The incidence of stress fractures is largely dependent upon the specific sporting activity, and the incidence in runners has been noted to be as high as 20% which accounts for 4.4% to 15.6% of all injuries in this athletic population (4,6). Moreover, bilateral stress fractures have been reported with relative frequency as this overuse injury can affect both sides of the body in at least 16% of cases (4).

Overall, approximately 95% of all stress fractures involve the lower extremities (7). Within the lower extremities, Matheson and coworkers specified that the tibia was the most common site of injury at 49.1% followed by the tarsal bones (25.3%), metatarsals (8.8%), femur (7.2%), and fibula (6.6%) (4). Bennell and colleagues corroborated these findings in a prospective study evaluating track and field athletes which reported that the most common stress fracture sites are the tibia (46%), navicular (15%), fibula (12%), metatarsal (8%), and other tarsal bones (4%) (8). Therefore, the bones that comprise the foot and ankle account for approximately 85% to 90% of all stress fractures in athletes (4,9).

Within the athletic population, certain sporting activities and individual athletes have been reported to be more susceptible to stress fractures. Johnson and colleagues, in fact, noted that injuries may be associated with specific sporting activities as track and field accounted for 64% of stress fractures in women and 50% in men (10). When evaluating stress fractures in 914 inter-collegiate athletes, the incidence varied according to sport with the highest rate in track and field (9.7%) followed by lacrosse (4.3%), crew (2.4%), and football (1.1%); however, no stress fractures were sustained in fencing, hockey, golf, softball, swimming, or tennis during the study period (10). Similar results were reported by Goldberg and Pecora who evaluated approximately 3,000 collegiate athletes over a 3-year period and found an increased incidence of stress fractures in softball (19%) followed by track and field (11%), basketball (9%), lacrosse (8%), baseball (8%), tennis (8%), and gymnastics (8%) (11,12).

When evaluating the incidence of stress fractures as related to gender, higher rates have been noted in female military recruits at 1.2 to 10 times the rate of their male counterparts (13–17). In the athletic population, this concept is somewhat controversial as men and women have been found to be at equal risk of sustaining a stress fracture when comparing the number of stress fractures per 1,000 training hours (8). As the elderly population is increasing participation in athletic activities, the occurrence of stress fractures within this subgroup should not be underestimated as they present unique challenges. Increased stress within the bone of elderly patients secondary to repetitive activities is further complicated by decreased bone quality from osteoporosis and other chronic medical conditions (18).

PATHOPHYSIOLOGY

Bone acts in accordance with Wolff's law as it represents a dynamic tissue with the capability to remodel in response to physiologic stress; therefore, bone remodeling after repetitive strain begins with osteoclastic resorption (19–21) which plateaus at 3 weeks (7,15) followed by immature, bone formation (over 3 months) (7,22) and subsequent maturation of the bone into normal lamellar layers (23). Bone can ultimately fail by two distinct mechanisms. The first mode of failure develops due to a single episode of loading where the strain exceeds the ultimate strength of the bone resulting in acute, catastrophic structural collapse (fracture). The second mode of failure develops from an accumulation of microdamage that occurs secondary to repetitive loading of the bone with submaximal failure strain loads (stress fracture).

Stress fractures result from these excessive, repetitive loads which cause an imbalance between bone formation and resorption; therefore, stress fractures may form as a result of an abnormal interaction between extrinsic (repetitive mechanical loading) and intrinsic factors (suboptimal bone biology). Consequently, a stress fracture of bone may develop from either excessive bone strain and microdamage with an inability to maintain adequate skeletal repair (fatigue fracture) or abnormal bone remodeling when undergoing normal strain loads (insufficiency fracture). The latter situation typically results in patients with suboptimal bony architecture, such as patients with metabolic bone disease, osteoporosis, and the elderly with chronic medical conditions. However, the former circumstance is normally the mode by which athletes, military recruits, and female athlete triad patients present to sports medicine offices with stress fractures.

In the athletic population, fatigue failure resulting in a stress fracture may occur over a period of time and classically progresses through three stages: Crack initiation, crack propagation, and final fracture (24). The exact phenomenon which results in the initiation of stress fractures remains controversial and is usually characterized by one of two theories. The first theory suggests that excessive forces are transmitted to the bone as the associated musculature becomes fatigued which consequently makes the bone susceptible to microfractures (25–27). The second theory proposes that the surrounding musculature contributes to the development of stress fractures by concentrating forces around a localized area of bone resulting in excessive mechanical insults above the stress-bearing capacity (28). Despite the inherent validity of each theory, the development of stress fractures is likely multifactorial with origins stemming from both extrinsic and intrinsic factors, including mechanical influences, athletic activities, nutritional deficiencies, hormonal imbalances, collagen abnormalities, and metabolic bone disorders.

CLINICAL EVALUATION

CLINICAL HISTORY

Establishing an early diagnosis is essential to avoid potential morbidity and allow for earlier return to play in the athletic population. The clinical presentation can vary which inherently makes the diagnosis difficult; however, a very thorough history can help differentiate stress fractures from other musculoskeletal conditions. The typical presentation consists of an insidious onset of pain during activity over a period of days to weeks. Initially, the pain will result from activity and resolve with rest; however, further activity will result in progression of pain which may not regress resulting in inability to participate in athletic activities. An initial clinical evaluation must include an assessment of the patient's trauma history, training or exercise programs, shoe wear, general health, medications, diet, occupation, women's menstrual history, and related activities as all of these factors may enhance the risk of stress fracture.

PHYSICAL EXAMINATION

On physical examination, tenderness directly over the bone of interest is the most obvious finding and represents the hallmark for diagnosing a stress fracture. Although many areas of the body are not in a subcutaneous position, the bones of the foot and ankle are almost universally superficial allowing for direct palpation. In addition, swelling over the affected bone may be evident. Matheson found that 66% of athletes had localized tenderness and 25% had swelling during physical examination (4). In addition, percussion of an area at a distance from the possible fracture site will typically cause transmission of pain if a stress fracture is present (29). Observation of gait and activity can also provide insight into the presence of a stress fracture as normal walking, walking on toes, running in place, and hopping on the affected extremity can often reproduce the patient's symptoms (6,30).

DIFFERENTIAL DIAGNOSIS

The differential diagnosis of a stress fracture is extensive and varies upon the anatomical location. Stress reactions of the bone represent areas of weakened, but not physically disrupted bone and can present in a similar fashion to stress fractures; however, infection, avulsion injury, nerve entrapment, tumor, compartment syndrome, arthritis, ligament or tendon injury, or stress syndromes must also be present on the differential. In the foot and ankle, the differential diagnosis is often greatly dependent upon the history and physical examination as the superficial position of the anatomic structures typically allows for direct palpation of the structures with assessment of secondary signs, such as swelling and ecchymosis.

IMAGING

Although clinical evaluation is crucial in the diagnosis of stress fractures, imaging is central to efficient and accurate diagnosis. This is often crucial in athletes with a necessity for return to play. Conventional radiographs are the mainstay of imaging in patients with musculoskeletal complaints; however, radiographic findings may not appear at the time of clinical presentation causing a delay in diagnosis (31). Therefore, additional imaging techniques are now available to help guide diagnosis and effectively allow for earlier treatment in the management of stress fractures, including bone scintigraphy, computed tomography (CT), and magnetic resonance imaging (MRI) (Fig. 20.1).

CONVENTIONAL RADIOGRAPHS

Conventional radiographs are important as a first-line imaging modality in the diagnosis of stress fractures as subtle osseous changes, especially in the small bones of the foot, can sometimes be differentiated. When a bone develops a stress fracture, it will progress through many stages from initial disruption to final healing. Early radiographic changes will typically include visualization of a faint but somewhat subtle radiolucency in the cortical bone; however, radiographs are often insensitive in the detection of stress fractures early in the disease process (32–35). As the bone remodels, the endosteum can become thickened, sclerotic, and ill-defined. Within 10 days after initial injury, periosteal new-bone formation on the cortical and endosteal surfaces will commonly occur with improved visualization of the osseous insult (33).

Thus, conventional radiographs are typically normal within the first 2 weeks after the onset of symptoms and may not reveal abnormalities for several months (36,37). In fact, stress fractures may be overlooked at least 85% of the time on initial radiograph and 50% of the time on second radiograph (38). Considering the subtle imaging findings at initial injury, the diagnosis of stress fractures using conventional radiographs may be difficult as the obvious signs of osseous injury are often delayed, often lending importance to additional imaging if warranted by clinical suspicion.

BONE SCINTIGRAPHY

Bone scintigraphy has long been considered the most sensitive method of diagnosing stress fractures in the early stages as it is typically abnormal within 6 to 72 hours of symptoms onset (4,16,31). Technetium-99m diphosphonate bone scintigraphy is optimally performed utilizing a three-phase technique. Acute stress fractures will characteristically demonstrate abnormal tracer activity within all three phases of the scan while soft-tissue injuries are differentiated upon the fact that increased uptake will only occur within the first two phases of the scan.

Although bone scintigraphy is highly sensitive for detecting stress fractures, it lacks specificity (39–41). Several limitations of bone scintigraphy include invasive testing, limited follow-up utility as abnormal tracer uptake may persist for months, and lack of tracer uptake in certain patients, including osteoporotic patients. Some authors have reported that 20% to 40% of stress fractures seen on bone scintigraphy are asymptomatic (42,43); yet, Gaeta and colleagues have reported that bone scintigraphy also failed to detect several cortical stress injuries which were identified on MRI or CT in athletes (44). Although additional imaging using computed tomography may allow for confirmation of fracture or help determine location, morphology, and state of fracture healing, it is not routinely obtained as it is inferior in sensitivity to bone scintigraphy and MRI (29,45). Therefore, a negative conventional radiograph and bone scintigraphy with a high clinical suspicion of stress fracture must guide further imaging through the utilization of MRI.

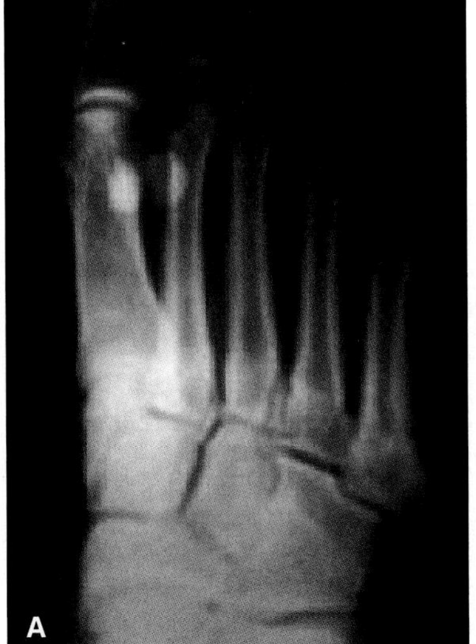

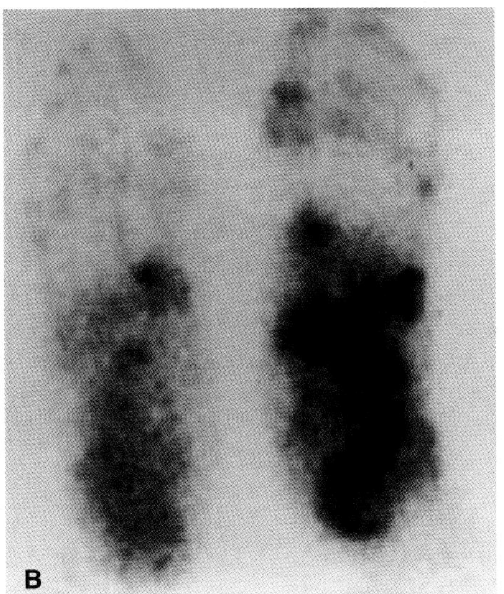

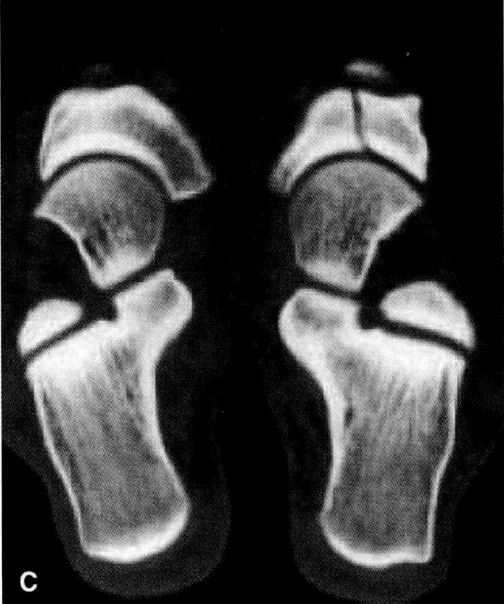

Figure 20.1. **A:** Standard anteroposterior radiograph of a professional basketball player with midfoot pain does not reveal a stress fracture. **B:** Bone scan reveals increased uptake in the navicular bone. **C:** CT scan demonstrates a complete navicular stress fracture. Reprinted from Boden BP, Osbahr DC. High-risk stress fractures. *J Am Acad Ortho Surg* 2000;8:344–353, with permission.

MAGNETIC RESONANCE IMAGING

When the clinical diagnosis is still unknown, MRI is an effective diagnostic tool to differentiate stress fractures from other injuries. Several studies support that MRI is the new gold standard for the evaluation of stress injuries (46,47). In fact, MRI allows for the discovery of abnormalities weeks before radiographs and has comparable sensitivity and superior specificity in comparison to radionuclide techniques for the detection of early osseous changes, including marrow edema and stress reactions (31,48,49).

In defining acute osseous abnormalities, MRI can also provide other invaluable information to aid in diagnosis and treatment. In fact, Niva and colleagues suggested that the early diagnosis and grading of stress fractures in the foot and ankle, especially the talus and calcaneus, is possible with the utilization of MRI (50). The cross-sectional imaging capabilities of MRI not only allow for the differentiation of subtle marrow changes but also afford detailed anatomic evaluation of the surrounding soft tissues which are in close association within the foot and ankle (45). Several classification systems have also been devised which aid in the categorization and treatment of stress fractures and will be explained later in this chapter while discussing classification-based treatment (43,46,47). MRI may also provide prognostic value as positive findings may be predictive of a longer symptomatic period indicating a more severe stress injury (51).

Although MRI has distinct advantages in the diagnosis and treatment of stress fractures, there are disadvantages that need to be considered during interpretation of this imaging modality which does not only relate to cost. Considering the high sensitivity of MRI in diagnosing stress reactions and bone marrow edema, MRI findings must be carefully interpreted in conjunction with the clinical presentation. In fact, bone marrow edema or stress reactions are not entirely specific to stress injury as early asymptomatic stress response to exercise may be a causative factor which must be considered. For example, asymptomatic runners have been shown to have stress reactions or bone marrow edema in the bones of the foot and ankle, and these areas of activity did not correlate with the risk of future development of stress fracture (52,53). Either way, the MRI finding of a discrete fracture line or stress reaction with corresponding clinical symptoms can be invaluable in the diagnosis of stress injuries in the foot and ankle.

PREVENTION

The foundation of stress fracture management involves prevention. For the successful establishment of preventative measures, especially in high-performance athletes, physicians must not only educate the athletes but also the parents, trainers, and coaches. Considering the unique environment of increased weight bearing in the foot and ankle, relatively small changes in biologic and environmental homeostasis can result in stress fractures. Many preventative measures can be established to avoid stress fractures; however, careful assessment must include an analysis of both intrinsic and extrinsic factors, particularly those that are modifiable.

In terms of modifiable intrinsic factors, patients should be assessed for eating disorders, nutritional deficiencies, metabolic bone disease, leg-length discrepancy, concomitant orthopedic injuries, foot type, shoe wear, and orthotic use. Eating disorders should be considered in all athletes with treatment focused on a multidisciplinary approach, including referral to a psychiatrist or psychologist. Nutrition is important as adequate intake must be assured to allow for the increased caloric requirements necessary for athletic activities. Optimal nutritional needs would be filled with low-fat and high-carbohydrate foods while avoiding phosphate-containing sodas. Metabolic bone diseases must also be assessed to assure that an underlying etiology does not exist which could be corrected through diet, supplementation, or other medications.

Leg-length discrepancy, concomitant orthopedic injuries, and foot type can also result in stress fractures by altering the normal mechanics of gait with a shift in load to other areas which cannot accommodate the increased forces. Proper shoe wear must also be considered to prevent as well as manage stress fractures. In fact, running shoes should be maintained in good condition and changed at least over 200 to 300 miles (54). Finally, orthotics should be considered when preventing overuse injuries in the foot and ankle as shock-absorbing insoles may reduce the incidence of lower extremity stress fractures in athletes and military recruits (55,56).

When considering modifiable extrinsic factors, patients should be evaluated for specific activities, volume and intensity of activities, and training surfaces. Stress fractures may occur at certain anatomical locations secondary to characteristic sporting activities. Recognition and attention to these aggravating factors allow for prevention prior to injury or treatment earlier in the disease process. Overtraining is an important cause of stress fractures as repetitive activities or an abrupt increase in activity may result in overuse injuries of the foot and ankle. When making alterations to a training routine, it is important to make gradual changes with periodic periods of rest to avoid overuse injuries. In fact, volume and intensity of training programs should be gradually increased to a period of weeks with high-level activities, requiring at least 6 weeks of graduated training (54).

Training surfaces must also be considered to prevent stress fractures. Activities should begin on surfaces that preferentially absorb forces with progression of activity to synthetic track, grass, and uneven terrain over a period of time (54). Considering that the foot and ankle are at constant risk of overuse injuries secondary to the continual transmission of load during repetitive activities, athletes should be monitored for all modifiable intrinsic and extrinsic risk factors to allow for appropriate modifications in training.

CLASSIFICATION-BASED TREATMENT

A successful classification system will provide direct information relating to treatment and prognosis. When discussing stress fractures, a descriptive analysis should provide information pertaining to its location as well as the classification. Several classification systems for stress fractures have been proposed based on risk assessment or grade of injury as dictated by imaging (25,46,47,57,58).

TREATMENT-BASED RISK STRATIFICATION

Overall, the bones of the foot and ankle are particularly prone to high loads from weight bearing; therefore, their inherent location makes them unique and challenging to manage, especially in athletes. Classification by risk stratification has been proposed by several authors and useful in the management of stress fractures (25,57–60). Risk stratification has been based on the classification of stress fractures as either high risk or low risk as previously proposed by Boden and Osbahr (25,57). An algorithm to guide treatment was defined for high-risk stress fractures by the same authors; however, we now present a modified algorithm for the classification-based treatment of stress fractures according to risk stratification relating to both high-risk and low-risk stress fractures (Fig. 20.2). This location-specific risk stratification allows the physician to understand the pathophysiology of the fracture and directly define management according to the associated risk for serious sequelae. This information directly aids in determining return to play guidelines.

High-risk Stress Fractures

High-risk stress fractures are generally loaded in tension and do not have a favorable natural history. Because of this mode of loading, high-risk stress fractures have a disadvantageous environment and may not heal properly with conservative management. In fact, a delay in diagnosis or less-aggressive treatment plan may result in complete fracture, delayed union, nonunion, necessity for operative management, and/or recurrence of fracture (25,57,58,60).

For most high-risk stress fractures of the foot and ankle, early diagnosis is crucial with the implementation of an aggressive non-operative management protocol consisting of immobilization with non–weight-bearing. This approach will often successfully treat these stress fractures; however, surgical intervention

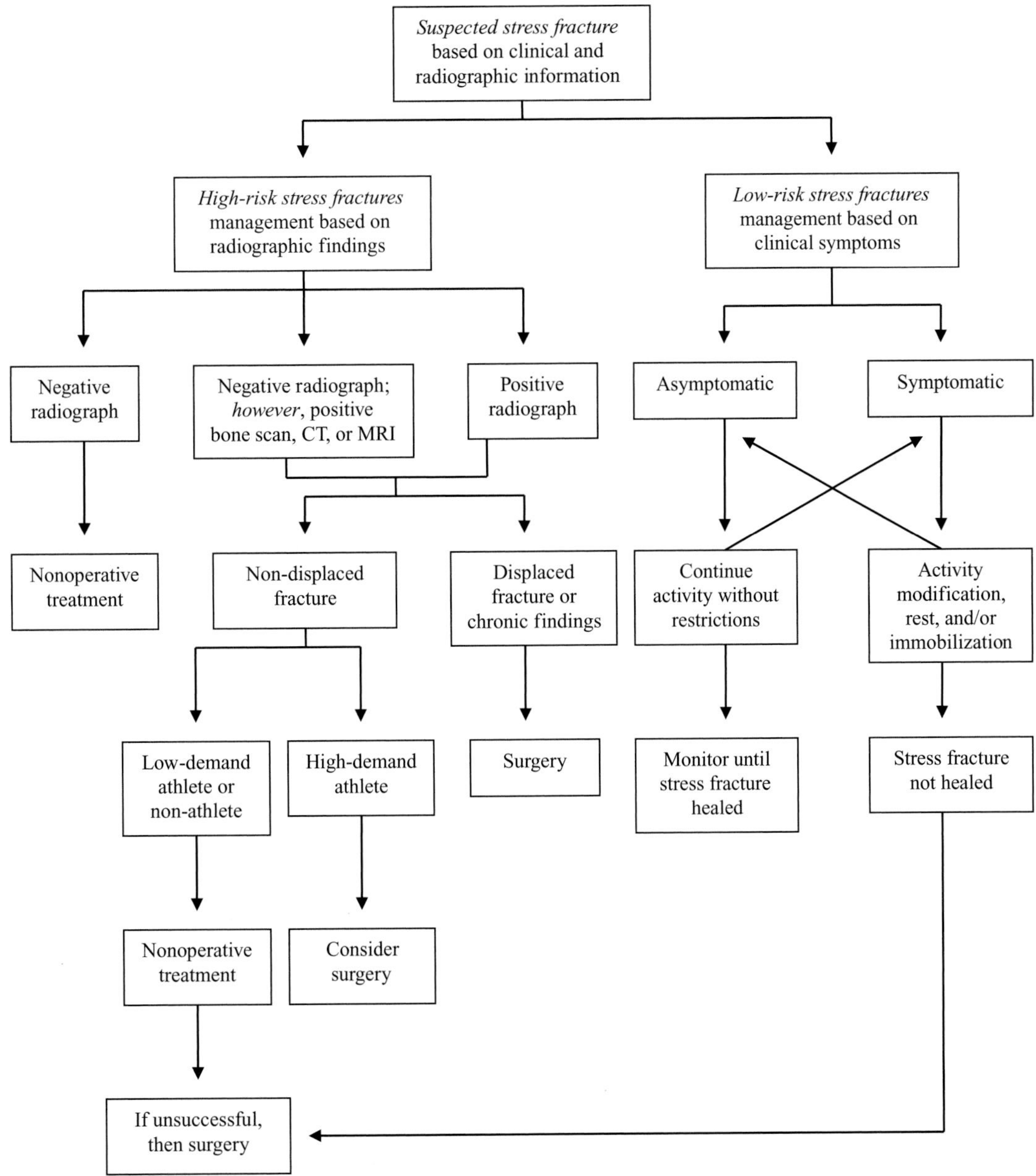

Figure 20.2. Classification-based treatment algorithm of stress fractures stratified by risk.

TABLE 20.1 Radiologic Grading System for Stress Fractures

Grade	Radiograph	Bone Scan	MR Imaging	Treatment
1	Normal	Mild uptake limited to one cortex	Normal or positive STIR image	3 wks rest
2	Normal	Moderate activity; larger lesion limited to unicortical area	Positive STIR and T2-weighted images	3–6 wks rest
3	Discrete line (+/−); periosteal reaction (+/−)	Increased activity (>50% bone width)	No definite cortical break; positive T1- and T2-weighted images	12–16 wks rest
4	Fracture or periosteal reaction	More intense bicortical uptake	Fracture line; positive T1- and T2-weighted images	16+ wks rest

Adapted from Arendt EA, Griffiths HJ. The use of MR imaging in the assessment and clinical management of stress reactions of bone in high-performance athletes. *Clin Sports Med* 1997;16:291–306, with permission.

may be warranted in individuals whose symptoms are refractive to non-operative management or high-performance athletes who require early return to sport (57,58). Numerous bones of the foot and ankle are classified as high-risk stress fractures: Anterior tibial cortex, medial malleolus, talus, tarsal navicular, fifth metatarsal, second metatarsal base, and great toe sesamoids (25,57,58,60,61).

Low-risk Stress Fractures

Low-risk stress fractures are usually loaded in compression and have a favorable natural history as they respond well to activity modification. Therefore, management of these injuries is typically guided primarily by symptoms. Considering that low-risk stress fractures occur in a more favorable environment, they are less likely to result in complete fracture, delayed union, necessity for operative management, and/or recurrence of fracture (25,57,58,60).

For most low-risk stress fractures of the foot and ankle, a non-operative management protocol consisting of rest followed by a gradual resumption of activity will often be successful in treating these injuries. In rare cases, surgical intervention may be warranted in an individual whose symptoms are refractive to non-operative management or high-performance athletes who require early return to sport (25,58). The following stress fractures are considered low risk in the foot and ankle: Tibial shaft, proximal and distal fibula, calcaneus, and first to fourth metatarsals (25,57,58,60,61).

TREATMENT-BASED GRADING SYSTEM

In addition to risk stratification, grading of stress fractures can be important in defining management and prognosis. Two main classification systems have been proposed which evaluate the spectrum of bone failure from stress reaction to fracture according to imaging modalities (46,47).

In reference to the foot and ankle, the classification system by Arendt and Griffiths has an improved profile considering it has already been utilized to describe stress fractures in the tibia, fibula, navicular, calcaneus, and forefoot and provides direct treatment recommendations. On the other hand, the classification system by Fredericson and colleagues has been developed and used only in the tibia (46,47).

Overall, both classification systems use a scale with increasing radiographic findings from grade 0 to grade 4 with grade 1 to grade 3 showing increasing periosteal changes and marrow edema, and grade 4 demonstrating a complete stress fracture (46,47). The classification system by Arendt and Griffiths is based on grading stress fractures utilizing findings from conventional radiographs, bone scintigraphy, and MRI (46) (Table 20.1). Depending upon the grade of stress fracture as defined by this classification system, treatment may be predicted based on the approximate time for healing with grade 3 and 4 injuries requiring a prolonged time interval to healing when compared to grade 1 and 2 injuries (46).

LOCATION-SPECIFIC STRESS FRACTURES

TIBIA

In athletes, the tibial shaft is the most common site for stress fracture with an incidence of 20% to 75% depending upon patient population (4). These stress fractures of the posteromedial tibial shaft are considered low risk in terms of progression to delayed union or nonunion (3). However, stress fractures may less commonly occur within the anterior cortex of the mid-tibia which portends a worse prognosis with poor healing and the requirement for an altered treatment algorithm. The differential diagnosis includes tibial shaft stress fracture, anterior cortex stress fracture, muscle strains, nerve entrapment syndromes, exertional compartment syndrome, infection, and tumor.

Posteromedial Tibial Shaft (Low Risk)

Tibial stress fractures may occur at any location along the shaft with injury site most often located in the posteromedial cortex or compression side of the tibia (47). These fractures can occur in athletes who participate in running sports, such as track, soccer, and football, with the highest prevalence in runners (4,8,47). The orientation of these fractures is typically transverse; however, longitudinal tibial shaft stress fractures have been described and often have an atypical presentation requiring an MRI for correct diagnosis (62,63).

Clinical assessment will reveal pain and tenderness at the stress fracture location which is readily palpable. Sometimes swelling may be appreciated secondary to early edema or late callous formation. Radiographs are typically normal at initial presentation, and clinical suspicion warrants close follow-up with additional imaging.

As tibial shaft stress fractures of the posteromedial cortex are considered low risk, they respond favorably to non-operative treatment with discontinuation of the inciting activity and gradual resumption of activity depending on symptoms. Most tibial stress fractures heal within 4 to 8 weeks with resumption of full sporting activities by 8 to 12 weeks. After a period of rest, the pain-free athlete may begin low-impact activities such as swimming or biking. If the athlete remains asymptomatic, then higher-impact activities may be gradually increased over a period of time as defined by symptoms.

No adequate studies have shown that weight bearing in the initial period alters healing or return to play; therefore, symptomatic management should help guide progression of weight bearing with return to activity. Symptomatic management utilizing a pneumatic brace has been shown to not only reduce pain but accelerate return to play (64–66). In fact, a randomized, prospective study by Swenson and colleagues found that the pneumatic brace treatment allowed return to full unrestricted activity in 21 days compared to 77 days in controls who were only treated with rest (65). In rare cases, tibial shaft stress fractures may not heal which may require surgical management often consisting of intramedullary fixation.

Anterior Tibial Cortex (High Risk)

As opposed to the typical posteromedial tibial stress fracture that is considered low risk, the anterior cortex tibial stress fracture is considered high risk with a much different risk profile. This tension-sided fracture with a hypovascular environment has shown a propensity for delayed healing. As opposed to compression-sided stress fractures which typically occur in runners, this tension-sided stress fracture commonly occurs in athletes who perform repetitive jumping and leaping activities, such as basketball players.

As with tibial shaft stress fractures, clinical assessment of anterior cortical stress fractures may reveal tenderness over the fracture site and possible swelling. However, this injury may also have an atypical presentation with minimal symptoms despite chronicity and possible nonunion (67). Radiographs are often initially normal but will subsequently show a characteristic "V"-shaped fracture pattern in the anterior tibial cortex which opens anteriorly (Fig. 20.3) (57). Callus formation is generally not present, and prolonged healing time has resulted in this stress fracture being named the "dreaded black line" by Hamilton in 1992 (30). With progression to nonunion, the cortex will become hypertrophic with a widened fracture fissure, and the decreased activity at the fracture site results in minimal activity on radionuclide imaging.

Despite the adverse environment that exists for this high-risk stress fracture, non-surgical management still plays a vital role with initial treatment focusing on a combination of rest, immobilization, electrical stimulation, and pneumatic leg brace for a minimum of 4 to 6 months. In fact, Rettig and colleagues found that anterior cortical stress fractures in basketball players may result in union with rest and electrical stimulation at an average time of 8.7 months with return to play by an average of 12.7 months (68). In a small case series, Batt and colleagues reported successful healing of stress fractures at a mean of 8 months in all three patients utilizing a pneumatic leg brace (69).

If chronic changes occur at the fracture site indicating progression to nonunion or high-performance athletes need to return to sport in an expedited fashion, then surgical management must be considered. Numerous surgical treatments have been proposed for treating anterior tibial stress fractures with delayed healing. Although healing has been shown to occur after excision and bone grafting, (70) intramedullary fixation has become the favored approach with good to excellent results being reported in patients treated with reamed, unlocked tibial nails (71).

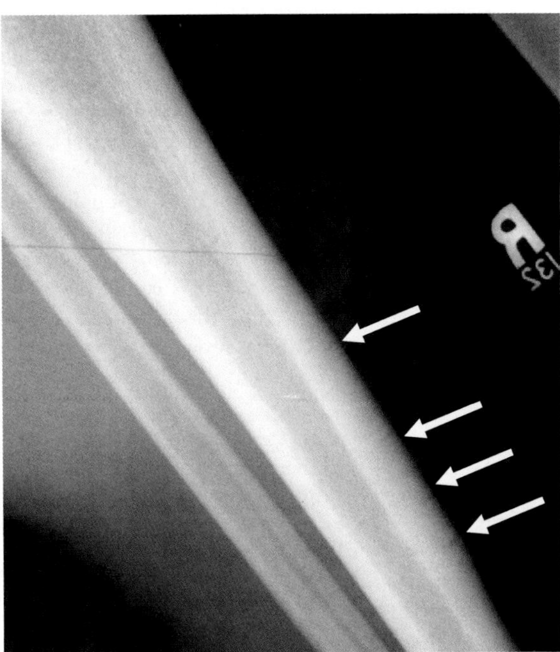

Figure 20.3. Multiple anterior cortical stress fractures in a 28-year-old professional football player.

FIBULA

Fibular stress fractures account for 4.6% to 21% of all stress fractures (72–74). Stress fractures of the fibula typically result from a combination of muscular traction and torsional forces as the fibula maintains a secondary role in weight bearing with load bearing varying from 2.3% to 10% of total load applied (75). Within the fibula, proximal bone stress fractures are much less common than those that occur distally; however, most epidemiologic studies do not distinguish between fracture sites making the true incidence according to location difficult. The differential diagnosis may include ankle sprain, syndesmosis injury, knee ligament injury, peroneal tendonitis or subluxation, ankle arthritis, exertional compartment syndrome, muscle strain, talar osteochondral lesions, neoplasm, or infection.

Proximal (Low Risk)

Proximal fibula stress fractures are considered low risk and routinely occur during intense jumping exercises with and without rotational motion (76). They have been described in several different athletic populations, including runners, dancers, and military recruits (76–78). Patients typically report diffuse proximal and lateral leg pain that is worsened by exercise and knee range of motion. Physical examination should include evaluation of the proximal and distal tibiofibular joints to rule out more severe problems, including knee and syndesmosis injuries which are known to occur in athletes.

Radiographic assessment typically reveals a transverse or oblique fracture line at the neck of the proximal fibula. If the fracture is in the healing phase, then periosteal new bone formation may be visualized as well. If radiographs are negative, MRI may be beneficial, especially if there is a clinical suspicion for injuries of the knee and/or ankle. Non-operative treatment utilizing a combination of rest and immobilization are typically successful. Resolution of symptoms usually occurs within 3 to 6 weeks after modifying activity. If symptoms do not resolve, then clinical suspicion should warrant further investigation into other associated injuries. When the patient is asymptomatic, a program instituting a gradual return to play may be commenced with progression dependent upon symptoms.

Distal (Low Risk)

Fibular stress fractures most often occur within the distal third of the bone. The location of fracture usually occurs just proximal to the inferior tibiofibular ligaments at the junction of the cortical and cancellous regions of bone (79,80). Although distal fibular stress fractures predominantly occur through cancellous bone in older, osteoporotic individuals, distance runners who train on hard surfaces are a population of athletic individuals who are also prone to this injury (80,81).

Clinical history typically includes a period of increased physical activity which precedes symptoms. Symptoms are usually insidious in onset associated with a gradual increase in pain occurring over several days to weeks which will be aggravated by activity and relieved by rest (80). On physical examination, pain and swelling may be localized over the distal fibula upon palpation with the potential for associated swelling. Ankle malalignment may indicate a more severe injury consisting of a displaced fracture and/or ankle fracture–dislocation.

In the early stages of healing, radiographic findings may not be visible as initial radiographs have been reported as negative in up to 70% of cases (82). The stress fracture may not appear for 2 to 4 weeks after injury as callous formation occurs with healing. For the most part, MRI has now supplanted bone scintigram in the diagnosis of distal fibular stress fractures if high clinical suspicion exists despite negative radiographs. MRI may differentiate between stress reaction and fracture as well as allowing for the detection of soft tissue abnormalities.

With early diagnosis, distal fibular stress fractures have an excellent prognosis with non-surgical management. Treatment typically consists of modified rest for a period of 3 to 6 weeks followed by gradual resumption of activity. With inadequate treatment, recovery may be delayed with symptoms persisting for 3 to 6 months (80). On the other hand, operative management is extremely rare with few reports documenting surgical treatment for delayed union of isolated distal fibular stress fractures (83).

MEDIAL MALLEOLUS (HIGH RISK)

First reported by Devas in 1975 (84), medial malleolus stress fractures have a reported incidence varying from 0.6% to 4.1% of all stress fractures (72,73). These stress fractures almost exclusively occur in athletes and are associated with running and jumping activities which have been proposed to result in repetitive impingement of the talus on the medial malleolus during ankle dorsiflexion and tibial rotation. Stress fractures of the medial malleolus typically have a characteristic oblique or vertical fracture line located at the level of the tibial plafond (85,86). These fractures have been proposed to arise from torsional forces and weight transmission; however, muscular forces likely do not play a significant role (84).

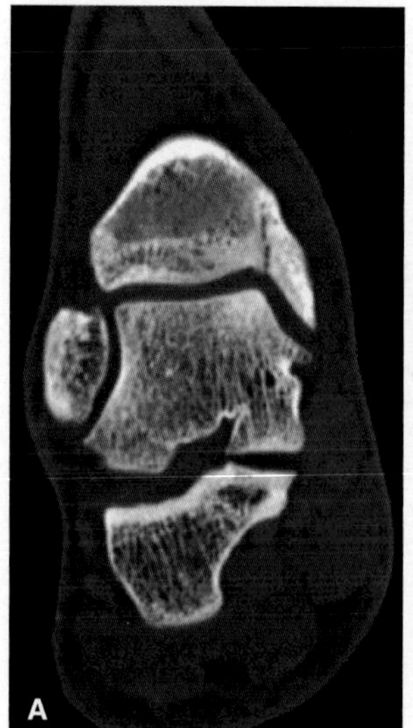

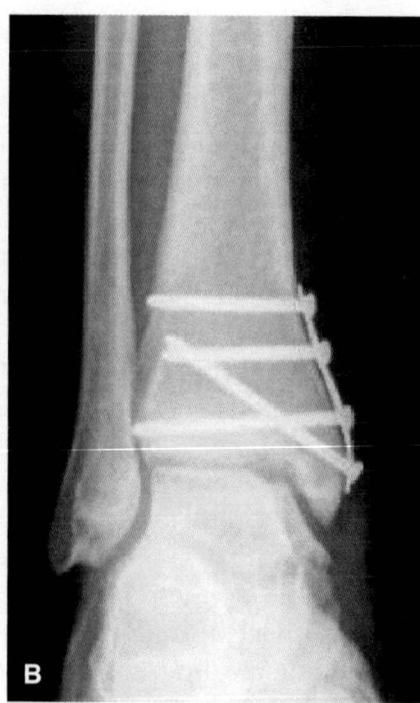

Figure 20.4. **(A)** Pre-operative CT scan and **(B)** post-operative x-ray of a medial malleolus stress fracture in a professional basketball player.

The differential diagnosis is similar to pathologies described for distal fibula fractures as previously described. The clinical presentation typically involves a prodrome of pain during activity lasting several weeks followed by an acute episode of pain prompting need for orthopedic care. Symptoms also increase with activity and are relieved with rest. As with stress fractures of the distal fibula at the lateral malleolus, tenderness may be localized directly over the medial malleolus with or without associated swelling. As with fractures of the proximal fibula, the sports-medicine physician must rule out a syndesmosis injury which may require a different treatment algorithm.

Clinical suspicion must help guide imaging as initial radiographs have been reported to be positive in less than 50% of patients (85,87,88). Therefore, bone scans and MRI must be utilized to diagnose these injuries as early diagnosis is crucial for successful treatment of these high-risk stress fractures. Patients who present with negative radiographs but a positive bone scan and/or MRI, treatment is guided by patient activity level.

Most patients may be treated with non-operative management using immobilization and rest; however, resolution of symptoms may take up to 4 or 5 months (89). On the other hand, fracture displacement and/or high-level athletes requiring early return to play may necessitate surgical management using percutaneous or internal fixation with possible bone grafting in chronic cases (Fig. 20.4) (85–87). Both operative and non-operative management typically result in good results with full return to play (85–87); however, complications have been noted, including delayed union, nonunion, and recurrent stress fracture (85,90,91).

TALUS (HIGH RISK)

Stress fractures in the talus are extremely rare and were first reported by McGlone in 1965 (92,93). There are relatively few

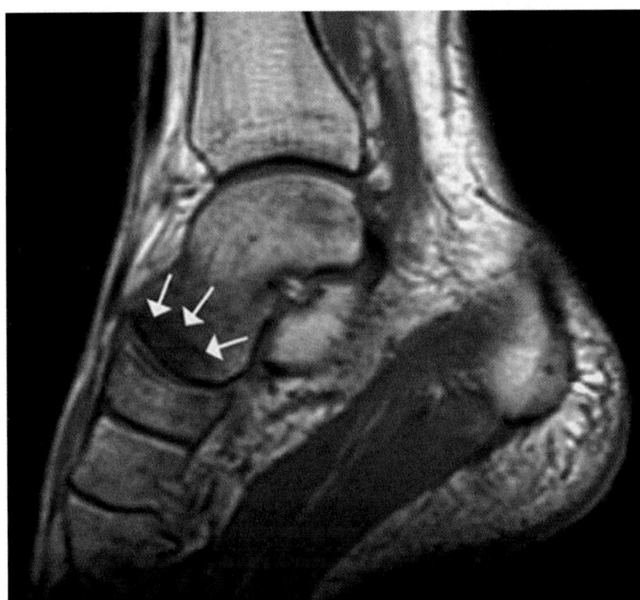

Figure 20.5. MRI of a stress fracture involving the talar head in a 19-year-old military recruit.

reports in the literature documenting talar stress fractures. When they do occur, the most common location involves the head of the talus followed by the body. Despite prior studies suggesting that these stress fractures were low risk (93,94), more recent studies suggest that they are likely high risk, considering their association with the potential for delayed healing and/or poor outcomes (57,92,95). In fact, case reports documenting necrosis of the talus after traumatic fractures have raised additional concern over the potential for avascular osteonecrosis (96,97).

The mechanism of injury typically involves excessive subtalar pronation and plantarflexion causing impingement of the lateral process of the calcaneus on the posterolateral corner of the talus or isolated foot supination concentrating forces of the lateral process of the talus (57). The clinical presentation typically involves lateral ankle or sinus tarsi pain with and without swelling, and the symptoms are usually exacerbated by activity. Conventional radiographs will often be negative requiring additional imaging using either CT and/or MRI. CT may be useful in identifying lesions in the posterolateral border of the talus; however, MRI may provide additional subtle findings, such as marrow edema and early signs of osteonecrosis (Fig. 20.5).

Overall, outcomes have been reported to be poor following talar stress fractures and have been attributed to delayed healing as well as continued pain in the setting of union (57,92,95). Non-operative and operative management has been used to treat talar stress fractures with varying results (92,95). Either way, a 6-week trial of non-operative treatment is warranted involving cast immobilization followed by rehabilitation and orthotics to correct excess pronation (57).

CALCANEUS (LOW RISK)

Calcaneal stress injuries are considered a relatively common source of heel pain in active populations, including long-distance runners, military recruits, and osteoporotic, elderly individuals (98). Most stress fractures of the calcaneus have been reported within the posterior aspect of the bone (50%) with the rest occurring in the anterior and middle portions of the calcaneus (99–101). These injuries are considered to be low risk for progression with no known documented studies detailing displaced fractures (25,49,100–102). However, stress fractures in the calcaneus have also been found in association with similar injuries to the surrounding bones of the foot and ankle (101).

Stress fractures of the calcaneus are frequently an unrecognized source of heel pain and require a high index of suspicion to distinguish from other pathologic diagnoses. The clinical history usually involves exercise-induced heel or ankle pain in active individuals, and examination will elicit pain associated with compression at the posterosuperior calcaneus just anterior to the apophyseal plate and/or tenderness to palpation directly over the calcaneus (25). To differentiate a calcaneal stress fracture from heel pain syndrome, a positive "squeeze" test may elicit pain when placing the calcaneus between both palms of the examiner and applying force (60). Calcaneal stress fractures have been historically diagnosed with conventional radiographs and are associated with a delay in diagnosis until the development of sclerosis about 2 weeks after injury. Therefore, MRI has become a critical diagnostic tool as it maintains high specificity and sensitivity for lower-grade injuries and provides improved documentation of stress injuries to the anterior and middle portions of the calcaneus (101). In addition, MRI can help exclude other diagnoses in the differential, including Achilles tendinopathy, plantar fasciitis, and retrocalcaneal bursitis.

Management of calcaneal stress fractures involves instituting non-operative measures, including rest, modification of activity, and rehabilitation. As these injuries are considered low risk, limitation of activity for 3 to 6 weeks will usually provide a favorable response. Once the painful symptoms have decreased, rehabilitation may begin focusing on orthotics and stretching exercises to help prevent recurrent disease and return to activity as tolerated. Most patients are able to return to activities by 8 weeks with recurrent symptoms commonly occurring after earlier return to full activity (98).

TARSAL NAVICULAR (HIGH RISK)

Stress fractures of the tarsal navicular have been previously considered relatively uncommon injuries, comprising only 0.7% to 2.4% of all stress fractures (103,104); however, more recent studies have suggested much higher occurrence rates, including up to 35% of all stress fractures (8,72,105). Although stress fractures may occur in several areas of the navicular bone, the central third of the bone is most susceptible considering the increased concentration of forces and decreased vascularity within this area (106–108). Despite numerous factors being implicated in the pathogenesis behind the development of navicular stress fractures, including shoe wear, decreased subtalar and ankle motion, medial talonavicular joint narrowing, metatarsus adductors, pes cavus, long second metatarsal, and short first metatarsal, no studies have demonstrated a significant association at this time (109–111).

A high index of suspicion is critical in correctly diagnosing navicular stress fractures. These injuries will typically occur during athletic activities, including sprinting, jumping, hurdling, and pushing off (111–113). They are characterized by insidious onset of midfoot pain which worsens during and following aggravating activities. Navicular stress fractures usually present with a paucity of physical examination findings, including absence of ecchymosis, swelling, and deformity. Initially, the pain is difficult to localize with vague symptoms along the longitudinal arch on the dorsolateral aspect of the foot. With disease progression, the pain will become focused to the dorsum of the navicular bone which can be localized on physical examination in 81% of patients ("N" spot) (105,111). Symptoms can also be reproduced by having the patient hop on the affected leg with the foot in an equinus position (112).

Conventional radiographs are the initial modality for diagnosing navicular stress fractures, including an anatomic anteroposterior radiograph with the foot inverted. Wilson and Katz have proposed a radiographic classification for navicular stress fractures utilizing four categories: (1) type I have a linear lucency, (2) type II have sclerosis of the fracture edges and callus formation, (3) type III have periosteal reaction and external callus, and (4) type IV have a mixed pattern. However, conventional radiographs often fail to initially demonstrate navicular stress fractures with a sensitivity as low as 24% to 33% as fractures may not reveal radiographic changes for 3 after injury or may be oriented in an oblique direction (103,114).

Therefore, clinical suspicion should warrant further imaging using bone scan, computed tomography, or MRI (Fig. 20.1) (103,109,111,112,115). Bone scans are highly sensitive for detecting stress fractures; however, they are nonspecific with an inability to distinguish between stress fractures and stress reactions (105,115,116). In addition, bone scans do not provide adequate information concerning the position or nature of the stress fracture, if present (117). Thin-sliced (1.5 mm) computerized tomography using three-dimensional reconstructions and MRI are more sensitive than bone scans in detecting the presence, position, and nature of the stress fracture. Although MRI can detect earlier pathologic changes within the navicular bone, including bone marrow edema, there have been no studies showing any advantages over computed tomography, including diagnostic ability and cost effectiveness (118). In addition, computed tomography is often necessitated and considered the gold standard in evaluating stress fractures as MRI may not be optimal in differentiating certain findings, including challenging fracture patterns, small ossicles associated with these injuries, and the distinction of stress fracture from osteonecrosis (116,119,120).

Management of navicular stress fractures is usually defined by aggressive non-operative or operative treatment considering these are high-risk injuries. Treatment algorithms support both non-operative and operative management but have been mostly based on small retrospective studies and case reports with only one known report evaluating these injuries prospectively (108,110–113,120–123). To guide treatment and predict healing, Saxena and colleagues designed a computerized tomography classification to subcategorize navicular stress fractures into three types: (1) type I includes a break in the dorsal cortex, (2) type II includes a break in the dorsal cortex and navicular body, and (3) type III includes a fracture that extends through another cortex (120). There initial results were confirmed by a more recent prospective study which found that navicular stress fractures may take 4 months to heal and more severe injuries, including fractures with cystic changes, sclerosis, or osteonecrosis, require longer healing time and are more likely to require surgery (123).

Non-operative treatment is most often successful with early diagnosis of partial, non-displaced navicular stress fractures (Saxena type I). These injuries have been shown to have high union rates when treated for 6 to 8 weeks of non–weight-bearing and cast immobilization (111,123). However, immediate operative intervention with internal fixation, especially in high-performance athletes, may be warranted in some non-displaced navicular stress fractures which extend into the navicular body (Saxena type II) or form a complete fracture (Saxena type III) (123,124).

Non-displaced fractures may be treated with percutaneous screw fixation with or without exposure of the fracture site (124). Displaced stress fractures, delayed unions, nonunions, or recurrent fractures are universally treated with open reduction internal fixation with one or two compression screws with or without bone grafting (112,123,124). Post-operative management typically consists of immobilization in a below-knee cast or boot with non–weight-bearing for 6 weeks followed by weight bearing in a boot for another 2 to 6 weeks depending on the absence of symptoms (123). Regardless of management, assessment of return to activity is based on the patient maintaining a pain-free functional status and may be expected to take as long as 4 to 8 months (111,119,123,125).

METATARSALS

The forefoot performs two specific functions: (1) provides a broad rigid platform to allow for weight bearing and (2) provides a mobile platform during ambulation to allow for uneven ground (126). Fractures involving the metatarsal bones can alter this platform and the functional biomechanics of gait resulting in inability to participate in activity. The metatarsal bones are a relatively common site of stress fracture (9% to 19% of all stress fractures) with the highest number occurring in the second and third metatarsals (80% of all metatarsal stress fractures) (4,37,127). The second metatarsal neck is the most common site of metatarsal stress fracture; however, less common locations include the base of the fifth metatarsal (i.e., basketball players), base of the second metatarsal (i.e., female ballet dancers), and the metatarsal heads (128–132). The differential diagnosis for metatarsal stress fractures includes metatarsalgia, Morton's neuroma, metatarsophalangeal instability, and Freiberg's infraction (133).

Although the first metatarsal endures approximately one-third of the body's weight, stress fractures are relatively rare as its relative size, strength, and mobility result in increased durability with lower rates of injury (126,134). The remaining four metatarsals (second to fifth) provide contact points that maintain a stable platform during gait with the force directly transmitted to specific areas at the plantar surface of each metatarsal. With progression from the second to fifth metatarsal, there is a gradual cascade in metatarsal length allowing for stress accommodation, and increasing mobility allows for the adaptability to uneven terrain. Although stress fractures of the metatarsals are known to result from excessive repetitive loads during activity without adequate rest periods, the exact mechanism is not clearly defined with a likely multifactorial etiology.

In fact, a short first metatarsal was originally targeted as the predisposing factor resulting in metatarsal stress fractures; however, several studies have shown that first metatarsal length does not directly correlate to the presence of a metatarsal stress fracture (135,136). Another hypothesis for the development of metatarsal stress fractures proposes that fatigue of the foot plantarflexors, especially the flexor digitorum longus, results in stress fracture by producing increased strain within the metatarsal (137). Either way, the location of stress fracture appears to be the most important factor in determining risk for delayed union, nonunion, or refracture (25,57).

Stress fractures of the metatarsal bones typically occur in the neck or shaft and are considered low risk; however, stress fractures within the base of the metatarsals are usually high risk with a propensity for delayed union, nonunion, or refracture (129–131,138–140). Although the base of the second and fifth metatarsal fractures are usually highlighted when discussing high-risk stress fractures of the metatarsals and will be discussed later in this section, the base of the fourth metatarsal fractures have also recently been proposed to be high-risk stress fractures with a tendency toward prolonged healing (139–141). With this in mind, these injuries require aggressive management, but typically respond to non-operative therapy consisting of a non–weight-bearing cast (139–141). Fractures of metatarsal heads have also been described with relative rarity and should be considered in the differential diagnosis when considering forefoot pain in active and osteoporotic individuals (128).

Distal Metatarsal (Low Risk)

Metatarsal shaft and neck stress fractures were considered the classic "march" fractures as they were initially described in military personnel (1,2). In addition, athletes are prone to these stress fractures which can occur with higher frequency in running, jumping, or dancing activities. These physically active patients are prone to sustaining this injury because training included repetitive exercise on hard surfaces. In fact, modifications in training including viscoelastic insoles in shoes and training on softer surfaces has shown to be successful in reducing the incidence of metatarsal stress fractures (142–144).

These particular stress fractures mostly occur in the distal metatarsal shaft as a result of excess, repetitive loads common during athletic activities. Patients typically present with a history of forefoot pain increased during weight-bearing activities. Physical examination findings may be variable; however, localized tenderness and/or occasional swelling may be apparent at the fracture site. It is important to evaluate each metatarsal separately to help isolate the symptoms and improve diagnosis. In addition, the increased load on the forefoot may present clinically with pain and callosity under the metatarsal head. Patients may also walk with a limp with inability to toe walk and exacerbation of symptoms upon running, jumping, or dancing activities.

Standard anteroposterior, lateral, and oblique radiographs should be evaluated for identification of stress fractures; however, initial radiographs within 10 days of symptom onset are typically negative. Radiographic findings may be subtle, including periosteal reaction, longitudinal cortical hypertrophy, and medullary canal narrowing, but new callous formation may not be visualized until 2 weeks after injury (Fig. 20.6). Therefore, radiographic diagnosis may be confirmed with serial radiographs although earlier diagnosis with bone scan or MRI may be preferred (25,134,145).

Distal metatarsal stress fractures of the shaft and neck may be effectively treated with non-operative treatment consisting of rest with restriction from aggravating activities. Symptomatic relief should be the goal of treatment with more severe pain or injuries requiring a short-leg walking boot or short-leg cast. With the progression of healing or the presence of less severe injuries, a stiff-soled shoe or carbon-reinforced bar in the shoe's sole may be utilized for symptomatic relief. Most metatarsal stress fractures heal 4 weeks after activity modification and immobilization; however, rare delayed unions, nonunions, or displaced stress fractures may require surgical management. Once symptoms have resolved with no localized tenderness at the fracture site, a graduated program may be commenced with return to full activity.

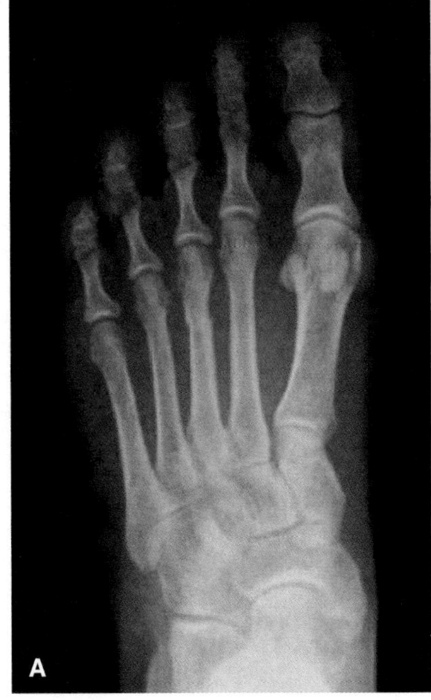

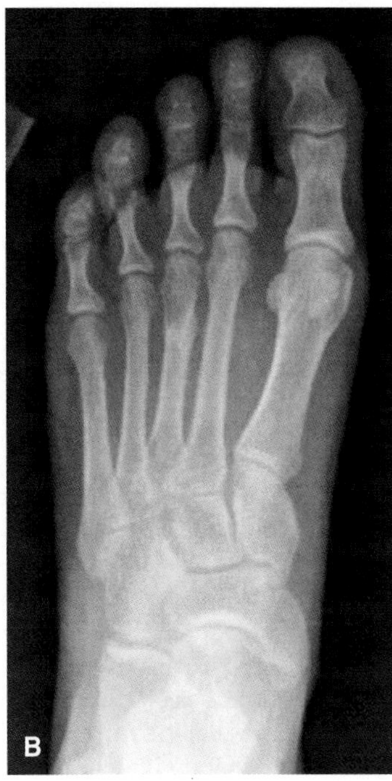

Figure 20.6. X-rays showing an **(A)** acute, and **(B)** healed stress fracture of the third metatarsal in a recreational runner.

Proximal Second Metatarsal (High Risk)

Proximal stress fractures in the second metatarsal are much less common than distal stress fractures involving the shaft or neck. Although distal second metatarsal stress fractures are considered low-risk stress fractures, proximal stress fractures are now regarded as high-risk stress fractures with a propensity for delayed union, nonunion, or refracture (57,129–131,138). The base of the second metatarsal fractures were previously believed to be isolated to ballet dancers, but more recent data indicates that other sporting activities may occasionally result in this injury, including running, basketball, golf, and football (138).

A high-index suspicion for this injury is warranted in ballet dancers and other athletes with more proximal pain along the metatarsal. A low volume of training has been associated with proximal versus non-proximal second metatarsal fractures (138). Other associated risk factors in differentiating proximal from non-proximal second metatarsal stress fractures include a longer duration of symptoms, shorter first metatarsal length, abnormal bone density, history of stress fracture, bilateral stress fractures, and Achilles tendon contracture (138).

In accordance with non-proximal second metatarsal stress fractures, initial radiographs of proximal stress fractures are important but typically fail to demonstrate abnormalities. Other imaging may be important for diagnosis as O'Malley and colleagues reported that only 34% of the base of the second metatarsal fractures were present on initial radiographs (131). In this same report, bone scans were positive in all patients with characteristic pain and negative initial radiographs. In addition, the authors argued that MRI is not a useful adjuvant as imaging rarely provided additional information.

Although proximal second metatarsal stress fractures have been deemed high risk, the treatment of these injuries is typically successful with aggressive non-operative management (129,131). Early recognition of these injuries with early treatment can minimize potential complications. Non-operative treatment should consist of rest and immobilization using a short-leg walking cast or stiff-soled shoe. Although return to activity is possible in ballet dancers, they should still be made aware that symptoms of pain and stiffness may persist in 14% of patients (131). There is little information pertaining to outcomes in athletes who are not ballet dancers, but some authors warn that inadequate and untimely management of these proximal injuries may result in poorer outcomes than non-proximal stress fractures of the second metatarsal (138).

Proximal Fifth Metatarsal (High Risk)

Sir Robert Jones was the first to describe proximal fifth metatarsal stress fractures in 1902 (146). Since this time, numerous research studies have been conducted analyzing the diagnosis, treatment, and outcomes of these injuries. As a result, proximal fifth metatarsal fractures have been subdivided according to the propensity for adverse outcomes, including delayed union and nonunion (147). Certain proximal fifth metatarsal fractures (metaphyseal–diaphyseal junction) are now considered high-risk injuries as blood supply to the proximal fifth metatarsal results in watershed in this area with vascular insufficiency potentially resulting in delayed union or nonunion (148,149).

Considering the high variability in outcomes for proximal fifth metatarsal stress fractures, this region has been classified into three fracture zones (150,151). Zone 1 is most proximal, including the metatarsocuboid articulation, insertion of the peroneus brevis, and insertion of the lateral plantar aponeurosis. These fractures are usually avulsion injuries related to acute inversion of the foot and can extend into the metatarsocuboid joint. Zone 2 includes injuries that occur at the metaphyseal–diaphyseal junction defined by the watershed area with decreased vascularity within the proximal fifth metatarsal. This zone corresponds to the classic "Jones" fracture and is characterized by a fracture line which begins in the distal portion of the tuberosity with extension transversely or obliquely into the fourth and fifth metatarsal articulation. These fractures typically result from a high load on the plantar aspect of the fifth metatarsal head and are considered high risk for progression to delayed union or nonunion. Finally, zone 3 includes the proximal portion of the diaphysis (approximately 1.5 cm), and these injuries occur secondary to a fatigue mechanism as excessive, repetitive loads are applied to the plantar surface of the fifth metatarsal head.

Torg and colleagues have proposed a classification system based on clinical and conventional radiographic criteria to differentiate the healing potential of proximal fifth metatarsal fractures regardless of location: (1) acute, (2) delayed union, and (3) nonunion (132). Type I (acute) fractures are clinically defined as acute and radiographically demonstrate sharp fracture margins with minimal or no periosteal reaction and/or cortical hypertrophy. Type II (delayed union) fractures are clinically defined by a history of previous injury or fracture and radiographically demonstrate widened fracture margins with some periosteal reaction and/or intramedullary sclerosis. Type III (nonunion) fractures are clinically defined by a history of repetitive trauma or recurrent symptoms and radiographically demonstrate blunted fracture margins and sclerosis obliterating the medullary canal.

Clinical history is usually defined by pain over the lateral aspect of the foot and may present acutely or after a period of time as symptoms persist. Pain is typically exacerbated by inversion of the foot and worsens with activities, especially running and jumping. Treatment is usually dependent upon the clinical presentation and radiographic findings with attention to the zone and type of injury as described above.

Zone 1 injuries, regardless of the Torg type, are usually treated successfully with non-operative treatment. Symptomatic care is the goal of managing these injuries as numerous reports document successful healing which is not affected by fragment size or degree of displacement (150,152). Non-operative management should consist of weight bearing as tolerated and immobilization using a hard-soled shoe or short-leg walker boot. Most fractures will heal within 6 to 8 weeks by bony union or an asymptomatic fibrous union with subsequent gradual return to activity (150,153,154). Operative management may be necessary for those stress fractures which are refractive to conservative management, including symptomatic nonunions and more significant stress fractures consisting of a large articular step-off (>2 mm) or greater than 30% of the articular surface (126,150,152,154).

The management of zone 2 (classic "Jones") or zone 3 (proximal diaphysis) stress fracture depends upon the Torg type and degree of displacement. For those fractures which are non-displaced or Torg type I may be treated non–weight-bearing in a short-leg boot or cast for 6 to 8 weeks with success (150,153–156). However, high-performance athletes requiring faster return to activity or those refusing non-operative treatment may be successfully treated using internal fixation with an interfragmentary screw, especially those patients with a classic zone 2 "Jones" fracture (157).

Zone 2 or 3 injuries which are displaced or present with radiographic findings indicative of Torg type II (delayed union) or III (nonunion) typically require early operative management, especially in high-performance athletes (150,153,154,156,157). Early operative management using closed reduction with intramedullary screw fixation or open reduction internal fixation using a plate and screws typically allow for good fixation and adequate healing to minimize the risk of delayed union, nonunion, and possible refracture and lead to earlier return to activity (126,150,154,157–160). Bone grafting may supplement fixation, especially in Torg type III stress fractures with evidence of chronic changes and nonunion; however, care must be taken if opening the fracture site as tentative blood supply in zone 2 may further compromise healing. Of note, excellent outcomes have been achieved with intramedullary screw fixation; however, surgeons and patients should be aware that complications have been documented, including refracture and symptomatic nonunion (159,160).

Overall, return to full activity may be achieved between 8 to 12 weeks after a graduated program with resolution of symptoms. High-performance athletes are able to achieve improved outcomes after operative management as radiographic union may be realized by 7.5 post-operative weeks with a full return to activity by 8.5 post-operative weeks (157). If there is concern about potential nonunion with a persistence of symptoms in the setting of equivocal conventional radiographs, then computerized tomography utilizing artifact subtraction software may be utilized to assess circumferential healing, especially in high-performance athletes (161).

GREAT TOE SESAMOIDS (HIGH RISK)

The great toe sesamoids allow for diminished forces through the first metatarsal head and provide a mechanical advantage for the flexor hallucis brevis. The great toe sesamoid bones experience increased loads during weight bearing as one-third of the body's weight is transferred through the two sesamoid bones underneath the first metatarsal head (126,134). Stress fractures of the great toe sesamoids are relatively uncommon. An increased incidence of stress fractures occurs in the medial sesamoid as increased loads are transferred across the medial side of the first metatarsal head. A diverse differential diagnosis must be considered when evaluating pain in the area of the first metatarsophalangeal joint, including sesamoiditis, metatarsophalangeal joint arthritis or synovitis, flexor hallucis brevis tendinitis, and metatarsalgia.

As the differential diagnosis is varied, one must consider the onset of symptoms and the mechanism of injury. Great toe sesamoid stress fractures usually occur with repetitive running or jumping activities which cause dorsiflexion of the great toe resulting in increased tensile forces through the sesamoid bones. Clinical history will include pain localized to the region of the first metatarsal head upon weight bearing, and this pain can be elicited during physical examination upon palpation directly over the plantar aspect of the metatarsophalangeal joint in the area of the sesamoids. Symptoms will usually increase with maximal dorsiflexion of the great toe, and the patient will have difficulty performing a push-off test with the great toe.

The great toe sesamoids may be multipartite in 5% to 30% of normal, asymptomatic individuals; therefore, clinical evaluation can be somewhat complicated, requiring imaging to confirm the diagnosis (162–165). Conventional radiographs should include anteroposterior and lateral weight-bearing views as well as the medial and lateral oblique sesamoid views. Conventional radiographs must be scrutinized to differentiate the jagged border of a stress fracture from the smooth cortical borders of a bipartite sesamoid. As bilateral bipartite sesamoids may occur in 25% of patients, radiographs of the opposite foot can evaluate for this occurrence (166). In fact, serial radiographs or CT may be necessary to diagnose a stress fracture by evaluating for an increased distance between fragments indicating a fracture (167). If conventional radiographs or CT do not allow for definitive diagnosis, then additional imaging with longitudinal bone scan or MRI can help differentiate the diagnosis and potentially provide for an earlier diagnosis (168).

As great toe sesamoid stress fractures are high risk for progression to delayed union, nonunion, or refracture, aggressive treatment is warranted. Acute stress fractures should be treated with initial non-operative management consisting of rest and immobilization. Immobilization should consist of a non–weight-bearing cast with toe plate preventing great toe dorsiflexion for 6 weeks. As symptoms resolve with evidence of radiographic union which typically occurs over 4 to 6 weeks, (27) immobilization may be discontinued with conversion to molded orthotics and progression of weight bearing. If symptoms are refractive to non-operative management for 6 to 8 weeks, surgery may be indicated.

Surgical management typically consists of complete or partial excision of the affected sesamoid with care not to disrupt the flexor hallucis brevis (169,170). Bone grafting without excision may also provide satisfactory results; however, this treatment is not typically preferred. In the case of chronic, displaced symptomatic sesamoid fractures, bone grafting may be indicated, especially in high-performance athletes, who require adequate strength of the capsulosesamoid apparatus (171). In a rare case of medial and lateral sesamoid stress fractures, the preferred treatment is partial sesamoidectomy. If possible, excision of both sesamoids should be avoided to prevent cock-up deformity. Post-operative management includes cast immobilization for 3 weeks followed by a graduated therapy program including gradual training at 6 to 8 post-operative weeks and a full return to activity by 3 to 6 months (169,170).

SPECIAL CONSIDERATIONS

FEMALE ATHLETE

More than 95% of all stress fractures occur in the lower extremity, and the highest incidence of stress fractures within the female athletic population occur in track and field (172). Despite a higher incidence of stress fracture occurring in the female athlete as opposed to their male counterparts, these differences have not been shown to be statistically significant (8). Thus, the apparent differences have been theorized to be associated with other intrinsic factors which can affect bone homeostasis, including diet, bone density, and menstrual history (173,174).

As the higher incidence of stress fractures noted in females have been linked to other gender-related factors, it is extremely important to screen all female athletes for associated abnormalities. Therefore, female athletes should be assessed for components of the female athlete triad which consists of eating disorders, amenorrhea, and osteoporosis. This disorder can manifest in several abnormalities, including stress fractures (175–177). The female athlete triad has a high incidence in athletes and has been noted to occur with higher rates in sporting activities where appearance is important (i.e., ballet, gymnastics, and figure skating) and/or low body fat is beneficial (i.e., distance runners) (173,175).

In the patient with signs of the female athlete triad, stress fractures are likely related to a combination of factors; consequently, diet, hormonal factors, and osteopenia play especially important roles and must be considered. Abnormal eating patterns may result in menstrual abnormalities and a hypoestrogenic state resulting in inadequate bone density (i.e., osteoporosis). These eating disorders may include food restriction, bingeing, purging, diet pills, and/or laxatives (178). The lack of estrogen has been theorized to cause an increased set point for bone remodeling resulting in a delayed bone repair mechanism with an associated decrease in bone mineral density and increase in stress fracture risk (174,178,179). The foot and ankle is especially at risk in these patients as altered bone homeostasis and repetitive, mechanical stress loading associated with athletic activities leads to a perfect storm resulting in stress reaction and subsequent stress fracture.

Management of stress fractures in female athletes must be directed at treatment as well as correction of the underlying abnormality in bone metabolism, if present. Treatments have produced varying results and have included nutritional counseling, parathyroid hormone, supplemental calcium and vitamin D, nonsteroidal anti-inflammatory drugs, bisphosphonates, testosterone, and oral contraceptives. Because of the hypoestrogenic state, oral contraceptives have presented an exciting avenue for treatment. Although oral contraceptive use has not been shown to significantly increase bone mineral density in athletes with hypoestrogenic amenorrhea and associated bone loss, several studies have shown that they may be protective against stress fractures (9,173,174,180,181). Either way, the best course of treatment is dictated by prevention with the identification of associated abnormalities before they manifest as musculoskeletal disease. Additional research is necessary concerning stress fractures in female athletes, and these studies should be directed at identifying risk factors and proposing treatments to alter the disadvantageous metabolic state of bone in these individuals.

PEDIATRIC ATHLETE

Prior to organized sports for children, stress fractures were extremely rare in these individuals; however, a recent increase in year-round youth sporting activities has resulted in an increase in stress fractures in this population, especially in the lower extremity (74,182). In fact, Orava and colleagues found that 9% of stress fractures occur in children under 15 years old and 32% occur in individuals between 16 and 19 years old (183). Although adult and pediatric athletes have a predominance of stress fractures occurring in the tibia (50%), there are apparent differences in the remaining distribution of pediatric stress fractures, including the fibula (20%) and pars interarticularis (15%) (184). However, pediatric stress fractures of the foot and ankle have also been noted in the metatarsals and tarsal navicular (183).

Bones of children and adolescents differ from adults in relation to their strength, elasticity, and healing. Children have increased elasticity and remodeling potential with an increased ability for healing which portends a good prognosis for most children with stress fractures. To date, studies relating to pediatric stress fractures have been confined to case reports and small, retrospective studies (127,185–188).

A more recent case series evaluated stress fractures in athletes with open physes and reported unsatisfactory outcomes with symptom duration for more than 6 months in 33% of patients (7 out of 21 cases) and symptom duration of more than 13 months in five patients (182). Six of the seven patients with unsatisfactory outcomes were noted to be associated with sports involving "bursts of speed interspersed with sudden stops" and four of these patients had fractures involving the tibial diaphysis (182). These findings were in opposition to a previous report by Bennell and colleagues indicating that tibial stress fractures typically occur in distance runners in adults as opposed to metatarsal and other foot fractures in explosive push-off activities. Heyworth and Green proposed that this finding in the pediatric population was likely related to an incomplete ossification process in long bones of children, such as the tibial shaft, as the high rotational and compressive forces in sporting activities with "sudden stops" result in these pediatric, tibial stress injuries (189).

Despite beneficial bone metabolism in pediatric athletes, these results underscore the importance of early, aggressive management in these patients to decrease potential morbidity, especially in injuries involving the tibial shaft (182). The associated differences between the pediatric and adult population highlights the importance of evaluating athletes with open physes separately as they may have distinct injuries that necessitate altered treatment algorithms and portend different prognoses. With an increased incidence of stress fractures now occurring in the pediatric population, additional studies are needed to further enhance our understanding of these injuries in this population and optimize diagnostic and treatment algorithms to improve outcomes.

SUMMARY

The bones of the foot and ankle are particularly prone to high loads from weight bearing; therefore, their inherent location makes them unique and challenging to manage, especially in athletes. Stress fractures have been encountered throughout the entire body; nevertheless, they are more common in the lower extremity, especially the foot and ankle, as these excessive, repetitive loads result in fatigue and subsequent fracture. A high index of suspicion is necessary in the early diagnosis of stress fractures and is based on a careful clinical history, physical examination, and directed imaging according to the location of interest.

Location-specific risk stratification according to high risk or low risk will subsequently enable the physician to understand the pathophysiology and determine the management of each particular stress fracture. The hallmark of stress fracture management should be prevention. After a stress fracture has occurred, the proposed classification-based treatment algorithm may be helpful in guiding management of high-risk and low-risk stress fractures; however, the clinician must determine an individualized treatment plan depending upon the environment of the patient as well as the fracture. An early diagnosis and well-designed treatment plan can result in the successful management of foot and ankle stress fractures by allowing for an earlier return to activity with a decreased probability of complications, such as delayed union, nonunion, or refracture.

REFERENCES

1. Breithaupt MD. Fur pathologie des menschlichen fusses. *Med Zeit* 1855;24:169–177.
2. Bernstein A, Stone JR. March fracture: a report of three hundred and seven cases and a new method of treatment. *J Bone Joint Surg Am* 1944;26(4):743–750.
3. Devas MB. Stress fractures of the tibia in athletes or shin soreness. *J Bone Joint Surg Br* 1958;40-B(2):227–239.
4. Matheson GO, Clement DB, McKenzie DC, et al. Stress fractures in athletes. A study of 320 cases. *Am J Sports Med* 1987;15(1):46–58.
5. Berger FH, de Jonge MC, Maas M. Stress fractures in the lower extremity. The importance of increasing awareness amongst radiologists. *Eur J Radiol* 2007;62(1):16–26.
6. Callahan LR. Stress fractures in women. *Clin Sports Med* 2000;19(2):303–314.
7. Sallis RE, Jones K. Stress fractures in athletes. How to spot this underdiagnosed injury. *Postgrad Med* 1991;89(6):185–188, 191–192.
8. Bennell KL, Malcolm SA, Thomas SA, et al. The incidence and distribution of stress fractures in competitive track and field athletes. A twelve-month prospective study. *Am J Sports Med* 1996;24(2):211–217.
9. Bennell KL, Malcolm SA, Thomas SA, et al. Risk factors for stress fractures in female track-and-field athletes: a retrospective analysis. *Clin J Sport Med* 1995;5(4):229–235.
10. Johnson AW, Weiss CB Jr, Wheeler DL. Stress fractures of the femoral shaft in athletes–more common than expected. A new clinical test. *Am J Sports Med* 1994;22(2):248–256.
11. Bennell KL, Brukner PD. Epidemiology and site specificity of stress fractures. *Clin Sports Med* 1997;16(2):179–196.
12. Goldberg B, Pecora C. Stress fractures: a risk of increased training in freshman. *Phys Sportsmed* 1994;22:68–78.
13. Brudvig TJ, Gudger TD, Obermeyer L. Stress fractures in 295 trainees: a one-year study of incidence as related to age, sex, and race. *Mil Med* 1983;148(8):666–667.
14. Jones BH, Bovee MW, Harris JM 3rd., et al. Intrinsic risk factors for exercise-related injuries among male and female army trainees. *Am J Sports Med* 1993;21(5):705–710.
15. Jones BH, Harris JM, Vinh TN, et al. Exercise-induced stress fractures and stress reactions of bone: epidemiology, etiology, and classification. *Exerc Sport Sci Rev* 1989;17:379–422.
16. Prather JL, Nusynowitz ML, Snowdy HA, et al. Scintigraphic findings in stress fractures. *J Bone Joint Surg Am* 1977;59(7):869–874.
17. Protzman RR, Griffis CG. Stress fractures in men and women undergoing military training. *J Bone Joint Surg Am* 1977;59(6):825.
18. Carpintero P, Berral FJ, Baena P, et al. Delayed diagnosis of fatigue fractures in the elderly. *Am J Sports Med* 1997;25(5):659–662.
19. Burr DB. Remodeling and the repair of fatigue damage. *Calcif Tissue Int* 1993;53(Suppl 1):S75–S80; discussion S80–S81.
20. Carter DR, Caler WE, Spengler DM, et al. Uniaxial fatigue of human cortical bone. The influence of tissue physical characteristics. *J Biomech* 1981;14(7):461–470.
21. Chamay A, Tschantz P. Mechanical influences in bone remodeling. Experimental research on Wolff's law. *J Biomech* 1972;5(2):173–180.
22. Frost HM. Some ABC's of skeletal pathophysiology. 5. Microdamage physiology. *Calcif Tissue Int* 1991;49(4):229–231.
23. Uhthoff HK, Jaworski ZF. Periosteal stress-induced reactions resembling stress fractures. A radiologic and histologic study in dogs. *Clin Orthop Relat Res* 1985;(199):284–291.
24. Fyhrie DP, Milgrom C, Hoshaw SJ, et al. Effect of fatiguing exercise on longitudinal bone strain as related to stress fracture in humans. *Ann Biomed Eng* 1998;26(4):660–665.
25. Boden BP, Osbahr DC, Jimenez C. Low-risk stress fractures. *Am J Sports Med* 2001;29(1):100–111.
26. McBryde AM Jr. Stress fractures in athletes. *J Sports Med* 1975;3(5):212–217.
27. Meyer SA, Saltzman CL, Albright JP. Stress fractures of the foot and leg. *Clin Sports Med* 1993;12(2):395–413.
28. Stanitski CL, McMaster JH, Scranton PE. On the nature of stress fractures. *Am J Sports Med* 1978;6(6):391–396.
29. Knapp TP, Garrett WE Jr. Stress fractures: general concepts. *Clin Sports Med* 1997;16(2):339–356.
30. Maitra RS, Johnson DL. Stress fractures. Clinical history and physical examination. *Clin Sports Med* 1997;16(2):259–274.
31. Sofka CM. Imaging of stress fractures. *Clin Sports Med* 2006;25(1):53–62, viii.
32. Anderson MW, Greenspan A. Stress fractures. *Radiology* 1996;199(1):1–12.
33. Daffner RH, Pavlov H. Stress fractures: current concepts. *AJR Am J Roentgenol* 1992; 159(2):245–252.
34. Greaney RB, Gerber FH, Laughlin RL, et al. Distribution and natural history of stress fractures in U.S. Marine recruits. *Radiology* 1983;146(2):339–346.
35. Spitz DJ, Newberg AH. Imaging of stress fractures in the athlete. *Radiol Clin North Am* 2002;40(2):313–331.
36. Engber WD. Stress fractures of the medial tibial plateau. *J Bone Joint Surg Am* 1977; 59(6):767–769.
37. Sullivan D, Warren RF, Pavlov H, et al. Stress fractures in 51 runners. *Clin Orthop Relat Res* 1984;(187):188–192.
38. Stafford SA, Rosenthal DI, Gebhardt MC, et al. MRI in stress fracture. *AJR Am J Roentgenol* 1986;147(3):553–556.
39. Fredericson M, Jennings F, Beaulieu C, et al. Stress fractures in athletes. *Top Magn Reson Imaging* 2006;17(5):309–325.
40. Keene JS, Lash EG. Negative bone scan in a femoral neck stress fracture. A case report. *Am J Sports Med* 1992;20(2):234–236.
41. Sterling JC, Webb RF Jr, Meyers MC, et al. False negative bone scan in a female runner. *Med Sci Sports Exerc* 1993;25(2):179–185.
42. Nielsen MB, Hansen K, Holmer P, et al. Tibial periosteal reactions in soldiers. A scintigraphic study of 29 cases of lower leg pain. *Acta Orthop Scand* 1991;62(6):531–534.
43. Zwas ST, Elkanovitch R, Frank G. Interpretation and classification of bone scintigraphic findings in stress fractures. *J Nucl Med* 1987;28(4):452–457.
44. Gaeta M, Minutoli F, Scribano E, et al. CT and MR imaging findings in athletes with early tibial stress injuries: comparison with bone scintigraphy findings and emphasis on cortical abnormalities. *Radiology* 2005;235(2):553–561.
45. Moran DS, Evans RK, Hadad E. Imaging of lower extremity stress fracture injuries. *Sports Med* 2008;38(4):345–356.
46. Arendt EA, Griffiths HJ. The use of MR imaging in the assessment and clinical management of stress reactions of bone in high-performance athletes. *Clin Sports Med* 1997; 16(2):291–306.
47. Fredericson M, Bergman AG, Hoffman KL, et al. Tibial stress reaction in runners. Correlation of clinical symptoms and scintigraphy with a new magnetic resonance imaging grading system. *Am J Sports Med* 1995;23(4):472–481.
48. Deutsch AL, Coel MN, Mink JH. Imaging of stress injuries to bone. Radiography, scintigraphy, and MR imaging. *Clin Sports Med* 1997;16(2):275–290.
49. Kiuru MJ, Niva M, Reponen A, et al. Bone stress injuries in asymptomatic elite recruits: a clinical and magnetic resonance imaging study. *Am J Sports Med* 2005;33(2):272–276.
50. Niva MH, Sormaala MJ, Kiuru MJ, et al. Bone stress injuries of the ankle and foot: an 86-month magnetic resonance imaging-based study of physically active young adults. *Am J Sports Med* 2007;35(4):643–649.
51. Yao L, Johnson C, Gentili A, et al. Stress injuries of bone: analysis of MR imaging staging criteria. *Acad Radiol* 1998;5(1):34–40.
52. Bergman AG, Fredericson M, Ho C, et al. Asymptomatic tibial stress reactions: MRI detection and clinical follow-up in distance runners. *AJR Am J Roentgenol* 2004;183(3):635–638.
53. Lazzarini KM, Troiano RN, Smith RC. Can running cause the appearance of marrow edema on MR images of the foot and ankle? *Radiology* 1997;202(2):540–542.
54. Beck BR. Tibial stress injuries. An aetiological review for the purposes of guiding management. *Sports Med* 1998;26(4):265–279.
55. Schwellnus MP, Jordaan G, Noakes TD. Prevention of common overuse injuries by the use of shock absorbing insoles. A prospective study. *Am J Sports Med* 1990;18(6):636–641.
56. Thacker SB, Gilchrist J, Stroup DF, et al. The prevention of shin splints in sports: a systematic review of literature. *Med Sci Sports Exerc* 2002;34(1):32–40.
57. Boden BP, Osbahr DC. High-risk stress fractures: evaluation and treatment. *J Am Acad Orthop Surg* 2000;8(6):344–353.
58. Diehl JJ, Best TM, Kaeding CC. Classification and return-to-play considerations for stress fractures. *Clin Sports Med* 2006;25(1):17–28, vii.
59. Brukner P, Bradshaw C, Bennell KL. Managing common stress fractures: let risk level guide treatment. *Phys Sportsmed* 1998;26(8):39–47.
60. Kaeding CC, Spindler KP, Amendola A. Management of troublesome stress fractures. *Instr Course Lect* 2004;53:455–469.
61. Kaeding CC, Yu JR, Wright R, et al. Management and return to play of stress fractures. *Clin J Sport Med* 2005;15(6):442–447.
62. Feydy A, Drape J, Beret E, et al. Longitudinal stress fractures of the tibia: comparative study of CT and MR imaging. *Eur Radiol* 1998;8(4):598–602.
63. Shearman CM, Brandser EA, Parman LM, et al. Longitudinal tibial stress fractures: a report of eight cases and review of the literature. *J Comput Assist Tomogr* 1998;22(2):265–269.
64. Dickson TB Jr, Kichline PD. Functional management of stress fractures in female athletes using a pneumatic leg brace. *Am J Sports Med* 1987;15(1):86–89.
65. Swenson EJ Jr, DeHaven KE, Sebastianelli WJ, et al. The effect of a pneumatic leg brace on return to play in athletes with tibial stress fractures. *Am J Sports Med* 1997;25(3):322–328.
66. Whitelaw GP, Wetzler MJ, Levy AS, et al. A pneumatic leg brace for the treatment of tibial stress fractures. *Clin Orthop Relat Res* 1991;(270):301–305.
67. Brukner P, Fanton G, Bergman AG, et al. Bilateral stress fractures of the anterior part of the tibial cortex. A case report. *J Bone Joint Surg Am* 2000;82(2):213–218.
68. Rettig AC, Shelbourne KD, McCarroll JR, et al. The natural history and treatment of delayed union stress fractures of the anterior cortex of the tibia. *Am J Sports Med* 1988; 16(3):250–255.
69. Batt ME, Kemp S, Kerslake R. Delayed union stress fractures of the anterior tibia: conservative management. *Br J Sports Med* 2001;35(1):74–77.
70. Green NE, Rogers RA, Lipscomb AB. Nonunions of stress fractures of the tibia. *Am J Sports Med* 1985;13(3):171–176.
71. Chang PS, Harris RM. Intramedullary nailing for chronic tibial stress fractures. A review of five cases. *Am J Sports Med* 1996;24(5):688–692.
72. Brukner P, Bradshaw C, Khan KM, et al. Stress fractures: a review of 180 cases. *Clin J Sport Med* 1996;6(2):85–89.

73. Iwamoto J, Takeda T. Stress fractures in athletes: review of 196 cases. *J Orthop Sci* 2003; 8(3):273–278.
74. Ohta-Fukushima M, Mutoh Y, Takasugi S, et al. Characteristics of stress fractures in young athletes under 20 years. *J Sports Med Phys Fitness* 2002;42(2):198–206.
75. Takebe K, Nakagawa A, Minami H, et al. Role of the fibula in weight-bearing. *Clin Orthop Relat Res* 1984;(184):289–292.
76. Symeonides PP. High stress fractures of the fibula. *J Bone Joint Surg Br* 1980;62-B(2):192–193.
77. Blair WF, Hanley SR. Stress fracture of the proximal fibula. *Am J Sports Med* 1980;8(3):212–213.
78. Strudwick WJ, Goodman SB. Proximal fibular stress fracture in an aerobic dancer. A case report. *Am J Sports Med* 1992;20(4):481–482.
79. Burrows HJ. Fatigue fractures of the fibula. *J Bone Joint Surg Br* 1948;30-B(2):266–279.
80. Devas MB, Sweetnam R. Stress fractures of the fibula; a review of fifty cases in athletes. *J Bone Joint Surg Br* 1956;38-B(4):818–829.
81. Burgess I, Ryan MD. Bilateral fatigue fractures of the distal fibulae caused by a change of running shoes. *Med J Aust* 1985;143(7):304–305.
82. Steinbronn DJ, Bennett GL, Kay DB. The use of magnetic resonance imaging in the diagnosis of stress fractures of the foot and ankle: four case reports. *Foot Ankle Int* 1994;15(2):80–83.
83. Guille JT, Lipton GE, Bowen JR, et al. Delayed union following stress fracture of the distal fibula secondary to rotational malunion of lateral malleolar fracture. *Am J Orthop* 1997;26(6):442–445.
84. Devas MB. *Stress Fractures.* New York, NY: Churchill Livingstone; 1975.
85. Orava S, Karpakka J, Taimela S, et al. Stress fracture of the medial malleolus. *J Bone Joint Surg Am* 1995;77(3):362–365.
86. Shelbourne KD, Fisher DA, Rettig AC, et al. Stress fractures of the medial malleolus. *Am J Sports Med* 1988;16(1):60–63.
87. Kor A, Saltzman AT, Wempe PD. Medial malleolar stress fractures. Literature review, diagnosis, and treatment. *J Am Podiatr Med Assoc* 2003;93(4):292–297.
88. Okada K, Senma S, Abe E, et al. Stress fractures of the medial malleolus: a case report. *Foot Ankle Int* 1995;16(1):49–52.
89. Reider B, Falconiero R, Yurkofsky J. Nonunion of a medial malleolus stress fracture. A case report. *Am J Sports Med* 1993;21(3):478–481.
90. Schils JP, Andrish JT, Piraino DW, et al. Medial malleolar stress fractures in seven patients: review of the clinical and imaging features. *Radiology* 1992;185(1):219–221.
91. Shabat S, Sampson KB, Mann G, et al. Stress fractures of the medial malleolus–review of the literature and report of a 15-year-old elite gymnast. *Foot Ankle Int* 2002;23(7):647–650.
92. Bradshaw C, Khan K, Brukner P. Stress fracture of the body of the talus in athletes demonstrated with computer tomography. *Clin J Sport Med* 1996;6(1):48–51.
93. McGlone JJ. Stress fractures of the talus. *J Am Podiatr Med Assoc* 1965;55:814–817.
94. Gilbert RS, Crawford AH, Rankin E. Stress fractures of the tarsal talus. *Sports Med* 1980;80:133–139.
95. Sormaala MJ, Niva MH, Kiuru MJ, et al. Outcomes of stress fractures of the talus. *Am J Sports Med* 2006;34(11):1809–1814.
96. Chiodo CP, Herbst SA. Osteonecrosis of the talus. *Foot Ankle Clin* 2004;9(4):745–755, vi.
97. Travlos J, Learmonth ID. Bilateral avascular necrosis of the talus following strenuous physical activity. *J Bone Joint Surg Br* 1991;73(5):863–864.
98. Leabhart JW. Stress fractures of the calcaneus. *J Bone Joint Surg Am* 1959;41-A:1285–1290.
99. Darby RE. Stress fractures of the os calcis. *JAMA* 1967;200(13):1183–1184.
100. Hullinger CW. Insufficiency fracture of the calcaneus similar to march fracture of the metatarsal. *J Bone Joint Surg Am* 1944;26:751–757.
101. Sormaala MJ, Niva MH, Kiuru MJ, et al. Stress injuries of the calcaneus detected with magnetic resonance imaging in military recruits. *J Bone Joint Surg Am* 2006;88(10):2237–2242.
102. Hopson CN, Perry DR. Stress fractures of the calcaneus in women marine recruits. *Clin Orthop Relat Res* 1977;(128):159–162.
103. Goergen TG, Venn-Watson EA, Rossman DJ, et al. Tarsal navicular stress fractures in runners. *AJR Am J Roentgenol* 1981;136(1):201–203.
104. Orava S, Puranen J, Ala-Ketola L. Stress fractures caused by physical exercise. *Acta Orthop Scand* 1978;49(1):19–27.
105. Khan KM, Brukner PD, Kearney C, et al. Tarsal navicular stress fracture in athletes. *Sports Med* 1994;17(1):65–76.
106. Golano P, Farinas O, Saenz I. The anatomy of the navicular and periarticular structures. *Foot Ankle Clin* 2004;9(1):1–23.
107. Kapandji IA. *The Physiology of the Joints.* Edinburgh, Scotland: Churchill Livingstone; 1970.
108. Orava S, Karpakka J, Hulkko A, et al. Stress avulsion fracture of the tarsal navicular. An uncommon sports-related overuse injury. *Am J Sports Med* 1991;19(4):392–395.
109. Pavlov H, Torg JS, Freiberger RH. Tarsal navicular stress fractures: radiographic evaluation. *Radiology* 1983;148(3):641–645.
110. Ting A, King W, Yocum L, et al. Stress fractures of the tarsal navicular in long-distance runners. *Clin Sports Med* 1988;7(1):89–101.
111. Torg JS, Pavlov H, Cooley LH, et al. Stress fractures of the tarsal navicular. A retrospective review of twenty-one cases. *J Bone Joint Surg Am* 1982;64(5):700–712.
112. Fitch KD, Blackwell JB, Gilmour WN. Operation for non-union of stress fracture of the tarsal navicular. *J Bone Joint Surg Br* 1989;71(1):105–110.
113. Hulkko A, Orava S, Peltokallio P, et al. Stress fracture of the navicular bone. Nine cases in athletes. *Acta Orthop Scand* 1985;56(6):503–505.
114. Sizensky JA, Marks RM. Imaging of the navicular. *Foot Ankle Clin* 2004;9(1):181–209.
115. Khan KM, Fuller PJ, Brukner PD, et al. Outcome of conservative and surgical management of navicular stress fracture in athletes. Eighty-six cases proven with computerized tomography. *Am J Sports Med* 1992;20(6):657–666.
116. Kiss ZS, Khan KM, Fuller PJ. Stress fractures of the tarsal navicular bone: CT findings in 55 cases. *AJR Am J Roentgenol* 1993;160(1):111–115.
117. Quirk R. Stress fractures of the navicular. *Foot Ankle Int* 1998;19(7):494–496.
118. Sanders TG, Williams PM, Vawter KW. Stress fracture of the tarsal navicular. *Mil Med* 2004;169(7):viii–xiii.
119. Lee A, Anderson R. Stress fractures of the tarsal navicular. *Foot Ankle Clin* 2004;9:85–104.
120. Saxena A, Fullem B, Hannaford D. Results of treatment of 22 navicular stress fractures and a new proposed radiographic classification system. *J Foot Ankle Surg* 2000;39(2):96–103.
121. Dennis L, Lombardi CM. Stress fracture of the tarsal navicular: two unusual case reports. *J Foot Surg* 1988;27(6):511–514.
122. Ostlie DK, Simons SM. Tarsal navicular stress fracture in a young athlete: case report with clinical, radiologic, and pathophysiologic correlations. *J Am Board Fam Pract* 2001; 14(5):381–385.
123. Saxena A, Fullem B. Navicular stress fractures: a prospective study on athletes. *Foot Ankle Int* 2006;27(11):917–921.
124. Jones MH, Amendola AS. Navicular stress fractures. *Clin Sports Med* 2006;25(1):151–158, x–xi.
125. Coris EE, Lombardo JA. Tarsal navicular stress fractures. *Am Fam Physician* 2003;67(1):85–90.
126. Early JS. Fractures and dislocations of the midfoot and forefoot. In: Buckholz RW, Heckman JD, eds. *Fractures in Adults.* Philadelphia, PA: Lippincott Williams and Wilkins; 2001:2215–2228.
127. Orava S. Stress fractures. *Br J Sports Med* 1980;14(1):40–44.
128. Chowchuen P, Resnick D. Stress fractures of the metatarsal heads. *Skeletal Radiol* 1998;27(1):22–25.
129. Harrington T, Crichton KJ, Anderson IF. Overuse ballet injury of the base of the second metatarsal. A diagnostic problem. *Am J Sports Med* 1993;21(4):591–598.
130. Micheli LJ, Sohn RS, Solomon R. Stress fractures of the second metatarsal involving Lisfranc's joint in ballet dancers. A new overuse injury of the foot. *J Bone Joint Surg Am* 1985;67(9):1372–1375.
131. O'Malley MJ, Hamilton WG, Munyak J, et al. Stress fractures at the base of the second metatarsal in ballet dancers. *Foot Ankle Int* 1996;17(2):89–94.
132. Torg JS, Balduini FC, Zelko RR, et al. Fractures of the base of the fifth metatarsal distal to the tuberosity. Classification and guidelines for non-surgical and surgical management. *J Bone Joint Surg Am* 1984;66(2):209–214.
133. DeLee JC. Fractures and dislocations of the foot. In: Mann R, Coughlin M, eds. *Surgery of the Foot and Ankle.* St. Louis, MO: Mosby Elsevier; 1993.
134. Shereff MJ. Complex fractures of the metatarsals. *Orthopedics* 1990;13(8):875–882.
135. Drez D, Jr, Young JC, Johnston RD, et al. Metatarsal stress fractures. *Am J Sports Med* 1980; 8(2):123–125.
136. Harris RI, Beath T. The short first metatarsal; its incidence and clinical significance. *J Bone Joint Surg Am* 1949;31A(3):553–565.
137. Sharkey NA, Ferris L, Smith TS, et al. Strain and loading of the second metatarsal during heel-lift. *J Bone Joint Surg Am* 1995;77(7):1050–1057.
138. Chuckpaiwong B, Cook C, Pietrobon R, et al. Second metatarsal stress fracture in sport: comparative risk factors between proximal and non-proximal locations. *Br J Sports Med* 2007;41(8):510–514.
139. Hetsroni I, Mann G, Dolev E, et al. Base of fourth metatarsal stress fracture: tendency for prolonged healing. *Clin J Sport Med* 2005;15(3):186–188.
140. Shearer CT, Penner MJ. Stress fractures of the base of the fourth metatarsal: 2 cases and a review of the literature. *Am J Sports Med* 2007;35(3):479–483.
141. Saxena A, Krisdakumtorn T, Erickson S. Proximal fourth metatarsal injuries in athletes: similarity to proximal fifth metatarsal injury. *Foot Ankle Int* 2001;22(7):603–608.
142. Gardner LI Jr, Dziados JE, Jones BH, et al. Prevention of lower extremity stress fractures: a controlled trial of a shock absorbent insole. *Am J Public Health* 1988;78(12):1563–1567.
143. Milgrom C, Burr DB, Boyd RD, et al. The effect of a viscoelastic orthotic on the incidence of tibial stress fractures in an animal model. *Foot Ankle* 1990;10(5):276–279.
144. Milgrom C, Giladi M, Kashtan H, et al. A prospective study of the effect of a shock-absorbing orthotic device on the incidence of stress fractures in military recruits. *Foot Ankle* 1985;6(2):101–104.
145. Gehrmann RM, Renard RL. Current concepts review: Stress fractures of the foot. *Foot Ankle Int* 2006;27(9):750–757.
146. Jones R. Fracture of the base of the fifth metatarsal bone by indirect violence. *Ann Surg* 1902;35(6):697–700.
147. Stewart IM. Jones's fracture: fracture of base of fifth metatarsal. *Clin Orthop* 1960;16:190–198.
148. Carp L. Fracture of the fifth metatarsal bone: with special reference to delayed union. *Ann Surg* 1927;86(2):308–320.
149. Smith JW, Arnoczky SP, Hersh A. The intraosseous blood supply of the fifth metatarsal: implications for proximal fracture healing. *Foot Ankle* 1992;13(3):143–152.
150. Dameron TB, Jr. Fractures of the proximal fifth metatarsal: Selecting the best treatment option. *J Am Acad Orthop Surg* 1995;3(2):110–114.
151. Dameron TB, Jr. Fractures and anatomical variations of the proximal portion of the fifth metatarsal. *J Bone Joint Surg Am* 1975;57(6):788–792.
152. Rettig AC, Shelbourne KD, Wilckens J. The surgical treatment of symptomatic nonunions of the proximal (metaphyseal) fifth metatarsal in athletes. *Am J Sports Med* 1992;20(1):50–54.
153. Quill GE Jr. Fractures of the proximal fifth metatarsal. *Orthop Clin North Am* 1995;26(2):353–361.
154. Rosenberg GA, Sferra JJ. Treatment strategies for acute fractures and nonunions of the proximal fifth metatarsal. *J Am Acad Orthop Surg* 2000;8(5):332–338.
155. Lawrence SJ, Botte MJ. Jones' fractures and related fractures of the proximal fifth metatarsal. *Foot Ankle* 1993;14(6):358–365.
156. Torg JS. Fractures of the base of the fifth metatarsal distal to the tuberosity. *Orthopedics* 1990;13(7):731–737.
157. DeLee JC, Evans JP, Julian J. Stress fracture of the fifth metatarsal. *Am J Sports Med* 1983; 11(5):349–353.
158. Kavanaugh JH, Brower TD, Mann RV. The Jones fracture revisited. *J Bone Joint Surg Am* 1978;60(6):776–782.
159. Larson CM, Almekinders LC, Taft TN, et al. Intramedullary screw fixation of Jones fractures. Analysis of failure. *Am J Sports Med* 2002;30(1):55–60.

160. Wright RW, Fischer DA, Shively RA, et al. Refracture of proximal fifth metatarsal (Jones) fracture after intramedullary screw fixation in athletes. *Am J Sports Med* 2000;28(5):732–736.
161. Fetzer GB, Wright RW. Metatarsal shaft fractures and fractures of the proximal fifth metatarsal. *Clin Sports Med* 2006;25(1):139–150, x.
162. Bizzaro AH. On the traumatology of the sesamoid structures. *Ann Surg* 1921;74:783–791.
163. Burman MS, Lapidus PW. The functional disturbances caused by the inconstant bones and sesamoids of the foot. *Arch Surg* 1931;22:936–975.
164. Hubay CA. Sesamoid bones of the hands and feet. *Am J Roentgenol Radium Ther Nucl Med* 1949;61(4):493–505.
165. Powers JH. Traumatic and developmental abnormalities of the sesamoid bones of the great toe. *Am J Surg* 1934;23:315–321.
166. Richardson DG, Donley BG. Disorders of hallux. In: Canale ST, Daugherty K, Jones L, eds. *Campbell's Operative Orthopaedics*. St. Louis, MO: Mosby-Year Book; 1998:1701–1706.
167. Frankel JP, Harrington J. Symptomatic bipartite sesamoids. *J Foot Surg* 1990;29(4):318–323.
168. Biedert R. Which investigations are required in stress fracture of the great toe sesamoids? *Arch Orthop Trauma Surg* 1993;112(2):94–95.
169. Biedert R, Hintermann B. Stress fractures of the medial great toe sesamoids in athletes. *Foot Ankle Int* 2003;24(2):137–141.
170. Hulkko A, Orava S, Pellinen P, et al. Stress fractures of the sesamoid bones of the first metatarsophalangeal joint in athletes. *Arch Orthop Trauma Surg* 1985;104(2):113–117.
171. Anderson RB, McBryde AM, Jr. Autogenous bone grafting of hallux sesamoid nonunions. *Foot Ankle Int* 1997;18(5):293–296.
172. Hame SL, LaFemina JM, McAllister DR, et al. Fractures in the collegiate athlete. *Am J Sports Med* 2004;32(2):446–451.
173. Barrow GW, Saha S. Menstrual irregularity and stress fractures in collegiate female distance runners. *Am J Sports Med* 1988;16(3):209–216.
174. Nattiv A, Armsey TD Jr. Stress injury to bone in the female athlete. *Clin Sports Med* 1997;16(2):197–224.
175. Nattiv A, Agostini R, Drinkwater B, et al. The female athlete triad. The inter-relatedness of disordered eating, amenorrhea, and osteoporosis. *Clin Sports Med* 1994;13(2):405–418.
176. Otis CL, Drinkwater B, Johnson M, et al. American College of Sports Medicine position stand. The female athlete triad. *Med Sci Sports Exerc* 1997;29(5):i–ix.
177. Yeager KK, Agostini R, Nattiv A, et al. The female athlete triad: disordered eating, amenorrhea, osteoporosis. *Med Sci Sports Exerc* 1993;25(7):775–777.
178. Zeni AI, Street CC, Dempsey RL, et al. Stress injury to the bone among women athletes. *Phys Med Rehabil Clin N Am* 2000;11(4):929–947.
179. Frost HM. A new direction for osteoporosis research: a review and proposal. *Bone* 1991;12(6):429–437.
180. Loucks AB, Horvath SM. Athletic amenorrhea: a review. *Med Sci Sports Exerc* 1985;17(1):56–72.
181. Marcus R, Cann C, Madvig P, et al. Menstrual function and bone mass in elite women distance runners. Endocrine and metabolic features. *Ann Intern Med* 1985;102(2):158–163.
182. Niemeyer P, Weinberg A, Schmitt H, et al. Stress fractures in adolescent competitive athletes with open physis. *Knee Surg Sports Traumatol Arthrosc* 2006;14(8):771–777.
183. Orava S, Jormakka E, Hulkko A. Stress fractures in young athletes. *Arch Orthop Trauma Surg* 1981;98(4):271–274.
184. Yngve DA. Stress fractures in the pediatric athlete. In: Sullivean JA, Grana WA, eds. *The Pediatric Athlete*. Park Ridge, IL: American Academy of Orthopaedic Surgeons; 1988.
185. Devas MB. Stress fractures in children. *J Bone Joint Surg Br* 1963;45:528–541.
186. DiFiori JP. Stress fracture of the proximal fibula in a young soccer player: a case report and a review of the literature. *Med Sci Sports Exerc* 1999;31(7):925–928.
187. Orava S, Puranen J. Exertion injuries in adolescent athletes. *Br J Sports Med* 1978;12(1):4–10.
188. Walker RN, Green NE, Spindler KP. Stress fractures in skeletally immature patients. *J Pediatr Orthop* 1996;16(5):578–584.
189. Heyworth BE, Green DW. Lower extremity stress fractures in pediatric and adolescent athletes. *Curr Opin Pediatr* 2008;20(1):58–61.

CHAPTER

21

Matthew H. Griffith
George Theodore

Hindfoot Injuries

INTRODUCTION

The hindfoot consists of the talus and calcaneus which make up the subtalar joint. The joint is stabilized by intrinsic ligaments including the cervical and interosseous ligaments and by extrinsic ligaments, the calcaneofibular ligament (CFL), the tibiocalcaneal portion of the deltoid ligament. The joint has a complex plane of motion that helps to stabilize the ankle when ambulating, especially on uneven surfaces. Hindfoot injuries in athletes are generally overuse in nature with plantar fasciitis being one of the most common causes. Acute injuries may also occur including subtalar joint sprain and fracture. Most conditions will respond to conservative treatment. Careful evaluation is necessary to ensure a correct diagnosis and treatment plan.

EVALUATION

Evaluation of the patient with a hindfoot injury begins with a thorough history. It is important to gather information regarding the onset of symptoms. If there was a prior injury, it is helpful to determine the mechanism, the foot position during injury and the severity of subsequent symptoms. The patient should be asked to localize the pain as specifically as possible. The presence of other complaints such as stiffness, instability or mechanical symptoms may help to narrow the differential diagnosis. It is important to inquire about a remote history of injury. An ankle sprain from years ago may result in subtle subtalar instability or cartilage injury that may present with symptoms long after recovery from the initial injury. If there is no history of injury, evaluate the patient's training and sports schedule. Recent changes in activities or increases in training may indicate an overuse syndrome. It is important to consider associated medical conditions such as diabetes or circulatory disorders, social issues such as tobacco abuse and psychological factors such as eating disorders that may play a role.

Physical examination begins with observation of gait and stance. Alignment of the entire limb should be evaluated as proximal abnormalities may affect foot biomechanics. Inspect the heel position in stance and with heel rise as well as the medial longitudinal arch. Single-leg stance with muscles relaxed will allow the hindfoot to fall into maximum valgus with leg internal rotation. Single-leg heel rise should result in leg external rotation, hindfoot varus and elevation of the medial arch. Inspect the skin for abnormalities including erythema, ecchymosis or swelling. Passive range of motion of the ankle, hindfoot and midfoot should be assessed and compared with the contralateral limb. Subtalar motion is tested by stabilizing the leg and grasping the heel. The calcaneus is inverted and everted and should have an arc of motion of about 20 degrees.

Focal tenderness can be very helpful in localizing the pathology and narrowing the differential diagnosis. Patients with acute injuries may present with significant swelling, ecchymosis, diffuse tenderness and limited motion. It is often valuable to provide initial symptomatic management and reevaluate the patient in 1 to 2 weeks when the examination is more specific. Stability of the ankle and subtalar joint is tested with the anterior drawer test and the lateral tilt test. Comparison is made to the normal foot.

Strength testing should be performed to assess dorsiflexion and plantarflexion strength. Posterior tibialis strength is tested by assessing inversion with the ankle plantarflexed. Motor strength is also tested in the flexor hallucis longus, peroneals, and extensor hallucis longus. A careful neurologic examination is performed to assess sensation and reflexes. Tinel's test may be performed over the course of sensory nerves if compression neuropathy is suspected. A vascular examination is performed by palpating the dorsalis pedis and posterior tibialis pulses and testing capillary refill.

This standard evaluation is performed for all patients with a foot injury and can provide a correct diagnosis in most cases. Radiographs are helpful in ruling out bony pathology and arthritis and can help to confirm the diagnosis.

DIFFERENTIAL DIAGNOSIS

The diagnosis can usually be made based on a thorough history and physical examination. If the patient can localize the symptoms or if there is focal tenderness, this can help to narrow the differential diagnosis (Table 21.1). It is important to consider systemic diseases and referred pain when evaluating the patient with hindfoot pain. Inflammatory conditions such as Reiter's syndrome and seronegative spondyloarthropathy may involve the hindfoot. Pain is usually bilateral in these conditions and inflammatory markers may be elevated. Nerve compression proximally in the spine or leg may be referred to the foot so a comprehensive history and physical examination is necessary.

TABLE 21.1 Differential Diagnosis

Location of Pain			
Plantar	***Posterior***	***Medial***	***Lateral***
Plantar fasciitis	Achilles tendon disorders	Plantar fasciitis	Peroneal tendonitis
Calcaneal stress fracture	Retrocalcaneal bursitis	Posterior tibialis tendonitis	Sinus tarsi syndrome
Baxter's nerve compression	Calcaneal stress fracture	Tarsal tunnel syndrome	Subtalar arthritis
Heel pad syndrome	Os trigonum	Deltoid ligament injury	Ankle/subtalar instability
	FHL tendonitis	Baxter's nerve compression	

PLANTAR FASCIITIS

Plantar fasciitis is a common cause of heel pain occurring in athletes and non-athletes. The most common etiology is overuse creating chronic pain and inflammation. However, rupture has been reported and must be suspected in the athlete with an acute injury resulting in heel pain with symptoms localized to the plantar fascia. The plantar fascia is a fibrous aponeurosis that originates from the anteromedial calcaneal tuberosity and divides into five bands. The bands insert distally on to the plantar aspect of the base of each proximal phalange. The fascia covers the intrinsic muscles and has fibers that connect to the skin, flexor tendon sheaths and transverse metatarsal ligament. It is an important part of the windlass mechanism that supports the longitudinal arch. As the metatarsophalangeal joints flex during gait with heel-rise and push-off, the plantar fascia tightens to support the arch.

The aponeurotic tissue is quite stiff and therefore leads to significant stress on the medial calcaneal tuberosity. This can lead to tensile overload of the fascia resulting in degeneration of the tissue and pain. Continued overuse and a delayed healing response may create a chronic problem. Pathologic studies of specimens from surgery performed for plantar fasciitis show myxoid degenerative changes and little inflammation similar to alterations seen in chronic tendinosis (1). Risk factors for plantar fasciitis include Achilles tendon tightness, obesity and a profession that involves spending most of the day standing (2). Riddle et al. showed that patient with ankle dorsiflexion of zero degrees or less with the knee extended have a significantly increased risk of developing plantar fasciitis. It has been shown that approximately 10 degrees of ankle dorsiflexion with the knee extended is required for normal gait (3). Individuals with limited ankle dorsiflexion may compensate by pronating the foot which has been shown to increase tension on the plantar fascia (4,5). Patients with plantar fasciitis generally complain of medial heel pain which is most severe when first arising in the morning. It is aggravated by activities and long periods of standing. Tenderness may be elicited within 1 cm of the medial calcaneal tuberosity and pain may be exaggerated by passive dorsiflexion of the metatarsophalangeal joints.

Acute rupture of the plantar fascia may occur and is most common in runners but also has been reported in tennis, volleyball, and basketball players (6–8). It is often an acute-on-chronic injury and is theorized to arise from overloading a weakened tissue. Tissue compromise that predisposes one to plantar fascia rupture may be secondary to long-term degenerative changes from chronic plantar fasciitis or prior steroid injections into the plantar fascia (6–10). Leach et al. reviewed six cases of rupture of the plantar fascia and noted that five of these patients had had several prior steroid injections into the origin of the plantar fascia (7). Similarly, Acevedo et al. noted that 44 of 51 patients with a rupture of the plantar fascia had a prior steroid injection (8).

Patients with rupture of the plantar fascia usually present with a history of prior symptoms of plantar fasciitis and an acute injury that includes sharp pain and often the sensation of tearing or a pop. There is usually swelling and ecchymosis at the calcaneal origin of the plantar fascia and tenderness in this area. Dorsiflexion of the metatarsophalangeal joint will tighten the plantar fascia which will worsen the patient's pain but also may make a defect palpable proximally. Radiographs are recommended in the acute injury to rule out a fracture but generally do not help with the diagnosis of plantar fasciitis. Magnetic resonance imaging or ultrasound may help confirm the diagnosis of rupture and may show thickening in cases of plantar fasciitis. In patients with plantar fasciitis, a bone spur is evident on the lateral radiograph in up to 50% but does not appear to affect the outcome of treatment (11,12). The bone spur is usually found at the origin of the flexor digitorum brevis and not the plantar fascia which accounts for why it is generally thought to have little clinical significance (13).

Treatment for plantar fasciitis is conservative and is effective in up to 90% of patients (14,15). Treatment options include anti-inflammatory medications, night splinting, orthotics, a stretching program and steroid injections. However, there have been few randomized controlled trials that support any of these modalities over non-treatment (16). More recently, data has suggested that a stretching program specifically designed to focus on the plantar fascia may be beneficial (15,17). Digiovanni et al. reported that 92% of the patients in their study who underwent their specific plantar fascia stretching protocol were satisfied with their outcome at 2 years (17).

Night splinting may be an effective addition to the conservative treatment of plantar fasciitis. The night splint prevents shortening of the fascia during sleep which is theorized to be the cause of the increased pain upon awakening seen in patients with plantar fasciitis. Several randomized controlled trials support the usage of night splints (18,19). Batt et al. report on a randomized controlled trial using a tension night splint in addition to Achilles stretching and anti-inflammatory medications and a heel cushion (18). The control group received similar treatment, excluding the night splint, for 8 to 12 weeks. At that point, 11 of 17 patients in the control group who had failed treatment were crossed over into the night splint group. Overall, they reported a 90% rate of success of their conservative approach including the tension night splint. Powell et al.

performed a randomized controlled crossover study using night splint for 1 month (19). They reported improvement in 80% when using night splinting alone.

Shoe inserts of various types have been used to help patients with plantar fasciitis. Little evidence has been found to support that this treatment alters the course of the disease (16). Landorf et al. performed a randomized controlled trial comparing sham orthotics, prefabricated orthotics and custom orthotics (20). They found that custom and prefabricated orthotics resulted in improved function at 3 months when compared to sham orthotics but this difference did not hold up at 1 year. There is little evidence to support expensive custom orthotics for the treatment of plantar fasciitis. Therefore, if shoe inserts are considered, an inexpensive prefabricated heel cushion is recommended.

There is controversy regarding the role of steroid injections for the treatment of plantar fasciitis. Many treating physicians use steroid injections in their treatment regimen for patients who are not progressing with other modalities. While evidence suggests short-term relief of symptoms, there is little to show that steroid injections provide long-term improvement compared with other conservative options (16,21). In addition, various complications have been reported after steroid injection including rupture of the plantar fascia, heel pad atrophy, and nerve injury (7,8,22). Pathologic analysis of the degenerative tissue shows myxoid degeneration and little inflammation which brings the role of steroid injections into question (1).

Extracorporeal shock wave therapy (ESWT) has been advocated as an alternative to surgery in refractory cases of plantar fasciitis. There are several methods used to concentrate and deliver energy including electromagnetic, electrohydraulic and piezoelectric (11). In addition, treatment protocols vary with respect to the amount of energy delivered and the number of treatment sessions required. The shock wave is delivered to the pathologic tissue to break up the degenerative poorly vascularized tissue, evoking inflammation and a healing response. Several randomized controlled trials have showed promising results using shock wave therapy to treat chronic plantar fasciitis (23–30). Patients seem to continue to experience progressive relief over the first year. Chuckpaiwong et al. studied 225 patients who underwent ESWT for recalcitrant plantar fasciitis and noted 70% successful results at 3 months and 77% at 12 months using validated outcome measures (31). In this study, the authors found that negative predictive factors include diabetes mellitus, advanced age and psychological issues. There was no difference in outcome based on body mass index, prior steroid injection, thickness of the plantar fascia, bilateral involvement or duration of symptoms. Longer-term studies have shown that good results are maintained over time. Wang et al. reported on 149 patients follow for over 5 years and showed 82.7% good and excellent results in the group treated with shock wave therapy compared with 55% in the control group. They noted an 11% recurrence rate of heel pain after shock wave therapy. From the literature available, ESWT appears to have a valuable role in the treatment of refractory cases of plantar fasciitis. This treatment modality has been shown to be safe with results comparable to surgical release without the risks related to surgery. It is recommended that at least 6 months of conservative treatment is attempted using at least five different modalities before ESWT is considered as the majority of patients will improve sufficiently over this time frame.

Surgical treatment for plantar fasciitis should only be considered in severe refractory cases after exhausting conservative options over a period of at least 6 to 12 months. Both open and endoscopic techniques have been described. The traditional open technique involves partial release of the medial aspect of the plantar fascia and decompression of the first branch of the lateral plantar nerve. Initially surgeons advocated debridement of the bone spur on the medial aspect of the calcaneus but this has fallen out of favor due to risk of calcaneus fracture and to the growing data suggesting that the bone spur may not be a source of pain (32). Endoscopic techniques involve using an arthroscope to perform partial release of the plantar fascia through a minimal approach. This technique does not allow the surgeon to decompress the lateral plantar nerve. Some reports suggest that recovery may be faster after endoscopic release compared with open surgery (33). In general, good results have been reported with both open (34–43) and endoscopic release (33,44–51) and no well-designed studies have been conducted to differentiate between the two. Most of the published outcomes studies are small case-series with short follow-up and success rates range from 49% to 100%. Daly et al. report medium-term follow-up at an average of 4.5 years (43). An open release was performed in 16 feet and good/excellent results were 71%. They noted sagging of the medial longitudinal arch secondary to the release. Woeffler et al. reported their results of open release in 33 feet at a follow-up of 5 years (41). The rate of patient satisfaction with the procedure was 91%; however, 5 of 30 patients had persistent complications. Ogilvie-Harris et al. reported on their results of endoscopic plantar fascia release in 65 patients with a minimum follow-up of 2 years (49). Eighty-nine percent of patients reported pain relief and 71% returned to unrestricted sports activities. O'Malley et al. performed 20 endoscopic plantar fascia releases and found 90% of patients in their study to have some pain relief however only nine patients reported complete relief. The one patient in their study with no improvement had bilateral involvement and they felt that this may be a risk for a poor outcome. Marafko et al. had 3 complications out of 83 endoscopic releases all of which occurred in obese patients (47).

Baxter et al. reported on the importance of releasing the first branch of the lateral plantar nerve in patients with heel pain (52). Careful preoperative evaluation is therefore necessary to assess for nerve involvement before deciding to proceed with endoscopic procedure. Endoscopic release has been criticized for this reason as well as for an increased risk of incomplete release and potential nerve injury due to difficulties with visualization. Regardless of technique used, it is important to consider that release of even a small portion of the plantar fascia alters the structure and kinematics of the foot (40,43,53–55). Clinical studies have shown sagging of the medial arch after plantar fascia release (40,43). This may lead to postoperative complications including medial pain and overloading of the lateral column (54). Lateral foot pain and even cuboid stress fractures have been reported due to the lateral overload (56). In a cadaveric study, Anderson et al. showed that sectioning of the plantar fascia increased tension in the supporting ligaments of the foot (53). The percentage increase was greatest after the first 25% of the plantar fascia was divided, indicating that partial plantar fascia release may alter foot biomechanics. Brugh et al. compared open and endoscopic plantar fascia release and found no difference in lateral column symptoms between groups (54). They did find a significant increase in symptoms when greater than 50% of the plantar fascia is divided.

Release of the plantar fascia should be reserved for patients with severe heel pain refractory to all forms of conservative treatment. Patients must be counseled that some degree of persistent pain is common and that the complication rate may be greater than 10%. Foot mechanics appear to be altered by even a partial release of the plantar fascia and the long-term sequelae of this are yet to be determined.

Acute plantar fascial ruptures should be treated conservatively (6,7). An initial period of immobilization in a walking boot non–weight-bearing is recommended depending on the patient's symptoms. As pain and swelling subside, weight bearing is progressed as tolerated. Saxena et al. described their experience in treating 18 athletes with a plantar fascia rupture at a mean follow-up of 42 months (6). They recommended 2 to 3 weeks of non–weight-bearing and then 2 to 3 weeks of weight bearing in a walking boot. The average time to return to activities was 9.1 months. Leach et al. reported on six athletes with rupture of the plantar fascia (7). Five patients responded to conservative treatment and one developed a painful swollen mass of fibroblastic tissue that responded to surgical excision and the patient was able to return to long-distance running.

HEEL PAD INJURY

The heel pad is a unique structure that cushions the heel during weight bearing. The heel pad consists of organized fibroelastic septae that divide the fat of the heel into vertical columns. The fibrous septae divide the adipose tissue into small chambers that resist compression and anchor the heel pad to the skin and underlying calcaneus. The unique organization of the heel pad allows it to resist shear and compression during weight-bearing activities. However, this tissue has a poor capacity for healing. The complex structure and organization that is critical for proper function is permanently lost if disrupted. The heel pad is capable of absorbing several times the body weight without sustaining damage. Usually, a fall from a significant height is required to disrupt the structure of the heel pad. However, repetitive trauma or a lower-energy injury may cause pain localized to the heel pad. Pain is generally diffuse across the plantar surface of the heel and may have associated signs of inflammation including erythema and swelling. More significant injury, especially when disruption of the fibrous architecture occurs, may present with fluctuance and ecchymosis. This may represent a separation of the heel pad from the calcaneus and hematoma formation.

Acute injuries are treated symptomatically and workup should include radiographs to rule out fracture. Cold therapy, splinting and limited weight bearing may be used initially as needed. Return to sports is slowly progressed once the pain and swelling has subsided. In more chronic situations, assessment of shoe wear and playing surface should be performed to look for factors that may be contributing to delayed recovery. In addition, the physical examination should focus on structural evaluation including arch height and tightness of the Achilles tendon. When significant disruption of the heel pad is suspected, diagnosis may be aided by ultrasound or MRI to evaluate for thinning or loss of the adipose tissue and formation of scar tissue. Rehabilitation should include an appropriate period of rest and cessation of aggravating activities, progressing to a program of stretching and strengthening. Soft shoe inserts and supportive shoe wear may also be beneficial in allowing return to activities without recurrence. Severe disruption of the heel pad may result in significant long-term functional limitations.

STRESS FRACTURE

Stress fractures occur relatively commonly in the hindfoot and usually follow an increase or change in level of training or activity. This condition represents a spectrum of injury ranging from edema seen on MRI to complete fracture evident on radiographs. Niva et al. reported on a series of athletes with stress fractures in the foot and ankle (57). They use MRI to diagnose the stress injury and found 88% to have low-grade injuries (edema on MRI) and 12% with high-grade (fracture line evident on MRI). In their series, the talus was involved in 39% and the calcaneus in 23%. More than one bone was involved in 63%. Evaluation begins with a history which should include the level of training and recent changes, shoe wear, dietary habits, and medical history. Physical examination may reveal swelling, focal tenderness and in the case of a calcaneal stress fracture, the "squeeze test" will elicit increased pain. This test is performed by squeezing or compressing the medial and lateral sides of the calcaneus. Radiographs should be obtained and may show a fracture line or sclerosis in the area of a healing fracture. However, many patients will have negative radiographs, especially early in the disease process, so a high index of suspicion for this condition is necessary. Additional imaging with a bone scan or MRI is helpful in confirming the diagnosis (Fig. 21.1). Studies have shown that magnetic resonance imaging is more specific than bone scan and also can show other pathology that may be contributing to the symptoms (53,58,59).

Treatment usually involves a period of non–weight-bearing in a cast or walking boot. When symptoms have resolved, slow progression back to walking followed by more strenuous activities is allowed. Potential factors contributing to the injury including improper shoe wear, nutrition, and training habits should be identified and addressed. Healing may be followed by radiographs or a repeat MRI (57). The follow-up MRI should show a resolution of edema and any fracture line that was previously seen. Recovery may take several months and recurrence of the stress injury is possible if return to activities is too aggressive. Controversy exists regarding the benefit of bone stimulators in the treatment of stress fractures. This topic is addressed further in Chapter 20.

SUBTALAR INSTABILITY

The subtalar joint includes the articulation of the talus and calcaneus. Stability is provided by the conforming bony articulations and the intrinsic and extrinsic ligaments (60). Cadaveric studies have demonstrated the importance of these ligaments in maintaining stability of the subtalar joint (61–68). The intrinsic ligaments between the talus and calcaneus include the interosseous and cervical ligaments. Extrinsic support is provided by the CFL and the tibio-calcaneal portion of the

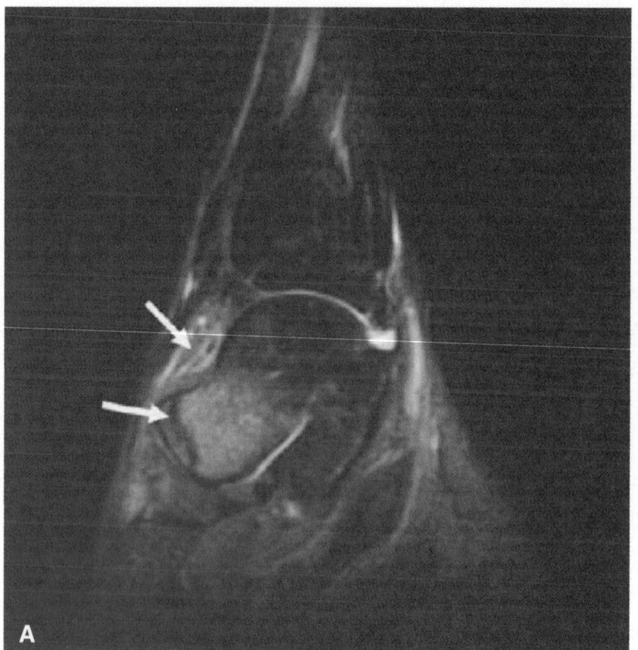

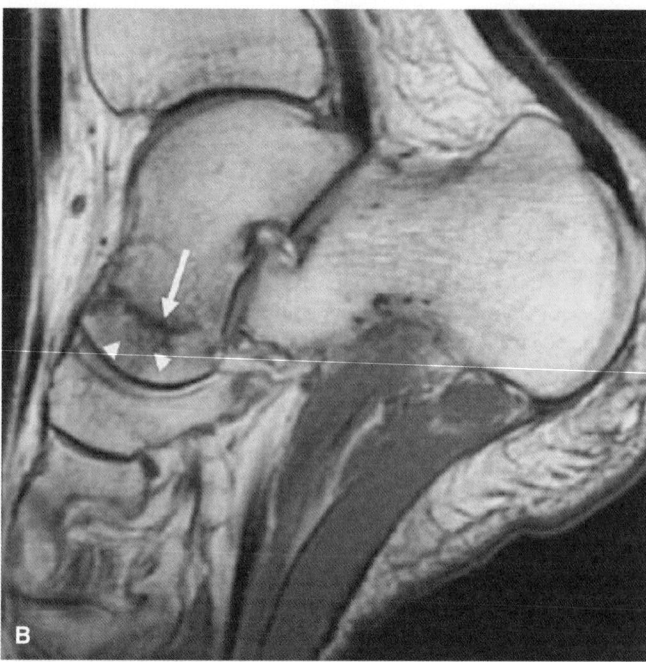

Figure 21.1. MRI images **(A, B)** demonstrating a talar stress fracture in a 19-year-old male with 20 days of ankle pain. Adapted from A: Niva MH, Sormaala MJ, Kiuru MJ, Haataja R, Ahovuo JA, Pihlajamaki HK.Bone stress injuries of the ankle and foot: an 86-month magnetic resonance imaging-based study of physically active young adults. *Am J Sports Med.* 2007 Apr;35(4):643–649. B: Rockwook, Green. *Fractures in Adults.* 4th ed., Figure 32–67. Lippincott Williams & Wilkins, April 1996.

deltoid ligament (66–68). The bony and ligamentous anatomy of the subtalar joint establishes a complex motion pattern that couples plantarflexion supination and inversion in one direction and dorsiflexion pronation and eversion in the other (69). Instability of the subtalar joint can range from subtle instability following chronic sprains to complete dislocation of the talocalcaneal and talonavicular joints.

Subtalar instability and subluxation may develop after multiple ankle sprains. Inversion- and supination-type injuries that stretch and tear the lateral ligaments may affect both the ankle and subtalar joints. The anterior talofibular ligament (ATFL) and CFL are commonly torn in ankle sprains and may have residual laxity after multiple injuries. Without the CFL to extrinsically support the subtalar joint, increased load may be placed on the intrinsic ligaments which may become attenuated over time. In a cadaveric study, Heilman et al. noted that sectioning of the CFL alone resulted in 5 mm of subtalar joint opening on stress radiographs (66). Additional release of the interosseous ligament increased the subtalar joint displacement to 7 mm. Tochigi et al. performed a cadaveric study to further evaluate the role of the interosseous talocalcaneal ligament (63). They noted that sectioning of the interosseous ligament increases laxity within the subtalar joint and multi-directional testing showed the axis of greatest displacement to be from lateral at the posterior border of the fibula, medially towards the center of the medial malleolus. Drawer testing should be performed in this direction to test for interosseous ligament integrity.

Patients with subtalar instability may present with a history of prior ankle sprains resulting in persistent pain and difficulty ambulating or running on uneven surfaces. A history of prior subtalar dislocation is less common but has been reported in athletes (70–74). A separate entity of subluxation of the subtalar joint has been reported in dancers. Menetrey et al. reported on 25 cases of subluxation of the subtalar joint in dancers while in the en pointe or demi-pointe position (75). They described a posteromedial subluxation of the joint when in a fully plantarflexed position. The dancers were found to have decreased subtalar motion and pain at the talonavicular and hindfoot joints. They were treated conservatively with a closed reduction and taping. The authors of this study hypothesized that subtalar subluxation in ballet dancers is related to the possibility that in the fully plantarflexed position, the main stabilizing ligaments are not oriented appropriately to resist axial loading.

Radiographic evaluation of subtalar subluxation begins with standard radiographs of the foot and ankle to rule out fixed subluxation, dislocation or fracture (Fig. 21.2). Stress radiographs have been shown to be beneficial in diagnosis (76–79). Broden's view with 40 degrees of cephalic tilt is taken with inversion stress applied to the calcaneus. In this view, the articular surfaces of the talus and calcaneus will appear parallel. With instability of the joint, opening will be evident on this stress radiograph. In addition, a standard lateral view of the ankle and subtalar joint may be taken with an applied anterior drawer load. This may show anterior translation of the ankle and subtalar joints. Comparison views of the normal side may help determine if the translation is pathologic. Authors have also reported on the value of arthrography in the diagnosis of subtalar instability (80,81). Sugimoto et al. used subtalar arthrography to assess for CFL injury and confirmed the diagnosis during surgery (81). They reported 92% sensitivity and 88% specificity for diagnosis of a CFL injury using their technique. MRI has become an increasingly popular diagnostic modality and may be helpful in evaluating ligament integrity. However, when evaluating subtalar instability, ligament injury alone as seen on MRI may not be enough to guide treatment. The majority of patients function very well after ankle and

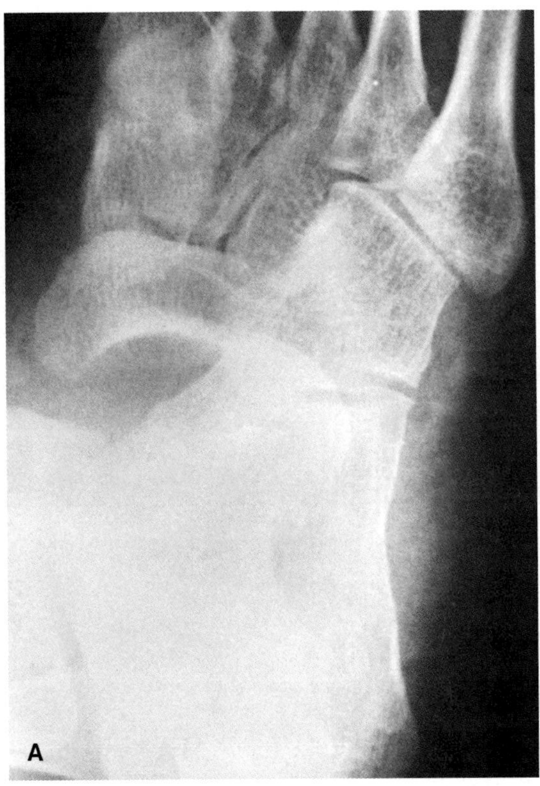

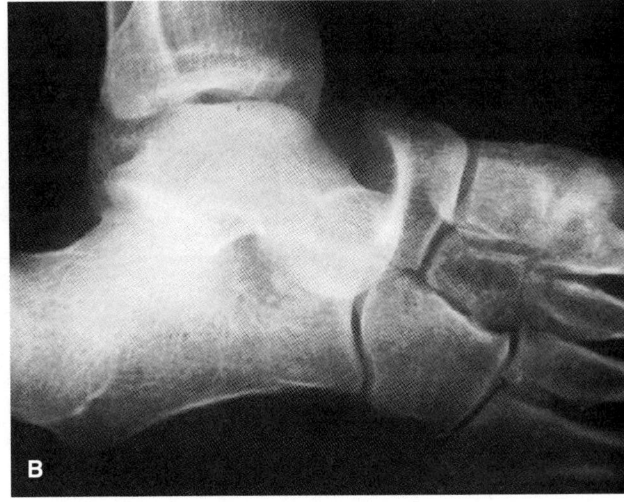

Figure 21.2. Anteroposterior and lateral radiographs **(A, B)** showing a medial subtalar dislocation. Adapted from Rockwook, Green. *Fractures in Adults.* 4th ed., 2319, Figure 32–67. Lippincott Williams & Wilkins, April 1996.

subtalar sprains. Diagnosing the functional instability as seen on stress radiographs or fluoroscopy is more valuable when considering ligament reconstruction (Fig. 21.3).

As with ankle sprains, the treatment of subtalar instability is primarily non-operative. Initial injuries should be treated symptomatically with ice, elevation, bracing and limited weight bearing. As symptoms subside, the patient is progressed to full

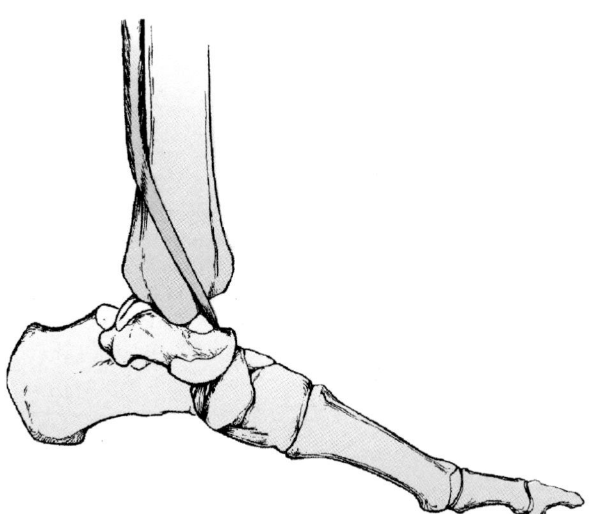

Figure 21.3. Lateral subtalar dislocation with interposed posterior tibialis tendon. Adapted from Rockwook, Green. *Fractures in Adults.* 4th ed., 2321, Figure 32–70.

weight bearing. In severe injuries or in patients with a history of recurrent sprains, a rehabilitation program may be of benefit before returning to sports. Stretching and strengthening as well as proprioceptive training are performed to enable safe return to play. In recurrent cases, ankle bracing, taping and shoe modification may be helpful in providing the athlete with an additional sense of support although there is little scientific evidence that this changes the natural history.

For patients who fail conservative treatment, reconstruction of the ligaments may be considered. Careful clinical and radiographic evaluation is critical to determine which structures are injured. In most cases, the ATFL is injured in addition to the CFL. When no prior surgery has been performed, a modified Brostrom procedure is usually sufficient to restore stability. In this procedure, a curved incision is made over the distal fibula, curving anteriorly towards the base of the fourth metatarsal (Fig. 21.4). Subcutaneous flaps are developed taking care not to violate the fibular periosteum or capsule distally. The ATFL, CFL and anterolateral capsule are released off of the fibular tip as a single sleeve taking care to release directly off bone, maintaining length and thickness of the tissue. The deep aspect of the CFL is released until the peroneal tendons are visualized. Next, a periosteal flap is elevated off the lateral surface of the fibula from distal to proximal. The bony surface is roughened to encourage healing. Two to three small bioabsorbable anchors loaded with number 2 non-absorbable sutures are inserted into the bone. The sutures are passed in a horizontal mattress fashion through the capsular flap and tied while holding an eversion force on the hindfoot. This reduces the ATFL, CFL and capsule down to bone. By passing

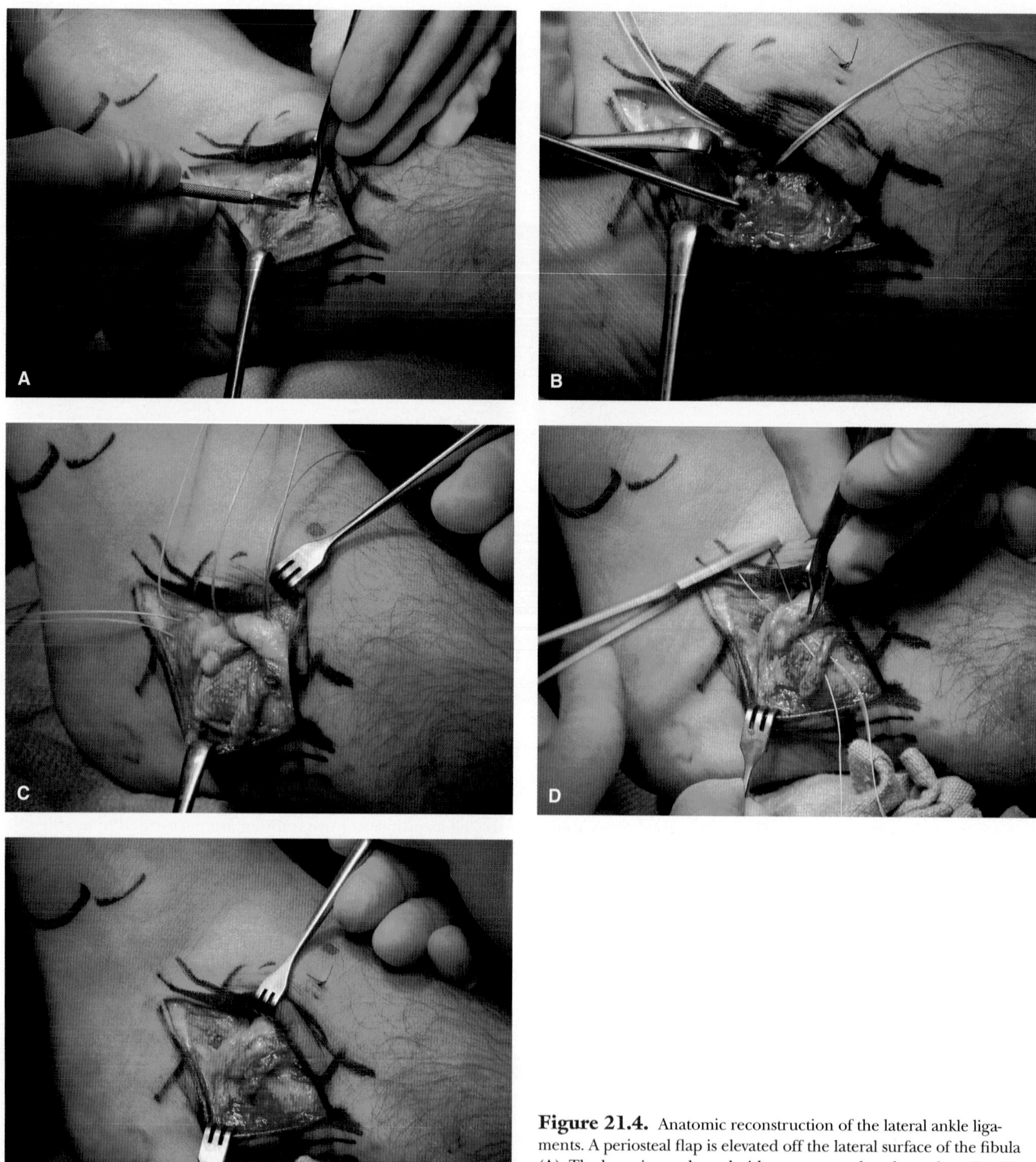

Figure 21.4. Anatomic reconstruction of the lateral ankle ligaments. A periosteal flap is elevated off the lateral surface of the fibula **(A)**. The bone is roughened with a curette and anchors place **(B)**. The sutures are passed through the sleeve of capsule including the ligaments in a horizontal fashion **(C)**. The proximal edge of the capsular sleeve is repaired to the flap of periosteum **(D)** completing the repair **(E)**.

the mattress sutures about 1 cm distal to the proximal edge of the capsular flap, the structures are effectively tightened. The proximal edge of the sleeve is then repaired to the periosteal flap with 2-0 absorbable sutures. We recommend routine ankle arthroscopy before ligament repair to allow for debridement of scar tissue and treatment of any cartilage lesion. After closure, the patient is placed in a plaster splint which is changed in the office to a walking boot. The patient is kept non–weight-bearing for 4 weeks. Weight bearing is then progressed using the walking boot and physical therapy is initiated. Return to sports that involve lateral cutting is allowed at 4 to 6 months after surgery. Karlsson et al. reviewed their results of treating a series of 22 patients with subtalar instability by imbricating the CFL and cervical ligament and reinforcing the repair with the inferior extensor retinaculum (82). They reported good or excellent results in 82% and noted injury to the lateral branch of the superficial peroneal nerve in three patients.

When patients have failed a prior anatomic repair and have persistent symptoms despite prolonged conservative treatment, a ligament reconstruction is indicated. Several techniques have been described to reconstruct the lateral ligaments (83–87). Graft options include the plantaris, a split peroneus brevis and allograft. Careful preoperative evaluation is required to determine which ligaments require reconstruction. Most patients will present with a combined ankle and subtalar instability where both the ATFL and CFL are insufficient. Based on the current literature, it is unclear which ligaments should be reconstructed when subtalar instability is seen on stress radiographs. The goal of reconstruction is to reproduce the ligamentous anatomy as closely as possible to restore stability without over-constraining the joint. Analysis of non-anatomic procedures such as the Chrisman–Snook reconstruction has shown that the subtalar joint motion may be limited which can lead to pain, dysfunction and arthritis (84,88).

Takao et al. described an anatomical reconstruction of the ATFL and CFL using a gracilis graft from the ipsilateral knee using interference screws for fixation (89). Four patients underwent reconstruction of both the ATFL and CFL in their series and they were found to have significantly an improved talocalcaneal angle on stress radiographs at 2 years. Authors have also recommended reconstructing the interosseous and/or cervical ligament in patients with subtalar instability (89,90). The decision to reconstruct these ligaments can be made intraoperatively. The CFL (and ATFL as indicated) is reconstructed and stress testing is then performed using fluoroscopy. If stress testing reveals persistent increased talar tilt, the cervical ligament is reconstructed. The graft is extended from the ATFL's distal docking site to the anterolateral calcaneus at the insertion of the cervical ligament.

Subtalar dislocations represent a serious injury and may have significant morbidity. Initial treatment is prompt closed reduction after radiographs are performed to rule-out fracture and to document the direction of dislocation. There have been several reports of subtalar dislocation in basketball players and this injury has been termed "basketball foot" in the past (70,71,91). Medial dislocation is most common in athletes and usually results from coming down from a jump with the foot in supination and inversion. The reduction maneuver is performed by bringing the ankle into plantarflexion and pulling traction on the foot. Next, the foot is pronated and dorsiflexed and a reduction should be felt. Post-reduction radiographs should be performed to confirm complete reduction and to rule out a fracture that may have been missed on the injury films. A short period of immobilization and limited weight bearing is recommended (2 to 3 weeks). Recurrence is rare but has been reported (71). Rehabilitation is performed with the goal of restoring full motion, strength and balance before returning to sport. Occasionally a subtalar dislocation may be irreducible. In medial dislocations, the most common cause is perforation of the talar head through the extensor digitorum brevis (92). In irreducible lateral dislocations, the posterior tibialis tendon is the most common block to reduction (Fig. 21.3). In either case, open treatment in the operating room is indicated to achieve congruent reduction. Postoperative treatment does not differ from the protocol described for rehabilitation after closed reduction.

SINUS TARSI SYNDROME

Sinus tarsi syndrome is a general term that describes pain localized to the tarsal sinus. The true etiology of this condition has yet to be determined and is most likely multifactorial. It may represent a subtle form of subtalar instability due to injury to the interosseous or cervical ligament (93–95). Other potential causes for pain localized to the sinus tarsi are synovitis, arthrofibrosis, soft tissue impingement, nerve alterations, injury to the extensor digitorum brevis and ganglion cyst formation. Patients complain of pain and have focal tenderness over the sinus tarsi. Some patients report an inversion injury preceding the onset of pain. Occasionally swelling will be present but very few other objective findings are common.

Radiographs are usually negative in this condition. MRI may show ligament injury, fibrosis, changes in the fatty tissue, synovitis or ganglion cyst formation (93). An injection of local anesthetic and steroid is a very useful diagnostic and therapeutic tool. Conservative treatment including shoe modification, anti-inflammatory medications, bracing, activity modification, physical therapy and steroid injections should be attempted before surgery is considered. Surgery should be avoided in patients who do not have temporary relief after injection into the sinus tarsi. Open debridement of the sinus tarsi may be performed by excising the fat pad and exposing the subtalar joint by elevating the extensor digitorum brevis. Joint pathology may be addressed and the interosseous and cervical ligaments may be directly assessed. Several authors have used subtalar arthroscopy in the diagnosis and treatment of sinus tarsi syndrome (93,94,96). Lee et al. reported on 31 patients (33 feet) treated arthroscopically for sinus tarsi syndrome with a mean follow-up of 24 months (94). They found partial interosseous ligament tears in 88% and synovitis in 55% of cases. Other pathology noted included partial tearing of the cervical ligament, arthrofibrosis and soft tissue impingement. They reported 87% good and excellent results based on American Orthopaedic Foot and Ankle Society (AOFAS) scores.

FRACTURE OF THE LATERAL PROCESS OF THE TALUS

Fracture of the lateral process of the talus should be suspected in athletes with acute injuries resulting in pain, swelling and ecchymosis localized to the lateral aspect of the ankle. This injury is most commonly seen in snowboarders and the mechanism of injury is felt to be axial loading in dorsiflexion–eversion (97,98). Lateral process fractures and stress injuries have also been reported in runners and dancers (98–102). It is important to have a high index of suspicion for this injury as they are often confused with ankle sprains. It has been reported that up to 40% of lateral process fractures are missed initially (97). Patients complain of lateral ankle pain, swelling and bruising and have focal tenderness over the lateral process which is found just distal and slightly anterior to the tip of the lateral malleolus. Radiographic evaluation includes anteroposterior, lateral and mortise views of the ankle as well as Broden's views

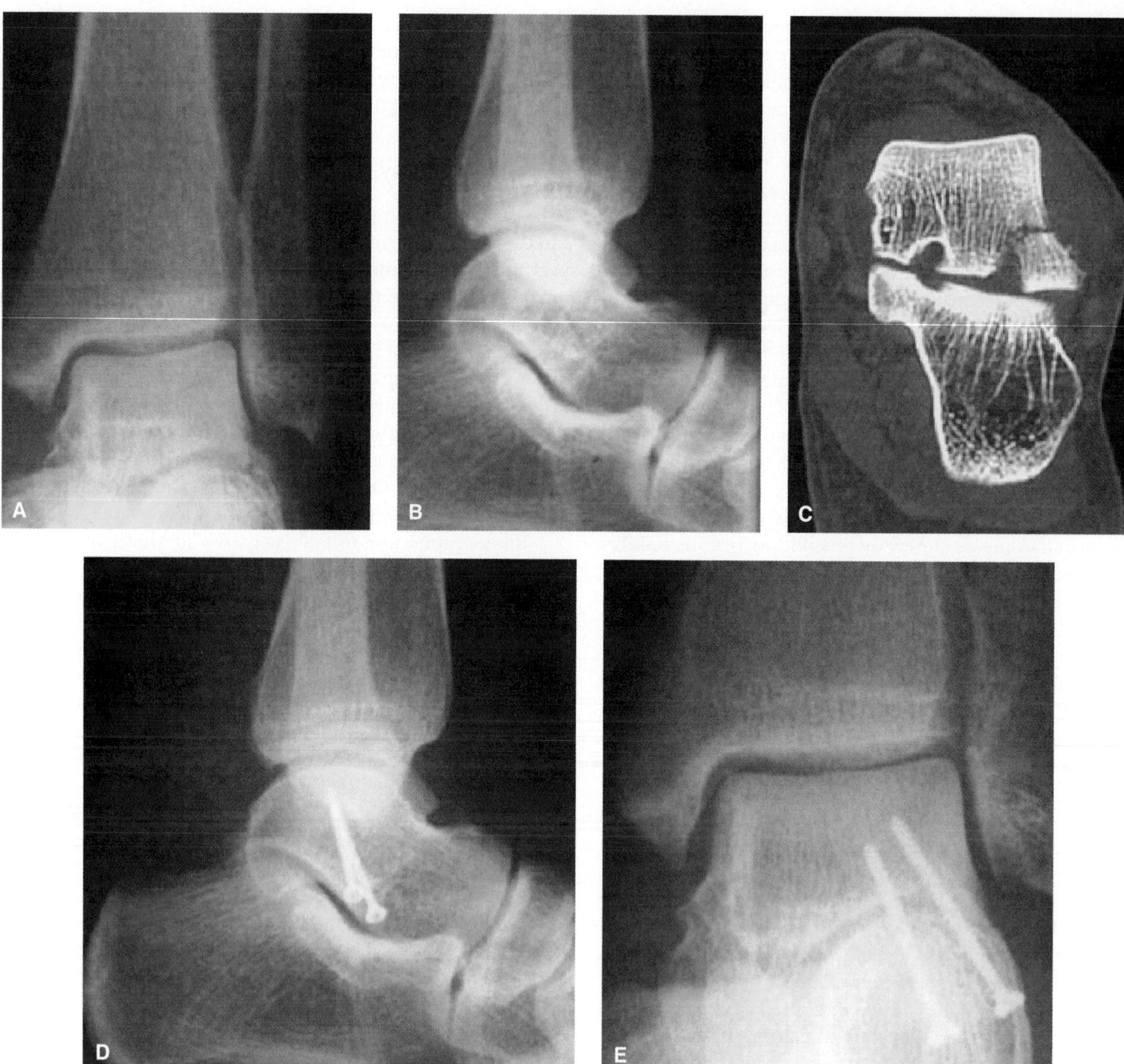

Figure 21.5. Anteroposterior **(A)** and lateral views **(B)** of the ankle showing a lateral process of the talus fracture in a snowboarder. A CT scan **(C)** clearly demonstrates the fracture. Postoperative radiographs show anatomic fixation with two small-fragment screws **(D, E)**. Adapted from Valderrabano V, Perren T, Ryf C, Rillmann P, Hintermann B. Snowboarder's talus fracture: treatment outcome of 20 cases after 3.5 years. *Am J Sports Med* Jun 2005;33(6):871–880. Epub 2005 Apr 12.

of the subtalar joint. Radiographic evaluation of fragment size and displacement is difficult and if a fracture is seen, a CT scan is usually obtained to further characterize the fracture.

Treatment is based on fracture-fragment size, articular involvement and degree of displacement. Non-operative treatment is recommended for small, non-displaced or comminuted extraarticular fragments. Larger fragments that are displaced more than 2 mm are treated operatively, especially if the articular surface is involved (98,103). When surgery is indicated, open reduction and internal fixation of t he fracture is performed if the fragment is large enough. Screw fixation is usually adequate to stabilize the fracture (Fig. 21.5). When there is significant comminution present, fixation may not be possible and debridement of the fragments may be performed to prevent painful non-union.

Despite prompt diagnosis and appropriate treatment, patients with these injuries often have persistent problems long term. Valderbanno et al. reported on 20 cases of lateral process fracture at 42-months follow-up (98). They found good or excellent results in 90% and found significantly better outcomes in patients treated surgically. Eighty percent were able to return to sports activities and 35% reported continued pain with demanding activities. In this series, 15% showed signs of subtalar arthritis on follow-up radiographs.

OS TRIGONUM

The os trigonum is an ossicle in the posterolateral ankle (Fig. 21.6). It is felt to represent a non-united portion of the posterior process of the talus. A general term, posterior

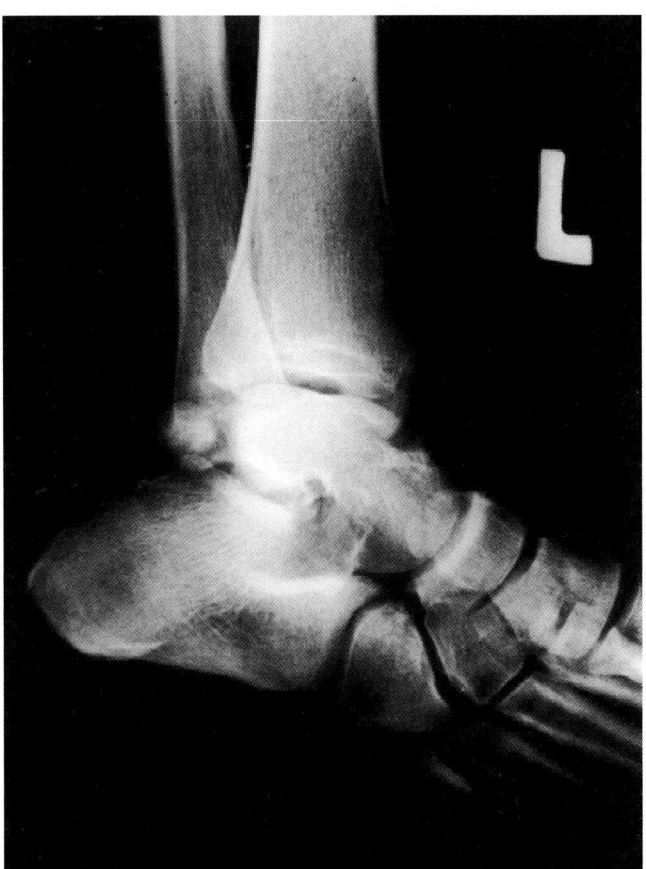

Figure 21.6. Lateral view of the ankle showing an os trigonum posterior to the talus. Adapted from Abramowitz Y. *J Bone Joint Surg Am* 2003;85:1051–1057 (on page 1052, Figure 1)

impingement, has been used to describe pain in the posterolateral ankle due to weight bearing in plantarflexion. This may include impingement of the posterior talus, an os trigonum or a Stieda process (a large posterior process of the talus representing a fused os trigonum) between the posterior tibia and calcaneus. This condition has most commonly been reported in ballet dancers due to the demi-pointe and en pointe positions (99). Tendonitis or stenosing tenosynovitis of the flexor hallucis longus is in the differential diagnosis and also may commonly coexist with posterior impingement. Patients with posterior impingement complain of pain in the posterolateral ankle and may have localized swelling. The condition is usually directly related to the aggravating activity that involves forced plantarflexion and period of rest may result in resolution of symptoms. Focal tenderness is present between the Achilles tendon and the peroneal tendons overlying the talus.

Standard ankle radiographs should be obtained. The lateral projection will show a well-circumscribed ossicle with smooth-appearing edges posterior to the talus in the case of an os trigonum. Careful assessment of the ossicle must be made so that a posterior process fracture is not missed. A CT scan may be helpful in ruling out a fracture. An injection of local anesthetic in the area of the ossicle may aid in diagnosis.

Treatment begins with rest and activity modification to avoid extreme plantarflexion. Bracing or casting may be helpful in more severe cases. After symptoms have resolved, return to activities is progressed. If prolonged immobilization is used, a period of rehabilitation may be beneficial before returning to activities to achieve full strength and normal proprioception. Steroid injections may also be considered in refractory cases. Care must be taken to avoid injecting the steroid into or around the nearby tendons due to the risk of rupture.

If symptoms persist and are limiting the patient's activities, surgery may be considered. Excision of the ossicle is performed through an incision posterior to the fibula. The sural nerve is identified and protected and the os trigonum or Stieda process is exposed and excised. The ossicle is localized just lateral to the fibro-osseous tunnel of the flexor hallucis longus. After excision of the os trigonum, the FHL should be inspected for damage. Postoperatively the patient is placed in a soft dressing and is non–weight-bearing. At follow-up, the patient is placed in a walking boot and weight bearing is progressed as tolerated. Physical therapy is initiated for early range of motion and progressing to strengthening as tolerated. Return to full activities may take up to 6 months (99).

Marotta et al. retrospectively reviewed their results of excision of an os trigonum in 15 dancers with a mean follow-up of 28 months (102). All patients reported improvement in their impingement symptoms although 67% still reported occasional pain with activities. The average return to full activities was 3 months in this series. Hamilton et al. published their results in treating 41 ankles in 37 dancers with posterior impingement (99). Twenty-six patients were treated for posterior impingement and FHL tendonitis, nine for only tendonitis and six for only posterior impingement. At 7-years follow-up, 75% had good or excellent results.

FLEXOR HALLUCIS LONGUS TENDONITIS

Tendonitis and stenosing tenosynovitis may be a cause of posterior ankle pain in athletes and is most commonly reported in ballet dancers (99). Pain is localized to the posteromedial ankle adjacent to the Achilles tendon. Swelling may be present in this area. Physical examination findings may include tenderness over the posteromedial ankle, pain with great toe extension and limited dorsiflexion of the great toe interphalangeal joint especially when the ankle is dorsiflexed. Triggering may occur with toe motion in some cases. Imaging studies are usually negative; however, MRI may demonstrate inflammation, partial tearing or thickening of the FHL.

Treatment options are similar to those described for posterior impingement. A period of immobilization and cessation of aggravating activities is usually helpful in managing painful FHL tendonitis. When the initial symptoms subside, stretching and strengthening is progressed. If the condition is due to an acute injury or inflammation from overuse, conservative treatment is often successful. However, if the pain is more chronic in nature and is due to tendinosis and tendon degeneration, results of treatment are less predictable. In these cases, return to ballet dancing or other high-demand activities may be difficult. Steroid injections are usually avoided due to the risk of tendon rupture or injury to the neurovascular bundle.

Surgical treatment is reserved for refractory cases. Preoperatively, evaluation for an os trigonum should be performed and assessed for symptoms because this may be easily addressed in the same surgical setting (99). The FHL is approached through a curved incision on the medial edge of the Achilles tendon that follows the posterior border of the neurovascular bundle. The FHL muscle belly is identified proximally adjacent to the Achilles tendon and is followed distally as it enters its fibro-osseous tunnel. Correct identification is confirmed by flexing and extending the great toe IP joint. The tendon is released down to the sustentaculum tali and is inspected for abnormalities. Partial tears may be repaired and myxoid-appearing degenerative tissue may be debrided. If an os trigonum is present and excision is planned, it may be approached from the same incision by dissecting laterally in the retrocalcaneal space deep to the Achilles. Hamilton et al. reported their results in treating ballet dancers with posterior ankle pain. Nine had surgical treatment of FHL tendonitis and 26 had treatment of FHL tendonitis and an os trigonum. At 7-years follow-up, 75% had good or excellent results and 88% were satisfied with their outcome.

SUMMARY

Hindfoot pain and injuries are common in athletes. Most conditions encountered are related to overuse and will respond to conservative treatment. Contributing factors such as aggravating activities, training schedule, shoe wear, playing surface and lower extremity alignment should be considered when formulating a treatment plan. In athletes with acute sprains or injuries, careful assessment must be performed so that instability or fracture is not overlooked.

REFERENCES

1. Lemont H, Ammirati KM, Usen N. Plantar fasciitis: a degenerative process (fasciosis) without inflammation. *J Am Podiatr Med Assoc* 2003;93(3):234–237.
2. Riddle DL, Pulisic M, Pidcoe P, et al. Risk factors for plantar fasciitis: a matched case-control study. *J Bone Joint Surg Am* 2003;85-A(5):872–877.
3. Inman VT, Ralston HJ, Todd F. *Human Walking.* Baltimore, MD: Williams and Wilkins; 1981.
4. Sarrafian SK. Functional characteristics of the foot and plantar aponeurosis under tibiotalar loading. *Foot Ankle* 1987;8(1):4–18.
5. Wright DG, Rennels DC. A study of the elastic properties of plantar fascia. *J Bone Joint Surg Am* 1964;46:482–492.
6. Saxena A, Fullem B. Plantar fascia ruptures in athletes. *Am J Sports Med* 2004;32(3):662–665.
7. Leach R, Jones R, Silva T. Rupture of the plantar fascia in athletes. *J Bone Joint Surg Am* 1978;60(4):537–539.
8. Acevedo JI, Beskin JL. Complications of plantar fascia rupture associated with corticosteroid injection. *Foot Ankle Int* 1998;19(2):91–97.
9. Herrick RT, Herrick S. Rupture of the plantar fascia in a middle-aged tennis player. A case report. *Am J Sports Med* 1983;11(2):95.
10. Sellman JR. Plantar fascia rupture associated with corticosteroid injection. *Foot Ankle Int* 1994;15(7):376–381.
11. Ogden JA, Alvarez RG, Levitt RL, et al. Electrohydraulic high-energy shock-wave treatment for chronic plantar fasciitis. *J Bone Joint Surg Am* 2004;86-A(10):2216–2228.
12. Lee GP, Ogden JA, Cross GL. Effect of extracorporeal shock waves on calcaneal bone spurs. *Foot Ankle Int* 2003;24(12):927–930.
13. Forman WM, Green MA. The role of intrinsic musculature in the formation of inferior calcaneal exostoses. *Clin Podiatr Med Surg* 1990;7(2):217–223.
14. Davis PF, Severud E, Baxter DE. Painful heel syndrome: results of nonoperative treatment. *Foot Ankle Int* 1994;15(10):531–535.
15. DiGiovanni BF, Nawoczenski DA, Lintal ME, et al. Tissue-specific plantar fascia-stretching exercise enhances outcomes in patients with chronic heel pain. A prospective, randomized study. *J Bone Joint Surg Am* 2003;85-A(7):1270–1277.
16. Crawford F, Thomson C. Interventions for treating plantar heel pain. *Cochrane Database Syst Rev* 2003;(3):CD000416.
17. Digiovanni BF, Nawoczenski DA, Malay DP, et al. Plantar fascia-specific stretching exercise improves outcomes in patients with chronic plantar fasciitis. A prospective clinical trial with two-year follow-up. *J Bone Joint Surg Am* 2006;88(8):1775–1781.
18. Batt ME, Tanji JL, Skattum N. Plantar fasciitis: a prospective randomized clinical trial of the tension night splint. *Clin J Sport Med* 1996;6(3):158–162.
19. Powell M, Post WR, Keener J, et al. Effective treatment of chronic plantar fasciitis with dorsiflexion night splints: a crossover prospective randomized outcome study. *Foot Ankle Int* 1998;19(1):10–18.
20. Landorf KB, Keenan AM, Herbert RD. Effectiveness of foot orthoses to treat plantar fasciitis: a randomized trial. *Arch Intern Med* 2006;166(12):1305–1310.
21. Miller RA, Torres J, McGuire M. Efficacy of first-time steroid injection for painful heel syndrome. *Foot Ankle Int* 1995;16(10):610–612.
22. Snow DM, Reading J, Dalal R. Lateral plantar nerve injury following steroid injection for plantar fasciitis. *Br J Sports Med* 2005;39(12):e41; discussion e41.
23. Ogden JA, Toth-Kischkat A, Schultheiss R. Principles of shock wave therapy. *Clin Orthop Relat Res* 2001;387(387):8–17.
24. Rompe JD, Schoellner C, Nafe B. Evaluation of low-energy extracorporeal shock-wave application for treatment of chronic plantar fasciitis. *J Bone Joint Surg Am* 2002;84-A(3):335–341.
25. Wang CJ, Wang FS, Yang KD, et al. Long-term results of extracorporeal shockwave treatment for plantar fasciitis. *Am J Sports Med* 2006;34(4):592–596.
26. Gerdesmeyer L, Frey C, Vester J, et al. Radial extracorporeal shock wave therapy is safe and effective in the treatment of chronic recalcitrant plantar fasciitis: results of a confirmatory randomized placebo-controlled multicenter study. *Am J Sports Med* 2008;36(11):2100–2109.
27. Theodore GH, Buch M, Amendola A, et al. Extracorporeal shock wave therapy for the treatment of plantar fasciitis. *Foot Ankle Int* 2004;25(5):290–297.
28. Rompe JD, Decking J, Schoellner C, et al. Shock wave application for chronic plantar fasciitis in running athletes. A prospective, randomized, placebo-controlled trial. *Am J Sports Med* 2003;31(2):268–275.
29. Malay DS, Pressman MM, Assili A, et al. Extracorporeal shockwave therapy versus placebo for the treatment of chronic proximal plantar fasciitis: results of a randomized, placebo-controlled, double-blinded, multicenter intervention trial. *J Foot Ankle Surg* 2006;45(4):196–210.
30. Gollwitzer H, Diehl P, von Korff A, et al. Extracorporeal shock wave therapy for chronic painful heel syndrome: a prospective, double blind, randomized trial assessing the efficacy of a new electromagnetic shock wave device. *J Foot Ankle Surg* 2007;46(5):348–357.
31. Chuckpaiwong B, Berkson EM, Theodore GH. Extracorporeal shock wave for chronic proximal plantar fasciitis: 225 patients with results and outcome predictors. *J Foot Ankle Surg* 2009;48(2):148–155.
32. Jerosch J. Endoscopic release of plantar fasciitis–a benign procedure? *Foot Ankle Int* 2000;21(6):511–513.
33. Kinley S, Frascone S, Calderone D, et al. Endoscopic plantar fasciotomy versus traditional heel spur surgery: a prospective study. *J Foot Ankle Surg* 1993;32(6):595–603.
34. Sinnaeve F, Vandeputte G. Clinical outcome of surgical intervention for recalcitrant infero-medial heel pain. *Acta Orthop Belg* 2008;74(4):483–488.
35. Conflitti JM, Tarquinio TA. Operative outcome of partial plantar fasciectomy and neurolysis to the nerve of the abductor digiti minimi muscle for recalcitrant plantar fasciitis. *Foot Ankle Int* 2004;25(7):482–487.
36. Brown JN, Roberts S, Taylor M, et al. Plantar fascia release through a transverse plantar incision. *Foot Ankle Int* 1999;20(6):364–367.
37. Sammarco GJ, Helfrey RB. Surgical treatment of recalcitrant plantar fasciitis. *Foot Ankle Int* 1996;17(9):520–526.
38. Lester DK, Buchanan JR. Surgical treatment of plantar fasciitis. *Clin Orthop Relat Res* 1984;(186):202–204.
39. Fishco WD, Goecker RM, Schwartz RI. The instep plantar fasciotomy for chronic plantar fasciitis. A retrospective review. *J Am Podiatr Med Assoc* 2000;90(2):66–69.
40. Jarde O, Diebold P, Havet E, et al. Degenerative lesions of the plantar fascia: surgical treatment by fasciectomy and excision of the heel spur. A report on 38 cases. *Acta Orthop Belg* 2003;69(3):267–274.
41. Woelffer KE, Figura MA, Sandberg NS, et al. Five-year follow-up results of instep plantar fasciotomy for chronic heel pain. *J Foot Ankle Surg* 2000;39(4):218–223.
42. Gormley J, Kuwada GT. Retrospective analysis of calcaneal spur removal and complete fascial release for the treatment of chronic heel pain. *J Foot Surg* 1992;31(2):166–169.
43. Daly PJ, Kitaoka HB, Chao EY. Plantar fasciotomy for intractable plantar fasciitis: clinical results and biomechanical evaluation. *Foot Ankle* 1992;13(4):188–195.
44. Urovitz EP, Birk-Urovitz A, Birk-Urovitz E. Endoscopic plantar fasciotomy in the treatment of chronic heel pain. *Can J Surg* 2008;51(4):281–283.
45. Lundeen RO, Aziz S, Burks JB, et al. Endoscopic plantar fasciotomy: a retrospective analysis of results in 53 patients. *J Foot Ankle Surg* 2000;39(4):208–217.
46. O'Malley MJ, Page A, Cook R. Endoscopic plantar fasciotomy for chronic heel pain. *Foot Ankle Int* 2000;21(6):505–510.
47. Marafko C. Endoscopic partial plantar fasciotomy as a treatment alternative in plantar fasciitis. *Acta Chir Orthop Traumatol Cech* 2007;74(6):406–409.
48. Boyle RA, Slater GL. Endoscopic plantar fascia release: a case series. *Foot Ankle Int* 2003;24(2):176–179.
49. Ogilvie-Harris DJ, Lobo J. Endoscopic plantar fascia release. *Arthroscopy* 2000;16(3):290–298.
50. Bazaz R, Ferkel RD. Results of endoscopic plantar fascia release. *Foot Ankle Int* 2007;28(5):549–556.
51. Hogan KA, Webb D, Shereff M. Endoscopic plantar fascia release. *Foot Ankle Int* 2004;25(12):875–881.
52. Baxter DE, Pfeffer GB. Treatment of chronic heel pain by surgical release of the first branch of the lateral plantar nerve. *Clin Orthop Relat Res* 1992;(279):229–236.
53. Anderson DJ, Fallat LM, Savoy-Moore T. Computer-assisted assessment of lateral column movement following plantar fascial release: a cadaveric study. *J Foot Ankle Surg* 2001;40(2):62–70.
54. Brugh AM, Fallat LM, Savoy-Moore RT. Lateral column symptomatology following plantar fascial release: a prospective study. *J Foot Ankle Surg* 2002;41(6):365–371.
55. Arangio GA, Chen C, Kim W. Effect of cutting the plantar fascia on mechanical properties of the foot. *Clin Orthop Relat Res* 1997;(339):227–231.
56. Yu JS, Spigos D, Tomczak R. Foot pain after a plantar fasciotomy: an MR analysis to determine potential causes. *J Comput Assist Tomogr* 1999;23(5):707–712.

57. Niva MH, Sormaala MJ, Kiuru MJ, et al. Bone stress injuries of the ankle and foot: an 86-month magnetic resonance imaging-based study of physically active young adults. *Am J Sports Med* 2007;35(4):643–649.
58. Kiuru MJ, Pihlajamaki HK, Hietanen HJ, et al. MR imaging, bone scintigraphy, and radiography in bone stress injuries of the pelvis and the lower extremity. *Acta Radiol* 2002;43(2):207–212.
59. Kiuru MJ, Pihlajamaki HK, Perkio JP, et al. Dynamic contrast-enhanced MR imaging in symptomatic bone stress of the pelvis and the lower extremity. *Acta Radiol* 2001;42(3): 277–285.
60. Sarrafian SK. Biomechanics of the subtalar joint complex. *Clin Orthop Relat Res* 1993;(290):17–26.
61. Weindel S, Schmidt R, Rammelt S, et al. Subtalar instability: a biomechanical cadaver study. *Arch Orthop Trauma Surg* 2008;130(3):313–319..
62. Jotoku T, Kinoshita M, Okuda R, et al. Anatomy of ligamentous structures in the tarsal sinus and canal. *Foot Ankle Int* 2006;27(7):533–538.
63. Tochigi Y, Amendola A, Rudert MJ, et al. The role of the interosseous talocalcaneal ligament in subtalar joint stability. *Foot Ankle Int* 2004;25(8):588–596.
64. Martin LP, Wayne JS, Owen JR, et al. Elongation behavior of calcaneofibular and cervical ligaments in a closed kinetic chain: pathomechanics of lateral hindfoot instability. *Foot Ankle Int* 2002;23(6):515–520.
65. Knudson GA, Kitaoka HB, Lu CL, et al. Subtalar joint stability. Talocalcaneal interosseous ligament function studied in cadaver specimens. *Acta Orthop Scand* 1997;68(5): 442–446.
66. Heilman AE, Braly WG, Bishop JO, et al. An anatomic study of subtalar instability. *Foot Ankle* 1990;10(4):224–228.
67. Kjaersgaard-Andersen P, Wethelund JO, et al. Stabilizing effect of the tibiocalcaneal fascicle of the deltoid ligament on hindfoot joint movements: an experimental study. *Foot Ankle* 1989;10(1):30–35.
68. Kjaersgaard-Andersen P, Wethelund JO, Helmig P, et al. The stabilizing effect of the ligamentous structures in the sinus and canalis tarsi on movements in the hindfoot. An experimental study. *Am J Sports Med* 1988;16(5):512–516.
69. Leardini A, Stagni R, O'Connor JJ. Mobility of the subtalar joint in the intact ankle complex. *J Biomech* 2001;34(6):805–809.
70. Sharda P, DuFosse J. Lateral subtalar dislocation. *Orthopedics* 2008;31(7):718.
71. Dendrinos G, Zisis G, Terzopoulos H. Recurrence of subtalar dislocation in a basketball player. *Am J Sports Med* 1994;22(1):143–145.
72. Kinik H, Oktay O, Arikan M, et al. Medial subtalar dislocation. *Int Orthop* 1999;23(6): 366–367.
73. Bak K, Koch JS. Subtalar dislocation in a handball player. *Br J Sports Med* 1991;25(1): 24–25.
74. Grantham SA. Medical subtalar dislocation: Five cases with a common etiology. *J Trauma* 1964;4:845–849.
75. Menetrey J, Fritschy D. Subtalar subluxation in ballet dancers. *Am J Sports Med* 1999; 27(2):143–149.
76. Senall JA, Kile TA. Stress radiography. *Foot Ankle Clin* 2000;5(1):165–184.
77. Yamamoto H, Yagishita K, Ogiuchi T, et al. Subtalar instability following lateral ligament injuries of the ankle. *Injury* 1998;29(4):265–268.
78. Louwerens JW, Ginai AZ, van Linge B, et al. Stress radiography of the talocrural and subtalar joints. *Foot Ankle Int* 1995;16(3):148–155.
79. Ishii T, Miyagawa S, Fukubayashi T, et al. Subtalar stress radiography using forced dorsiflexion and supination. *J Bone Joint Surg Br* 1996;78(1):56–60.
80. Meyer JM, Garcia J, Hoffmeyer P, et al. The subtalar sprain. A roentgenographic study. *Clin Orthop Relat Res* 1988;(226):169–173.
81. Sugimoto K, Takakura Y, Samoto N, et al. Subtalar arthrography in recurrent instability of the ankle. *Clin Orthop Relat Res* 2002;(394):169–176.
82. Karlsson J, Eriksson BI, Renstrom P. Subtalar instability of the foot. A review and results after surgical treatment. *Scand J Med Sci Sports* 1998;8(4):191–197.
83. Keefe DT, Haddad SL. Subtalar instability. Etiology, diagnosis, and management. *Foot Ankle Clin* 2002;7(3):577–609.
84. Thermann H, Zwipp H, Tscherne H. Treatment algorithm of chronic ankle and subtalar instability. *Foot Ankle Int* 1997;18(3):163–169.
85. Colville MR, Marder RA, Zarins B. Reconstruction of the lateral ankle ligaments. A biomechanical analysis. *Am J Sports Med* 1992;20(5):594–600.
86. Lui TH. Arthroscopic-assisted lateral ligamentous reconstruction in combined ankle and subtalar instability. *Arthroscopy* 2007;23(5):554.e1–e5.
87. Chrisman OD, Snook GA. Reconstruction of lateral ligament tears of the ankle. An experimental study and clinical evaluation of seven patients treated by a new modification of the Elmslie procedure. *J Bone Joint Surg Am* 1969;51(5):904–912.
88. Schmidt R, Benesch S, Friemert B, et al. Anatomical repair of lateral ligaments in patients with chronic ankle instability. *Knee Surg Sports Traumatol Arthrosc* 2005;13(3):231–237.
89. Takao M, Oae K, Uchio Y, et al. Anatomical reconstruction of the lateral ligaments of the ankle with a gracilis autograft: a new technique using an interference fit anchoring system. *Am J Sports Med* 2005;33(6):814–823.
90. Karlsson J, Eriksson BI, Renstrom PA. Subtalar ankle instability. A review. *Sports Med* 1997;24(5):337–346.
91. St Pierre RK, Velazco A, Fleming LL, et al. Medial subtalar dislocation in an athlete. A case report. *Am J Sports Med* 1982;10(4):240–244.
92. Heck BE, Ebraheim NA, Jackson WT. Anatomical considerations of irreducible medial subtalar dislocation. *Foot Ankle Int* 1996;17(2):103–106.
93. Lee KB, Bai LB, Park JG, et al. Efficacy of MRI versus arthroscopy for evaluation of sinus tarsi syndrome. *Foot Ankle Int* 2008;29(11):1111–1116.
94. Lee KB, Bai LB, Song EK, et al. Subtalar arthroscopy for sinus Tarsi syndrome: arthroscopic findings and clinical outcomes of 33 consecutive cases. *Arthroscopy* 2008;24(10):1130–1134.
95. Brunner R, Gachter A. Sinus tarsi syndrome. Results of surgical treatment. *Unfallchirurg* 1993;96(10):534–537.
96. Tasto JP. Arthroscopy of the subtalar joint and arthroscopic subtalar arthrodesis. *Instr Course Lect* 2006;55:555–564.
97. Funk JR, Srinivasan SC, Crandall JR. Snowboarder's talus fractures experimentally produced by eversion and dorsiflexion. *Am J Sports Med* 2003;31(6):921–928.
98. Valderrabano V, Perren T, Ryf C, et al. Snowboarder's talus fracture: treatment outcome of 20 cases after 3.5 years. *Am J Sports Med* 2005;33(6):871–880.
99. Hamilton WG, Geppert MJ, Thompson FM. Pain in the posterior aspect of the ankle in dancers. Differential diagnosis and operative treatment. *J Bone Joint Surg Am* 1996;78(10): 1491–1500.
100. Black KP, Ehlert KJ. A stress fracture of the lateral process of the talus in a runner. A case report. *J Bone Joint Surg Am* 1994;76(3):441–443.
101. Hontas MJ, Haddad RJ, Schlesinger LC. Conditions of the talus in the runner. *Am J Sports Med* 1986;14(6):486–490.
102. Marotta JJ, Micheli LJ. Os trigonum impingement in dancers. *Am J Sports Med* 1992; 20(5):533–536.
103. Hawkins LG. Fracture of the lateral process of the talus. *J Bone Joint Surg Am* 1965;47: 1170–1175.

CHAPTER

22

Michael J. Trepal
Thomas M. DeLauro
Elynor Giannin Perez

Forefoot Injuries

As the distal-most portion of the lower extremity, it is no surprise that the forefoot would suffer frequent injury during sports-related activities. At times these injuries may generate chronic effects that pose lifelong morbidity, necessitating early recognition and treatment.

NAIL TRAUMA

Trauma to the nail and surrounding structures (Fig. 22.1) is common due to ill-fitting shoes and faulty biomechanics. In athletes it is dependent on the magnitude of speed, intensity of play, and side-to-side motion (1). Fractures to the distal phalanx (Fig. 22.2) can also occur with high-energy force. Any pathology can result in onycholysis, onychocryptosis, discoloration, nail plate thickening, and infection (2,3).

The nail unit consists of (4):

Nail plate—fully keratinized multilayer sheet of cornified cells—3 layers: Superficial, intermediate, and ventral. >5 mm of onycholysis within the lunula will disrupt adherence to nail bed.
Proximal nail fold.
Nail matrix—proliferative epithelium keratinized without a granular layer: Responsible for superficial and intermediate aspect of the nail plate.
Nail bed—highly vascularized subcutaneous layer which links the nail bed to the periosteum of the distal phalanx. Responsible for the ventral aspect of the nail plate.
Hyponychium—distal free edge of nail plate

The lunula is half-moon shaped and the only visible portion of the nail matrix. The hyponychium and eponychium (proximal to the lunula) are anatomical barriers against the environment and microbes. Since, the distal phalanx is intimately related with the nail matrix; infection including osteomyelitis (OM) can spread if these barriers are altered (1).

Complete regeneration of a toenail can take anywhere between 7 and 10 months as the rate of growth ranges from 1.3 to 1.8 mm/month (4).

PHYSICAL EXAMINATION

Trauma will cause subungual hematomas (SH) as the nail bed integrity is violated. When patients present with a SH involving greater than 25% of the nail bed, there is a 20% to 25% chance of an associated distal phalanx fracture (3) (Figs. 22.1, 22.2).

CLASSIFICATION

With open fractures, tetanus and antibiotic prophylaxis is indicated. The Gustilo and Anderson classification provides useful information (2).

Nail Bed Injuries: Rosenthal classification (2):

Zone I: Distal to distal phalanx—usually allowed healing by secondary intention.
Zone II: Distal to the lunula—local advancement of flap, either Atasoy V-Y flap or Kutler biaxial medial and lateral V flap advancements.
Zone III: Proximal to distal end of lunula—matrix excision is recommended due to nail bed reconstruction not being possible. Partial digital amputation usually performed at distal interphalangeal joint level.

TREATMENT

Decompression of a SH is imperative to minimize damage to the nail matrix along with pain relief. The integrity of the nail folds will determine how decompression is performed. If the nail folds are stable and SH is less than 25% drainage can be accomplished by a hand-cautery unit, 18G needle, 11 bayonet blade, or a small bur to pierce the nail plate. Saline irrigation, application of a topical antibiotic and dry sterile dressing should be applied (2,3). SH >25% of the nail plate or if there is damage to the medial/lateral/proximal nail fold, the nail must be avulsed as a nail bed laceration is very likely. A digital anesthetic block is performed to properly manipulate the digit. Upon avulsion, saline or dilute iodine solution is used for irrigation. Nail bed lacerations are repaired with 5-0 absorbable suture tapered needle in a simple interrupted manner. Non-adherence gauze is placed over the nail bed and underneath the proximal nail fold in order to maintain the cul de sac nature of the proximal nail groove. The sutures are removed 10 to 14 days after the procedure and monitoring of the emerging nail plate should continue until fully re-grown (3).

In open fractures, small unstable bone fragments externally exposed or distally far displaced should be removed during the initial debridement. If the wound is heavily contaminated, repeat surgical debridement and delayed closure is advisable. Large unstable fragments can be stabilized with a K wire, however, if the patient is less than 18 years old—assess the distal phalangeal physis.

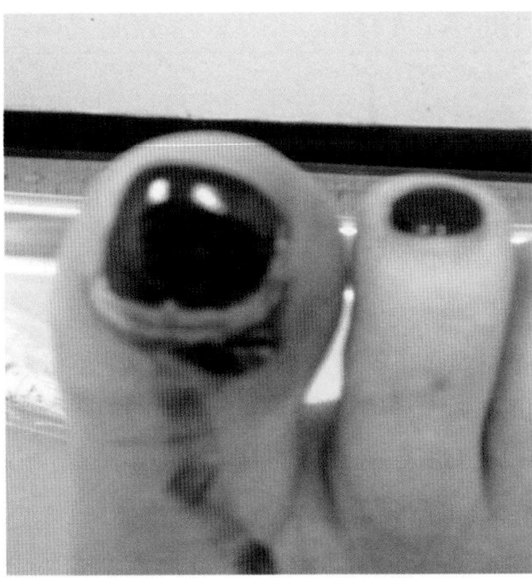

Figure 22.1. Impaction injury to nail complex from soccer.

Any trauma to the nail unit can result in nail plate dystrophy and later are susceptible to infections. Infected toenails should be removed by a partial or total nail avulsion and treated with a week of antibiotics. Usually, the most common organism is *Staphylococcus aureus*. Thereafter, once a day daily soaks with dilute povidone-iodine or peroxide are done for the tissue to drain and remain clean. Prior to any treatment, patients should be aware of complications as dystrophy occurs as the nail plate grows back, if at all.

NEUROMAS

The term neuroma is actually a misnomer because it is not a neoplastic or proliferate process but a degenerative one and in most cases due to entrapment of the nerve. Histology slides of the nerve show demyelination of the nerve fibers with fibrosis of the epineurium, endoneurium, and Renaut bodies (densely packed whorls of collagen) (5).

The most common neuroma in the foot occurs within the third intermetatarsal space (IMS) at the communicating branch between the lateral and medial plantar nerve passing deep to the transverse metatarsal ligament (TML) and was named after Morton who described it in 1876. The anatomist Civinini from the University of Pisa in 1835 was the first to actually identify a fusiform swelling in the common digital nerve of the third interspace and the Queens's surgeon-chiropodist Lewis Durlacher initially described the symptoms (5,6).

Many theories have been proposed for the actual cause of this condition, which include pronation, trauma, a bursa, mechanical impingement of the nerve by the deep intermetatarsal ligament and ischemia.

Neuromas can occur in any of the IMS and have been named from first to fourth IMS: Heuter's, Hauser's, Morton's, and Islen's, respectively. Joplin in 1971 described a neuroma on the medial aspect of the hallux (5–7).

PHYSICAL EXAMINATION

Chief complaint will be pain localized to the plantar forefoot between the metatarsal heads. Symptoms of pain are typically described as sharp, stabbing, burning, tingling, and radiating to the toes. Application of mediolateral pressure to the metatarsal heads with a mechanical sensation of a clunk or click—Mulder's sign—is supportive of an interdigital neuroma (6) Side to side motion seen in sports will elicit pain in the athlete however, it is more commonly seen with tight-fitting shoes. Local anesthetics (diagnostic injection) are useful in confirming the diagnosis (6).

IMAGING

Usually a clinical diagnosis is confirmed with the aid of an injection. Radiographs rule out any osseous pathology. Controversy surrounds MRIs and ultrasound (US) for diagnosing interdigital neuromas. MRIs may find incidental non-symptomatic neuromas but can rule out any other differential diagnosis (Fig. 22.3). Low signal intensities on T1- and T2-weighted images are seen due to the fibrous content of a neuroma. US can serve as guidance for injections and will show a hypoechoic

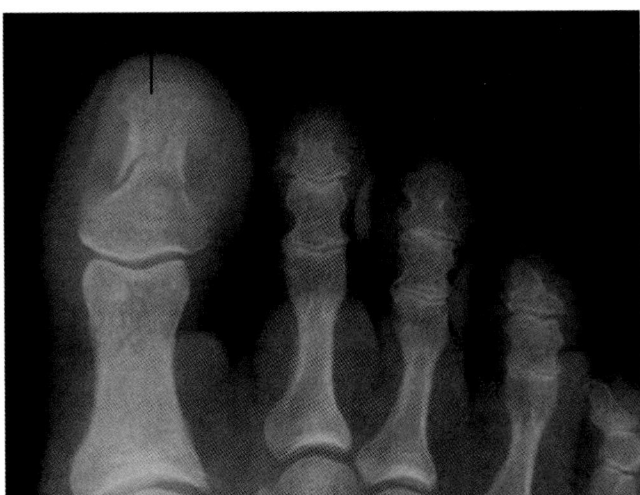

Figure 22.2. Fracture of distal phalanx on the hallux secondary to soccer injury.

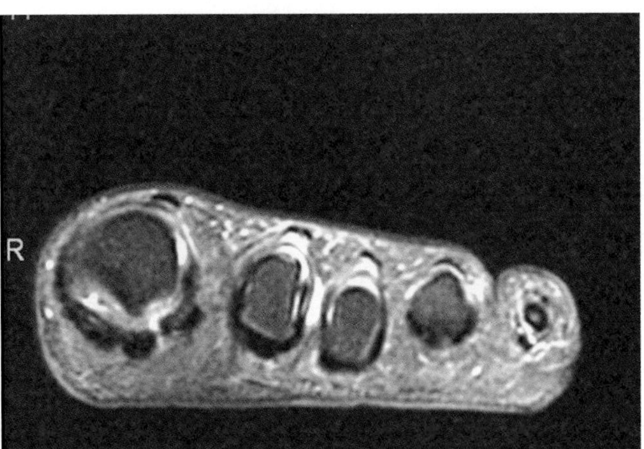

Figure 22.3. MRI with contrast demonstrating second interspace neuroma.

ovoid mass parallel to the long axis of the metatarsal; however, they are highly operator dependent (7,8).

CLASSIFICATION

There is currently no classification system for neuromas.

TREATMENT

Conservative treatments include metatarsal pads placed proximal to the metatarsal heads distributing the pressure. Oral NSAIDs are used to decrease pain and inflammation. A mixture of corticosteroid and local anesthetic injections can also be given, typically no more than three, and the success rates vary greatly between studies. There are however, some complications with injections—fat pad atrophy, telangiectasia, and hypopigmentation.

Sclerosing agents such as 4% alcohol or a combination of the alcohol with a corticosteroid can also be used. Extracorporeal shockwave therapy has been described with some relief (6).

SURGICAL INTERVENTION

Sixty percent to seventy percent of patients continue on to surgical treatment after exhausting conservative treatment. Neurectomy is commonly performed and the incision can be made dorsal or plantar (Fig. 22.4). A plantar incision is discouraged due to fear of a hypertrophic scar on the weight-bearing area however the exposure is excellent. Currently, there are no studies showing advantages of one incision over the other (5,6). The proximal stump of the nerve is implanted into the adjacent intrinsic muscle in order to prevent a stump neuroma.

Cryogenic neuroablation has also been described as a minimally invasive procedure using temperatures of −50°C to −70°C applied to the nerve causing demyelination followed by Wallerian degeneration (5). Post operatively, the patient is allowed to weight bear on the heel with a surgical shoe. Within 2 weeks, the patient is allowed to increase forefoot weight bearing and a compressive wrap is continued for at least 5 weeks (8).

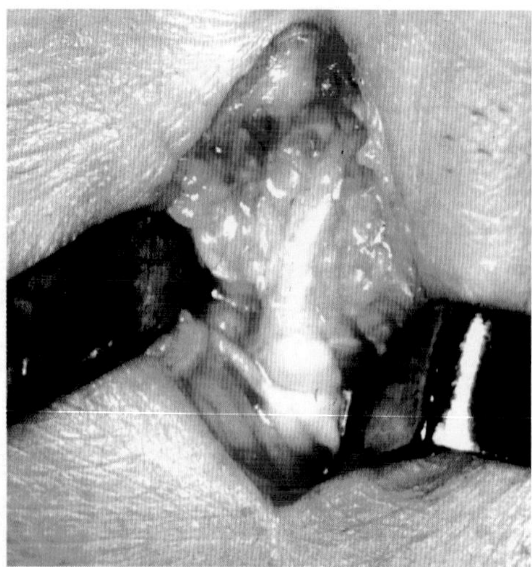

Figure 22.4. Intra-operative visualization of neuroma from dorsal incision.

THE GREAT TOE

Injuries to the great toe are under appreciated and often missed which can be detrimental to an athlete. Such injuries can lead to functional disability including persistent pain, loss of push off, and deformity ultimately leading to joint degeneration.

Bowers and Martin originally described turf toe on football players in 1976. The game was played on artificial surfaces and the mechanism of injury occurred as delivering an axial load to a foot that is fixed in equinus driving the hallux metatarsophalangeal joint (MTPJ) into hyperextension and therefore disrupting or attenuating the plantar joint complex. A strain or sprain can occur on the plantar structures as well as frank dorsal dislocation of the hallux, which can damage the dorsal cartilage on the metatarsal head.

Stability of the first MTPJ is provided by the capsuloligamentous and tendinous structures surrounding it, since the joint itself is not deep enough to resist forces in any direction. Specifically, abductory stresses are resisted by the abductor hallucis tendon, the medial joint capsule and ligaments, and the medial metatarsosesamoidal ligament. Adductory forces are resisted by the conjoined tendon of the adductor hallucis, the lateral joint capsule and ligaments, and the lateral metatarsosesamoidal ligament. Plantarflexory stresses are resisted only by the dorsal joint capsule, the small extensor hallucis brevis tendon, and the extensor hallucis longus tendon. Anatomically, the greatest structural support seems to be provided plantarly in an effort to protect against excessive dorsiflexion: The plantar capsule and its thickened plantar plate, the flexor hallucis longus tendon, and the flexor hallucis brevis tendons strengthened by the sesamoidal apparatus. Despite these additional structural supports, the term "turf toe" has come to be associated with the constellation of injuries resulting from greater-than-normal first MTPJ dorsiflexion, specifically a tearing of the plantar plate (9,10).

Although isolated case reports of medial, lateral, and dorsal (also known as "sand toe") capsuloligamentous tears have appeared in the sports medicine literature, true turf toe (i.e., plantar tears) were relatively unknown until the introduction of artificial turf playing surfaces (hence its name). This has led to much speculation as to the true etiology of the injury but most clinicians agree that the combination of a fixed foot (made more likely by the use of turf cleat shoes) and the flexibility of these shoes contribute to hyperdorsiflexion (hyperextension) injuries either by the athlete in motion or by another athlete falling upon an already dorsiflexed joint (9,10).

As one would surmise, injuries range from simple sprains of the plantar structures to frank dislocation of the first MTPJ with sesamoidal fracture. The extent of the injuries, imaging changes, treatments, and return to activity recommendations may be found in Table 22.1 (10,11).

Unfortunately, long-term sequelae of these injuries include permanent reduction of range of motion, hallux rigidus, and impaired push-off. Only slightly more than half of patients surveyed are satisfied with the overall outcome (9,10).

SESAMOID INJURIES

Galen (129 to 200 AD) is credited with coining the term "sesamoids" due to their resemblance to sesame seeds. It has been argued that perhaps it was castor oil seeds from the plant *ricinus*

TABLE 22.1 First Metatarsophalangeal Joint Injuries

Grade/type	Structures Involved	Clinical Findings	Imaging Results	Treatment	Prognosis
Grade 1	Plantar capsuloligamentous stretching	Minimal tenderness, no ecchymosis, minimal edema, minimal loss of motion	Radiographs negative, MRI reveals only edema, tendonitis, and synovitis	Tape hallux in plantarflexion	Often can continue playing
Grade 2	Plantar capsuloligamentous tearing without articular damage	More tenderness, edema, and loss of motion. Ecchymosis evident. Symptoms worsen over 24 h	Same	Immobilize in postoperative shoe × 2 wks	Restrict play for 2 wks
Grade 3	Complete plantar tearing with/without sesamoid fracture or diastasis, dorsal joint compression injury	Severe pain plantarly and dorsally, severe ecchymosis and swelling, unable to bear weight medially	Radiographs may reveal sesamoid fracture, diastasis, or proximal migration	Non—weight-bearing × 1–3 days, below-knee casting with hallux in 10 degree plantarflexion	No play for 2–6 wks or until hallux can be dorsiflexed 90 degree. Protect with taping.
Type I first MTPJ dislocation	Dislocation of hallux with sesamoids. Plantar plate resting dorsal to metatarsal head	No intersesamoid ligament disruption; irreducible	First MTPJ dorsal dislocation with distal displacement of sesamoids	Open reduction required	Same as Grade 3 above
Type IIA first MTPJ dislocation	Same as Type I but sesamoids separated	Intersesamoid ligament ruptured; irreducible	Same as Type I but sesamoids distal and separated mediolaterally	Open reduction required	
Type IIB first MTPJ dislocation	Partial sesamoid fracture	Partial plantar plate rupture; reducible	Dislocation with sesamoid fracture	Closed reduction only	
Type IIIA first MTPJ dislocation	Dislocation with proximal sesamoid migration	Complete avulsion of plantar plate from proximal phalanx	Dislocation with proximal sesamoid migration	Closed reduction only	
Type IIIB first MTPJ dislocation	Dislocation, sesamoid fracture, proximal sesamoid migration	Complete avulsion of plantar plate with sesamoid fracture	Dislocation with proximal sesamoid migration and sesamoid fracture	Closed reduction only	

that was the reference due to the word sesamum. Sesamoids in general are not always composed of bone and can be a mixture of cartilage and fibrous tissue along with bone (12).

The sesamoids are imbedded within the plantar plate and the tendons of flexor hallucis brevis. They suspend from the metatarsal head by the medial and lateral sesamoidal ligaments (9,12–14). The sesamoid complex is made up of seven muscles, eight ligaments, and two sesamoids (15). All these structures create a stirrup-type arrangement that contributes to the gliding function of the joint as well as shock absorbers and fulcrums of the hallux (9,12–14). The complex transmits 50% of the body weight and greater than 300% during push off, leaving vulnerable to many pathologies, which include, sesamoiditis, stress fractures/fractures, non-unions, avascular necrosis and chondromalacia (12).

Ossification occurs between 7 and 10 years of age with the fibular sesamoid ossifying first. Bipartite sesamoids result from multiple ossification centers—tibial 10% (bilateral 25%) and rarely the fibular (14). Three sesamoids are associated with the great toe—two constant and one inconstant. When the third inconstant sesamoid is present, it is located underneath the interphalangeal joint (IPJ). Compared to the fibular sesamoid, the tibial is larger, ovoid, and elongated predisposing it to greater pathology (12).

Vascular supply is of great importance in sesamoidal injury, healing, and surgical procedures. Blood is supplied by the plantar artery in 25% of the cases, 25% stems from the plantar arch and 50% from both sources. The distal aspect of the sesamoids are the least vascularized obtaining their blood supply from the capsule alone explaining disorders such as non-union and osteonecrosis (12).

Sesamoid disorders account for 9% of foot injuries and 1.2% of running injuries and diagnosis will vary with mechanism of injury. Acute fractures are usually transverse or stellate shaped and caused by falls, landing from jumps (ballerinas), forced dorsiflexion of the hallux, and crush injuries. Stress fractures are due to overuse and are common in athletes.

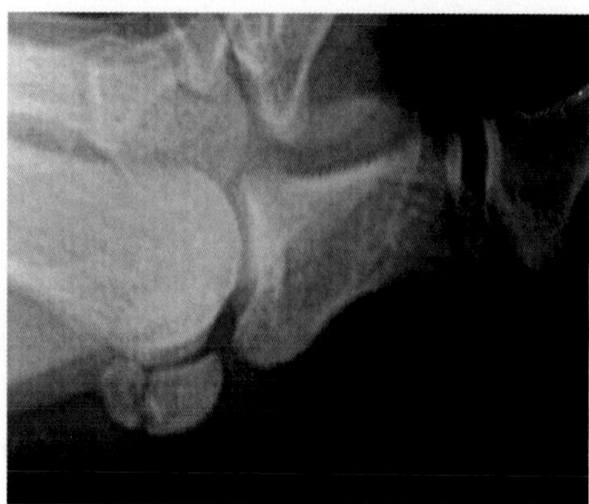

Figure 22.5. Oblique view demonstrating tibial sesamoid fracture.

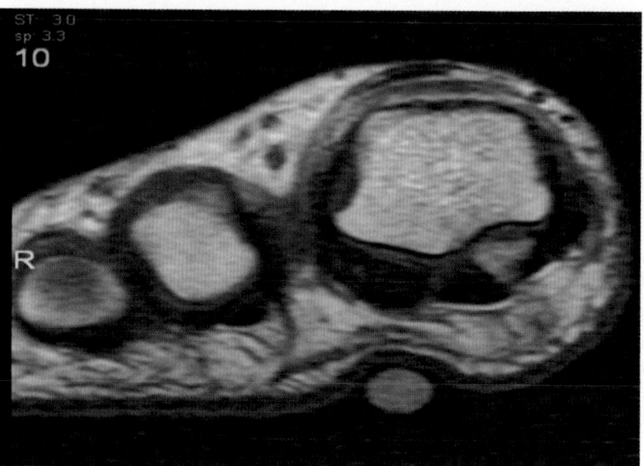

Figure 22.6. MRI demonstrating AVN of fibular sesamoid.

PHYSICAL EXAMINATION

Pain will be localized at the plantar aspect of the MTPJ when weight bearing and while placing the joint through full range of motion, especially during dorsiflexion of the hallux. If grinding with pain is felt upon compression then arthritis is usually the culprit. The presence of swelling, warmth, ecchymosis, and erythema should all be noted and if a plantarflexed first ray is noticed, consider intractable plantar keratosis (IPK) or sesamoiditis.

IMAGING

AP radiographs will illustrate bipartite sesamoids and fractures (9,11–15). A lateral oblique view will stress the fibular sesamoid where the medial oblique will stress the tibial sesamoid (Fig. 22.5). A sesamoidal axial view allows for inspection of the cristae, sesamoids, and position of the sesamoidal apparatus. This view is also beneficial for focal arthrosis, bony prominences, and plantar osteophytes. Contralateral views will rule out bipartite sesamoids; however, if the uninvolved foot does not have a partite sesamoid—one cannot confirm a fracture.

CT scan is more sensitive and specific for detection of fractures. It allows visualization of periostitis, articular irregularity, sub and articular collapse of osteonecrosis, pseudocyst formation, and early stress fractures.

MRIs differentiate between bone and soft tissue abnormalities and extremely useful in determining vascularity of fragments in non-unions (Fig. 22.6). However, they are reserved for when CT scans are unrevealing of an occult fracture, early osteonecrosis or chondromalacia.

A three phase bone scan with pinhole images is useful in differentiating between medial and lateral sesamoidal pain.

CLASSIFICATION

Currently there is no accepted grade system for fractures of the sesamoids.

TREATMENT

Conservative treatment involves a period of a non–weight-bearing cast with a toe plate followed by protected weight bearing in a surgical shoe. Later on, custom orthosis with a metatarsal pad are used. The literature is limited and there are no specific recommendations for non-operative treatment. Complete relief of symptoms can take up to 6 months.

SURGICAL INTERVENTION

There is one report by Pagenstert et al. on open reduction internal fixation for two chronic non-unions of the tibial sesamoid in conjunction with HAV deformity. Both cases went on to clinical and radiologic unions (Level V evidence). There are no other reports on open reduction internal fixation (16).

Bone grafting and partial sesamoidectomy of the distal fragment have been described for chronic fractures refractory to conservative treatment. Removal of the distal fragment allows portion of the sesamoid for weight bearing. A medial incision is used for the tibial and a dorsal or plantar incision for the fibular sesamoidectomy (often more challenging). Minimal dissection is recommended to preserve the blood supply (9,14). Complete excision is performed if symptoms persist but it is not without complications. In this case the sesamoid should be shelled out and the void sutured closed. If both sesamoids are involved, every effort should be undertaken to not excise both as it would completely disrupt function and mechanics. Postoperative management is 4 weeks of non—weight-bearing in a below the knee cast followed by range of motion exercises and physical therapy. The patient can return to their sport after 8 weeks with taping and a steel shoe insert.

PLANTAR PLATE TEARS

Second metatarsal joint instability is usually associated with ill-fitting shoes in the female population due to high-heeled shoes that hyperextend the second MTPJ leading to elongation and weakening of the capsule and plantar aponeurosis. In time instability of the second MTPJ and plantar plate (PP) rupture ensues. PP tears have also been noticed in the young athletic population who participate in running, tennis, aerobic exercises, and walking at a high level (17).

The main static stabilizers of the second MTPJ are the PP and the medial and lateral collateral ligaments. Dynamic stabilization is provided by the intrinsic flexors (18). Shape of the PP is rectangular or even trapezoidal. Distally, it inserts into the base of the proximal phalanx and proximally, it originates on the metatarsal head through a thin synovial attachment. Important structures attach at this level, such as the collateral ligaments, TMLs, interosseous tendons, fibrous sheath of the flexor tendons, and the distal fibers of the plantar fascia. The intrinsic musculature of the second toe is unique: Only one lumbrical tendon inserting medially, two dorsal interossei (no plantar interossei), and all structures pass plantar to the axis of rotation of the MTPJ (17–19).

Coughlin in 1986 coined the term "crossover toe" and in 1987 Thompson and Hamilton explained the "positive Lachman"/Drawer test (18). The examination consists of grasping the proximal phalanx between your thumb and forefinger and attempting to dorsally displace it. A positive test exists if more than 2 mm of dorsal displacement is achieved during the examination indicating a PP tear. The physician should be aware of false positives in patients with ligamentous laxity (18–20).

The thickness of the PP ranges from 2 mm to 5 mm with the borders being thicker than the central aspect. The width is between 8 and 13 mm and is 16 to 23 mm in length. The PP is composed of 75% Type 1 collagen followed by 21% of Type 2 collagen. Poor healing capacity might be attributed to the amount of Type 1 collagen. Pathology occurs when chronic hyperextension forces are applied to the MTPJ leading to overstretching/attenuation of the PP and capsule therefore decreasing the stabilization of the second MTPJ (19,20).

Diagnosis of PP tears are commonly missed or confused with fat pad atrophy, neuromas, Freiberg's infarction, inflammatory or degenerative arthritis, and metatarsalgia.

PHYSICAL EXAMINATION

Patients will present with focal pain underneath the second toe at the level of the MTPJ. The pain has been described as "walking on a marble" (18). The area is usually swollen (capsular swelling) with malalignment or dorsal dislocation of the proximal phalanx on the metatarsal. Tenderness will surround the MTPJ depending on the location of capsular disorder. As the disease progresses, the second toe will deviate medially and eventually cross over the hallux (17–21).

IMAGING

Diagnosis is a clinical one but radiographs should be obtained to rule out any fractures. On an AP view, 2 to 3 mm of clear space between the MTPJ (articular cartilage) should be seen, and will disappear as the base of the proximal phalanx subluxes (Fig. 22.7.). Subluxation is best appreciated on the lateral view. The metatarsal protrusion distance should also be assessed and the first metatarsal should be +/−2 mm compared to the second. A short first or long second metatarsal is predisposed to a PP tear and subsequent second MTPJ dislocation (17–19,22).

MR arthrography is useful although invasive but has been used at the second MTPJ in order to detect PP and joint capsular tears. One to two milliliters of a 4 mmol preparation of gadopentetate dimeglumine diluted into saline, and iopromide mixed with 1% of lidocaine plain is used. The mixture in injected into a 20 to 30 degree plantarflexed MTPJ joint. Capsular tears can be distinguished clearly from PP tears since contrast will be disseminated into the tendon sheath in the latter (23).

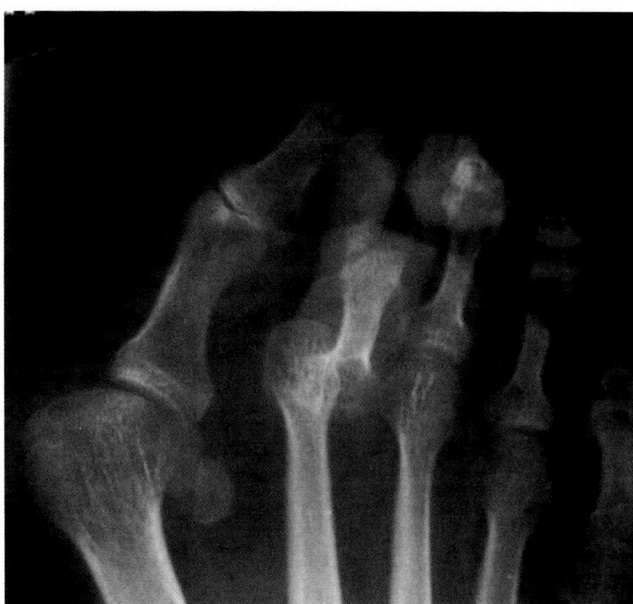

Figure 22.7. DP x-ray demonstrating subluxed second MTPJ.

MRIs are an alternative to arthrography and will show increased signal intensity in the PP distally at the base of the proximal phalanx. They are helpful in differentiating between articular and non-articular diagnoses.

US, although operator dependent has the advantage of being dynamic and the operator can move the toe as well as compare the PP to adjacent ones. Pathology will show a loss of homogenicity with focal areas of hypoechoic defects (11).

CLASSIFICATION

Anatomic grading of plantar plate tears (19)

Grade 0: Plantar plate or capsular attenuation/discoloration
Grade 1: Transverse distal tear <50% at insertion into proximal phalanx and/or mid-substance tear <50%
Grade 2: Transverse distal tear >50% and/or mid-substance tear <50%
Grade 3: Transverse and/or longitudinal extensive tear (collaterals may be involved)
Grade 4: Extensive tear with button hole (dislocation); combination transverse and longitudinal plate tear.

TREATMENT

Conservative treatment is successful at the beginning stages and will slow the progression of the disease but will not stop it. In a dislocated joint, surgical treatment is advisable. NSAIDs will alleviate symptoms and taping will maintain the toe in neutral position but may lead to chronic edema and ulceration. A metatarsal pad will disperse the weight on the plantar surface and should be placed proximal on the metatarsal head. There are two schools of thought in regard to orthotics. Offloading the area by making a "U" cutout at the level of the MTPJ or restricting motion across the joint as in carbon fiber footplate. Injections will eliminate symptoms temporarily but should not be used repetitively due to potential attenuation and further dislocation of the joint (18,19).

SURGICAL INTERVENTION

Incision placement can vary; a dorsal approach over the second web space with a longitudinal capsulotomy is performed inferior to the tendons in order to expose the second MTPJ. A miniature joint distractor is used in order to visualize the plantar plate, which is then inspected and graded. Grade 3 tears are repaired with non-absorbable suture in an interrupted fashion. Grade 1 and 2 tears are attached to the plantar edge of proximal phalanx with the suture passed from plantar to dorsal and tied dorsally on the base of the proximal phalanx. A Weil osteotomy along with repair of the lateral collateral ligaments can be added to the procedure in an already medially deviating toe (18,19).

The plantar step-down approach is described as a distal longitudinal arm over the lateral aspect of the involved digital base and the proximal longitudinal arm over the first interspace or the interdigital space medial to the involved toe. The transverse arm is at the sulcus of the involved toe. Transverse tears of the plantar plate are elliptically excised removing necrotic tissue and end-to-end repair is performed with a 3-0 absorbable suture. Mitek mini anchors are used to reattach tears at the base of the proximal phalanx (18,21,22).

Dressing changes are performed weakly and discontinued at 2 weeks. Compression wraps are then applied and the patient can ambulate—heel weight only—in a surgical shoe. Passive range of motion is started at 2 weeks along with physical therapy (18,19,22).

STRESS FRACTURES

Fifth metatarsal stress fractures were first described in marching Prussian soldiers as an overuse injury in 1855 and are now commonly known as "march fractures." The advent of radiography 40 years later would confirm the diagnoses. Devas in 1958 however, was the first to describe this injury in athletes (24). Stress fractures are common in athletes who engage in sports with repetitive motion such as running, football, basketball, soccer, and lacrosse. It is the repetitive motion or marked increase in load to a bone that causes stress fractures rather than from a single high force load and the shape of the foot also plays a role.

The etiology of stress fractures is multifactorial and includes high serum parathyroid hormone level, polymorphism of vitamin D receptor, low serum levels of 25(OH)-vitamin D, low bone mineral/density content, iron deficiency, gender, and smoking. Corticosteroid use and chronic medical conditions such as metabolic bone disease and rheumatoid arthritis patients are also at an increased risk of stress fractures (25,26).

Stress fractures can occur in any bone—tibia being the most common followed by the tarsals and metatarsals (26). There are intrinsic and extrinsic factors that can explain cause and determine treatment options for stress fractures. Intrinsic factors include leg-length discrepancy, forefoot varus, hormonal factors, bone density, and increased high arch. Extrinsic factors include shoe wear, training regimen (fatigue), type of equipment, and diet. There is a higher incidence in female athletes and it can be attributed to the "female athlete triad" which consists of disordered eating, amenorrhea, and osteoporosis (25).

There are two different types of categories for stress fractures (27):

1. Low risk: Good prognosis is generally associated with these stress fractures as in the calcaneus and second metatarsal.
2. High risk: Delayed/non-union/progression to complete fracture and dislocation is increased in these stress fractures. Talus, navicular, fifth metatarsal metaphyseal fracture—"Jones' fracture," and medial malleolar are included in this group.

SECOND METATARSAL STRESS FRACTURES

Occur more commonly in the neck region and diaphyseal aspect but in ballet dancers they are common at the base of the second metatarsal. Studies have shown that the second metatarsal sustains the highest amount of shear forcers and bending strain during running (25).

PHYSICAL EXAMINATION

Presentation is variable but there is localized pain and swelling. Patient will present with a limp unable to bear weight on the forefoot. Usually there has been an increase in activity or an abrupt change in training regimen.

IMAGING

X-rays are often negative as it takes about 2 weeks for stress fractures to be seen. Standard views should be obtained. Tech 99 scan can be useful to diagnose, as it is sensitive but not specific. An isolated increase in uptake is suggestive of a stress fracture. MRI is preferred due to its high sensitivity and specificity. It can differentiate between synovitis, bone stress reaction, and a stress fracture. A CT scan will determine if the fracture is complete or incomplete (27).

TREATMENT

Most stress fractures of the second metatarsal can be managed conservatively. A short leg cast for 6 to 8 weeks. Surgical intervention may be necessary in order to remove necrotic bone on neglected stress fractures.

FIFTH METATARSAL STRESS FRACTURES

Fractures at the metaphyseal–diaphyseal junction commonly known as "Jones Fracture" are common in young athletes. The name comes from British orthopedic surgeon Sir Robert Jones, who sustained this fracture while dancing. Patients with high arched cavovarus feet and those with limited hindfoot eversion are most at risk since repetitive force to the lateral aspect of the foot is increased.

CLASSIFICATION

The Torg classification (28) is a radiologic classification for fifth metatarsal stress fractures that evaluates the medullary canal in order to assess the need for bone grafting procedures.

Type I: Acute fracture, no cortical hypertrophy, and no intramedullary sclerosis.

Type II: Delayed union, fracture line involves cortices, periosteal new bone formation, and evidence of intramedullary sclerosis.

Type III: Non-unions, history of repetitive trauma, recurrent symptoms, and obliteration of the medullary canal by sclerotic bone.

TREATMENT

A Type-I fracture can be treated with a below the knee non–weight-bearing cast. Type II can be treated conservatively but can also be treated as a Type III. This involves medullary curettage and bone grafting in order to expedite healing for the athlete.

NAVICULAR STRESS FRACTURES

The boat-shaped navicular bone is susceptible to stress fractures, especially the central one-third aspect of the bone. This center zone is devoid of direct blood supply; medially the navicular receives blood from the medial plantar artery and laterally from the dorsalis pedis, therefore it renders the central zone relative avascular—watershed area and predisposed to stress fractures (29).

PHYSICAL EXAMINATION

Unfortunately, a delay in diagnoses of navicular stress fractures is common. Patients usually present with vague and subtle symptoms. The pain will be felt dorsally on the midfoot and only when engaging in sports that require rapid changes in direction, jumping, and sprinting. Commonly, no/minimal symptoms are felt during rest. The term "N Spot" has been used to identify the midportion of the navicular where the focal point of pain is felt.

IMAGING

Standard x-rays should be obtained although radiographs can appear normal. There is no order in which imaging should be done next, but a bone scan, CT scan, or MRI must be obtained. A CT scan has demonstrated to be more sensitive than an MRI and typically it demonstrates an incomplete oblique fracture line extending from dorsomedial to plantar lateral (25,27,29).

CLASSIFICATION

Saxena and Fullen created a classification system based on frontal plane CT scans (30).

Type I: Involves only the dorsal cortex
Type II: Extending to the body
Type III: Extends the whole body of the navicular breaking the plantar cortex.

TREATMENT

Conservative treatment of casting and non–weight-bearing for at least 6 weeks followed with slow return to pre-fracture activities is recommended. However, internal fixation is usually the treatment of choice for athletes having sustained a Type-II or Type-III fracture. Two percutaneous cannulated screws are placed from lateral to medial on the navicular under fluoroscopy. Bone grafts and a bone stimulator can be used for non/delayed unions.

Patients are then casted for 4 weeks non—weight-bearing and the cast is discontinued at 6 weeks when activities are gradually resumed (11,30).

PREVENTION

Sports-related injuries have obvious economic and social impacts (31). Especially amongst children, a number of articles cite the use of protective equipment, rule changes and enforcement, improved coaching and training, and an increased awareness of the possibility of injury as paramount to successful injury prevention (32–34).

The rationale that foot structure, shoe design, and weight-bearing surface can individually or collectively influence the incidence of sports-related injuries is well-documented (35–42). Turf toe injuries were virtually unknown before the introduction of artificial playing surfaces, but no study has been able to implicate artificial turf conclusively. The switch from rigid long-cleat shoes (which provided little traction on artificial turf) to more flexible, short-cleat ones has also been studied as the cause of turf toe, but the few studies that are available seem to contradict one another. The addition of a Morton's extension

TABLE 22.2 Forefoot Injuries Reported in Specific Sports

Sport	Reported Forefoot Injury (Excluding Fractures)
Basketball	Sesamoiditis, FHL tenosynovitis, hallux rigidus (44)
Bicycling	Hallux amputation (shoeless passengers on rear carrier) (45)
Racquet sports	Hallux rigidus, subungual hematoma ("tennis toe") (46,47)
Soccer	Contusions (48,49)
Windsurfing	Contusions, lacerations (50)
Cerebral palsy-disabled athletes	Metatarsalgia (51)
Expedition-length adventure racing	Blisters (52)
Dance	Hallux rigidus (53), toenail avulsion and hematoma, Freiberg's infarction, sesamoiditis, and MTPJ subluxation (54)
Running	Morton's neuroma, metatarsalgia, sesamoiditis, blisters, hallux rigidus, second MTPJ subluxation (55,56,57), and toenail avulsion and hematoma (especially the lateral toes) (57)
Taekwondo	Open first IPJ lateral collateral ligament injury (58)

to an orthosis used in a flexible turf shoe, by slightly restricting first MTPJ motion, could conceivably reduce the incidence of turf toe injuries. Custom-made or prefabricated insoles reduced the number of *ankle* injuries in military recruits, but forefoot injuries were not studied (43).

SPORTS-SPECIFIC FOREFOOT INJURIES

Sport-specific surveys of foot and ankle injuries have been described, but they are sparse in number. As an aid to the reader, they are summarized in Table 22.2.

Forefoot injuries in sports are commonplace yet difficult to prevent. Early recognition, prompt and accurate diagnosis, and proficient treatment are the best measures for returning the injured to the playing field.

REFERENCES

1. Eisele SA. Conditions of the toenails. *Orthop Clin North Am* 1994;25:183–188.
2. Malay DS. How to address nail bed injuries. *Podiatr Today* 2006;19:38–44.
3. Tucker DJ, Jules KT, Raymond F. Nailbed injuries with hallucal phalangeal fractures. *J Am Podiatr Med Assoc* 1996;86(4):170–173.
4. Baran R, Hay RJ, Haneke E. Eds. Onychomycosis: The Current Approch to Diagnosis and Therapy, 2nd ed. Boca Raton: Taylor & Francis, 2006:13–15.
5. Adams WR. Morton's neuroma. *Clin Podiatr Med Surg* 2010;27:535–545.
6. Stamatis ED, Karabalis C. Interdigital neuromas: current state of the art-surgical. *Foot Ankle Clin* 2004;9:287–296.
7. Mann RA, Reynolds JC. Interdigital neuroma: a critical clinical analysis. *Foot Ankle* 1983; 3:238–243.
8. Peters PG, Adams AB, Schon LC. Interdigital neuroma. *Foot Ankle Clin* 2010;16:305–315.
9. Maskill JD, Bohay DR, Anderson JG. First ray injuries. *Foot Ankle Clin* 2006;11:143–163.
10. Pontell D, Hallivis R, Dollard MD. Sports injuries in the pediatric and adolescent foot and ankle: common overuse and acute presentations. *Clin Podiatr Med Surg* 2006;23:209–231.
11. Umans HR. Imaging sports medicine injuries of the foot and toes. *Clin Sports Med* 2006;25:763–780.
12. Boike A, Schirring-Judge M, McMillin S. Sesamoid disorders of the first metatarsophalangeal joint. *Clin Podiatr Med Surg* 2011;28:269–285.
13. McCormick JJ, Anderson RB. The great toe: failed turf toe, chronic turf toe and complicated sesamoid injuries. *Foot Ankle Clin* 2009;14:135–150.
14. Kadakia AR, Molloy A. Current concepts review: traumatic disorders of the first metatarsophalangeal joint and sesamoid complex. *Foot Ankle Int* 2011;8(32):834–839
15. Lee DK, Mulder GD, Schwartz AK. Hallux, sesamoid, and first metatarsal injuries. *Clin Podiatr Med Surg* 2011;28:43–56.
16. Pagenstert GI, Valderrabano V, Hintermann B. Medial sesamoid nonunion combined with hallux valgus in athletes: a report of two cases. *Foot Ankle Int* 2006;27(2):135–140.
17. Coughlin MJ. Second metatarsophalangeal joint instability in the athlete. *Foot Ankle* 1993; 14:309–319.
18. Baravarian B, Thompson J, Nazarian D. Plantar plate tears: a review of the modified flexor tendon transfer repair for stabilization. *Clin Podiatr Med Surg* 2011;28:57–68.
19. Coughlin MJ, Baumfeld DS, Nery C. Second MTP joint stability: grading of the deformity and description of surgical repair of capsular insufficiency. *Phys Sportsmed* 2011;39(3):132–141.
20. Coughlin MJ, Schutt SA, Hirose CB, et al. Metatarsophalangeal joint pathology in crossover second toe deformity: a cadaveric study. *Foot Ankle Int* 2012;33:133–140.
21. Nery C, Coughling MJ, Baumfeld D, et al. Lesser metatarsophalangeal joint instability: prospective evaluation and repair of plantar plate and capsular insufficiency. *Foot Ankle Int* 2012;33:301–311.
22. Bouche RT, Heit EJ. Combined plantar plate and hammertoe repair with flexor digitorum longus tendon transfer for chronic, severe sagittal plane instability of the lesser metatarsophalangeal joints: preliminary observations. *J Foot Ankle Surg* 2008;47(2):125–137.
23. Kier R, Abrahamian H, Caminear D, et al. MR arthrography of the second and third metatarsophalangeal joints for the detection of tears of the plantar plate and joint capsule. *Am J Roentgenol* 2010;194:1079–1081.
24. Glenn WR, Hergan DJ. Treatment of stress fractures: the fundamentals. *Clin Sports Med* 2006;25:29–36.
25. Gehrmann RM, Renard RL. Current concepts review: Stress fractures of the foot. *Foot Ankle Int* 2006;9(27):750–757.
26. Iwamoto J, Sato Y, Takeda T, et al. Analysis of stress fractures in athletes based on our clinical experience. *World J Orthop* 2011;1(2):7–12.
27. Anderson RB, Hunt KJ, McCormick JJ. Management of common sports-related injuries about the foot and ankle. *J Am Acad Orthop Surg* 2010;18:546–556.
28. Torg JS, Balduini FC, Zelko RR, et.al. Fractures of the base of the fifth metatarsal distal to the tuberosity. Classification and guidelines for non-surgical and surgical management. *J Bone Joint Surg* 1984;66:209–214.
29. Mann JA, Pedowitz DI. Evaluation and treatment of navicular stress fractures, including nonunions, revision surgery, and persistent pain after treatment. *Foot Ankle Clin* 2009;14:187–204.
30. Saxena A, Fullem B, Hannaford D. Results of treatment of 22 navicular stress fractures and a new proposed radiographic classification system. *J Foot Ankle Surg* 2000;39:96–103.
31. Knowles SB, Marshall SW, Miller T, et al. Cost of injuries from a prospective cohort study of North Carolina high school athletes. *Inj Prev* 2007;13:416–421.
32. Twellaar M, Verstappen FTJ, Huson A. Is prevention of sports injuries a realistic goal? A four-year prospective investigation of sports injuries among physical education students. *Am J Sports Med* 24(4): 528–534, 1996.
33. Flynn JM, Lou JE, Ganley TJ. Prevention of sports injuries in children. *Curr Opin Pediatr* 2002;14(6):719–722.
34. Demorest RA, Landry GL. Prevention of pediatric sports injuries. *Curr Sports Med Rep* 2003;2 (6):337–343.
35. Kaufman KR, Brodine SK, Shaffer RA, et al. The effect of foot structure and range of motion on musculoskeletal overuse injuries. *Am J Sports Med* 1999;27:585–593.
36. Mundermann A, Nigg BM, Humble RN, et al. Foot orthotics affect lower extremity kinematics and kinetics during running. *Clin Biomech* 2003;18:254–262.
37. Williams BE, Yakel JD. Clinical uses of in-shoe pressure analysis in podiatric sports medicine. *J Am Podiatr Med Assoc* 2007;97(1):49–58.
38. Busseuil C, Freychat P, Guedj EB. et al. Rearfoot-forefoot orientation and traumatic risk for runners. *Foot Ankle* 1998;19(1):32–37.
39. Michelson JD, Durant DM, McFarland E. The injury risk associated with pesplanus in athletes. *Foot Ankle* 2002;23(7):629–633.
40. Murphy DF, Connolly DAJ, Beynnon BD. Risk factors for lower extremity injury: a review of the literature. *Br J Sports Med* 2003;37:13–29.
41. Van der Putten EP, Snijders CJ. Shoe design for prevention of injuries in sport climbing. *Appl Ergon* 2001;32:379–387.
42. Ford KR, Manson NA, Evans BJ, et al. Comparison of in-shoe loading patterns on natural grass and synthetic turf. *J Sci Med Sport* 2006;9:433–440.
43. Aaltonen S, Karjalainen H, Heinonen, A, et al. Prevention of sports injuries: systematic review of randomized controlled trials. *Arch Intern Med* 2007;167(15):1585–1592.
44. McDermott EP. Basketball injuries of the foot and ankle. *Clin Sports Med* 1993;12(2):373–393.
45. Subrahmanyam M. Bicycle injury pattern among children in rural India. *Trop Geogr Med* 1984;36:243–247.
46. Zecher SB, Leach RE. Lower leg and foot injuries in tennis and other racquet sports. *Clin Sports Med* 1995;14(1):223–239.
47. Bylak J, Hutchinson MR. Common sports injuries in young tennis players. *Sports Med* 1998;26(2):119–132
48. Wong P, Hong Y. Soccer injury in the lower extremities. *Br J Sports Med* 2005;39:473–482.
49. Giza E, Fuller C, Junge A, et al. Mechanisms of foot and ankle injuries in soccer. *Am J Sports Med* 2003;31:550–554.
50. Nathanson AT, Reinert SE. Windsurfing injuries: results of a paper- and internet-based survey. *Wilderness Environ Med* 1999;10:218–225.
51. Klenck C, Gebke K. Practical management: common medical problems in disabled athletes. *Clin J Sport Med* 2007;17(1):55–60.
52. Townes DS, Taibot TS, Wedmore IS, et al. Event medicine: injury and illness during an expedition-length adventure race. *J Emerg Med* 2004;27(2):161–165.
53. Garrick JG, Lewis SL. Career hazards for the dancer. *Occup Med* 2001;16(4):609–618.
54. Prisk VR, O' Loughlin PF, Kennedy JG. Forefoot injuries in dancers. *Clin Sports Med* 2008;27:305–320.
55. Lilich JS, Baxter DE. Common forefoot problems in runners. *Foot Ankle* 1986;7(3):145–151.
56. Watson AS. Running injuries – knees to toes. *Aust Fam Physician* 1988;17(2):99–103.
57. Scher RK. Jogger's toe. *Int J Dermatol* 1978;17(9):719–720.
58. Shin YW, Choi IH, Rhee NK. Open lateral collateral injury of the interphalangeal joint of the great toe in adolescents during taekwondo. *Am J Sports Med* 2008;36(1):158–161.

Keith R. Reinhardt
Moira McCarthy
Dean G. Lorich

CHAPTER 23

Forefoot Trauma

INTRODUCTION

Injuries to the metatarsals, phalanges, and surrounding structures of the forefoot occur commonly in athletes. Forefoot injuries result in significant time lost from sports, surpassed only by injuries to the knee and ankle (1). While in the general population these injuries are often considered minor in comparison to those of the midfoot and hindfoot, in athletes they take on greater importance and occur more frequently. The reason for this is because the forces normally seen by the forefoot during normal stance and gait can be tripled in athletes during running and jumping maneuvers. This is especially true of the hallux, which bears twice the load of the lesser toes (2). Proper recognition and management of injuries to the forefoot is therefore important in avoiding chronic disability given the amount of load this part of the foot experiences with everyday walking.

RELEVANT ANATOMY

An understanding of the anatomy and biomechanics of particular aspects of the forefoot is crucial to correctly diagnosing and treating injuries to this area. For example, the first metatarsophalangeal (MTP) joint is anatomically complex and derives its stability from both its osseous and soft tissue components. The articulation consists of the concave base of the proximal phalanx and the convex head of the first metatarsal, and is supported by collateral ligaments and the plantar plate. Biomechanically, the collateral ligaments become taut with flexion of the first MTP joint, whereas the plantar plate becomes tight in extension. The plantar plate, which is part of the capsuloligamentous complex that affords the joint stability, is a thick fibrocartilaginous structure that has strong attachments to the proximal phalanx but relatively weak attachments to the metatarsal. Knowing this, it is then easy to recognize why hyperdorsiflexion of the first MTP joint often results in rupture of the plantar plate from the relatively weaker attachment site, the metatarsal neck (3). This will be discussed in more detail later in the chapter.

Like our knowledge of the biomechanics of the forefoot, familiarity with its neurovascular supply will also help guide our diagnosis and treatment of injuries to this area. For example, vascular insufficiency of the proximal fifth metatarsal was first recognized as a potential cause of delayed unions by Carp in 1927 (4). Since then the blood supply and its implications for fracture healing have been elucidated. The unique blood supply to the proximal aspect of the fifth metatarsal poses important challenges in treating fractures involving this region. The fifth metatarsal derives its blood supply from three sources: Metaphyseal arteries from surrounding soft tissues, periosteal arteries, and the nutrient artery (Fig. 23.1). The nutrient artery enters the bone of the fifth metatarsal from the medial side at the junction of the middle and proximal third of the diaphysis. Proximally the nutrient artery divides into terminal branches before reaching the proximal metaphysis. This creates a "watershed" area devoid of robust blood supply at the proximal metaphyseal–diaphyseal junction, which creates a potential for nonunion or delayed union of fractures at this location (5). Knowledge of this vascular anatomy provides insight into proper management of fractures of the proximal fifth metatarsal. Whereas fractures both proximal and distal to the watershed area can be treated more conservatively because of a higher tendency to unite uneventfully, true "Jones" fractures, especially in athletes, require a more aggressive approach as we will discuss.

FRACTURES AND FRACTURE-DISLOCATIONS OF THE GREAT TOE

Great Toe Phalangeal Fractures

Great toe phalangeal fractures are relatively common because the great toe forms the medial border of the foot. Transverse or comminuted fractures occur because of a direct impact on an unprotected foot. Spiral or oblique fractures occur because of a stubbing injury with axial load and varus or valgus force. Adolescent athletes may have physeal fractures through the proximal phalanx that result from a plantarflexion injury (6). Fractures are evident by soft tissue swelling and ecchymosis. Radiographs of the toe in the AP, lateral, and oblique plane are sufficient for diagnosis. If radiographs appear normal despite high clinical suspicion, an MRI is indicated to evaluate for stress reactions, bone edema, and osteochondral defects. Osteochondral defects are common in repetitive kicking athletes. Phalangeal fractures that are left unreduced may heal with plantar angulation due to a stronger flexion force than an extensor force on the fracture. In the athlete, this can result in significant pain and shoe-wearing difficulty.

These fractures are treated more aggressively than fractures of the lesser phalanges. Nondisplaced extra-articular fractures are generally treated with at least 4 weeks of buddy-taping, hard-soled shoes, and protected weight bearing. Fractures

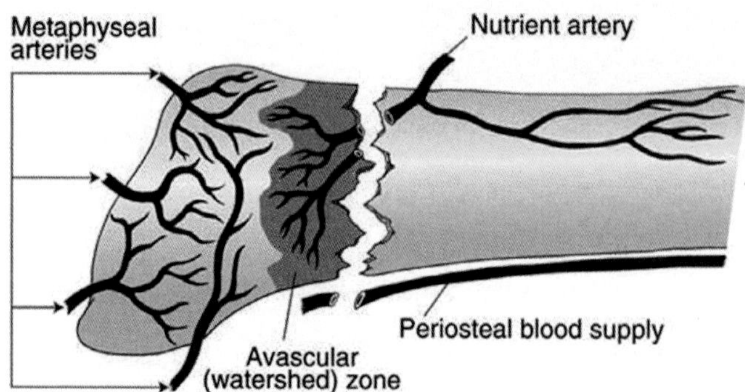

Figure 23.1. Illustration of the vascular supply to the proximal fifth metatarsal demonstrating the avascular, or watershed, zone in the metaphyseal–diaphyseal region. Modified and reprinted with permission from: Smith JW, Arnoczky SP, Hersh A. The intraosseous blood supply of the fifth metatarsal: Implications for proximal fracture healing. *Foot Ankle Int.* 1992;13(3), Figure13, page 151.

demonstrating displacement and instability are treated with closed reduction and percutaneous pinning. Intra-articular fractures are treated with anatomic reduction and internal fixation. Post-operative rehabilitation includes 4 to 6 weeks of protected weight bearing in a short leg cast. Surgical treatment of osteochondral defects, including excision, debridement, and microfracture of the defect, has been shown to be effective in returning 85% of 81 beach soccer players to their sport (7).

Great Toe Interphalangeal (IP) Dislocations

Dislocations of the great toe IP joint are due to an axial load on the terminal end of the digit. Presentation is that of a hyperextended joint with inability to flex the IP joint. This correlates with a dorsal dislocation. Diagnosis is by radiographs in the AP, lateral, and oblique plane to rule out a concomitant fracture.

Simple dislocations of the great toe IP joint are reduced with longitudinal traction. If the reduction is achieved and stable throughout range of motion, the toe can be splinted or buddy-taped for 3 weeks with gradual return to weight bearing as tolerated. An irreducible IP dislocation may occur because of interposition of either the FHL, plantar plate, or sesamoid (8). In irreducible cases or cases of gross instability, fracture-dislocation, or residual joint incongruity after reduction, open reduction and internal fixation is necessary. Though a medial or lateral surgical approach to the IP joint, depending on the injury, the joint and fracture fragments are reduced anatomically and stabilized with K-wires.

A complication of fractures and dislocations of the great toe that is worth considering is stiffness of the IP joint. The normal physiologic range of motion of the IP joint is from 20 to 60 degrees. This is generally well-tolerated as patients can compensate through motion at the MTP joint. If the MTP joint is also injured or ankylosed, then IP stiffness may be more disabling in terms of pain and ability return to play.

Additional considerations with great toe fractures and dislocations are the surrounding soft tissues and the nailbed. Subungual hematomas constituting at least 25% of the toenail should be evacuated. Controversy exists over treatment of hematomas of 50% or greater with an associated phalangeal fracture. Some authors recommend treatment of the open fracture with irrigation and nailbed laceration repair (9) while others report that evacuation only, regardless of the size of the hematoma, is the appropriate treatment (10).

FIRST MTP JOINT INJURIES

Physiologic gait relies on mobility at the MTP joint. Hallux MTP joint injuries can be debilitating injuries in athletes, especially if the severity of the injury is not appreciated or treatment is delayed (11). MTP joint stability relies on the complex capsuloligamentous anatomy made up of the plantar plate, collateral ligaments, the FHB, the adductor hallucis, and the abductor hallucis. Physiologic MTP motion ranges from 40 to 100 degrees of dorsiflexion to 3 to 45 degrees of plantarflexion. Injuries to the MTP joint can range from mild sprains to severe sprains (turf toe) to dislocations. Various combinations of fractures, dislocations, and subluxations can occur.

Dislocations of the first MTP are relatively rare with the reported incidence ranging from 0.0008% to 0.004% and generally occur as a result of high-energy axial load with the foot in equinus resulting in a hyperextension injury (3,12,13,14) Dorsal dislocations are most common (Fig. 23.2), whereas plantar or lateral dislocations occur less frequently (12). The classification for dorsal dislocations was originally developed by Jahss and has since been modified (Fig. 23.3). Type IA involves disruption of the proximal sesamoid attachment and the plantar plate with the sesamoids incarcerated within the MTP joint. Type IB involves disruption of the sesamoid complex more distally. Type II dislocations disrupt the inter-sesamoidal ligament allowing either divergence of the sesamoids (IIA), transverse fracture of one of the sesamoids (IIB), or a combination of both (IIC). Radiographic confirmation of the dislocation with anteroposterior as well as lateral views should be performed when this is suspected.

Treatment of these dislocations requires prompt attention to avoid soft tissue compromise. Closed reduction with a digital block should be attempted initially. If the joint is unstable or incongruent after successful closed reduction, or if it is irreducible, then open reduction internal fixation is required. These

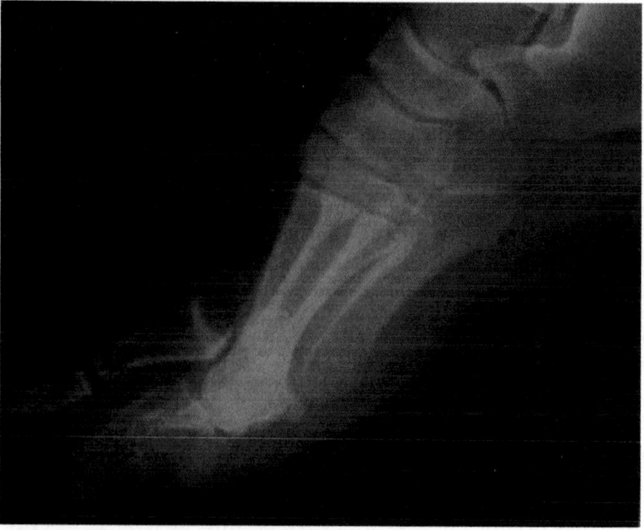

Figure 23.2. Lateral radiograph demonstrating a dorsal dislocation of the first MTP joint. Reprinted with permission from: Berquist. Imaging of the foot and ankle. 3rd ed.; 2011:309.

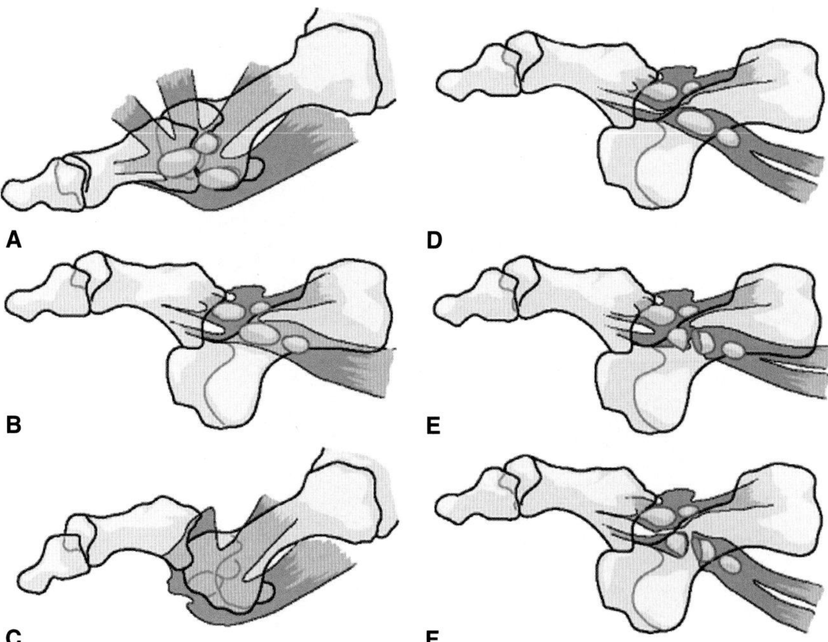

Figure 23.3. Classification of dorsal dislocations of the first MTP joint according to involvement of the plantar plate and sesamoid complex. **(A)** Normal anatomy; **(B)** Type IA dislocation; **(C)** Type IB dislocation; **(D)** Type IIA dislocation; **(E)** Type IIB dislocation; **(F)** Type IIC dislocation. Modified and reprinted with permission from: Mittlmeier T, Haar, P. Sesamoid and toe fractures. *Injury* 2004;35(2):Suppl 1:87–97.

dislocations have been reported to be irreducible secondary to the metatarsal head buttonholing through the sesamoid-short flexor mechanism with the inter-sesamoid ligament remaining intact (15). Open reduction through a dorsal-medial approach at the first webspace is performed followed by K-wire immobilization.

In most cases the closed reduction technique is successful. If the joint is stable to range of motion and congruent on radiographs, the patient can weight bear as tolerated with restricted dorsiflexion for 4 weeks followed by progressive return to sports. Following open reduction, the patient is immobilized in a non–weight-bearing cast for 2 to 3 weeks followed by gradual weight bearing, range of motion and strengthening before return to play is allowed. The prognosis for return to full function is generally favorable. When reduced early, these dislocations do not result in prolonged disability or degenerative joint disease. When treatment is delayed, however, they can become potentially career-ending if complicated by residual pain, stiffness, instability, hallux rigidus, and/or hallux valgus.

FRACTURES OF THE SESAMOIDS

The sesamoid complex consists of two bones centered over the plantar aspect of the MTP joint of the great toe. The tibial sesamoid is within the medial head of the flexor hallucis brevis while the smaller fibular sesamoid is within the lateral head. The two sesamoids are connected by the inter-sesamoid ligament which helps make up the plantar plate of the first MTP joint (16). The sesamoids increase the moment arm of the flexors as well as cushion the MTP joint and thereby protect the flexor tendon (16). The complex transmits as much as 50% of body weight and can experience loads of greater than 300% of body weight during push-off (17). The arterial blood supply to the sesamoids arises from the plantar arch in 25%, from the medial plantar artery in 25%, and from both in 50% (18) (Fig. 23.4).

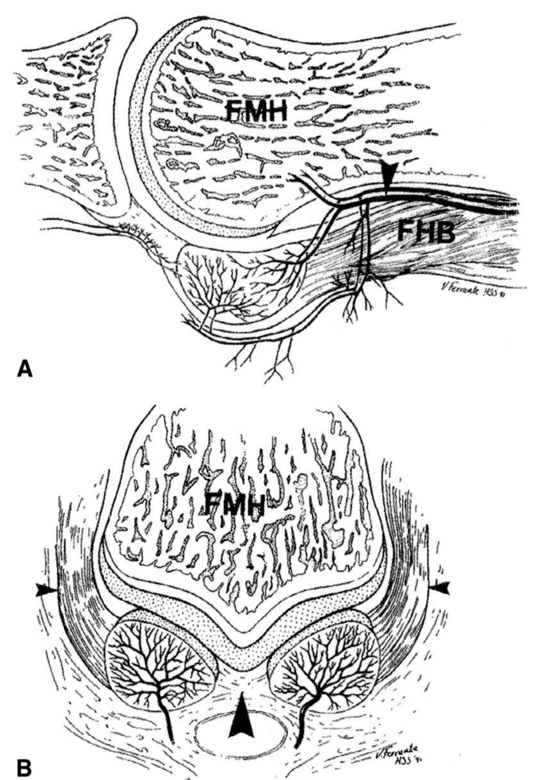

Figure 23.4. **A:** Sagittal section through the tibial sesamoid demonstrating the typical blood supply. The proximal and plantar supply is from branches of the first metatarsal artery (*arrow*). Distal blood supply is limited. **B:** Coronal section showing the rich plantar blood supply and absence of vascularity through the capsule (*small arrows*) and inter-sesamoid ligament (*large arrow*). FMH, first metatarsal head; FHB, flexor hallucis brevis.Copyright C 2011 by the American Orthopaedic Foot and Ankle Society, Inc., originally published in *Foot Ankle Int.*, 13(6):361 and reproduced here with permission.

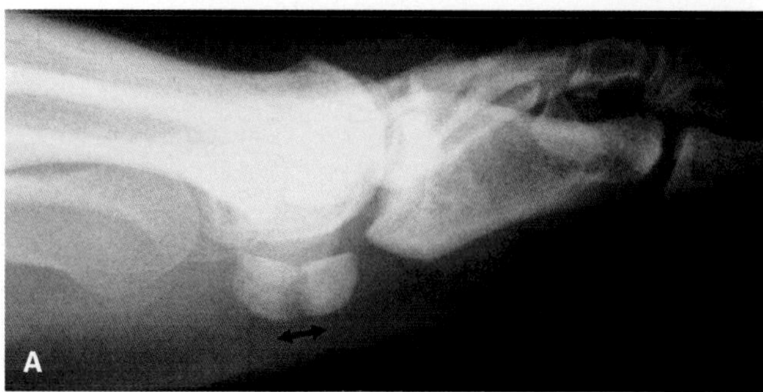

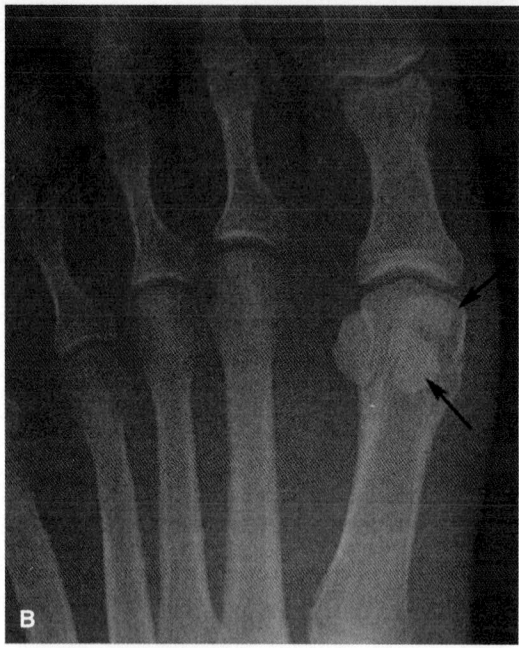

Figure 23.5. Radiographs demonstrating an acute sesamoid fracture **(A)** indicated by the irregular borders at the fracture site, and a bipartite medial sesamoid (*arrows*). **(B)**. Modified and reprinted with permission from: Berquist. Imaging of the foot and ankle. 3rd ed.; 2011:193.

Sesamoid injuries include stress fractures (40%), sesamoiditis (30%), and acute fractures (10%) (17). Stress fractures are common in dancers and runners and result from repetitive loading of the first MTP joint. They are most common in the tibial sesamoid (19). Acute sesamoid fractures resulting from hyperdorsiflexion injuries of the MTP are transverse and usually involve the larger tibial sesamoid while those resulting from direct impact as in jumpers are usually stellate (20). Distinguishing between bipartite sesamoids and an acute fracture can be difficult (Fig. 23.5). Bipartite sesamoids occur in 7.8% to 35.5% of the population with bilateral bipartite sesamoids occurring in 85% of those patients (21). Acute fractures have irregular and unequal sesamoid fragments, absence of similar contralateral findings, and callus formation on follow-up radiographs whereas bipartite sesamoids typically do not (20). Lateral radiographs taken with the MTP dorsiflexed can reveal displacement of acute fractures that may go unnoticed with the MTP in neutral position.

Evaluation of the sesamoids is critical for diagnosis as well as treatment. Radiographs should include standing anteroposterior and lateral views, a lateral 40 degree oblique view for the fibular sesamoid, and a medial 40 degree oblique view for the tibial sesamoid. An axial view of the first MTP offers detail of the joint and the sesamoids. As discussed above, a dorsiflexed lateral view is indicated to reveal displacement. Further imaging includes radionuclide scans, CT scans with 1 mm cuts, and MRI. MRI is most helpful for diagnosing other conditions of the MTP joint in addition to sesamoid pathology.

The mainstay of treatment for sesamoid injuries remains conservative. Rest, ice, nonsteroidal anti-inflammatory medications, and orthoses are first-line. Stress fractures and nondisplaced acute fractures are casted for 6 to 8 weeks followed by 6 weeks of protected activity, and long-term orthosis treatment. Prolonged recovery, at least 4 to 6 months and possibly up to 1 year, can be expected with fractures in athletes. Non-athletes may be given more time with conservative treatment. For displaced fractures and those that do not respond to conservative treatment after 6 months, the primary surgical interventions are bone grafting or partial or complete excision of one or both sesamoids (16). Excision of both sesamoids should be avoided except in extreme conditions because of the resultant cock-up deformity of the great toe (16). In addition, sesamoid excision may result in first MTP joint instability which can result in decreased performance for some dancers and other athletes who require repetitive lift-off from the great toe (22). Percutaneous screw fixation as well as open reduction internal fixation of the sesamoids have recently been described (23,24).

Excision of a single sesamoid is the mainstay of treatment and is generally well tolerated. Return to activity may occur as early as 7.5 weeks after surgery (25). Biedert et al. reported on six sesamoid stress fractures in five athletes who had all failed conservative treatment and underwent proximal partial sesamoidectomy. All athletes had no complications and returned to full sports activities within 6 months. At final follow-up, one patient had restricted activity but all were rated good–excellent (26). A recent case report of one patient who underwent ORIF of an acute fracture resulted in complete radiographic healing at 14 weeks and complete return to function at final 36-month follow-up (27). Percutaneous screw fixation has been shown to result in return to function within 3 months (23). Hulkko et al. reported on 15 stress fractures of the sesamoids in athletes. Ten were treated conservatively and five were treated with excision. There were no complications and athletes returned to training in 8 weeks. Seven of the conservatively treated athletes and all of the surgically treated athletes returned to full function and had good outcomes, with the remaining conservatively treated athletes having mild residual symptoms (28).

Post-operative rehabilitation generally consists of a non–weight-bearing short leg cast for at least 3 weeks. Passive MTP flexion and mobilization of the IP joint may begin at 3 weeks. Progressive range of motion and weight bearing may begin after 6 weeks, depending on the initial degree of fracture displacement. The earliest time for removal of the cast is generally 6 weeks followed by a post-operative shoe for approximately 2 weeks or until the patient can bear weight without pain.

Complications from sesamoid fractures and operative treatment are varied and generally depend on the degree of displacement as well as pre-existing hallux deformities. Non-operative treatment can result in delayed union or nonunion. With excision, particularly of the tibial sesamoid, increases in hallux valgus deformities can occur. This can be limited but not completely prevented by MTP capsular repair. Hallux varus deformity has also been described following fibular sesamoid excision (21). Excision of both sesamoids can result in decreased push-off strength, cock-up deformities of the great toe, and transfer metatarsalgia (16). Chronic pain resulting from either a neuroma or an incision directly over the sesamoids is common and should not be confused with a stress fracture.

METATARSAL FRACTURES

Metatarsal fractures are among the most common injuries in the foot. An epidemiologic study of these fractures found that the fifth is the most commonly fractured metatarsal and that 7.9% of all metatarsal fractures occur with athletics (29). Another study reported that approximately 9% of all metatarsal fractures were from athletics with soccer being the most common sport (30). The typical mechanisms of injury include direct force, a fall, or a crush injury. Torque injuries such as twisting on a planted foot can also result in metatarsal fractures, especially of the fifth. Finally, avulsion fractures of the metatarsals can occur with plantarflexion or inversion moments due to ligamentous and tendinous attachments (29). Classification of metatarsal fractures is simply by anatomic location: Base, shaft, neck, or head.

The treatment of metatarsal fractures includes both conservative and operative management. Guidelines for operative management include 10 degrees or more of angulation, 3 to 4 mm of fracture displacement, rotational derangement of the toes, or shortening that alters the parabolic relationship of the metatarsal heads (31).

Non-operative treatment includes immobilization and restricted weight bearing for at least 3 to 5 weeks. Depending on the stability of the fractures, weight bearing can begin immediately or after 1 to 2 weeks. Immobilization devices include a supportive shoe, an arch support to unload the metatarsal heads, a short leg cast, or a cast shoe. Fractures usually heal within 6 weeks and a return to normal function can be expected (31).

Closed reduction can be attempted for displaced fractures, yet the reduction is rarely maintained without internal fixation. Closed reduction and K-wire fixation is often sufficient for non-comminuted fractures. Open reduction internal fixation techniques include K-wire fixation, lag screw fixation for long spiral or oblique fractures, and bridge plating for comminuted fractures. Periarticular fractures of either the head or the base can be treated with locking periarticular plates (32). Fractures of the first metatarsal must be corrected in the sagittal plane to restore normal weight bearing and in the transverse plane to prevent deformity such as hallux valgus (Fig. 23.6) (33). Fractures of the second through fifth metatarsals require restoration of length and sagittal plane alignment to evenly distribute weight bearing in the forefoot (33).

Post-operative rehabilitation includes splinting the foot but allowing immediate active and passive range of motion of the MTP joints unless K-wires are traversing the joint. At 2 to 3 weeks a short leg cast or CAM walker is placed and toe-touch weight bearing is initiated. K-wires are removed between 4 and 6 weeks and progressive weight bearing with range of motion of the ankle, foot, and toes is started. Healing usually takes place by 3 months and patients are changed to a supportive shoe.

Complications include malunion, transfer metatarsalgia, nerve compression, and difficulty with shoe wear secondary to deformity. Prolonged pinning can lead to MTP stiffness.

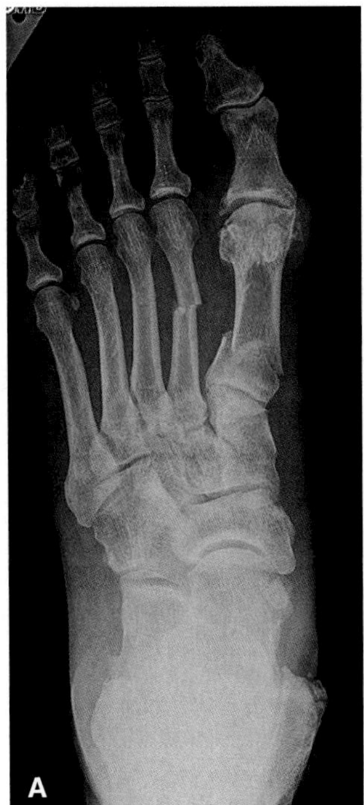

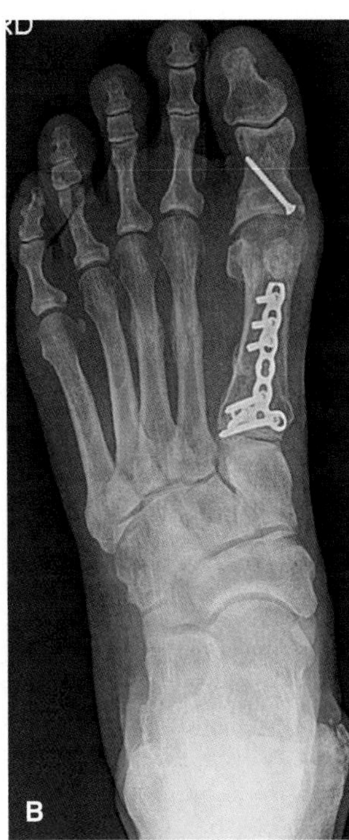

Figure 23.6. AP radiographs showing **(A)** first, second, and third metatarsal fractures in a patient with hallux valgus, and **(B)** healing of the first metatarsal fracture following plate fixation and correction of the hallux valgus including an Akin osteotomy of the proximal phalanx of the first toe. Note the healing of the second and third metatarsals treated without internal fixation. Images courtesy of Matthew M. Roberts, MD.

Plates can irritate extensor tendons and may require hardware removal.

Few studies have examined the outcomes of metatarsal shaft fractures. One study reported no significant difference in outcome with K-wire fixation versus casting (34). A randomized controlled trial evaluating casting versus elastic bandaging showed less pain during treatment in the elastic bandaging group while all healed at 3 months (35).

FRACTURES AND FRACTURE-DISLOCATIONS OF THE LESSER TOES

Fractures of the phalanges of the lesser four toes usually occur from blunt trauma and rarely occur in athletes. When they do occur they typically are treated satisfactorily by simple taping to the adjacent toe and a hard-soled shoe for comfort during ambulation (36). Return to play is guided by resolution of symptoms. Open reduction is usually not necessary for these fractures, unless they are associated with a dislocation as discussed below.

Traumatic dislocations of the lesser metatarsophalangeal joints (LMTPJ) occur less frequently than their counterpart in the great toe (37). The development of artificial playing surfaces has been cited by some as the herald of these injuries (11). Like the first MTP joint, the lesser MTP joints are stabilized by a similar bony articulation and capsuloligamentous complex consisting of collateral ligaments and a plantar plate. Therefore, the LMTPJ's, like the great toe, are susceptible to hyperextension injuries and rupture of the plantar plate from the metatarsal neck ("turf toe"). This has been attributed to the interface between lightweight, flexible shoes, and stiff artificial playing surfaces. The flexible shoes allow hyperextension at the forefoot, making players who wear them susceptible to dorsal dislocations of the MTPJ's. These injuries, however, occur infrequently especially with recent awareness and attention paid to optimizing the shoe–surface interface with modifications in shoe manufacturing.

Patients or players who present with dislocations of the LMTPJ's should undergo an attempt at closed reduction. Often with athletes this will be performed by the team physician or trainer on the field or sideline at the time of injury. If this is done radiographs should be obtained to rule out associated fractures and confirm restoration of alignment. Most commonly the proximal phalanx is dislocated dorsally on the metatarsal (37). Reduction should include hyperdorsiflexion of the MTP joint, longitudinal traction, and plantar-directed pressure on the base of the proximal phalanx. In the vast majority of cases closed reduction is successful and results in a stable articulation. However, in rare cases they are irreducible by closed means. This is usually due to button-holing of the metatarsal head through the plantar capsule and interposition of the plantar plate between the base of the proximal phalanx and the metatarsal head. Rarely, associated metatarsal head fractures can cause persistent instability of the joint after attempted reduction. In these cases open reduction is required with or without temporary pin fixation for grossly unstable joints.

Following closed reduction, if it is stable, taping to adjacent toes or a dorsal splint may be initially applied. A stiff-soled shoe is helpful in avoiding forefoot extension and providing a comfortable platform for weight bearing. If open reduction was required and instability of the joint required temporary K-wire fixation, this should be removed by 3 weeks and joint mobilization initiated to prevent stiffness (37). Regardless of treatment, flexion and extension of the joint should be started by 3 weeks post-injury at the latest, and preferably by 2 weeks. Return to play is usually permitted when the player's symptoms allow. Cross-taping and the use of a stiffer shoe or orthotic can provide protection during the transition back to play. Long-term results of these injuries are scarce because typically with resolution of symptoms patients have no long-term sequelae and no need to return for follow-up. Failure to treat MTP dislocations with appropriate reduction, however, can lead to long-term pain and discomfort requiring surgical intervention later (37).

FRACTURE OF THE DISTAL SHAFT OF THE FIFTH METATARSAL: "DANCER'S FRACTURE"

The forefoot of a ballet dancer is subjected to extraordinary forces during highly demanding positions of dance, and is therefore susceptible to acute traumatic injuries. One of the more common acute injuries occurs when a dancer rolls over the lateral border of the foot in the demi pointe position, resulting in a spiral fracture of the distal diaphysis of the fifth metatarsal (38). This has been termed the "dancer's fracture," and it is characteristically oriented from proximal-medial to distal-lateral on the AP radiograph, and proximal-dorsal to distal-plantar on the lateral (38) (Fig. 23.7).

Historically, these fractures were treated with anatomic reduction and fixation, but more recently non-operative management has become the mainstay for these injuries even in high performance athletes. This likely relates to the relative mobility of the fifth metatarsal and its allowance for malunion without changing the biomechanics of the forefoot (39). Immobilization in a CAM walker or weight-bearing short leg cast with protected weight bearing for comfort has been shown to be an effective strategy in getting these fractures to heal (38). Based on the results of this treatment, patients and athletes can reasonably expect to walk pain-free around 6 weeks following the injury. Professional ballet dancers can be expected to return to barre exercises (weight-bearing exercises while holding onto a horizontal bar) by 12 weeks and full performance by 19 weeks (38). Dancers whose fractures have significant displacement may be expected to take a few weeks longer in returning to full performance. Nonetheless, long-term functional sequelae or residual symptoms do not seem to be prevalent following this injury when treated non-operatively, and return to high-performance dancing can be expected.

FRACTURES OF THE PROXIMAL FIFTH METATARSAL

Fractures of the proximal aspect of the fifth metatarsal occur more commonly than do fractures to the other metatarsals, with up to 70% involving the fifth metatarsal (40). There are three anatomic fracture zones of the base of the fifth metatarsal: Zone 1 = tuberosity, zone 2 = metaphyseal–diaphyseal junction, zone 3 = proximal diaphysis (Fig. 23.8) (41). This distinction is important because fractures in each zone have different healing properties and require different treatment strategies. In addition, with the origins of the abductor digiti minimi and flexor digiti minimi brevis muscles on the metatarsal base, the insertions of the peroneus brevis and lateral band of the plantar fascia on the tuberosity, and the insertion of the peroneus tertius on the proximal diaphysis, a number of considerable deforming forces act upon the proximal fifth metatarsal (Fig. 23.9) (41). This, along with the unique blood supply to the proximal fifth metatarsal as already discussed, represent unique challenges to the effective treatment and healing of injuries involving this area.

Fifth Metatarsal Tuberosity Fractures

Fractures of the tuberosity (Zone I) often result from a mechanism of foot inversion whereby the peroneus brevis tendon insertion on the tuberosity is avulsed along with an osseous fragment. Tuberosity avulsion fractures typically do not extend into the 4–5 intermetatarsal articulation, but they can extend to the fifth metatarsocuboid joint. However, regardless of extension to the articular surface or even fracture displacement, these fractures heal with non-operative therapy (42). As noted previously, the tuberosity of the fifth metatarsal receives its vascular supply predominantly from metaphyseal arteries from the surrounding soft tissues (5), which is likely responsible for the high rate of healing seen with this patient population. Patients with these fractures can be placed in a hard-soled shoe or short leg cast and allowed to bear weight as tolerated. Fracture healing even in athletes can be expected by 6 weeks post-injury with this treatment (43,44). With treatment with only a hard-soled shoe, 85% of patients can expect to return to their pre-injury functional level by 6 months following the injury, and nearly 100% by 1 year (42).

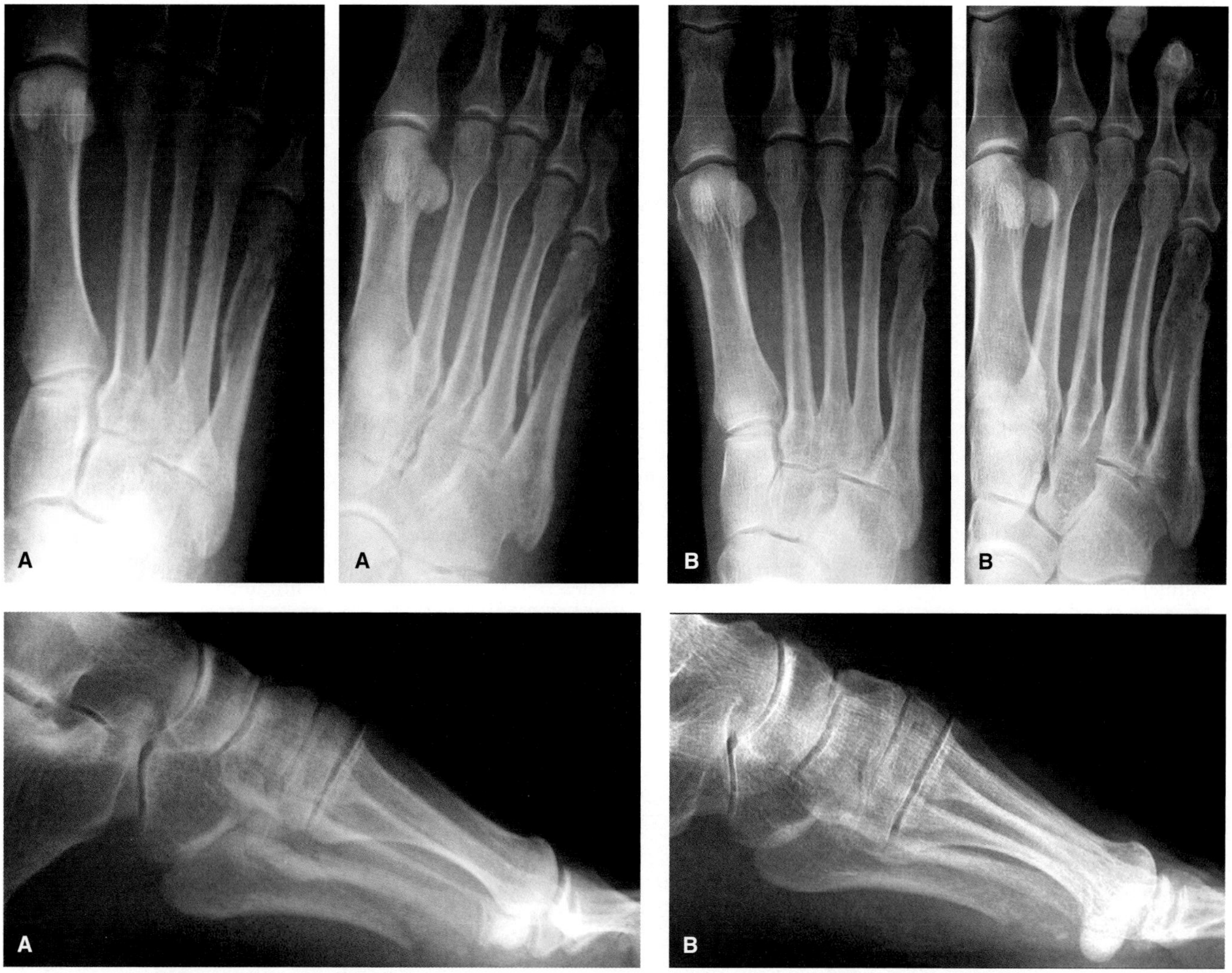

Figure 23.7. Anteroposterior, lateral, and oblique radiographs of a fifth metatarsal shaft fracture with fracture pattern characteristic of a "dancer's fracture," both at the time of injury **(A)** and 3 months later after healing with non-operative treatment **(B)**. Images courtesy of Matthew M. Roberts, MD.

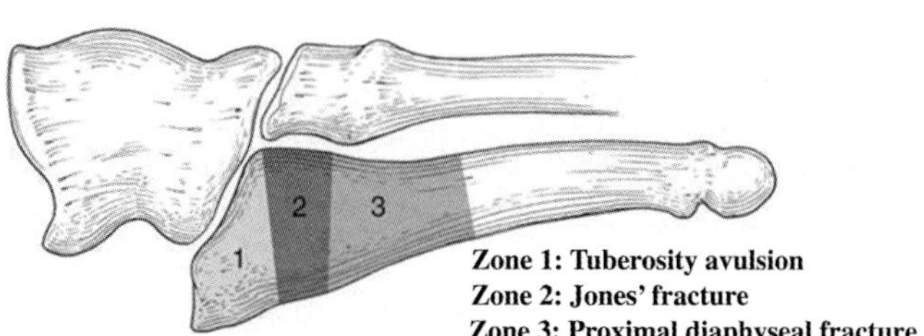

Figure 23.8. Schematic illustrating the three "fracture zones" of the proximal fifth metatarsal i.e., Zone 1: Tuberosity avulsion, Zone 2: Jones' fracture, Zone 3: Proximal diaphyseal fracture (stress fracture). Modified and reprinted with permission from: Lawrence SJ, Botte MJ. Jones' fractures and related fractures of the proximal fifth metatarsal. *Foot Ankle Int.* 1993;14(6), Figure 3, page 360.

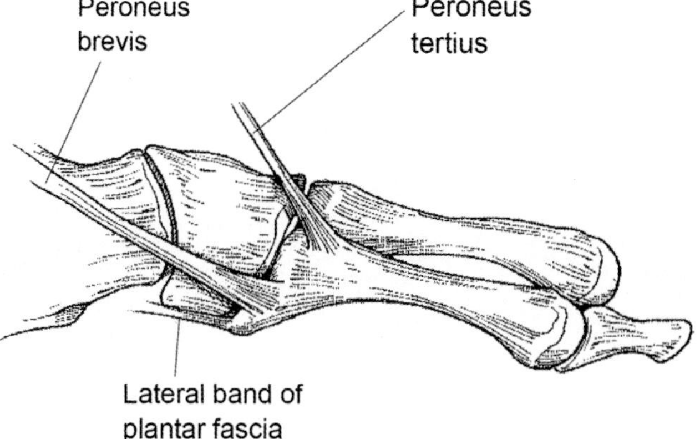

Figure 23.9. Illustration of lateral forefoot anatomy demonstrating the various structures inserting on the proximal fifth metatarsal. Modified and reprinted with permission from: Lawrence SJ, Botte MJ. Jones' fractures and related fractures of the proximal fifth metatarsal. *Foot Ankle Int.* 1993;14(6), Figure 4, page 360.

Jones' Fractures

Fractures of the metaphyseal–diaphyseal junction (Zone 2) of the proximal fifth metatarsal have received much clinical and basic science research attention given the difficulty these fractures pose to treatment and successful healing, especially in athletes. As they have been termed, a true "Jones' fracture," is an acute fracture at the metaphyseal–diaphyseal junction with extension to, or adjacent to, the 4–5 inter-metatarsal articulation medially, but without extension distal to this articulation (45). These fractures typically occur with the ankle plantarflexed, during which a large adduction force on the forefoot, such as that during a pivoting or cutting maneuver, with the body weight on the metatarsal heads, causes the bone to fail at the metaphyseal–diaphyseal junction (46).

Acute, nondisplaced Jones' fractures may be treated in a low demand patient with non–weight-bearing in a short leg cast for 6 to 8 weeks (41,47,48). However, biologic impairments to healing (as discussed), compounded by an athlete's schedule that demands expeditious treatment and faster return to play, do not bode well for non-operative treatment of these fractures in athletes. In high-level and recreational athletes treated conservatively with a short leg cast and non–weight-bearing for differing periods of time, Kavanaugh et al. saw 9 of the 16 patients develop a delayed or nonunion (46). Clapper et al. showed that after non-operative management, 18 of 25 (72%) patients achieved union, but not until an average 21 weeks following the injury (43). These patients required 8 weeks of non–weight-bearing in a short leg cast, and an additional 12 weeks in a weight-bearing cast in order to achieve union. The seven patients in that study who underwent operative internal fixation all healed by 12 weeks after surgery (43). In a recent large series, Jones fractures treated by 4 to 6 weeks with a non–weight-bearing cast or boot, followed by 4 to 8 weeks in a functional orthotic, demonstrated similar time to radiographic fracture union as those treated operatively (49). However, athletes in this cohort treated operatively returned to sports at an average of 15 weeks whereas those non-operatively managed did not return to sports until 30 weeks following the injury (49). This has left many surgeons seeking more aggressive treatment options for this fracture, especially in athletes where time to healing is of great importance.

The alternative to conservative management is operative fixation, which is currently recommended for high-performance athletes in the acute setting, and for recreational or non-athletes with delayed or nonunions that have failed conservative treatment (43,46,47,50). A number of fixation methods have been described, but percutaneous intramedullary fixation with a partially threaded screw has become favored by most authors because of its ability to provide compression without disrupting the biology of healing by avoiding exposure at the fracture site (46,50–52) (Fig. 23.10). In skeletally mature patients, it is

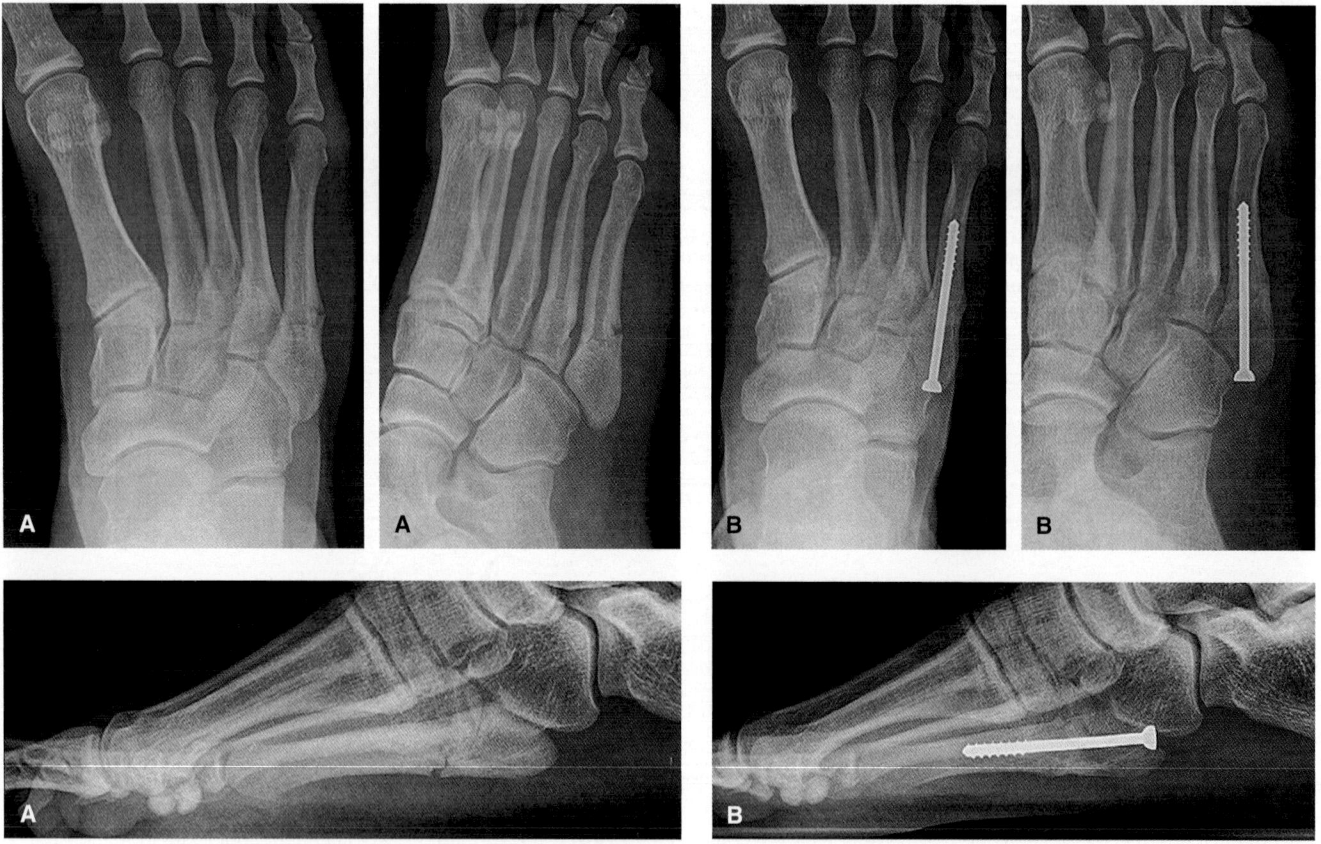

Figure 23.10. Anteroposterior, lateral, and oblique radiographs of the foot demonstrating a Jones' fracture in a 19-year old male patient at the time of injury **(A)** and after intramedullary screw fixation and healing 3 months later **(B)**. Also note the bipartite medial and lateral sesamoids. Images courtesy of Matthew M. Roberts, MD.

suggested to use at least a 4.5 mm screw that is long enough that the threads pass the fracture site (53). Some suggest that the metatarsal can accommodate a 6.5 mm screw which provides greater pullout strength (54). Porter et al. compared 4.5 mm cannulated screws to 5.5 mm cannulated screws in 50 Jones' fractures and found no differences in refracture rates, although three patients did demonstrate bending of the 4.5 mm screws, but this occurred without clinical significance (55). The other point of contention has been regarding whether cannulated screws are biomechanically inferior to the traditionally used 4.5 mm malleolar solid screws. Biomechanical testing has not shown a significant advantage of one 4.5 mm screw over the other, leaving the choice of cannulated or solid to the treating surgeon (56). Nonetheless, at a minimum, the largest screw permitted by the anatomy of the metatarsal should be used to maximize medullary canal thread purchase and screw pull-out strength.

Intramedullary screw fixation has been successful in the timely treatment of athletes, even at the professional level. Basketball players treated with solid intramedullary screw fixation all healed within 3 months of surgery in one series (50). Low et al. reviewed the outcomes of Jones fractures treated in elite football players (collegiate and NFL). Regardless of whether their fracture occurred during the season or during the off-season, of 46 patients treated surgically only 7% developed a nonunion, whereas 20% of the 40 fractures treated non-operatively developed a nonunion (57). When only "in-season" athletes were analyzed, all Jones fractures were treated with intramedullary screw fixation and 94% healed uneventfully (57).

In the NFL, return to competition is allowed by most surgeons by 6 to 12 weeks. However, there is still no universally agreed upon protocol for weight bearing following screw fixation, with half of NFL team physicians allowing immediate weight bearing and half making their athletes non–weight-bearing for 4 to 6 weeks (57). Return to play should be permitted with caution. Early re-fracture has been seen in athletes allowed to return to sport despite even radiographic and clinical evidence of healing, suggesting the possible need for CT or MRI confirmation of complete healing prior to clearance for return to competition (58,59).

SUMMARY

Injuries to the metatarsals, phalanges, and surrounding structures of the forefoot occur commonly in athletes and can result in significant time lost from sports. For many of these injuries, when discussing athletes, the outcomes of non-operative treatment must be considered in the context of time to return to play. This at times will alter the treatment algorithm in favor of operative treatment, as illustrated for example by the tendency for operative fixation of Jones' fractures in athletes. Regardless of treatment chosen, prompt attention to forefoot injuries is critical to minimizing the risk of long-term disability. Furthermore, for many athletes with a forefoot injury, ultimate return to play can be expected following appropriate and timely orthopedic management as discussed in this chapter.

REFERENCES

1. Clanton TO, Butler JE, Eggert A. Injuries to the metatarsophalangeal joints in athletes. *Foot Ankle* 1986;7(3):162–176.
2. Stokes IA, Hutton WC, Stott JR, et al. Forces under the hallux valgus foot before and after surgery. *Clin Orthop Relat Res* 1979;(142):64–72.
3. Giannikas AC, Papachristou G, Papavasiliou N, et al. Dorsal dislocation of the first metatarso-phalangeal joint. Report of four cases. *J Bone Joint Surg Br* 1975;57(3):384–386.
4. Carp L. Fracture of the fifth metatarsal bone: With special reference to delayed union. *Ann Surg* 1927;86(2):308–320.
5. Smith JW, Arnoczky SP, Hersh A. The intraosseous blood supply of the fifth metatarsal: Implications for proximal fracture healing. *Foot Ankle* 1992;13(3):143–152.
6. Maffulli N. Epiphyseal injuries of the proximal phalanx of the hallux. *Clin J Sport Med* 2001;11(2):121–123.
7. Altman A, Nery C, Sanhudo A, et al. Osteochondral injury of the hallux in beach soccer players. *Foot Ankle Int* 2008;29(9):919–921.
8. Banerjee R, Bradley MP, Bluman EM, et al. Clinical pearls: Locked great toe. *Acad Emerg Med* 2003;10(8):878–880.
9. Simon RR, Wolgin M. Subungual hematoma: Association with occult laceration requiring repair. *Am J Emerg Med* 1987;5(4):302–304.
10. Seaberg DC, Angelos WJ, Paris PM. Treatment of subungual hematomas with nail trephination: A prospective study. *Am J Emerg Med* 1991;9(3):209–210.
11. Bowers KD Jr, Martin RB. Turf-toe: A shoe-surface related football injury. *Med Sci Sports* 1976;8(2):81–83.
12. Jahss MH. Traumatic dislocations of the first metatarsophalangeal joint. *Foot Ankle* 1980; 1(1):15–21.
13. Gurd FB. The treatment of complete dislocation of the outer end of the clavicle: A hitherto undescribed operation. *Ann Surg* 1941;63:1094–1098.
14. Lervick GN. Direct arthroscopic distal clavicle resection: A technical review. *Iowa Orthop J* 2005;25:149–156.
15. Brunet JA. Pathomechanics of complex dislocations of the first metatarsophalangeal joint. *Clin Orthop Relat Res* 1996;(332):126–131.
16. Barber FA. Coplaning of the acromioclavicular joint. *Arthroscopy* 2001;17(9):913–917.
17. McBryde AM Jr, Anderson RB. Sesamoid foot problems in the athlete. *Clin Sports Med* 1988;7(1):51–60.
18. Pretterklieber ML, Wanivenhaus A. The arterial supply of the sesamoid bones of the hallux: The course and source of the nutrient arteries as an anatomical basis for surgical approaches to the great toe. *Foot Ankle* 1992;13(1):27–31.
19. Kay SP, Ellman H, Harris E. Arthroscopic distal clavicle excision. Technique and early results. *Clin Orthop Relat Res* 1994;(301):181–184.
20. Henry MH, Liu SH, Loffredo AJ. Arthroscopic management of the acromioclavicular joint disorder. A review. *Clin Orthop Relat Res* 1995;(316):276–283.
21. Snyder SJ, Banas MP, Karzel RP. The arthroscopic mumford procedure: An analysis of results. *Arthroscopy* 1995;11(2):157–164.
22. Aper RL, Saltzman CL, Brown TD. The effect of hallux sesamoid excision on the flexor hallucis longus moment arm. *Clin Orthop Relat Res* 1996;(325):209–217.
23. Blundell CM, Nicholson P, Blackney MW. Percutaneous screw fixation for fractures of the sesamoid bones of the hallux. *J Bone Joint Surg Br* 2002;84(8):1138–1141.
24. Riley J, Selner M. Internal fixation of a displaced tibial sesamoid fracture. *J Am Podiatr Med Assoc* 2001;91(10):536–539.
25. Novak PJ, Bach BR Jr, Romeo AA, et al. Surgical resection of the distal clavicle. *J Shoulder Elbow Surg* 1995;4(1 Pt 1):35–40.
26. Flatow EL, Duralde XA, Nicholson GP, et al. Arthroscopic resection of the distal clavicle with a superior approach. *J Shoulder Elbow Surg* 1995;4(1 Pt 1):41–50.
27. Bigliani LU, Nicholson GP, Flatow EL. Arthroscopic resection of the distal clavicle. *Orthop Clin North Am* 1993;24(1):133–141.
28. Gartsman GM, Combs AH, Davis PF, et al. Arthroscopic acromioclavicular joint resection. An anatomical study. *Am J Sports Med* 1991;19(1):2–5.
29. Slawski DP, Cahill BR. Atraumatic osteolysis of the distal clavicle. Results of open surgical excision. *Am J Sports Med* 1994;22(2):267–271.
30. Renfree KJ, Riley MK, Wheeler D, et al. Ligamentous anatomy of the distal clavicle. *J Shoulder Elbow Surg* 2003;12(4):355–359.
31. Petersson CJ. Resection of the lateral end of the clavicle. A 3 to 30-year follow-up. *Acta Orthop Scand* 1983;54(6):904–907.
32. Walsh WM, Peterson DA, Shelton G, et al. Shoulder strength following acromioclavicular injury. *Am J Sports Med* 1985;13(3):153–158.
33. Ellman H. Arthroscopic subacromial decompression: Analysis of one- to three-year results. *Arthroscopy* 1987;3(3):173–181.
34. Gartsman GM. Arthroscopic resection of the acromioclavicular joint. *Am J Sports Med* 1993;21(1):71–77.
35. Zenios M, Kim WY, Sampath J, et al. Functional treatment of acute metatarsal fractures: A prospective randomised comparison of management in a cast versus elasticated support bandage. *Injury* 2005;36(7):832–835.
36. Anderson L. Injuries of the forefoot. *Clin Orthop Relat Res* 1977;(122):18–27.
37. Brunet JA, Tubin S. Traumatic dislocations of the lesser toes. *Foot Ankle Int* 1997;18(7):406–411.
38. O'Malley MJ, Hamilton WG, Munyak J. Fractures of the distal shaft of the fifth metatarsal. "Dancer's fracture". *Am J Sports Med* 1996;24(2):240–243.
39. Prisk VR, O'Loughlin PF, Kennedy JG. Forefoot injuries in dancers. *Clin Sports Med* 2008; 27(2):305–320.
40. Petrisor BA, Ekrol I, Court-Brown C. The epidemiology of metatarsal fractures. *Foot Ankle Int* 2006;27(3):172–174.

41. Lawrence SJ, Botte MJ. Jones' fractures and related fractures of the proximal fifth metatarsal. *Foot Ankle* 1993;14(6):358–365.
42. Egol K, Walsh M, Rosenblatt K, et al. Avulsion fractures of the fifth metatarsal base: A prospective outcome study. *Foot Ankle Int* 2007;28(5):581–583.
43. Clapper MF, O'Brien TJ, Lyons PM. Fractures of the fifth metatarsal. Analysis of a fracture registry. *Clin Orthop Relat Res* 1995;(315):238–241.
44. Wiener BD, Linder JF, Giattini JF. Treatment of fractures of the fifth metatarsal: A prospective study. *Foot Ankle Int* 1997;18(5):267–269.
45. Stewart I. Jones fracture: Fracture of the base of the fifth metatarsal. *Clin Orthop* 1960; 16:190–198.
46. Kavanaugh JH, Brower TD, Mann RV. The Jones fracture revisited. *J Bone Joint Surg Am* 1978;60(6):776–782.
47. Torg JS, Balduini FC, Zelko RR, et al. Fractures of the base of the fifth metatarsal distal to the tuberosity. Classification and guidelines for non-surgical and surgical management. *J Bone Joint Surg Am* 1984;66(2):209–214.
48. Quill GE. Fractures of the proximal fifth metatarsal. *Orthop Clin North Am* 1995;26(2):353–361.
49. Chuckpaiwong B, Queen RM, Easley ME, et al. Distinguishing Jones and proximal diaphyseal fractures of the fifth metatarsal. *Clin Orthop Relat Res* 2008;466(8):1966–1970.
50. Fernandez Fairen M, Guillen J, Busto JM, et al. Fractures of the fifth metatarsal in basketball players. *Knee Surg Sports Traumatol Arthrosc* 1999;7(6):373–377.
51. Den Hartog BD. Fracture of the proximal fifth metatarsal. *J Am Acad Orthop Surg* 2009; 17(7):458–464.
52. Fetzer GB, Wright RW. Metatarsal shaft fractures and fractures of the proximal fifth metatarsal. *Clin Sports Med* 2006;25(1):139–150, x.
53. DeLee JC, Evans JP, Julian J. Stress fracture of the fifth metatarsal. *Am J Sports Med* 1983; 11(5):349–353.
54. Kelly IP, Glisson RR, Fink C, et al. Intramedullary screw fixation of Jones fractures. *Foot Ankle Int* 2001;22(7):585–589.
55. Porter DA, Rund AM, Dobslaw R, et al. Comparison of 4.5- and 5.5-mm cannulated stainless steel screws for fifth metatarsal Jones fracture fixation. *Foot Ankle Int* 2009;30(1): 27–33.
56. Pietropaoli MP, Wnorowski DC, Werner FW, et al. Intramedullary screw fixation of Jones fractures: A biomechanical study. *Foot Ankle Int* 1999;20(9):560–563.
57. Low K, Noblin JD, Browne JE, et al. Jones fractures in the elite football player. *J Surg Orthop Adv* 2004;13(3):156–160.
58. Wright RW, Fischer DA, Shively RA, et al. Refracture of proximal fifth metatarsal (Jones) fracture after intramedullary screw fixation in athletes. *Am J Sports Med* 2000;28(5): 732–736.
59. Larson CM, Almekinders LC, Taft TN, et al. Intramedullary screw fixation of Jones fractures. analysis of failure. *Am J Sports Med* 2002;30(1):55–60.

Iftach Hetsroni
Mark Drakos
Pete Draovitch
Bryan Kelly

CHAPTER

24

Inter-relations Between Foot and Hip Mechanics in Athletes

INTRODUCTION

Athletes can acquire a variety of hip-related problems, but among the most common is femoroacetabular impingement (FAI). FAI is a relatively recent concept championed by Reinhold Ganz and rapidly gaining acceptance as a distinct pathologic entity in contemporary orthopedics (1). In essence, deviation from a round, circular femoral head and a round, semi-circular acetabulum may lead to high stresses and shear forces over the anterior-superior labrum and acetabulum as well as the femoral head–neck junction. Some authors have espoused that such alterations in morphology may be a precursor of osteoarthritis. To alter the natural history of FAI, many have advocated a femoral neck debridement and in some cases acetabuloplasty to improve the kinematics of the hip joint and alleviate the impingement. However, at present we have only short term results which demonstrate improvement in symptoms, but little data to support a change in the ultimate course of the disease. Furthermore, there is a paucity of literature on the effectiveness of non-surgical modalities to combat the less severe presentations of FAI in which patients may benefit from subtle changes in muscle balance. The focus of this chapter will be the potential of foot mechanics and morphology to alter the kinematics of the lower extremity and ultimately to alleviate or exacerbate FAI and other hip pathologies.

FAI is an increasingly recognized diagnosis in orthopedic surgery. This concept describes how abnormalities of the femoral head/neck junction and acetabulum cause abnormal contact in the hip joint that lead to degenerative changes and eventually osteoarthritis (1). Two general categories of impingements exist; Cam and Pincer impingements (1).

In Cam impingement, abnormally decreased offset between the femoral head/neck region results in damage to the hip joint as the prominent head/neck abuts against the acetabular cartilage. It has been suggested that subtle untreated abnormalities that result from conditions such as Perthes disease and slipped capital femoral epiphysis cause this bony anomaly (2). Cam impingement generally leads to chondral damage at the transition zone of the hip between the labrum and articular cartilage. Cartilage cleavage injury in the acetabulum occurs as the abnormal femoral head shears off cartilage on the acetabulum in the transition area between the cartilage and labrum. The damage starting with this process eventually leads to more global and generalized damage to the entire hip as proposed by Beck et al. (3).

Pincer impingement occurs due to linear or global over coverage of the hip joint by the acetabular rim. In this scenario, the normal femoral head/neck junction abuts against the prominent acetabular rim. The first structure to fail is the labrum as a result of its repetitive crushing between the femoral head/neck and acetabular rim. Intra substance degeneration and fissuring of the labrum occurs and with time this degenerated labrum can ossify. Cartilage damage of the femoral head occurs later in the process in the form of a contrecoup lesion or damage to the posterior inferior femoral head cartilage (3).

Labral tears from FAI have been subdivided by Seldes into Types I and II (4). Type I tears or labral detachment from the cartilage layer in the transition zone are associated with Cam impingement. Pincer impingement is associated with Type II labral tears or intra substance degeneration. Middle-aged women more commonly present with Pincer impingement while younger males present with Cam impingement. New studies are also shedding light on the patterns of labral and chondral damage consistent with Seldes' concept (4). However, most hips exhibit a combination of these deformities to produce their impact on the hip joint. Once the degenerative process starts, altering its course is the focus of ongoing research. Current surgical treatment aims at correcting the subtle deformities before the degenerative cascade starts while improving the quality of life (5).

Mechanical characteristics of the hip joint are primarily the result of articular congruency, depth of the acetabular socket, and orientation of the acetabulum and the proximal femur. The direct mechanical effects on the hip joint can be divided into dynamic and static factors. Dynamic factors include altered femoral head morphology (Cam lesions), femoral retroversion, femoral varus, and acetabular overcoverage (Pincer lesions). These dynamic factors lead to a decrease in hip internal rotation and adduction, and result in a dynamic derangement of the joint cartilage when the hip is brought into a flexed position. The static factors include acetabular undercoverage (classic dysplasia), femoral anteversion, and femoral valgus. These static factors lead to a static overload of the anterior and superior portions of the hip joint with weight bearing. In addition to these direct effects on hip joint, alterations in the mechanics of adjacent and distal articulations along the lower limb may also indirectly affect hip mechanics during locomotion.

Heel strike is the earliest part of the stance phase, followed immediately by foot pronation. The contribution of altered mechanics in this complex motion to the development of overload injuries along the lower limb has drawn much attention in the orthopedic sports literature. Since hindfoot pronation is related to internal rotation of the tibia and the femur, it has been hypothesized that alterations in hindfoot mechanics could be related to overuse injuries in the knee and the hip joint (6,7).

This short review summarizes the basics of current knowledge regarding these articular inter-relations, and provides a rationale for future research.

HIP/FOOT MECHANICS

Areas of research that may shed light on the relationship between foot and hip mechanics may start with a comprehensive review of pediatric hip disorders. Specifically, conditions that affect the hip early in childhood can lead to adaptive changes in gait that ultimately have an impact on foot function. Yoo et al. completed a CT and gait analysis on nine patients with late presenting Perthes disease (8). Five patients with an out-toeing gait pattern were noted to have an anteriorly deviated hump deformity of the femoral head. Four patients with an in-toeing gait had a laterally deviated hump deformity on the femoral head. It was postulated that this gait pattern was a result of compensatory rotation of the proximal femur and pelvis to avoid hip impingement (8). By moving the femoral hump to the relatively deficient anterolateral aspect of the hip joint, painful impingement and potential wear of the joint is minimized. It follows that this adaptive or compensatory change noted in gait shows the inter-related nature of the mechanics of the entire lower extremity.

In slipped capital femoral epiphysis, the proximal capital epiphysis of the femoral head slip posterior and inferiorly relative to the metaphysis in a growing adolescent. Subsequently, the patient presents with pain, decreased internal rotation and an out-toed gait. This adaptation in gait helps reduce the extent of impingement and facilitates pain-free hip motion. It has been postulated as well that residual yet subtle deformities from this condition contributes to the development of FAI and later osteoarthritis (2,9).

Torsional or rotational deformities of the lower extremity in pediatric orthopedics also provide further examples of this connection. Young patients who have more internal rotation than external rotation of the hip joint generally have increased femoral anteversion resulting in an in-toeing gait. An out-toeing gait is associated with external torsion of the tibia or femur and other disorders of the hip including slipped capital femoral epiphysis, coxa vara, hip dysplasia. Severe cases of out-toeing are associated with pes planus deformity of the foot (10). Although not causative in relationship, further research in this area can help delineate the extent of inter-relation between conditions affecting the hip and their manifestation in the lower extremity, specifically in the foot.

Both pes planus and cavus have been implicated in lower extremity overuse injury. Pes cavus is a structural abnormality of the foot characterized by high arch. Weight bearing in this condition is distributed unevenly among the metatarsal heads and the lateral border of the foot which may lead to symptoms. This condition can further be divided into flexible and rigid types depending on the ability of the foot arch to adapt when weight bearing. Due to a smaller contact area with which to distribute load, the cavus foot is susceptible to both heel pain and stress fractures (11). The kinematics of the cavus foot is coupled with excessive subtalar inversion and forefoot supination. This leads to varus deformity of the knee and external rotation of the femur. The external rotation moment of the femur may lead to an alleviation of the mechanical effects of dynamic impingement morphology and an exacerbation of anterior–superior static overload of the hip joint. Orthotics is usually targeted at improving load distribution along the arch with soft, flexible materials.

Pes planus (flatfoot deformity) is characterized by loss of the medial arch due to a medially and plantar-displaced head of the talus. This stretches both the posterior tibial tendon and the spring ligament. This can be either rigid or flexible as indicated by restoration of the arch when standing upon the toes. Patients often have a flat-footed gait characterized by a pronated foot and shortening of the foot evertors (11). This gait abnormality can lead to weakened push-off, hypothetically leading to an increase in psoas/hip flexor demand required during the swing phase of gait ultimately resulting in increased anterior hip stress. The arthrokinematics and structure of the subtalar joint controls the motion of the LE. Therefore, if the subtalar joint does not allow for appropriate pronation, deceleration is compromised, causing increased forces up the kinetic chain. Furthermore, a foot that stays supinated throughout the stance phase will not allow for efficient absorption of ground reaction forces that takes place with normal pronation. These increased ground reaction forces will be transmitted up the kinetic chain.

Pronation of the hindfoot is a complex triplanar motion that consists of eversion, abduction, and dorsiflexion (12). Maximum pronation is normally reached during the first half of the stance phase (13–16). Since the first description of abnormal foot pronation by Sgarlato (17), as either that which functions about an abnormally pronated position or that which moves in the direction of pronation when normally it should be supinating, numerous studies investigated the association between this abnormality and the development of overuse injuries along the lower limb. It is believed that abnormal hindfoot pronation may be correlated with lower limb overuse injuries through two major mechanisms: One is the role of hindfoot pronation in ground impact load attenuation after heel strike (12,18,19), and the other relates to the coupling of closed chain pronation with internal rotation of the tibia and femur (12,20–23).

The effects of abnormal hindfoot mechanics can be accentuated during the running motion. During the normal running gait, the foot makes initial contact in a slightly supinated position (rearfoot inversion/subtalar supination). The subtalar joint then pronates (calcaneus eversion, talus plantarflexion and adduction), and the tibia and the femur internally rotate. The femur also moves from a slightly abducted position into slight adduction. This movement continues as the foot moves toward midstance where maximum pronation and limb internal rotation occurs. As the foot proceeds past foot flat and into heel rise, the toe-off motion reverses resulting in the subtalar joint to move back toward a supinated position creating a rigid lever for push off (calcaneus inversion, talus dorsiflexion and adduction). In preparation for push off, the tibia externally rotates and the femur externally rotates with slight abduction.

In the case of someone who has a foot type that leads to excessive pronation, or a mechanical deviation of hindfoot mechanics resulting in prolongation of the pronation phase (after midstance), the femur may remain in an internally rotated and adducted position as the limb moves into the extension phase. This hip joint position will lead to a natural aggravation of hip joint overload if there is any underlying FAI morphology.

Until recently, abnormal foot pronation has been most frequently correlated with abnormal mechanics of the patellofemoral joint, stating that excessive internal rotation of the shank in "abnormal" pronators could result in overloading of the lateral patellar facet (12,24,25). On this ground, some investigators even advocated the use of wedged orthotic devices to "correct" excessive pronation in the treatment of patellofemoral pain (26–30). Although few studies doubted any significant clinical correlation between abnormal foot pronation and patellofemoral symptoms in healthy athletic populations (13,31), it seems that current literature provides reasonable basis for clinical decision making in this respect.

Recent data also suggests that deviations in foot structure, specifically the alignment of the hindfoot during standing and during walking in seemingly normal, young, athletic populations, could be correlated with overuse injuries proximal to the knee, namely stress fractures of the femur (14), and intermittent low back pain (32). Since these observations suggest a correlation between alterations in foot mechanics and the expression of overuse injuries both proximal and distal to the hip joint, it would be intuitive to suspect that overuse symptoms in and around the hip joint may also be correlated with altered foot mechanics. However, this has never been investigated in symptomatic athletic populations. Although biomechanical models suggested a theoretical correlation between alterations in foot mechanics and the appearance of femoroacetabular symptoms through rotational effects on the femur (6,7,33), evidence to support a clinically significant relationship does not exist. Studies that evaluated the inter-relations between foot and hip mechanics examined usually healthy asymptomatic populations which were exposed to over-pronation by artificial means as wedged orthoses or wedged platforms (22,33,34).

In a study evaluating 35 healthy subjects, over-pronation was induced by wedges that everted the foot to 10, 15, and 20 degrees (22). With the 20 degrees wedged platform, the hindfoot eversion angle increased by 7 degrees as compared to standing on flat flour, the tibia internal rotation increased by 5 degrees, but the femur internally rotated by only 3 degrees. It seems therefore, that significant increase in foot eversion resulted in a minor effect on femoral rotation compared to the effect on the tibia and the knee. However, the pelvis anterior tilt in the sagittal plane increased in this scenario by a mean of 2 to 3 degrees in 40% of the participants. Therefore, the sum effect of increased foot eversion on the hip joint included both femur internal rotation and pelvis anterior tilt. This combined femoral and acetabular effect as a result of increased hindfoot eversion could theoretically aggravate hip symptoms that are related to anterosuperior femoroacetabular impingement. Still, the clinical significance of these findings has not been investigated in this study.

In another study evaluating the effect of 10 degrees medially wedged and 10 degrees laterally wedged foot orthoses in healthy asymptomatic individuals, the effects of the orthoses were most consistent at the hindfoot complex, with a highly statistically significant effect on the transverse plane kinematics (34). However, at the knee there were small angular changes in the transverse plane but none was statistically significant and all angular changes at the hip and pelvis were small, and none were statistically significant. Kinetic measurements demonstrated in this study that moments at the knee and hip were also not significantly different between medial and lateral wedged orthoses.

Although alterations in foot mechanics are most frequently induced in studies by either medial or lateral hindfoot wedges, joint inter-relations have been recently investigated also in response to a unique rockered shoe wear (35). Running kinematics and kinetics in response to this intervention demonstrated that this major deviation in sole geometry did not induce any significant alterations in moments and motions in the knee and hip articulations, and therefore clinical relevance to knee and hip symptoms in the face of this unique alteration in foot mechanics is unlikely.

Viewing the findings of these studies could emphasize the normal immediate effect of altered hindfoot mechanics on inter-segmental relationship, but this does not necessarily reflect prolonged adaptive effect. Thus, applying these mechanical inter-relations between the foot and the hip joints to symptomatic populations with hip symptoms remains questionable.

FAI AND FOOT MECHANICS

Current knowledge supports the inter-segmental mechanical relationships between the foot and more proximal segments along the lower limb. The over-pronated foot in this respect may contribute to internal rotation of the shank and thigh, and affect pelvic orientation, theoretically contributing to FAI hip symptoms. Intuitively, compared to mechanical inter-relations between the foot and the knee, since the hip is farther apart from the foot, it is expected that larger deviations from normal foot mechanics would be required to create clinically significant symptoms in this joint.

The effects of FAI can be influenced by all foot deformities. The location of the impingement will determine what motions will be most affected or most limited. If the impingement limits IR of the hip (typical anterolateral cam lesion), excessive pronation will be a problem since coupled internal rotation of the limb will bring the hip forcefully to the end of its available range of motion. If the impingement limits abduction (less common superolateral cam lesion), then a supinated foot is going to cause a problem since coupled external rotation of the limb will cause the femur to forcefully reach its end point. Alteration of the position of the pelvis over the hip joint can further complicate the relationships. Either anterior inclination or pelvic tilt can lead to further aggravation of underlying impingement and increase the possibility of the labrum being incarcerated between the acetabular rim and the cam lesion.

Other mechanical hip joint alterations may equally be affected by foot mechanics. For example, excessive femoral anteversion will lead to increased hip IR and retroversion will lead to increased hip ER. Therefore anteversion will better accommodate a supinated foot structure and retroversion will better accommodate a pronated foot structure. Excessive anteversion can cause increased medial knee problems while retroversion can increase retropatellar pain especially along the medial facet. Sports and activities requiring more lateral movement or increased hip abduction could cause increased pain in the setting of FAI.

There is a relative paucity of good scientific evidence on the effect of the foot on hip mechanics. Many of the lower extremity injury clinical and motion analysis studies do not specifically look at the hip. Given the inherent complexities of the foot and hip inter-relation, one may question the ability to prophylactically treat foot morphology to avoid chronic lower extremity injury or exacerbation of a current injury. To the authors' knowledge, there is no study which has clinically looked at the effects of foot type on the incidence of hip pathology or how foot morphology may affect FAI. The effect of foot type on chronic overuse injury of the lower extremity has been well studied with multiple reports that both pes cavus and planus are risk factors for injury. It has been proposed that pes planus may lead to excessive internal rotation and expose the hip adductors to injury as well as exacerbate the effects of underlying FAI morphology. We were unable to find any support for either of these hypotheses in a clinical study. Unfortunately, what is lacking are quality-controlled studies looking at interventions and how they may affect the mechanics and chronic overuse injury. Prospective studies are desperately needed to evaluate the effects of various non-invasive modalities such as orthotics, stretching and target muscle group strengthening for both the prevention and treatment of lower extremity injury. Future research should include descriptive data and prospective designs to evaluate the inter-relations between foot and hip mechanics in symptomatic populations before practical clinical recommendations can be withdrawn.

In conclusion, it is likely that foot mechanics do play a role in the development of hip pathology particularly in the young, active patient. However, to what extent is at this point unknown. We would encourage those evaluating these patients to perform a thorough examination of the entire lower extremity with specific attention to alignment and possible foot and knee deformity. If identified, these abnormalities may be a potential target area for therapy in order to comprehensively treat the hip pathology.

REFERENCES

1. Ganz R, Leunig M, Leunig-Ganz K, et al. The etiology of osteoarthritis of the hip: an integrated mechanical concept. *Clin Orthop Relat Res* 2008;466(2):264–272.
2. Harris WH. Etiology of osteoarthritis of the hip. *Clin Orthop Relat Res* 1986;(213):20–33.
3. Beck M, Kalhor M, Leunig M, et al. Hip morphology influences the patterns of damage to the acetabular cartilage: femoroacetabular impingement as a cause of early osteoarthritis of the hip. *J Bone Joint Surg Br* 2005;87(7):1012–1018.
4. Seldes RM, Tan V, Hunt J, et al. Anatomy, histologic features, and vascularity of the adult acetabular labrum. *Clin Orthop Relat Res* 2001;(382):232–240.
5. Beaule PE, LeDuff MJ, Zaragoza E. Quality of life following femoral head-neck osteochondroplasty for femoroacetabular impingement. *J Bone Joint Surg Am* 2007;89(4):773–779.
6. Tiberio D. Pathomechanics of structural foot deformities. *Phys Ther* 1988;68:1840–1849.
7. Tiberio D. The effect of excessive subtalar joint pronation on the patellofemoral mechanics: a theoretical model. *J Orthop Sports Phys Ther* 1987;9:160–165.
8. Yoo WJ, Choi IH, Cho TJ, et al. Out-toeing and in-toeing in patients with Perthes disease: role of the femoral hump. *J Pediatr Orthop* 2008;28(7):717–722.
9. Loder RT, Aronsson DD, Dobbs MB, et al. Slipped capital femoral epiphysis. *Instr Course Lect* 2001;50:555–570.
10. Lincoln TL, Suen PW. Common rotational variations in children. *J Am Acad Orthop Surg* 2003;11(5):312–320.
11. Franco AH. Pes cavus and pes planus. Analyses and treatment. *Phys Ther* 1987;67(5):688–694.
12. James SL, Bates BT, Osternig LR. Injuries to runners. *Am J Sports Med* 1978;6:40–50.
13. Hetsroni I, Finestone A, Milgrom C, et al. A prospective biomechanical study of the association between foot pronation and the incidence of anterior knee pain among military recruits. *J Bone Joint Surg Br* 2006;88-B:905–908.
14. Hetsroni I, Finestone A, Milgrom C, et al. The role of foot pronation in the development of femoral and tibial stress fractures: A prospective biomechanical study. *Clin J Sport Med* 2008;18:18–23.
15. Neely FG. Biomechanical risk factors for exercise: related lower limb injuries. *Sports Med* 1998;26:395–413.
16. McPoil T, Cornwall MW. Relationship between neutral subtalar joint position and pattern of rearfoot motion during walking. *Foot Ankle Int* 1994;15:141–145.
17. Sgarlato TE. *A Compendium of Podiatric Biomechanics.* San Francisco, CA: California College of Podiatric Medicine; 1971:265–281.
18. Freychat P, Belli A, Carret JP, et al. Relationship between rearfoot and forefoot orientation and ground reaction forces during running. *Med Sci Sports Exerc* 1996;28:225–232.
19. Perry SD, Lafortune MA. Influences of inversion/eversion of the foot upon impact loading during locomotion. *Clin Biomech (Bristol, Avon)* 1995;10:253–257.
20. Czerniecki JM. Foot and ankle biomechanics in walking and running. A review. *Am J Phys Med Rehabil* 1988;67:246–252.
21. Nigg BM, Cole GK, Nachbauer W. Effects of arch height of the foot on angular motion of the lower extremities in running. *J Biomech* 1993;26:909–916.
22. Khamis S, Yizhar Z. Effect of feet hyperpronation on pelvic alignment in a standing position. *Gait Posture* 2007;25(1):127–134.
23. Cornwall MW, McPoil TG. Footwear and foot orthotics effectiveness research: a new approach. *J Orthop Sports Phys Ther* 1995;21:337–344.
24. Duffey MJ, Martin DF, Cannon DW, et al. Etiologic factors associated with anterior knee pain in distance runners. *Med Sci Sports Exerc* 2000;32:1825–1832.
25. Moss RI, Devita P, Dawson ML. A biomechanical analysis of patellofemoral stress syndrome. *J Athl Train* 1992;27:64–69.
26. Johnston LB, Gross MT. Effects of foot orthoses on quality of life for individuals with patellofemoral pain syndrome. *J Orthop Sports Phys Ther* 2004;34:440–448.
27. Saxena A, Haddad J. The effect of foot orthoses on patellofemoral pain syndrome. *J Am Podiatr Med Assoc* 2003;93:264–271.
28. Gross MT, Foxworth JL. The role of foot orthoses as an intervention for patellofemoral pain. *J Orthop Sports Phys Ther* 2003;33:661–670.
29. Eng JJ, Pierrynowski MR. Evaluation of soft foot orthotics in the treatment of patellofemoral pain syndrome. *Phys Ther* 1993;73:62–68.
30. Pitman D, Jack D. A clinical investigation to determine the effectiveness of biomechanical foot orthoses as initial treatment for patellofemoral pain syndrome. *J Prosthet Orthot* 2000;12:110–117.
31. Powers CM, Chen PY, Reischl SF, et al. Comparison of foot pronation and lower extremity rotation in persons with and without patellofemoral pain. *Foot Ankle Int* 2002;23:634–640.
32. Kosashvili Y, Fridman T, Backstein D, et al. The correlation between pes planus and anterior knee or intermittent low back pain. *Foot Ankle Int* 2008;29:910–913.
33. Lafortune MA, Cavanagh PR, Sommer HJ 3rd, et al. Foot inversion-eversion and knee kinematics during walking. *J Orthop Res* 1994;12:412–420.
34. Nester CJ, Van Der Linden ML, Bowker P. Effects of foot orthoses on the kinematics and kinetics of normal walking gait. *Gait Posture* 2003;17:180–187.
35. Boyer KA, Andriacchi TP. Changes in running kinematics and kinetics in response to a rockered shoe intervention. *Clin Biomech* 2009;24:872–876.

CHAPTER

25

Brian Halpern

Leg Pain in Runners

The lower leg designates an area from the knee to the ankle, composed of the bony tibia and fibula with all the soft tissue surrounding the structures. Injuries to this site account to up to 30% of sports medicine clinic patients (1,2).

Evaluating and treating patients with lower leg symptoms evolve around a careful history and physical examination, supplemented only when necessary with various imaging modalities. Many of these injuries are self-limiting with relative rest, but this is often difficult in the competitive athletic population.

Distinguishing these entities as acute trauma versus atraumatic overload helps direct the initial assessment and treatment. Overuse injuries account for the greatest percentage of lower leg complaints. These usually begin from the repetitive microtrauma of foot strike with dorsi/plantarflexion at the ankle. Excessive pronation/supination also contributes greatly to specific overload medially and laterally of the lower leg. In this regard, malalignment of the lower extremity/ankle/foot suggest specific methods of overload.

Following the repetitive microtrauma, the tissue fatigues to the point of initiating the inflammatory cascade with recruitment of leukotrienes, macrophages, and growth factors. Platelets degranulate to assist in healing of the tissue and pain begins as the symptom to designate injury is occurring.

The pain functions as the signal to stop activity, enabling the tissue to recover. The pain and inflammation lead to a decreased muscular performance. If this acute process is not averted by relative rest or cross training to incorporate other muscle groups, then fibrous degeneration can occur with further tissue damage and progression to a chronic tendinopathy with scar formation. At this stage, evidence of acute inflammatory mediators is no longer evident and a chronic overuse-injury pattern evolves. The acute and chronic overuse injuries collectively include mostly tendonitis and tendinopathy, stress fractures and exertional compartment syndromes.

SHIN SPLINT/MEDIAL TIBIAL STRESS SYNDROME

This entity traditionally occurs in any sport that requires running as in track, soccer, baseball, lacrosse, basketball, football, and others. Pain is located over the posteromedial tibia diffusely from the mid to distal third. Training errors, with a change in intensity, duration, or frequency, precipitate this problem. Poor footwear and malalignment issues are also significant contributors, as well as specific muscle imbalances. Irritation at the insertion of the soleus on the posteromedial tibia has been suggested to be the source of the pain (3). MRI imaging has at times, confirmed this postulate. Three-phase bone scans as well, show a characteristic pattern of uptake, different from a stress fracture (4–11). There is diffuse uptake of the radionuclide material along the posterior aspect of the tibia on delayed images. Phase I radionuclide angiograms and phase II blood pool images are usually normal (12) (Table 25.1). Routine plain x-rays (AP and lateral) are usually normal. They may occasionally show hypertrophy of the posteromedial cortex of the tibia (12).

Although imaging is helpful in distinguishing shin splints from stress fractures, the diagnosis can usually be made without the cost of these studies. The pain is diffuse in this entity, along the posteromedial tibial shaft, whereas more localized in a stress fracture. It is not uncommon to occur bilaterally and often associated with hyperpronation of the foot and/or pes planus. Orthotics, ice, and NSAIDs help ameliorate the problem. Continued participation can also be helped by certain lower leg taping techniques and/or cross training. It is rare to be forced to stop the activity completely while treating this entity of medial tibial stress syndrome.

STRESS FRACTURE OF THE LOWER LEG

Medial/tibial stress syndrome can sometimes mimic an early stress fracture on clinical examination. Runners can reach incidents of stress fractures as high as 16% (13,14). "A stress fracture is a partial or complete fracture of a bone resulting from its inability to withstand nonviolent stress that is applied in a rhythmic, repeated subthreshold manner" (12). The pathophysiology of stress fractures evolves from muscle fatigue to bone failure, and ultimately fracture. Beyond a certain yield strength, the bone is irreversibly deformed, which leads to a breaking point, and ultimate collapse in compression or being torn apart in tension. Tension stress fractures are much more difficult to heal than the compressive type. In the lower leg, tension-type stress fractures occur at the anterior tibia and medial malleolus while compression-type fractures occur at the proximal tibia and tibial shaft posteromedially and the fibular shaft.

Etiology of stress fractures occurs, especially in runners, from either excessive mileage, intense workout, rapid increase of mileage, inadequate warm up, abnormal running surface,

TABLE 25.1 Bone Scan Appearance of Medial Tibial Stress Syndrome Versus Stress Fracture

	MTSS	Stress Fracture
Phase	Only positive on delayed images	Any phase can be positive
Shape	Linear/vertical	Round/fusiform
Location	Posteromedial tibia	Anywhere in the lower leg
Intensity	1+ to 3+ with varying uptake along length	Can be 1+ or 3+
Length	Nearly one-third of the bone	Less than 20% of the bone

Source: Adapted from Matire JR. The role of nuclear medicine scans in evaluating pain in athletics injuries. *Clin Sports Med* 1987;6:713–737; and Rupani H, Holder L, Espinole D, et al. Three phase radionuclide bone imaging in sports medicine. *Radiology* 1985;156:187–196.

bad shoes, lower limb malalignment, osteoporosis, and/or eating disorders. In a recent study done on 240 collegiate track athletes for 5 years prospectively, the majority of stress fractures were found to occur in the tibia in this population, the mid tibia being the most common skeletal location (15).

TIBIAL STRESS FRACTURE

The tibia represents up to 10% of the injuries that present to a sports medicine clinic (16). The most common area of tibial stress fractures are at the posteromedial aspect of the tibia, females having a higher incidence than males, Caucasians greater than Afro-Americans, and with reference to tibial width, the greater the width, the lesser the risk (17). Biomechanical risk is suggested by a rigid high-arched foot, which is unable to absorb the load; or by an excessive flatfoot that may perpetuate muscle fatigue (18).

In the early phases of overuse, stress fracture can mimic medial tibial stress syndrome; but if the athletic endeavor persists, the athlete begins to note increasing pain at the end of exercise. This progresses to pain during the entire exercise and can even occur with activities of daily living. Focal point tenderness becomes prominent over the tibia.

Imaging of suspected stress fractures should begin with a routine lower leg x-ray, a plain AP and lateral. Two-thirds of initial x-rays are negative and other findings are variable as at least 2 to 3 weeks of symptoms are required for bone changes to be observed (19,20). Initial findings include subtle blurring of trabecular margins, and small, fluffy densities corresponding to new bone formation (21,12). As a stress fracture matures, periosteal thickening and occasionally a fracture line can be seen. Eventually, periosteal new bone formation occurs with endosteal thickening and cortical hypertrophy (12).

If the initial x-rays are negative, the physician can manage clinically and/or repeat x-rays in 2 weeks to see if bony changes have occurred. It can take up to 10 to 21 days for a positive bone scan lesion to show up on standard x-rays (20,21).

If you clinically suspect a stress fracture, you can begin the treatment again or better document with a bone scan or MRI.

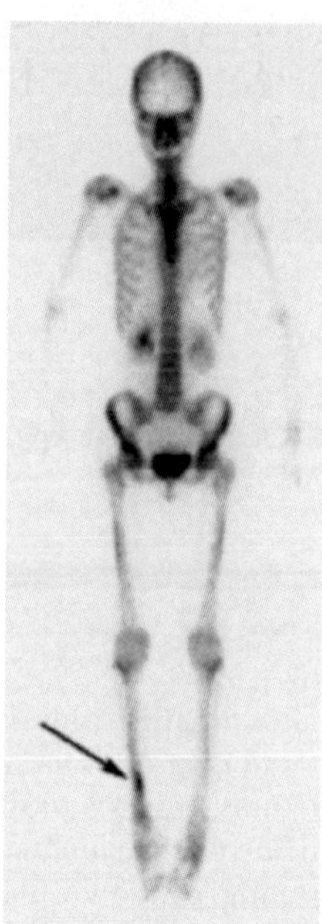

Figure 25.1. Distal tibial stress fracture. Frontal whole-body bone scan image in a patient shows increased uptake (*arrow*) in the medial aspect of the right lower leg reflecting stress fracture.

The bone scan can be positive as early as 6 hours after symptoms, but usually it takes 2 to 8 days (13,20,22,23). The bone scan can show focal fusiform uptake, different from a linear diffuse uptake of medial tibial stress syndrome (24) (Fig. 25.1). Often multiple areas of increased uptake are seen on the bone scan. Studies document that up to 40% of these positive findings are not symptomatic, (7,10), probably representing stress remodeling (8,25,26). They can go on to a true symptomatic stress fracture if the repetitive loading is not altered or they may never be symptomatic. Bone scans do expose the patient to radiation, which is why MRI, except for cost, is now the imaging of choice.

Stress fractures on MRI show focal marrow edema, characterized by decreased signal on T1-weighted images with corresponding increased signal intensity on T2-weighted or fat-suppressed images (27–30).

Once the diagnosis of posteromedial stress fracture is made, multiple treatment options follow. The simplest is to stop the offending activity for 6 to 8 weeks, which allows the bone to heal, followed by gradual reintroduction of activity with continued cross training like biking and swimming. Applying an Air Leg Brace often allows the athlete to continue running with a little bit longer healing time.

This treatment focuses on increased venous pressure through the Air Leg Brace with perhaps some effect on nitrous oxide and electrical gradients (31). Running with these braces often causes skin breakdown around the foot piece, so applying moleskin here is helpful.

ANTERIOR TIBIAL STRESS FRACTURE

Pain along the anterior tibial spine in a runner may signify an anterior tibial stress fracture. The etiology proposed is repetitive forceful contractions of the flexor leg muscles; this occurs

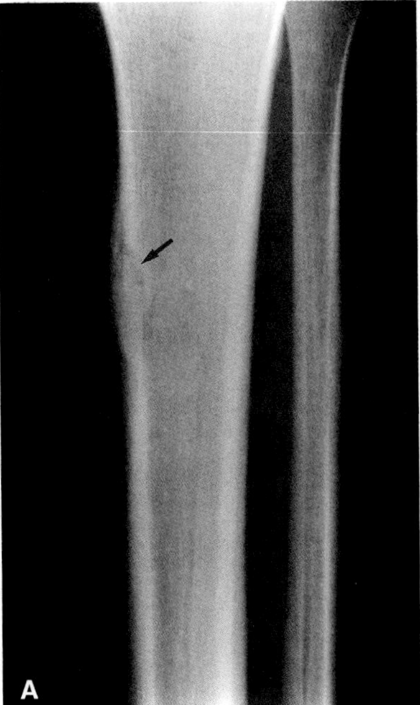

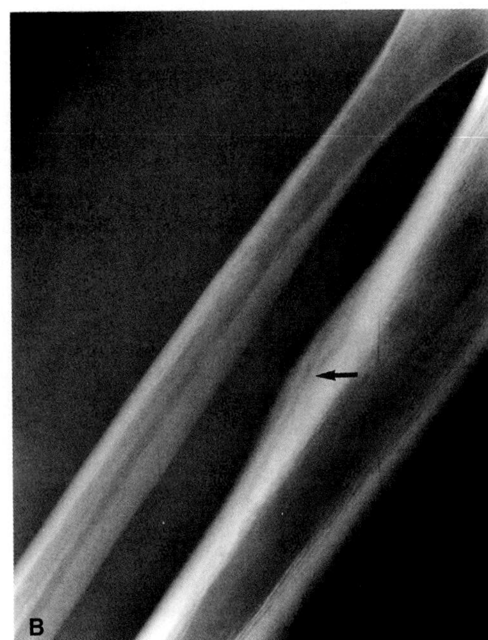

Figure 25.2. Tibial *stress fracture* in a runner. **A:** Detail of a frontal radiograph of the tibia shows the fracture along the medial cortex (*arrow*). Laminated periosteal reaction indicates the patient continued to run despite the pain. **B:** Lateral view shows the fracture involves the posterior cortex (*arrow*). This is the typical site for a *stress fracture* caused by running.

mostly in jumping athletes (1,32,33). These are tension-type stress fractures with poor vascular supply and difficult healing. It is not unusual for the fractures to go on to a nonunion and require surgical tibial rodding. The "dreaded black line" of the horizontal fracture may be evident on the x-ray.

Pain along the area of the pes bursa in the younger patient may actually represent a proximal anterior medial stress fracture of the tibia (Fig. 25.2). Limiting activity allows healing and occasionally a short leg walking cast is prescribed.

Medial malleolus stress fractures are also difficult to heal, being a tension-type fracture. Unloading completely early with crutches and a non–weight-bearing cast is helpful. Fixation surgery is sometimes necessary.

FIBULAR STRESS FRACTURES

The fibula accounts for between 6% and 20% of all stress fractures (13,16). They typically occur at the distal third, approximately 5 cm above the lateral malleolus (34). They tend to heal quickly. Air Leg Braces work as well as limiting activity does.

CHRONIC EXERTIONAL COMPARTMENT SYNDROME

Compartment syndromes are acute (a traumatic event as in a high-velocity tibial fracture), or chronic, (progressive lower leg pain with activity). By definition, compartment syndrome occurs when elevated tissue pressure in a closed fascial space results in a reduced capillary blood perfusion and compromised neurologic function (1,27,35).

Compartment syndrome of the lower extremities is defined within four and sometimes five fascial compartments of the lower leg (1,27,35). The classic four compartments are the anterior, lateral, superficial posterior, and deep posterior. The fifth compartment is sometimes considered alone comprised solely of the tibialis posterior (1,27,35). These compartments are defined by the fascial planes that encompass them and all have their own sensory/motor nerves and muscles groups that occupy the compartment (See Table 25.2). The anterior/lateral compartments are more often affected.

The pathophysiology is thought to be pain and limitation as a result of relative ischemia in the particular compartment with activity. As the tissue pressure increases in the compartment with activity, the fascia does not respond in its normal fashion secondary to a decrease in elasticity, and therefore acts as a strangulation of the neuromuscular components of the compartment. As activity stops and pressures normalize in the compartment, so do the signs and symptoms resolve. This is a relative simplistic model to explain this complex syndrome. Probably, there are multiple cellular-level dynamics that accompany this syndrome.

Patients complain of pain with prolonged activity, specifically running when using the muscles in the affected compartment. Numbness and weakness in the distribution of the nerve of the affected compartment is also often noted (12). There is usually not a loss of distal pulses, but swelling and tightness in the compartment can be observed. Some patients present with fascial herniations of the affected compartment, which signifies the body's attempt at auto compartment release. The patient is often able to direct the physician by the location of pain to the involved compartment. Sometimes all four compartments are involved and bilateral signs and symptoms are not unusual.

The work up should include imaging with plain x-rays and/or MRI to rule out a stress fracture first, although both diagnoses can coexist. The definitive diagnosis is made with compartment pressure measurements in the compartment. It has been recommended to perform resting, exercise, and post-exercise measurements, but I think this is excessive with unnecessary needle sticks. My method is to skip the resting measurements as it often offers no important information

TABLE 25.2 Main Lower Leg Compartments

Compartment	Muscles	Nerve	Deficit
Anterior	Extensors (TA, EDL, EHL)	Deep peroneal	Weak ankle and toe extension; decreased sensation over first web space
Lateral	Peroneals	Superficial peroneal	Weak ankle eversion; decreased sensation, lateral leg
Superficial posterior	Gastrocnemius–soleus	Sural	Decreased ankle plantarflexion; decreased sensation, lateral foot
Deep posterior	Flexors (FHL, FDL)	Tibial	Decreased toe flexion; decreased sensation, sole of foot
Posterior tibialis		Tibial	Decreased ankle inversion

Source: Adapted from Monaco R, Halpern B. Lower leg injuries. *Imaging in Musculoskeletal & Sports Medicine,* Blackwell Science; 1997.

not achieved with exercise, symptomatic measurements. If the pressures are elevated greater than 30 mm Hg during or immediately post-exercise, I then do not perform 5-minute post-exercise testing as usual. If pressures are normal or still not elevated with exercise, then I perform the 5-minute post-exercise measurements as pressures may still be on their way up. Criteria for a positive test are variable. In a recent survey of 55 orthopedic surgeons in the United Kingdom, 42% used a maximum intracompartmental pressure during exercise greater than 35 mm Hg and 35% use a modified criteria by Pedowitz (35). One must fulfill at least one of the following Pedowitz criteria:

1. Pre-exercise pressure greater than or equal to 15 mm Hg.
2. One minute post-exercise pressure greater than or equal to 30 mm Hg.
3. Five minutes post-exercise pressure greater than or equal to 20 mm Hg (35).

If the increased pressure correlates with the symptoms, then this confirms the diagnosis.

In the past, we measured all four compartments of both legs, symptomatic or not, but it is hard to recommend surgery for an asymptomatic compartment, so now we only measure what appears to be the symptomatic compartments. As the anterior and lateral compartments are by far the most commonly involved, we test both when signs and symptoms point to either one. We only test the posterior compartments of the patient if the patient complains of calf symptoms. One reason for this is that the posterior compartment surgical releases do not have as good an outcome as the anterior lateral releases. Another reason is that the deep posterior compartment should probably be measured under ultrasound imaging such as not to traumatize any major blood vessels with this measurement.

Following a positive test, surgical release of the compartment through a superficial fasciectomy (36) is the most dependable treatment. Cessation of the causative activities will usually alleviate the pain, but requires restriction of activities. Massage therapy, physical therapy, and/or orthotics may be helpful and worth an attempt for alleviation of symptoms, but do not usually resolve the pain. At times, following the actual compartment testing, the symptoms abate. There is unknown etiology for this outcome.

The surgical release should include the entire compartment involved. Post-surgical scarring can at times lead to recurrent symptoms when a fasciectomy may be necessary (36).

POPLITEAL ARTERY ENTRAPMENT SYNDROME/NERVE ENTRAPMENT SYNDROMES

Exertional compartment syndrome creates symptoms that are sometimes similar to a much rarer entity, popliteal artery entrapment syndrome. In this case, the popliteal artery becomes compressed most commonly from hypertrophy of the gastrocnemius muscle (37). Symptoms include cramping and paresthesias during activity. MRI angiography is becoming the imaging of choice with surgery as the best treatment option (37).

Other common entrapments in the lower leg can involve any of the six nerves: Sural, common peroneal, superficial peroneal, deep peroneal, tibial, and saphenous. Surgical decompression may be required to resolve the signs and symptoms from the affected nerve (37).

ACUTE INJURIES

Muscle-strain injury is common in the lower leg. They usually are partial or complete tears of the musculotendinous unit (12). A forceful contraction, usually from eccentric load with muscle lengthening causes this problem (38). This is felt as a sudden acute pain, sometimes with an audible or palpable pop.

GASTROCNEMIUS STRAINS

This injury can simulate someone being shot in the back of the leg or feel like you were hit by a ball in the back of the leg. The medial gastrocnemius is one of the most common areas of injury (39,40). Rarely is the plantaris involved as previously believed (27,41).

The patients may present with swelling and ecchymosis. Imaging is rarely needed. Treatment involves unloading the calf with crutches and/or heel lifts, ice and NSAIDs as needed. Complete resolution is common within a few weeks. This injury

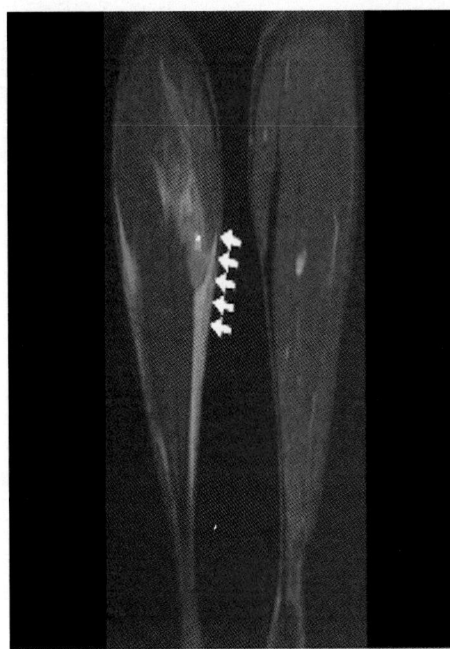

Figure 25.3. Muscle tendon tear of the medial gastrocnemius (tennis leg). Coronal short tau inversion recovery (STIR) MR image of both lower legs showing acute right sided tear of the gastrocnemius (*short arrows*). Hematoma (h) fills the gap.

can mimic a DVT if a good history is not obtained and in these instances, a venous Doppler is prudent. MRI as well will identify the muscular injury (Fig. 25.3).

CONTUSIONS

Blunt trauma to the lower leg can result in hemorrhage, inflammation, and disruption of muscle fibers (42). This mainly affects the muscle belly whereas strains occur more commonly at the musculotendinous junction. X-rays will rule out a fracture. Occasionally, a seroma will result, which if symptomatic, can be aspirated under ultrasound guidance. Another potential complication is myositis ossificans, which may present as a firm, hard mass palpable between 2 and 4 weeks after injury. By the third or fourth week, x-rays will demonstrate a soft-tissue density. Active range of motion is important, not passive, and it can take 6 months or more for this calcification to mature.

REFERENCES

1. Andrish JT. The leg. In: DeLee JC, Drez D, eds. *Orthopedic Sports Medicine Principles and Practices*. Vol 2. Philadelphia, PA: WB Saunders; 1994:1603.
2. Deveraux MD, Lachmann SM. Athletes attending a sports injury clinic-a review. *Br J Sports Med* 1983;1:137–142.
3. Michael RH, Holder LE. The soleus syndrome; a cause of medial tibial stress (shin splints). *Am J Sports Med* 1985;13:87–94.
4. Milgrom C, Giladi M, Stein M, et al. Medial tibial pain. *Clin Orthop* 1986;213:167–171.
5. Norfray J, Schlachter L, Kemahan W Jr, et al. Early confirmation of stress fractures in joggers. *JAMA* 1980; 243:1647–1649.
6. Nusbaum A, Treves S, Micheli L. Bone stress lesions in ballet dancers: scintigraphic assessment. *AJR* 1988;150:851–855.
7. Rosen FR, Micheli L, Treves S. Early scintigraphic diagnosis of bone stress and fractures in athletic adolescents. *Pediatrics* 1982:70:11–15.
8. Roub LW, Gunnerman LW, Hanley EN, et al. Bone stress: a radionuclide imaging perspective. *Radiology* 1979;131:431–438.
9. Rupani H, Holder L, Espinole D, et al. Three phase radionuclide bone imaging in sports medicine. *Radiology* 1985;156:187–196.
10. Zwas S, Elkanovitch R, Frank G. Interpretation and classification of bone scintigraphic findings in stress fractures. *J Nucl Med* 1987;28:452–457.
11. Holder LE, Michael RH. The specific scintigraphic pattern of "shin splints" in the lower leg. *J Nucl Med* 25:865–869.
12. Monaco R, Halpern B, et al. *Lower leg injuries. Imaging in Musculoskeletal & Sports Medicine*, Blackwell Science; 1997. 236–249.
13. Matheson GO, Clement DB, McKenzie DC, et al. Stress fractures in athletes: a study of 320 cases. *Am J Sports Med* 1987;15:46–48.
14. Orava S, Hulkko A. Stress fracture in athletes. *Am J Sports Med* 1987;8:221–226.
15. Touhy J, Nativ, A. A prospective analysis of tibial stress fracture incident distribution, and risk factors in collegiate track athletes. *Abstract Clin J Sports Med* 2008;18(2):186.
16. McBryde AM. Stress fractures in athletes. *Am J Sports Med* 1976;5:212–217.
17. Giladi M, Milgrom C, Simkin A, et al. Stress fractures in tibial bone width. A risk factor. *J Bone Joint Surg Br* 1987;69(2):326–329.
18. Wilder RP, Sethi S. Overuse Injuries: Tendinopathies, stress fractures, compartment syndrome, and shin splints. *Clin Sports Med* 2004;23(1):55–81, vi.
19. Devas M. *Stress fractures*. London: Churchill-Livingstone; 1975:56–91.
20. Greaney RB, Gerber FH, Laughlin RL, et al. Distribution and natural history of stress fracture in US Marine recruits. *Radiology* 1983;146:339–346.
21. Berquist TH. Tibia, fibula, and calf. *Imaging of sports injuries*. Gaitherberg, MD: Aspen; 1992:155–165.
22. Siddiqui AR. Bone scans for early detection of stress fracture. *N Engl J Med* 1978;298:1033.
23. Wilcox JR Jr, Moniot AL, Green JP. Bone scanning in the evaluation of exercise-related stress injuries. *Radiology* 1977;123:699–703.
24. Manire JR. The role of nuclear medicine scans in evaluating pain in athletic injuries. *Clin Sports Med* 1987;6:713–737.
25. Matheson GO, Clement DB, McKenzie DC, et al. Scintigraphic uptake of technetium at nonpainful sites in athletes with stress fractures: the concept of bone strain. *Sports Med* 1987;4:65–75.
26. Chisin R, Milgrom C, Giladi M, et al. Clinical significance of nonfocal scintigraphic findings in suspected tibial stress fractures. *Clin Orthop Relat Res* 1987;220:200.
27. Bachner EJ, Friedman MJ. Injuries to the leg. In: Hershman EB, Nicholas JA, eds. *The lower extremity and spine in sports medicine*. Vol 1. St Louis, MO: Mosby; 1995:523–581.
28. Lee JK, Yao L. Stress fractures: MR imaging *Radiology* 1988,169:217–220.
29. Avendt EA, et al. The MR spectrum of stress injury to bone and its clinical relevance. *Am J Sports Med* (in press).
30. Nugler JB, Murphy WA. Bone marrow imaging. *Radiology* 1968;168:679.
31. Date PA. Fracture healing with elevated venous pressure, *Orthopaedic Research Society, 35th Annual Meeting* Feb 6, 1984,590–591.
32. Reting A, Shelbourne D, McCarroll J, et al. The natural history and treatment of delayed union stress fractures of the anterior cortex of the tibia. *Am J Sports Med* 1988;16:250–255.
33. Green N, Rogers R, Lipscomb B. Nonunions of stress fractures of the tibia. *Am J Sports Med* 1985;13:171–176.
34. Blair WF, Marley SR. Stress fractures of the proximal fibula. *Am J Sports Med* 1980;8: 212–213.
35. Pedowitz RA, Hargens A, Mubarak S, et al. Modified criteria for the objective diagnosis of chronic syndrome of the leg. *Am J Sports Med* 1990;18:35–40.
36. Tzortziou V, Maffulli N, Padhiar N. Diagnosis and management of chronic exertional compartment syndrome (CECS) in the UK. *Clin J Sport Med* 2006;16(3):209–213.
37. Pell RF 4th, Khanuja HS, Cooley GR. Leg pain in the running athlete. *J Am Acad Orthop Surg* 2004;12(6):396–404.
38. Garrett WE. Basic science of musculotendinous injuries. In: Nicholas JA, Hershman BB eds. *The lower extremity and spine in sports medicine*. St. Louis, MO: Mosby, 1986.
39. Sutro CJ, Sutro WH. The medial head of the gastrocnemius: a review of the basis for the partial rupture and for intermittent claudication. *Bull Hosp Jt Dis Orthop Inst* 1985;45:150–157.
40. Frominson A. Tennis leg. *JAMA* 1969;209:415–416.
41. Speer KP, Lohnes J, Garrest WE. Radiographic imaging of muscle strain injury. *Am J Sports Med* 1993;21:89–96.
42. Garrett WE, Lohnes J. Cellular and matrix response to mechanical injury myotendinous junction. In: Leadbetter WB, Buckwalter JA, Gordon SI, eds. *Sports-induced inflammation*. Park Ridge, IL: American Academy of Orthopedic Surgeons; 1990:215–224.

CHAPTER

26

Hannah N. Ladenhauf
Shevaun M. Doyle
Gilbert Chan
John S. Blanco
Daniel W. Green

Foot and Ankle Conditions in Athletic Children and Adolescents

INTRODUCTION

Foot and ankle conditions in the child and adolescent are wide and varied. These conditions range from various congenital and developmental diagnoses to traumatic injuries as well as overuse conditions. The development of these conditions is influenced by rapid growth and physiologic changes, which are seen in the growing child. These changes commonly include increased muscle strength, body mass, and decreased flexibility. In addition, there is greater involvement of young children in competitive sports and activities. The intensity of training in increasingly younger athletes may result in unique childhood injury patterns. Foot and ankle injuries represent the second most common problem in the young athlete. Another consideration is the anatomic difference between the growing and the mature skeleton. This is best exemplified by the difference in strength between a child's ligaments and bones. Due to growth plates at the end of long bones, a child's bone is more likely to be harmed than the surrounding ligaments. In contrast, adults with similar mechanisms of injury are more likely to sustain a ligament injury than a fracture. An understanding of the specific physiologic and anatomic differences in the growing athletic child will allow the physician to counsel families, formulate plans aimed at injury prevention, and establish appropriate treatment protocols for the pediatric athlete.

EPIDEMIOLOGY

Each year, more than 775,000 children younger than 15 years old are treated in hospital emergency rooms in the United States for sports-related injuries. In the young athlete, foot and ankle problems represent the second most common reason why children visit their primary care physician (1). Children and adolescents are involved in more frequent and intense sporting events, which are predicted to increase the incidence of injuries.

Almost all foot and ankle injuries in children are related to sports activities, especially basketball, football, baseball, and soccer (2). Injuries are not unique to competitive sports; bicycling, skateboarding, roller-skating, and in-line skating are some of the more common individual sports that predispose the pediatric population to foot and ankle ailments.

CLINICAL EVALUATION

The clinical evaluation, particularly in the very young child, may be a challenge. Oftentimes it is impossible to obtain an accurate history to verify the mechanism of the injury. The history is often second-hand information provided by the caregiver, who may not have witnessed the incident. A complete physical examination is essential to determine the nature and severity of the injury. Evaluation of the entire lower extremity is performed to uncover swelling, ecchymoses, deformity, and/or tenderness.

A thorough intake of the child's birth, past medical, and surgical history as well as a detailed review of systems are mandatory to rule out associated medical or congenital conditions that might compromise or mimic signs and symptoms of a musculoskeletal injury. Signs and symptoms of pain, particularly those that are chronic in nature, point to conditions such as juvenile inflammatory arthritis or metabolic bone disease. A history of fever would raise the suspicion of an infectious or neoplastic focus such as osteomyelitis, septic arthritis, or leukemia.

DIAGNOSTIC EVALUATION

Plain radiographs of the affected area are usually adequate to assess the injury or condition. Anteroposterior (AP), lateral, and oblique views are obtained for the foot and AP, lateral, and mortise views are taken for the ankle. Specific conditions of the calcaneus, navicular or sesamoid bones may warrant special views including the Harris heel view, the Saltzmann view, external oblique and sesamoid view. Radiographs of the unaffected contralateral limb may delineate normal anatomic findings. In cases where the injury may not be clear on initial radiographic evaluation, or where the cause of the pain is poorly localized, a whole body bone scan with AP and lateral foot views may localize the lesion. Computed tomography (CT) may further define bony anatomy, which is invaluable for the preoperative plan, especially in fracture treatment. Magnetic resonance imaging (MRI) defines the extent of soft-tissue and articular cartilage damage, which is useful for the evaluation and management of osteochondral lesions.

CONGENITAL AND DEVELOPMENTAL CONDITIONS

TARSAL COALITION

A tarsal coalition (TC) is an abnormal bridging between tarsal bones, which may cause pain and restricted motion. This abnormal connection may be cartilaginous, osseous, or fibrous in origin; and it is thought to result from a failure of differentiation and segmentation of the primitive mesenchyme. Previous reports in the literature report an autosomal dominant pattern of inheritance (3). The actual incidence of tarsal coalition is still unresolved; values of less than 1% to 3% of the entire population are reported in the literature (4,5). More recent studies show a higher incidence. Solomon et al. evaluated 100 cadaver feet and found a 12.7% incidence of non-osseous coalitions (6). Nalaboff and Schweitzer reviewed 667 consecutive MRIs performed on 640 patients and found that the incidence of tarsal coalition may be as high as 11% (7). Calcaneonavicular and talocalcaneal coalitions are reported to be the most common types. Stormont et al. reported the most common type of coalition to be calcaneonavicular (53%) followed by talocalcaneal (37%) (4). Solomon et al. likewise showed that calcaneonavicular coalitions are the most common type (6). Similarities exist in Nalaboff's study where calcaneonavicular coalition was found to be the most common type (71%) (7).

The physical examination findings are a rigid flat foot and tenderness in the anterolateral aspect of the hindfoot with maximum ankle plantarflexion. The rigidity is due to the loss of motion in the subtalar joint, which is typically more severe in talocalcaneal coalitions compared to talonavicular coalitions. Pain is the most common presenting complaint; many patients with tarsal coalitions are not symptomatic. Leonard showed that only 24% of cases were symptomatic (3). The pain typically manifests during adolescence between 8 and 16 years. This is due to a progressive increase in activity and loss of flexibility of the foot as the coalition begins to ossify. The pain is theorized to result from microfractures, which may respond favorably to immobilization (8). Other causes of pain include ligamentous strain, muscle spasm, and irritation of the sinus tarsi and subtalar joint (9). Pain is more often located in the midfoot or medial aspect of the hindfoot. On examination, these patients have a rigid planovalgus deformity; the medial longitudinal arch fails to reconstitute with ankle plantarflexion or standing on tip toe. This occurs because the coalition blocks heel inversion. In addition, tarsal coalition must be a consideration in patients who present with recurrent ankle sprains or distal fibular physeal fractures (10,11).

Often radiographs suffice to establish the diagnosis of tarsal coalition, particularly those that are ossified. Tarsal coalitions are best viewed with specific radiographs. On lateral radiographs, talar beaking, known as the "anteater sign", and the "C sign" may indicate the presence of a coalition (12–15). A calcaneonavicular coalition is best seen on the internal oblique radiograph with an osseous coalition. There is a characteristic bony bar. A cartilaginous or fibrous coalition may show a narrow distance between the calcaneus and navicular with irregular borders (Fig. 26.1). Talocalcaneal coalitions are more difficult to evaluate with plain films.

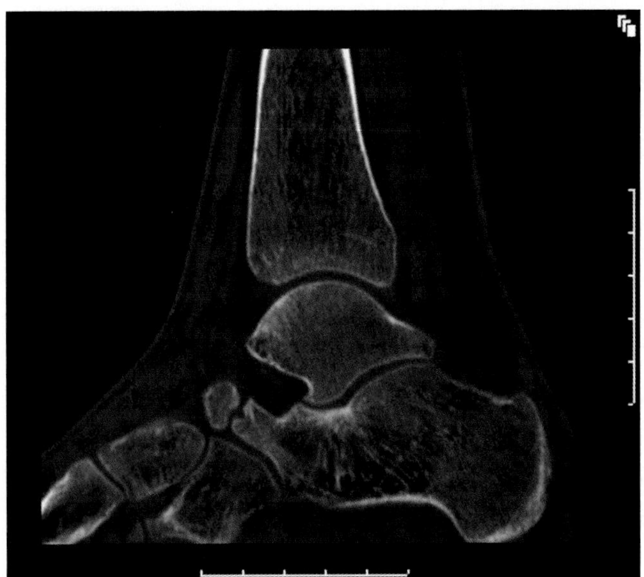

Figure 26.1. CT scan image of a 15-year-old male showing calcaneonavicular coalition. The irregularity between the calcaneus and navicular is indicative of a classic fibrocartilaginous coalition.

These coalitions most commonly involve the middle facet of the calcaneus (16). The best radiographic view to demonstrate a talocalcaneal coalition is the Harris or axial heel view (5). When radiographs are not sufficient to fully evaluate a coalition, particularly one that is cartilaginous or fibrous, CT and MRI provide additional details to not only clarify the diagnosis, but also detect additional coalitions. CT and MRI are useful tools to ensure an appropriate preoperative plan. The advantage of the CT scan is that it provides greater bony detail of osseous coalitions, particularly at the level of the subtalar joint (17,18). MRI is also an accepted alternative; however, it may require sedation in the younger child. The advantage of MRI is that it demonstrates better soft-tissue detail with non-osseous coalitions and avoids radiation exposure. Wechsler et al. compared CT and MRI in the evaluation of tarsal coalitions and found that CT scans did not depict fibrous coalitions as well as MRI (19). El Rassi et al. also presented a series of 19 patients with restricted subtalar motion and pain over the anterolateral aspect of the foot. Imaging studies were non-diagnostic except for bone scan studies that showed increased uptake. Intra-operative findings in these cases showed arthrofibrosis, which should be considered when imaging studies are negative (20).

Pain is the main indication for surgical management; however, prior to any surgical intervention, a trial of conservative management should be instituted. Conservative management consists of temporary immobilization with a cast, followed by physical therapy with emphasis on muscle stretching and ankle strengthening, and possibly orthotics. Patients who do not respond to these recommendations require surgery. The key to successful treatment is complete resection of the coalition. The goal of surgical management is to achieve pain relief and restore hindfoot motion. Studies have shown that surgical intervention does not restore the foot to its normal osseous alignment, but better post-operative function does correlate with better results (21,22). Hestroni et al. evaluated plantar pressures before and after resection of symptomatic tarsal coalitions. In their series, they found significant correction of increased midfoot pressures (23). Surgical intervention typically consists of complete resection of the coalition with fat or muscle interposition (24–26). Results of surgical management are more predictable with calcaneonavicular coalitions compared to talocalcaneal coalitions. For cases with severe valgus deformity, a calcaneal osteotomy may be performed. Subtalar arthrodesis may be indicated for patients with large bars and degenerative changes.

ACCESSORY NAVICULAR BONE

The accessory navicular is the most common accessory bone of the foot (27). It is most often bilateral and more common in females. This condition is considered a normal variant, and three types have been described (28). Type 1 is a sesamoid bone found within the body of the tibialis posterior tendon. Type 2 is an ossicle connected to the body of the navicular bone through a synchondrosis. A type 3 is a large cornuate navicular bone, which many believe to be a fusion of a type 2 accessory navicular bone. These usually present as a prominence on the plantar medial aspect of the foot. Planovalgus feet may accompany the condition, but there is no clear correlation between flat feet and accessory navicular bones (29). Pain and tenderness are the most common presenting complaints. Grogan and colleagues performed a histologic study and found areas of microfracture through the cartilaginous synchondrosis (30). A painful prominence may also be seen. Plain radiographs of the foot, which include the external oblique view, are used to establish the diagnosis (Fig. 26.2) (30). Conservative management with orthotics or cast immobilization is effective for most symptomatic accessory navicular bones. Surgery may be needed for adequate pain relief when conservative management fails (31). Simple excision of the prominence provides satisfactory results with adequate pain relief (29,32). Alternatively, percutaneous drilling has been reported for symptomatic type 2 accessory navicular bones with good results (33).

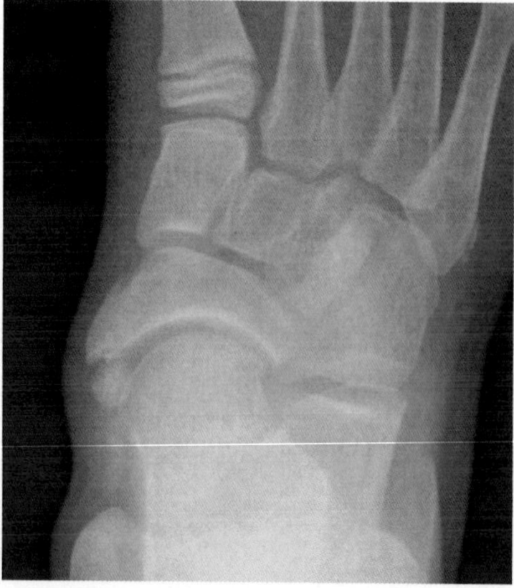

Figure 26.2. Frontal view of the right mid-foot of an 11-year-old male demonstrates an accessory navicular.

TRAUMATIC CONDITIONS

ANKLE SPRAINS

Most ankle injuries in the skeletally immature athlete occur during sports activities. Ankle sprains are the most common traumatic sports injury with an incidence of seven sprains per year per 100 persons in the United States. Unlike younger children, who usually injure their distal physes, older children and adolescents often present with ankle sprains. Sprains account for 85% of ankle injuries, with 85% of these affecting the lateral ankle. The most common mechanism of injury is inversion and plantarflexion of the foot (34). Medial ankle sprains are less common and more likely to be associated with injury of the syndesmosis. Children most commonly complain about pain, swelling, and tenderness. Conservative treatment is used first for stable injuries, with good to excellent functional outcomes. Conservative treatment includes functional support or immobilization of the injured ankle during the acute phase of injury. Functional support is preferable over complete immobilization, as the former is achieved through bracing, elastic bandages, tape, or a soft cast. Nevertheless, jumping, pivoting, or participation in any sports competition should not be performed until pain resolves and the patient has restored full mobility, strength and proprioception. The patient should be able to run and hop on the injured limb without any discomfort or instability before returning to sports. Chronic ankle instability may be prevented through an appropriate physical therapy regimen. When the ankle is not amenable to rehabilitation, surgical ligament reconstruction may be necessary to restore stability. The surgeon must protect the open physes in the skeletally immature patient.

FRACTURES

There are multiple factors that influence the nature and character of a pediatric injury. The age of the patient is one of the most important factors, as it directly influences the structure and size of the bone. This determines the response to forces applied to the bone either directly or indirectly. Another consideration is the physis with its variable stages of ossification throughout growth. This variability may dictate the pattern of injury. Finally, the nature of the traumatic incident, the amount of force involved, and the mechanism of injury will determine the ultimate injury pattern.

PEDIATRIC ANKLE FRACTURES

Ankle fractures account for 5% of all pediatric fractures. They also account for 15% of all physeal injuries (35–37). The ossific nuclei of the distal tibia generally appear between 6 months and 2 years of age. The medial malleolus ossifies by the seventh or eighth year of life. The distal fibula ossific nucleus (lateral malleolus) appears by 18 to 20 months. The distal tibial physis provides 20% of growth of the lower extremity, which contributes approximately 3 to 4 mm of growth annually. A severe injury affecting the ankle may result in a growth arrest with a significant limb-length discrepancy or malalignment of the ankle joint (Fig. 26.3A–D).

Classifications of pediatric ankle fractures have been designed to aid in the management of these injuries. Classification schemes are based on the anatomy and/or the mechanism of

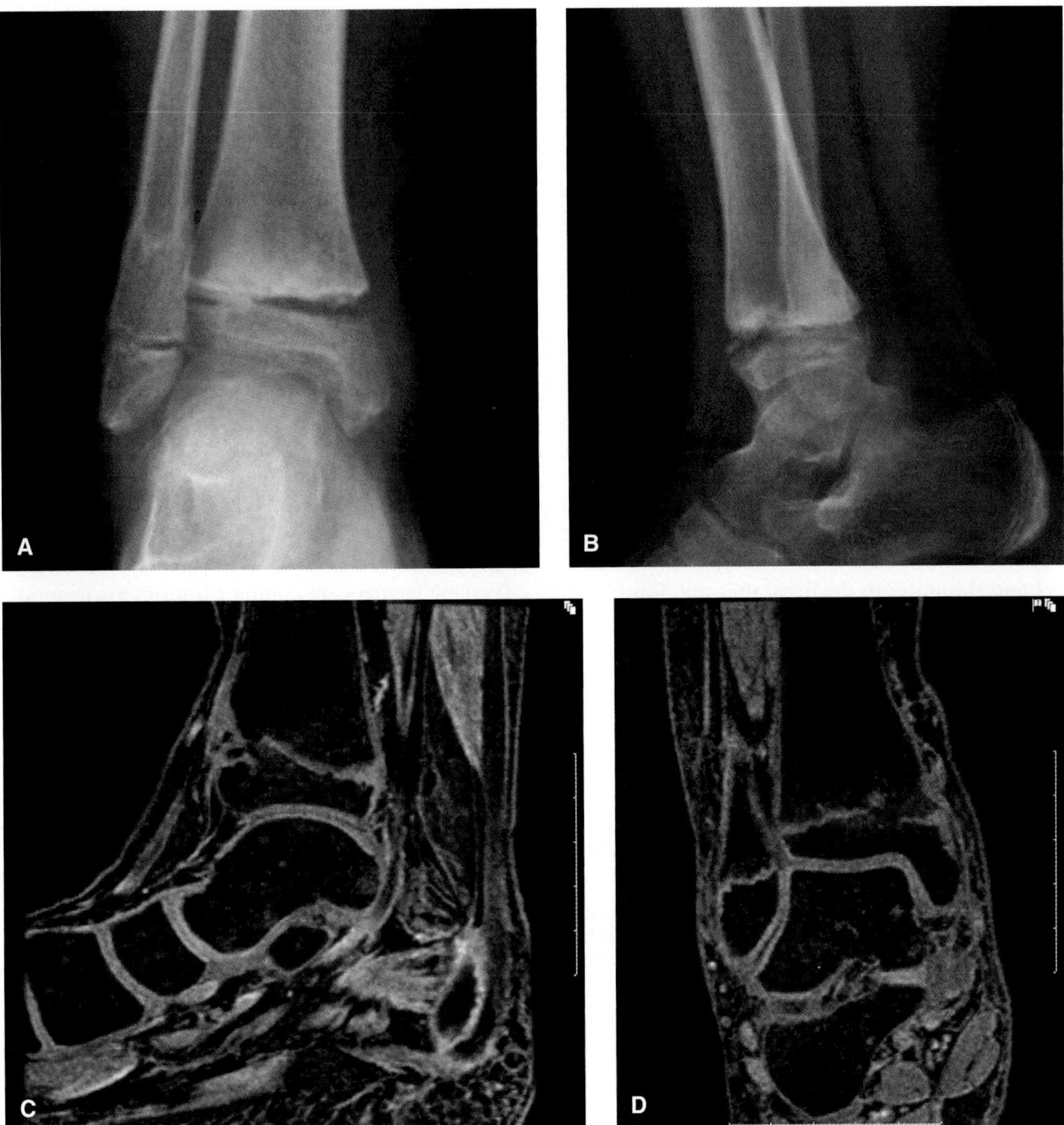

Figure 26.3. **A–D:** This 8-year-old female suffered a Salter–Harris II fracture of the right ankle, resulting in growth arrest of the right distal tibial physis. On AP and lateral x-rays 2 months after the injury the growth plate of the distal tibia is widened. MRI images show partial ossification bridging across the growth plate.

injury. The Salter–Harris classification of physeal injuries is the most commonly used anatomic classification scheme (38). It has a distinct advantage of simplicity and provides prognostic information about the injury. Other classification schemes are based upon the mechanism of injury, such as the Lauge and Hansen classification established in 1950 (39,40). This scheme was later modified by Diaz and Tachdjian for children and incorporated the Salter–Harris classification (41). The classification describes the position of the foot during injury and the direction of the force applied. The goal of the classification is to aid reduction of the fracture by reversing the mechanism of injury. The complexity of the classification makes it difficult to implement. Vahvanen et al. proposed to simplify the classification of pediatric ankle fractures by dividing it into two basic types: A low-risk type comprised of avulsion fractures and epiphyseal separation injuries and a high-risk group comprised of injuries through the growth plate (42).

LOW-RISK ANKLE FRACTURES

Salter–Harris (SH) type I and II injuries occur through the zone of hypertrophy and carry a good prognosis as well as long-term outcome. Salter–Harris I injuries to the distal tibia are not common. Salter–Harris I injuries to the distal fibula are much more common in children with open growth plates. Sankar et al. reviewed a series of children who sustained an acute ankle injury and found an 18% incidence of Salter–Harris I injuries to the distal fibula (43). The exact incidence of Salter–Harris I injuries to the distal tibia is reported to be 15% of physeal injuries (35,36). Salter–Harris II injuries to the distal tibia are more common, and account for 40% of injuries to the distal tibia (35,36). The main difference between a type I and a type II injury is that a type I injury occurs as a pure epiphyseal separation, while a type II injury begins through the epiphysis and exits through the metaphysis. The metaphyseal extension is called a Thurston–Holland fragment. It is important to note that in a type II injury, the periosteal tear is opposite to the Thurston–Holland fragment. The periosteum may interpose between the fracture fragments and block an anatomic reduction.

These injuries are often managed with conservative measures. A gentle closed reduction under anesthesia with cast application for 4 to 6 weeks is often all that is required. It is imperative that minimal attempts at reduction are performed on displaced growth plate fractures to avoid undue damage to the growth plate. When an adequate closed reduction cannot be achieved, it is necessary to perform an open reduction to achieve anatomic alignment of the fracture fragments. Soft-tissue interposition usually prevents the reduction. Once these blocks to reduction are removed, a good anatomic reduction is obtained. In those cases where reduction is unstable, it may be necessary to stabilize the fracture fragments by using 3.5 mm or 4.0 mm cannulated screws. If fracture stability may only be achieved by crossing the growth plate, it is imperative that smooth pins are used. Rohmiller et al. reviewed their series of Salter–Harris I and II injuries to the distal tibia and found that a pronation–abduction injury is more likely to develop premature physeal closure (PPC) in a supination–external rotation injury. Furthermore, they found that post-reduction displacement is the most important determinant of PPC (44). Once the fracture is treated, the child is followed regularly for maintenance of reduction and signs of healing. Once healed, the patient is followed at regular intervals for any signs of growth arrest. This is usually done for a 2-year-period post-injury. A full growth arrest may result in significant limb-length discrepancy, while a partial arrest may result in an angular deformity. A growth of arrest of the tibia may also result in significant overgrowth of the fibula, which may result in lateral impingement of the ankle.

HIGH-RISK ANKLE FRACTURES

Salter–Harris III and IV fractures typically constitute high-risk injuries due to the intraarticular displacement associated with these injuries. These injury patterns involve the articular surface (SH III and IV), which in the presence of significant displacement will necessitate an anatomic reduction of not only the articular surface, but of the growth plate to ensure optimal results. Less than anatomic reduction in these patterns of injury may result in significant degenerative changes and growth arrest.

Salter–Harris type III injuries accounts for 25% of injuries across the ankle (35,36). The fracture exits through the epiphysis and is usually intraarticular in nature. These fractures are exemplified by medial malleolus or Tillaux fractures in children. The incidence of Salter–Harris type IV fractures is reported to be 25% (35,36). These fractures exit through the articular surface and are metaphyseal, epiphyseal, and physeal. These fractures are exemplified by triplane fractures, as well as shear fractures. Given the articular nature of these fractures, an anatomic reduction is required to prevent long-term complications.

Closed reduction may be attempted. Displaced fractures with an articular step off greater than 2 mm post-reduction must be opened to align the fracture fragments. The fracture is stabilized with screws or smooth pins. Crossing the physis with threaded implants is to be avoided unless the child is very close to skeletal maturity. Screw fixation is usually performed percutaneously, with the screw placed parallel to the physis. Alternatively, a bioabsorbable screw may be used to obviate the need for screw removal. In a series by Podeszwa et al. they compared two groups diagnosed preoperatively with either Salter–Harris III or IV injuries of the distal tibia treated with a standard metal screw and those treated with a bioabsorbable screw. They found a comparable return to full activity and fewer complication rates in the bioabsorbable screw group (45). Kling et al. reported on a series of 29 SH III and IV fractures of the distal tibia. Only 1 in 20 cases treated with an open reduction developed a partial growth arrest, in contrast to 5 in 9 children who developed growth disturbance after closed reduction of the fracture (46).

SPECIFIC FRACTURE PATTERNS

Triplane Fractures

Triplane factures are complex injuries involving the distal tibia in the coronal, sagittal, and transverse planes. Although most distal tibia fractures in the growing child can be classified by the Salter–Harris (SH) classification, the complex nature of the deformity prevents it from fitting into one simple category. All three planes must be considered prior to treatment. Typically, the triplane fracture consists of two to four parts with the vast majority being intraarticular fractures. Though rare, there are reports of extraarticular fractures. The classic description of the triplane fracture is a three-part fracture which consists of an SH III fracture pattern in the anteroposterior plane (similar to the juvenile Tillaux fracture), a SH IV fracture pattern on the lateral view with a metaphyseal spike with the Thurston–Holland tibial fragment. The triplane fracture is a transitional fracture; it occurs in individuals who are approaching skeletal maturity. It occurs slightly earlier in girls (12 to 14 years) than in boys (13 to 15 years), since girls tend to reach skeletal maturity at an earlier age. The incidence of triplane fractures is 6% of pediatric ankle fractures (47). Triplane fractures are best seen on CT. The CT clearly delineates the entire fracture and the amount of displacement particularly at the articular surface (Fig. 26.4A–D) (48,49). Brown et al. reviewed their findings on 51 cases of triplane fractures. They found that two-part fractures are the most common; plafond injuries are more common than malleolar injuries, but medial malleolar extension of the fracture is more common than previously recognized (49). CT scans are essential for the pre-operative plan.

Treatment of triplane fractures is aimed at obtaining an anatomic reduction particularly at the articular surface. Non-displaced fractures may be treated non-operatively. The prerequisite for non-operative treatment is intraarticular displacement of less than 2 mm. A post-reduction CT scan may be obtained to assess the adequacy of reduction. Ertl et al. showed that residual displacement greater than 2 mm can lead to pain and is directly related to activity (50). Open reduction and fixation of lateral fractures may be performed through an anterolateral approach; medial fractures are best approached anteromedially. The order of fixation is largely dependent upon the fracture configuration, whether the metaphyseal fragment or the epiphyseal fragment is fixed first. It is usually best to restore the intraarticular surface and then proceed to the metaphyseal

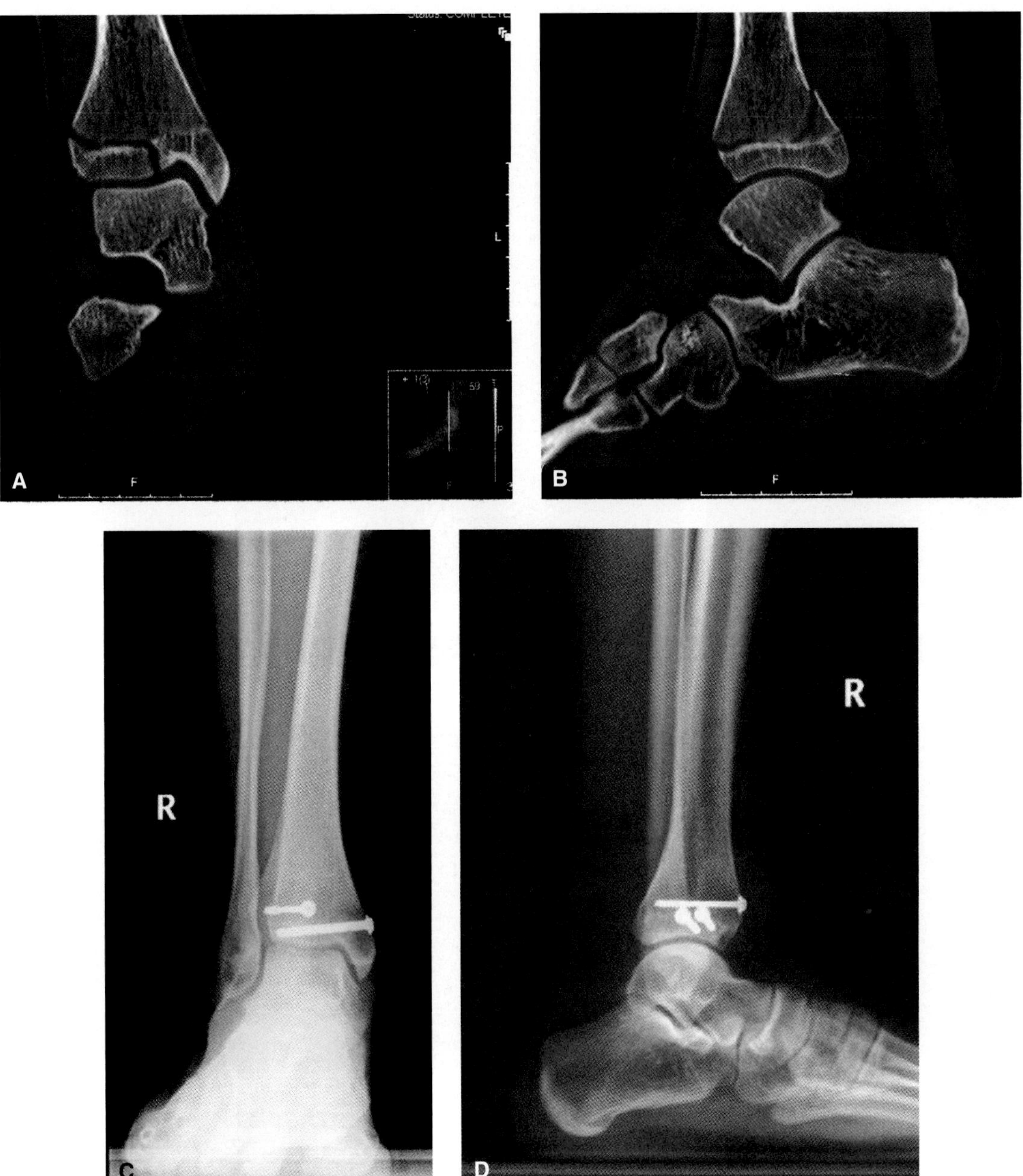

Figure 26.4. **A–D:** CT scan images of a 15-year-old male in sagittal and coronal view of the ankle showing a triplane fracture. This was treated with closed reduction and percutaneous screw fixation with good post-operative results.

fixation. In younger children with at least 2 years of growth, crossing the physis should be avoided if at all possible as this may cause possible growth disturbance. Cannulated systems have allowed for better placement of fixation without compromising the physis. Smooth pins may be used to achieve fixation if crossing the physis cannot be avoided.

Tillaux Fractures

Juvenile Tillaux fractures are SH III fractures of the distal tibial epiphysis which account for 3% of pediatric ankle fractures (51,52). These fractures occur in older children between 12 and 14 years of age due to the sequence of distal tibial physeal closure (Fig. 26.5A–F). The injuries result from supination and external rotation, resulting in an avulsion of the anterolateral distal tibial epiphysis by the anterior inferior tibiofibular ligament. Occasionally, the injury will be accompanied by a concomitant fibular fracture. Treatment of the injury is guided by the amount of fracture displacement and articular step-off. Often, it is necessary to obtain a CT scan of the fracture to delineate the amount of fracture displacement. Horn et al. showed that a CT scan was more sensitive than plain radiographs in detecting fractures with greater than 2 mm of displacement (53). Treatment is aimed at obtaining an anatomic reduction particularly of the articular surface. A closed reduction may be attempted. If displacement greater than 2 mm is

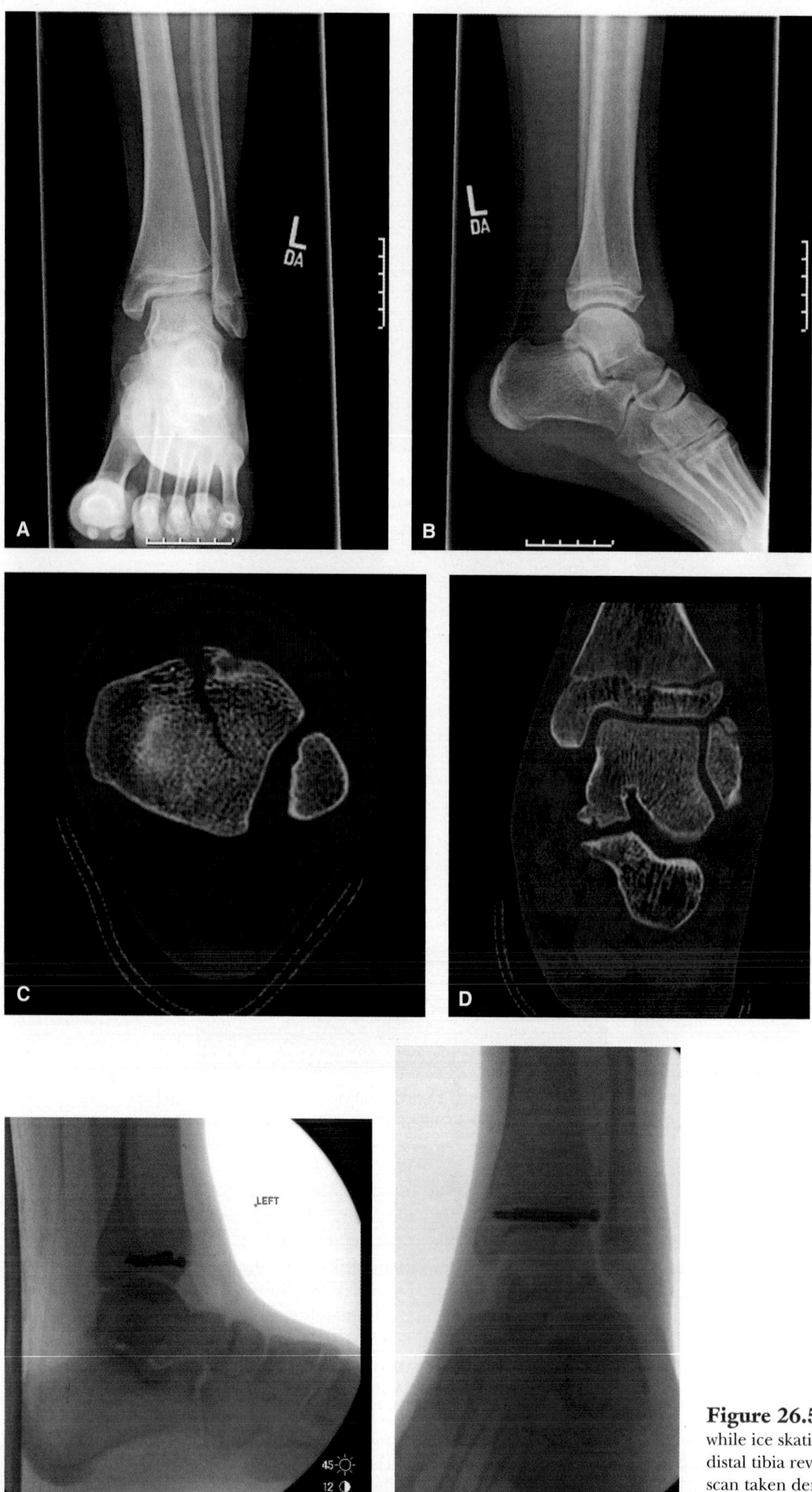

Figure 26.5. **A–F:** This 15-year-old male fell while ice skating. AP and lateral radiographs of the distal tibia reveal a displaced Tillaux fracture. CT scan taken demonstrates 3 mm displacement. This was treated operatively with an open reduction and screw fixation of the Tillaux fragment.

noted, open reduction is performed and the joint is reduced. Usually the anterolateral approach is used to access the joint. Once reduced, the fracture is stabilized with cannulated screws parallel to the physis. In the child close to skeletal maturity, fracture fixation across the physis is acceptable. Alternatively, arthroscopic visualization and fixation of the fracture may be performed. Multiple reports using this technique have shown good outcomes with good visualization and reduction of the fracture (54–56).

OSTEOCHONDRAL INJURIES TO THE TALUS

Ankle pain after a traumatic event is reported to be the most common presenting complaint in children with an osteochondral injury to the talus. The incidence of a traumatic injury to the ankle with an osteochondral injury is reported to be as high as 63% (57). These lesions tend to be located anterolaterally or posteromedially. In a large review, Elias and colleagues found that the most common location of talar osteochondral lesions was the medial talar dome (58). Canale and Belding performed a retrospective review of 31 cases. They found that lateral lesions were thinner (like a wafer), associated with inversion or inversion–dorsiflexion trauma, and more likely to be displaced. Medial lesions were cup shaped and deeper (59). Berndt and Harty found that combined inversion and dorsiflexion produced lateral lesions, while eversion and plantarflexion produced medial lesions (60).

The classification of osteochondral injuries to the talus was proposed by Berndt and Henry in 1959. Type 1 lesions are undetached areas of subchondral compression, type 2 lesions are partially detached, type 3 lesions are detached but not displaced, and type 4 lesions are completely displaced (60). Children manifest with pain and swelling after a traumatic event, such as an inversion injury. Radiographic evaluation is performed with the use of plain radiographs, which will often reveal the lesion (Fig. 26.6). MRI is useful in evaluating the articular cartilage, determining the extent of osteochondral injury, defining the exact location of the lesion, and aiding in the surgical plan. Treatment of talar osteochondral lesions depends upon the amount of displacement. Type 1 and 2 lesions are managed conservatively with immobilization in a short leg non–weight-bearing cast for a period of 6 to 8 weeks. This may be followed by a period of protected weight bearing and activity modification for an additional 2 to 3 months until the patient is completely asymptomatic and pain free. In patients who are still symptomatic despite conservative management or those with type 3 or type 4 lesions, arthroscopically guided drilling and fixation of the osteochondral fragment is indicated. Large loose bodies are removed. Outcomes in skeletally immature children are better than adults.

OSTEOCHONDROSES

Osteochondroses are a group of disorders that may affect any bone in the body due to an abnormality in endochondral ossification. These are idiopathic conditions resulting from unknown etiology. Each specific disorder has been well defined in the literature with its course and natural history well documented.

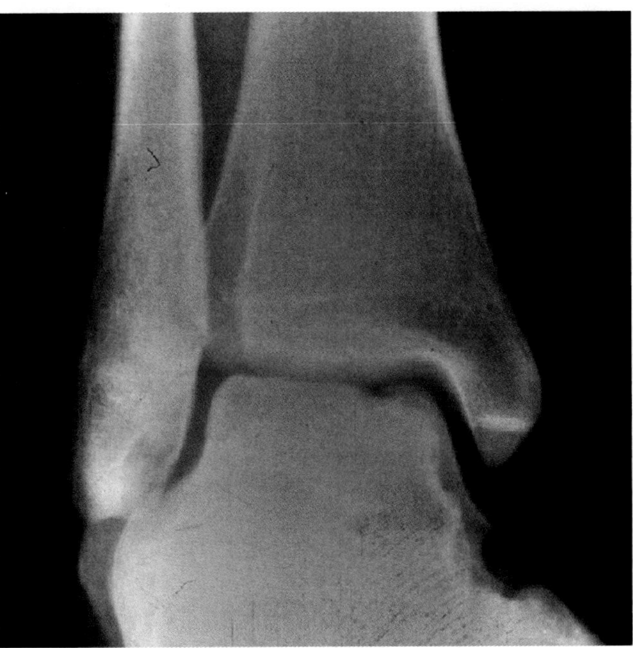

Figure 26.6. Frontal view of the ankle, obtained with the patient standing, demonstrates lucency of the medial talar dome consistent with osteochondritis dissecans.

FREIBERG INFARCTION

Freiberg infarction or Freiberg disease is an osteochondrosis which manifests as an osteonecrosis of the lesser metatarsal heads. Originally described by Freiberg in 1914 (61), this condition most commonly affects the second metatarsal, though the other metatarsals may be involved. The pathologic mechanism is thought to be repetitive stress across the involved area, which results in microfractures and vascular compromise. This condition usually manifests during adolescence. The patients present with pain localized to the affected metatarsal head, which is usually more severe with weight-bearing activity. Initial evaluation with plain radiographs may yield negative results early in the course of the condition. Subsequent radiographs may demonstrate widening of the metatarsophalangeal joint space with subchondral collapse and sclerosis (Fig. 26.7). Other imaging studies, such as bone scans, may be useful to localize the lesion. MRI may show findings consistent with avascular necrosis of the metatarsal head. Initial treatment is conservative with rest and immobilization in a short leg cast until resolution of symptoms. This is usually done for a period of at least 4 to 6 weeks. Orthotics may be employed to optimize foot position to alleviate pressure on the involved metatarsal head. Steroid injections may be used to relieve pain. Rarely surgery is indicated when patients do not respond to conservative treatment. Joint debridement, synovectomy, and a metatarsal dorsiflexion osteotomy are the main components of surgical treatment (62,63). Treatment of late-stage Freiberg disease with osteochondral plug transplantation has also been described with good results (64).

KOHLER DISEASE

Commonly described as osteonecrosis of the tarsal navicular bone, this condition is defined as an osteochondrosis that was first described by Kohler in 1908. This condition typically

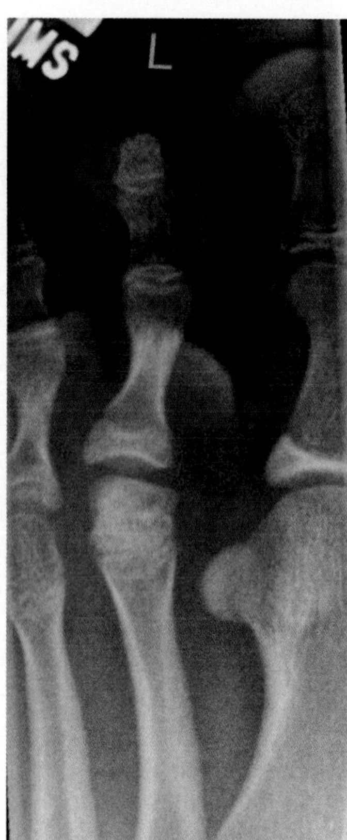

Figure 26.7. AP radiograph image of the foot showing sclerosis and collapse of the second metatarsal head consistent with Freiberg's infarction.

affects children between the ages of 2 and 10 years (65,66). The exact etiology of this condition remains unclear. Though multiple factors are implicated, trauma with subsequent disruption of the vascular supply appears to be the most plausible theory. The delay in ossification of the navicular bone puts it at risk for mechanical compression by the already ossified talus, which may disrupt the blood supply to the navicular bone. Children with Kohler disease present with a limp and midfoot pain. Radiographically, the condition may manifest as either thinning or flattening of the navicular bone into a wafer shape with irregularity of the ossification center or increased density in a normally shaped navicular bone. Occasionally, a bone scan may show areas of decreased uptake, suggestive of avascular necrosis (67). Treatment is conservative. Activity restriction and nonsteroidal anti-inflammatory medication may be used to afford relief. In more symptomatic cases, treatment in a short leg cast for a period of 4 to 6 weeks alleviates the pain. The clinical course is benign with no long-term sequelae.

OVERUSE INJURIES

STRESS FRACTURES

Stress fractures result from repetitive stress and trauma, which results in bone fatigue. This eventually leads to structural failure and stress fractures. The submaximal stress is normally well tolerated; however repetitive stress applied too forcefully may lead to injury. This injury occurs in individuals involved in high-intensity physical activity or those who are involved in repetitive physical training. These patients present with localized pain over the fracture site. This pain may be elicited or aggravated by weight-bearing or physical activity. Radiographs may or may not show a radiolucent line indicative of a fracture. Repeat radiographs 2 to 3 weeks post-injury usually will reveal a periosteal reaction. In cases where the radiographs are negative, a bone scan is useful in identifying the area of injury. Advanced imaging studies such as CT scans or MRIs may also be used to identify and delineate the injury. Management is usually directed at minimizing or abstaining from the implicated physical activity. Immobilization with a short leg cast for a period of 6 to 8 weeks usually is sufficient to relieve pain and allow the bone to heal. Depending upon the site, some fractures may be subject to delayed healing. Once healing is documented, a gradual return to physical activity and sports may be facilitated.

ISELIN'S DISEASE

This condition was first described by Iselin in 1912 as a traction apophysitis of the fifth metatarsal tuberosity. This condition occurs in older children and adolescents and coincides with the time of appearance of the fifth metatarsal apophysis (10 years in females and 12 years in males). The apophysis appears as a fleck of bone on the lateral plantar aspect of the fifth metatarsal tuberosity, parallel to the shaft of the metatarsal. This is found embedded in the peroneus brevis tendon. Iselin's disease should be differentiated from an avulsion fracture of the base of the fifth metatarsal. The distinction is made by the pattern of the radiolucent band, which is usually perpendicular to the axis of the fifth metatarsal in avulsion injuries.

Iselin's disease occurs in patients who are active in sports. Activities that involve running, jumping, or cutting movements may cause a sudden inversion stress on the forefoot. These patients present with pain in the lateral aspect of the foot with weight-bearing activity. They will also be tender in the proximal fifth metatarsal, especially with resisted eversion of the forefoot. Other injuries such as fractures of the base of the fifth metatarsal should be ruled out. AP, lateral, and oblique radiographs of the foot should be obtained. On radiographs, these injuries may show fragmentation of the ossification center. Bone scans are usually positive. Treatment is conservative. Immobilization with a short leg cast until the patient is asymptomatic is the mainstay of treatment. Once the patient is pain free, physical therapy may be instituted for stretching and strengthening of the peroneal tendons.

SEVER'S APOPHYSITIS

Sever's apophysitis or Sever's disease is one of the most common overuse injuries in children. The incidence of this condition has been reported to be as high as 8% of all overuse injuries in children (68). It is reported to be bilateral in 61% of cases (69). This condition is thought to result from repetitive shear stress on the calcaneal apophysis. Ogden and colleagues reported that the condition results from repetitive microtrauma to the calcaneus, rather than being a result of inflammation as was previously reported (70). Radiographically, the secondary ossification center of the calcaneus shows greater fragmentation when compared to normal controls on lateral radiographs; this supports the mechanical etiology of this condition (71). Patients present with pain localized to the heel. Discomfort in this area is aggravated by physical activity. Examination reveals pain on palpation of the plantar calcaneus extending to the insertion of the Achilles tendon. Localized swelling and erythema are absent. Tightness of the Achilles tendon is typically seen. Management is conservative and generally consists of activity modification and relieving stress over the calcaneal apophysis in the acute stages of Sever's disease. This is usually achieved by physical therapy which consists of Achilles tendon stretching and strengthening of ankle dorsiflexors. Non-steroidal anti-inflammatory agents, orthotics, and heel cups may alleviate symptoms. Casting may be performed in more severe cases. Patients return to sports within 2 months of treatment (69).

PREVENTION OF FOOT AND ANKLE INJURIES IN CHILDREN AND ADOLESCENTS

The number of children and adolescents participating in organized, competitive sports steadily increases worldwide. Despite this trend, a significant decrease in fitness levels of children is observed (70,71). Subsequently reduced coordination skills, joint instability, loss of flexibility, muscle strength, and obesity all seem to be significant risk factors for injuries in the skeletally immature athlete. There is increasing awareness that muscle–tendon imbalance and a lowered proprioceptive skill level put the young athlete at risk for ankle or foot injury, especially in competitive sports, such as soccer or basketball. Ankle injury is a common occurrence, often followed by residual symptoms like pain, instability, crepitus, and weakness which affects future sports performances. Therefore, development of preventive strategies needs to be emphasized in youth sports.

The implementation of regular training programs with agility and neuromuscular skills helps to decrease the rate of injury in young athletes. A study by Passanen and colleagues conducted in 2008 showed that neuromuscular training programs which focus on motor skill and body control enhancement were able to reduce the risk of leg injury by 66%. The risk of non-contact ankle and knee ligament injury was reduced by 65% (72). In sports activities like basketball or volleyball, correct landing techniques and body-movement strategies may reduce the rate of ankle injury (73). Further injury prevention can be achieved through good body flexibility, improved core muscle strength, and regular warm ups before sports which include jogging, walking lungs, butt kicks, zig-zag runs, and jumps.

The importance of protection of a young athlete who is recently injured cannot be underestimated. Premature return to competition after a foot and ankle injury may lead to re-injury. Rehabilitation after a previous foot and ankle injury with good neuromuscular control is therefore essential to return to competition.

REHABILITATION AFTER FOOT AND ANKLE INJURY IN CHILDREN

Athletes with a history of ankle sprains are at high risk for recurrent ankle injury. McKay et al. revealed that the incidence rate of re-injury in basketball players is almost five times higher than in children without previous injury (74).

Slow, supervised return to competitive sports is advised, once the athlete is pain free and has restored full range of motion and strength. Return to sports before a complete recovery is strongly discouraged. An intermediate to high level of fitness should be established before a young athlete may return to competitive sports. Athletes should be able to do single calf raises, squats, leg dips, jumps, and hops in all directions. They should also be able to perform diagonal runs and cuts before getting clearance for competitive sports activities. Weekly neuromuscular training with the use of wobble boards and coordination regimens improves hyperlaxity of ligaments of the ankle which are essential for rehabilitation from an ankle injury. Integration of targeted balance and muscle-strengthening exercises, together with agility training for the ankle and calf region, help stabilize the ankle joint and protect the athlete from recurrent injuries.

Sports trainers and athletes have to be educated about the benefits of rehabilitation and other preventive measures such as bracing, ankle taping, or proper-quality footwear during play. Injury prevention is important and includes body-weight control, neuromuscular training, overall body fitness, regular warming up before sports, and fair play in competitive sports activities.

CONCLUSION

Foot and ankle problems in the child and adolescent comprise a wide range of conditions. Awareness of various congenital and developmental diagnoses is essential. The development of these conditions is often related to rapid growth changes or overuse conditions. In the young athlete, foot and ankle injuries represent the second most common problem with ankle sprains being the leading cause for athletes to present to their primary care physician. Clinical evaluation can be a challenge in the pediatric setting, but often hints to the correct diagnosis are obtainable. Special attention needs to be placed on the distal tibial growth plate and injuries of the physes must be treated with special care. A severe fracture of the ankle may result in growth arrest of tibia and/or fibula resulting in significant limb-length discrepancy or malalignment of the ankle joint.

Prevention of injuries of the ankle or foot in children and young athletes should be taken seriously and may be achieved by regular neuromuscular training regimens that include balance, proprioception, and strengthening exercises. Athletic trainers must be educated to provide rehabilitation programs that maximize recovery and return to sport readiness.

REFERENCES

1. Stanish WD. Lower leg, foot and ankle injuries in young athletes. *Clin Sports Med* 1995; 14(3):651–668.
2. Waterman BR, Davey S, Zacchilli MA, et al. Epidemiology of ankle sprains in the United States. *J Bone Surg Am* 2010;92(13):2279–2284.
3. Leonard MA. The inheritance of tarsal coalition and its relationship to spastic flat foot. *J Bone Joint Surg Br* 1974;56B(3):520–526.
4. Stormont DM, Peterson HA. The relative incidence of tarsal coalition. *Clin Orthop Relat Res* 1983;(181):28–36.
5. Harris RI, Beath T. Etiology of peroneal spastic flat foot. *J Bone Joint Surg Br* 1948; 30B(4):624–634.
6. Solomon LB, Ruhli FJ, Taylor J, et al. A dissection and computer tomograph study of tarsal coalitions in 100 cadaver feet. *J Orthop Res* 2003;21(2):352–358.
7. Nalaboff KM, Schweitzer ME. MRI of tarsal coalition: frequency, distribution, and innovative signs. *Bull NYU Hosp Jt Dis* 2008;66(1):14–21.

8. Sullivan JA. Ankle and foot injuries in the pediatric athlete. *Instr Course Lect* 1993;42: 545–551.
9. Mosier KM, Asher M. Tarsal coalitions and peroneal spastic flat foot. A review. *J Bone Joint Surg Am* 1984;66(7):976–984.
10. Elkus RA. Tarsal coalition in the young athlete. *Am J Sports Med* 1986;14(6):477–480.
11. O'Neill DB, Micheli LJ. Tarsal coalition. A followup of adolescent athletes. *Am J Sports Med* 1989;17(4):544–549.
12. Conway JJ, Cowell HR. Tarsal coalition: clinical significance and roentgenographic demonstration. *Radiology* 1969;92(4):799–811.
13. Lateur LM, Van Hoe LR, Van Ghillewe KV, et al. Subtalar coalition: diagnosis with the C sign on lateral radiographs of the ankle. *Radiology* 1994;193(3):847–851.
14. Resnick D. Talar ridges, osteophytes, and beaks: a radiologic commentary. *Radiology* 1984; 151(2):329–332.
15. Sakellariou A, Sallomi D, Janzen DL, et al. Talocalcaneal coalition. Diagnosis with the C-sign on lateral radiographs of the ankle. *J Bone Joint Surg Br* 2000;82(4):574–578.
16. Jayakumar S, Cowell HR. Rigid flatfoot. *Clin Orthop Relat Res* 1977;(122):77–84.
17. Sarno RC, Carter BL, Bankoff MS, et al. Computed tomography in tarsal coalition. *J Comput Assist Tomogr* 1984;8(6):1155–1160.
18. Wechsler RJ, Karasick D, Schweitzer ME. Computed tomography of talocalcaneal coalition: imaging techniques. *Skeletal Radiol* 1992;21(6):353–358.
19. Wechsler RJ, Schweitzer ME, Deely DM, et al. Tarsal coalition: depiction and characterization with CT and MR imaging. *Radiology* 1994;193(2):447–452.
20. El Rassi G, Riddle EC, Kumar SJ. Arthrofibrosis involving the middle facet of the talocalcaneal joint in children and adolescents. *J Bone Joint Surg Am* 2005;87(10):2227–2231.
21. Lyon R, Liu XC, Cho SJ. Effects of tarsal coalition resection on dynamic plantar pressures and electromyography of lower extremity muscles. *J Foot Ankle Surg* 2005;44(4):252–258.
22. Chambers RB, Cook TM, Cowell HR. Surgical reconstruction for calcaneonavicular coalition. Evaluation of function and gait. *J Bone Joint Surg Am* 1982;64(6):829–836.
23. Hetsroni I, Ayalon M, Mann G, et al. Walking and running plantar pressure analysis before and after resection of tarsal coalition. *Foot Ankle Int* 2007;28(5):575–580.
24. Gonzalez P, Kumar SJ. Calcaneonavicular coalition treated by resection and interposition of the extensor digitorum brevis muscle. *J Bone Joint Surg Am* 1990;72(1):71–77.
25. Morgan RC Jr, Crawford AH. Surgical management of tarsal coalition in adolescent athletes. *Foot Ankle* 1986;7(3):183–193.
26. Olney BW, Asher MA. Excision of symptomatic coalition of the middle facet of the talocalcaneal joint. *J Bone Joint Surg Am* 1987;69(4):539–544.
27. Shands AR Jr, Wentz IJ. Congenital anomalies, accessory bones, and osteochondritis in the feet of 850 children. *Surg Clin North Am* 1953:1643–1666.
28. Zadek I, Gold AM. The accessory tarsal scaphoid. *J Bone Joint Surg Am* 1948;30A(4): 957–968.
29. Sullivan JA, Miller WA. The relationship of the accessory navicular to the development of the flat foot. *Clin Orthop Relat Res* 1979;(144):233–237.
30. Grogan DP, Gasser SI, Ogden JA. The painful accessory navicular: a clinical and histopathological study. *Foot Ankle* 1989;10(3):164–169.
31. Lawson JP, Ogden JA, Sella E, et al. The painful accessory navicular. *Skeletal Radiol* 1984; 12(4):250–262.
32. Veitch JM. Evaluation of the Kidner procedure in treatment of symptomatic accessory tarsal scaphoid. *Clin Orthop Relat Res* 1978;(131):210–213.
33. Nakayama S, Sugimoto K, Takakura Y, et al. Percutaneous drilling of symptomatic accessory navicular in young athletes. *Am J Sports Med* 2005;33(4):531–535.
34. Hertel J. Functional anatomy, pathomechanics, and pathophysiology of lateral ankle instability. *J Athl Train* 2002;37:364–375.
35. Mizuta T, Benson WM, Foster BK, et al. Statistical analysis of the incidence of physeal injuries. *J Pediatr Orthop* 1987;7(5):518–523.
36. Peterson HA, Madhok R, Benson JT, et al. Physeal fractures: Part 1. Epidemiology in Olmsted County, Minnesota, 1979–1988. *J Pediatr Orthop* 1994;14(4):423–430.
37. Worlock P. Supracondylar fractures of the humerus. Assessment of cubitus varus by the Baumann angle. *J Bone Joint Surg Br* 1986;68(5):755–757.
38. Salter RB, Harris WR. Injuries involving the epiphyseal plate. *J Bone Joint Surg Am* 1963; 45(3):587–622.
39. Lauge N. Fractures of the ankle; analytic historic survey as the basis of new experimental, roentgenologic and clinical investigations. *Arch Surg* 1948;56(3):259–317.
40. Lauge-Hansen N. Fractures of the ankle. II. Combined experimental-surgical and experimental-roentgenologic investigations. *Arch Surg* 1950;60(5):957–985.
41. Dias LS, Tachdjian MO. Physeal injuries of the ankle in children: classification. *Clin Orthop Relat Res* 1978;(136):230–233.
42. Vahvanen V, Aalto K. Classification of ankle fractures in children. *Arch Orthop Trauma Surg* 1980;97(1):1–5.
43. Sankar WN, Chen J, Kay RM, et al. Incidence of occult fracture in children with acute ankle injuries. *J Pediatr Orthop* 2008;28(5):500–501.
44. Rohmiller MT, Gaynor TP, Pawelek J, et al. Salter-Harris I and II fractures of the distal tibia: does mechanism of injury relate to premature physeal closure? *J Pediatr Orthop* 2006; 26(3):322–328.
45. Podeszwa DA, Wilson PL, Holland AR, et al. Comparison of bioabsorbable versus metallic implant fixation for physeal and epiphyseal fractures of the distal tibia. *J Pediatr Orthop* 2008;28(8):859–863.
46. Kling TF Jr, Bright RW, Hensinger RN. Distal tibial physeal fractures in children that may require open reduction. *J Bone Joint Surg Am* 1984;66(5):647–657.
47. Cooperman DR, Spiegel PG, Laros GS. Tibial fractures involving the ankle in children. The so-called triplane epiphyseal fracture. *J Bone Joint Surg Am* 1978;60(8):1040–1046.
48. Jones S, Phillips N, Ali F, et al. Triplane fractures of the distal tibia requiring open reduction and internal fixation. Pre-operative planning using computed tomography. *Injury* 2003;34(4):293–298.
49. Brown SD, Kasser JR, Zurakowski D, et al. Analysis of 51 tibial triplane fractures using CT with multiplanar reconstruction. *AJR Am J Roentgenol* 2004;183(5):1489–1495.
50. Ertl JP, Barrack RL, Alexander AH, et al. Triplane fracture of the distal tibial epiphysis. Long-term follow-up. *J Bone Joint Surg Am* 1988;70(7):967–976.
51. Dias LS, Giegerich CR. Fractures of the distal tibial epiphysis in adolescence. *J Bone Joint Surg Am* 1983;65(4):438–444.
52. Spiegel PG, Cooperman DR, Laros GS. Epiphyseal fractures of the distal ends of the tibia and fibula. A retrospective study of two hundred and thirty-seven cases in children. *J Bone Joint Surg Am* 1978;60(8):1046–1050.
53. Horn BD, Crisci K, Krug M, et al. Radiologic evaluation of juvenile tillaux fractures of the distal tibia. *J Pediatr Orthop* 2001;21(2):162–164.
54. Leetun DT, Ireland ML. Arthroscopically assisted reduction and fixation of a juvenile Tillaux fracture. *Arthroscopy* 2002;18(4):427–429.
55. Miller MD. Arthroscopically assisted reduction and fixation of an adult Tillaux fracture of the ankle. *Arthroscopy* 1997;13(1):117–119.
56. Ono A, Nishikawa S, Nagao A, et al. Arthroscopically assisted treatment of ankle fractures: arthroscopic findings and surgical outcomes. *Arthroscopy* 2004;20(6):627–631.
57. Higuera J, Laguna R, Peral M, et al. Osteochondritis dissecans of the talus during childhood and adolescence. *J Pediatr Orthop* 1998;18(3):328–332.
58. Elias I, Zoga AC, Morrison WB, et al. Osteochondral lesions of the talus: localization and morphologic data from 424 patients using a novel anatomical grid scheme. *Foot Ankle Int* 2007;28(2):154–161.
59. Canale ST, Belding RH. Osteochondral lesions of the talus. *J Bone Joint Surg Am* 1980; 62(1):97–102.
60. Berndt AL, Harty M. Transchondral fractures (osteochondritis dissecans) of the talus. *J Bone Joint Surg Am* 1959;41-A:988–1020.
61. Freiberg A. The infraction of the second metatarsal bone. *Surg Gynecol Obstetr* 1914;19: 191–193.
62. Kinnard P, Lirette R. Freiberg's disease and dorsiflexion osteotomy. *J Bone Joint Surg Br* 1991;73(5):864–865.
63. Lee SK, Chung MS, Baek GH, et al. Treatment of Freiberg disease with intra-articular dorsal wedge osteotomy and absorbable pin fixation. *Foot Ankle Int* 2007;28(1):43–48.
64. Miyamoto W, Takao M, Uchio Y, et al. Late-stage Freiberg disease treated by osteochondral plug transplantation: a case series. *Foot Ankle Int* 2008;29(9):950–955.
65. Sinclair GG, Uhlman RE, Zeichner AM. Osteochondrosis of the tarsal navicular bone: Kohler's disease. *J Am Podiatry Assoc* 1981;71(2):77–80.
66. Williams GA, Cowell HR. Kohler's disease of the tarsal navicular. *Clin Orthop Relat Res* 1981;(158):53–58.
67. Khoury J, Jerushalmi J, Loberant N, et al. Kohler disease: diagnoses and assessment by bone scintigraphy. *Clin Nucl Med* 2007;32(3):179–181.
68. Maffulli N, Wong J, Almekinders LC. Types and epidemiology of tendinopathy. *Clin Sports Med* 2003;22(4):675–692.
69. Micheli LJ, Ireland ML. Prevention and management of calcaneal apophysitis in children: an overuse syndrome. *J Pediatr Orthop* 1987;7(1):34–38.
70. Kuntzelman CT, Reiff GG. The decline in American children's fitness levels. *Res Q Exerc Sport* 1992;63:107–111.
71. Tomkinson GR, Olds TS, Gulbin J. Secular trends in physical performance of Australian children. Evidence from the Talent Search program. *J Sports Med Phys Fitness* 2003;43: 90–98.
72. Pasanen K, Parkkari J, Pasanen M, et al. Neuromuscular training and the risk of leg injuries in female floorball players: cluster randomised controlled study. *BMJ* 2008;337(7661): 96–99.
73. Bahr R, Lian O, Bahr IA. A twofold reduction in the incidence of acute ankle sprains in volleyball after the introduction of an injury prevention program: a prospective cohort study. *Scand J Med Sci Sports* 1997;7:172–177.
74. McKay GD, Goldie PA, Payne WR, et al. Ankle injuries in basketball: injury rate and risk factors. *Br J Sports Med* 2001;35:103–108.

CHAPTER

27

Bethany Gallagher
Robert H. Brophy

Sports-specific Injury Prevention

TRAINING PROGRAM

Injuries to the foot and ankle are a common complaint among high-performance athletes and may be detrimental to both their current level of participation as well as their potential for future play. A broad spectrum of treatments ranging from conservative symptomatic management to operative intervention exists. These treatments, however effective, require a prolonged recovery period of inactivity and limited playing time. In order to protect athletes at risk, there may be a role for preventative training programs to reduce the incidence of injury or re-injury to the foot and ankle. These preventative protocols often include balance and proprioception, range of motion, strengthening, and functional exercises.

Prevention of ankle injuries potentially plays an important part in longevity of participation for high-performance athletes. According to Freeman, functional ankle instability results from the loss of appropriate articular neural feedback from the injured ankle ligaments (1,2). Improvement of balance and coordination may positively affect the sensorimotor system and reduce the proprioceptive deficits that lead to ligamentous ankle instability. The use of ankle disc training has routinely been clinically shown to improve balance, reduce ankle symptoms, and decrease re-injury. The balance board or tilt table programs start with initial simplistic exercises with the eyes open and no additional distractions (Fig. 27.1A) (3). These slowly progress over the course of weeks to more technical exercises with the incorporation of activities such as single-leg stance, dribbling a ball, catching objects, and eliminating visual input (Fig. 27.1B–D) (4–6). Rehabilitation protocols typically incorporate 15 to 45 second repetitions for 10 to 15 minutes several times per week (Table 27.1). The preventative protocols should be initiated and carefully supervised. Several studies have shown significant reduction in re-injury with supervised physiotherapy as compared to a home program (4,5,6).

There is a paucity of information concerning the specific mechanism by which balance board training improves ankle stability. One purposed mechanism is training on a balance board or ankle disc decreases time of onset of activity for muscle groups around the ankle (2). The muscle reaction times of the peroneals, specifically in previously injured ankles, showed marked improvement after only 2 months of balance training (7). This may yield a protective mechanism to stabilize the ankle and prevent injury. Unfortunately, it is unclear whether this more rapid reaction time is sufficient for protection against injury.

Studies have evaluated the efficacy of balance and proprioception training protocols citing a fourfold increased risk of injury for athletes who did not participate in balance training (4). The beneficial effects are most consistently seen in those participants with a history of previous ankle injury. Within 1 year post-injury, these individuals are two times more prone to re-injury (5). In the previously injured athlete, use of an ankle disc protocol during the competitive season yields a significant reduction in subsequent ankle injuries of up to 60% to 76% (6). There are several controlled randomized trials supporting the utility of proprioception and balance board training for high-risk populations. Tropp evaluated three groups of soccer players (n = 450) in a randomized controlled trial focusing on the benefit of a balance and proprioceptive training regimen. Those participants in the coordination program with history of ankle injury showed a significant decrease in recurrent injury. The incidence of ankle sprains in this population approached the number of those without injury history (4). Verhagen demonstrated a trend toward decreased risk of injury in at-risk volleyball players with a balance board program (5). Even in the more contact-intensive sports of basketball and soccer, McGuine showed a reduction in recurrent ankle sprains with the incorporation of balance board training (5). In addition to the randomized trials, McHugh supported this finding in a cohort study of high-school–varsity football players participating in balance intervention training. The patients were placed in study groups stratified by risk of injury based on BMI and a history of previous ankle sprain(s). With these subsets, this study demonstrated that coordination training dramatically reduced the risk of recurrent injury in a high-risk population by 77% (6). Little support exists for the integration of a proprioception training regimen in those athletes without prior history of injury. However, there is substantial support for this practice in the high-risk athlete with prior ankle injuries.

Some studies have combined interventions within the training programs. For example, a combination of proprioceptive, strength training, and technical education protocols have been implemented for preventative/rehabilitative measures (8). Strength training is important to address the weakness in the evertor muscle group, which, in combination with diminished proprioception, may be the primary underlying cause for ankle instability and recurrent injury. Wedderkopp combined both

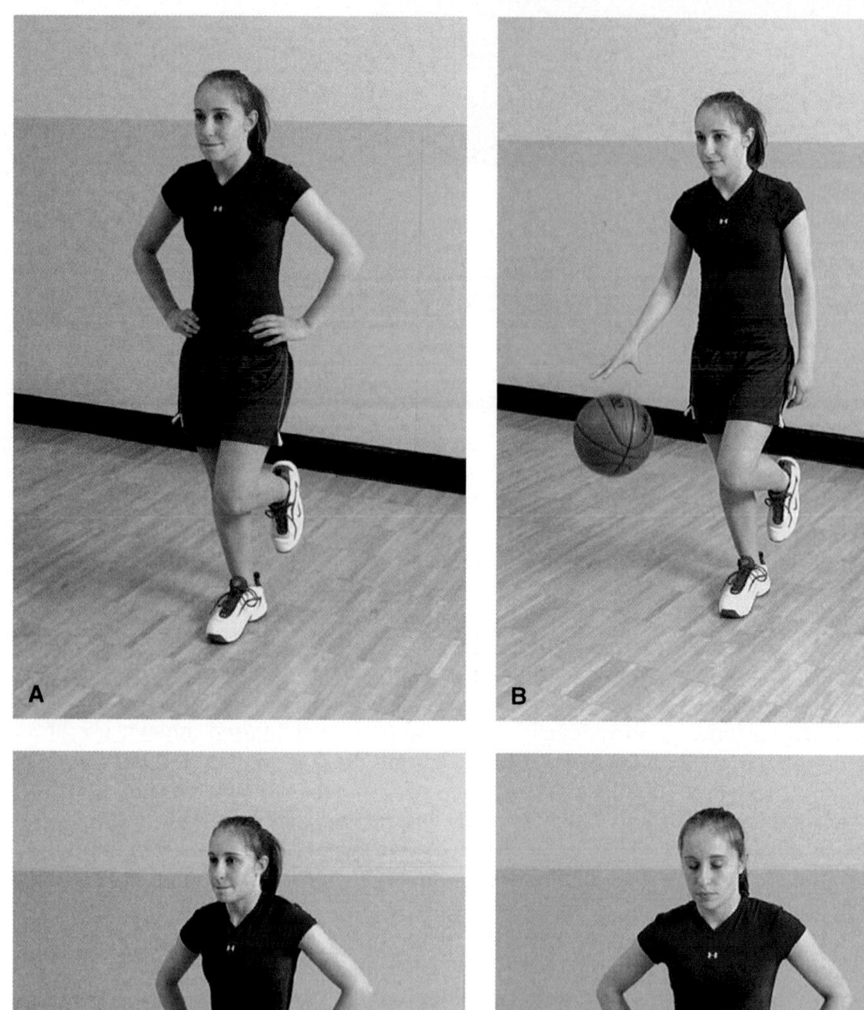

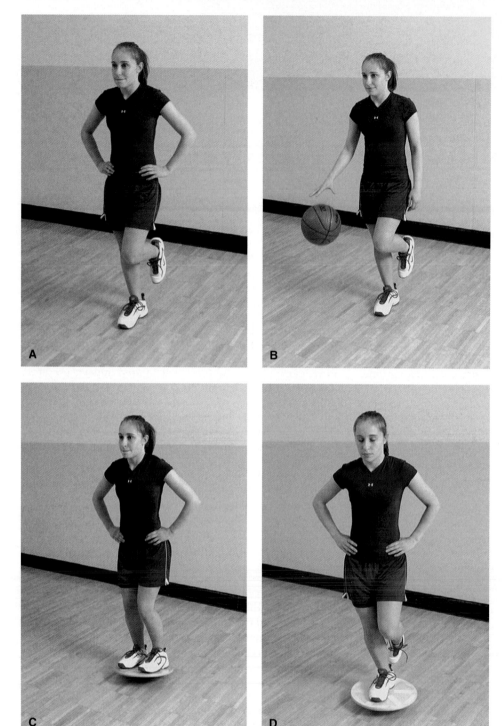

Figure 27.1. **A–D:** Illustration of balance board training. **A**-Balancing without board. **B**-Balancing while performing functional activities (dribbling). **C**-Double-leg stance while rotating the board. **D**-Balancing on the board while the eyes are closed.

functional strengthening with balance training (8). The combined program reduced ankle re-injury risk significantly more than isolated functional strengthening (8). Bahr, focusing on multi-intervention volleyball-specific technical training, athlete education, and proprioceptive training, showed a decrease in ankle injury by 47%; however, the prophylactic benefit in uninjured athletes was only revealed after at least 2 years of the injury prevention training. Athletes participating in short-term preseason training protocols with an ankle disc or balance board and no prior history of ankle injury had minimal change in injury risk; whereas athletes predisposed to recurrent injury to the ankle require a significantly shorter duration of training to yield beneficial effects (9). These studies fail to identify the specific mechanism(s) for risk reduction, but clearly illustrate the benefit from intervention for the previously injured athlete.

There is little evidence to demonstrate any benefit with the integration of specific stretching exercises and functional activities in reducing the incidence of foot and ankle injury.

TABLE 27.1 The Balance Training Program[a]

Phase	Surface	Eyes	Exercise
I	Floor	Open	Single-leg stance
Week 1		Open	Single-leg stance while swinging the raised leg
		Open	Single-leg squat (30–45°)
		Open	Single-leg stance while performing functional activities (dribbling, catching, kicking)
II	Floor	Closed	Single-leg stance
Week 2		Closed	Swinging the raised leg
		Closed	Single-leg squat (30–45°)
III	Board	Open	Single-leg stance
Week 3		Open	Swinging the raised leg
		Open	Single-leg squat (30–45°)
		Open	Double-leg stance while rotating the board
IV	Board	Closed	Single-leg stance
Week 4		Open	Swinging the raised leg
		Open	Single-leg squat (30–45°)
		Open	Single-leg stance while relating the board
V	Board	Closed	Single-leg stance
Week 5+		Open	Single-leg squat (30–45°)
		Open	Single-leg stance while rotating the board
		Open	Single-leg stance while performing functional activities (dribbling, catching, kicking)

[a]Phases I through IV were performed 5 days per week. Phase V was performed 3 days per week for the rest of the season. Each exercise was performed for a duration of 30 seconds per leg, and legs were alternated during a rest period of 30 seconds between repetitions.

Reprinted from McGuine TA, Keene JS. The effect of a balance training program on the risk of ankle sprains in high school athletes. *Am J Sports Med* 2006;34:1103–1111, with permission (3).

Stretching theoretically reduces muscle stiffness and reduces the force transmission through the musculotendinous unit. This increased tensile strength may play a protective role. Although a trial incorporating a program emphasizing flexibility and agility for soccer players in Sweden demonstrated a reduction of ankle injuries (7), this study had additional interventions including ankle taping and leg guards. However, others have described stretching as having a detrimental effect on performance secondary to decreased joint stability and energy absorption as well as reducing muscle unit strength. Theoretically, stretching of the Achilles tendon significantly increases ankle dorsiflexion and reduces plantarflexion strength. Increased motion in these planes increases the relative risk of overuse injury, up to eight times greater in the hyper-flexible individual (10). The efficacy in stretching is controversial and requires further well-controlled studies to delineate the actual role of isolated stretching on injury prevention (11,12).

Currently, the method of choice for preventative protocols incorporates both a regimen of strengthening and balance training. Overwhelming evidence exists supporting the use of these measures in high-performance athletes with prior history of injury. At this time, few studies support the use of prophylactic training programs for the uninjured athlete unless the training regimen is continued over several competitive seasons. Further well-designed studies are needed to truly isolate the benefits of these programs for sports-specific activities.

TAPING AND BRACING

In addition to incorporating a thorough preventative training regimen, many programs have adopted the use of external ankle bracing and taping as a means to further prevent injuries in the high-risk athlete. There are many explanations for the efficacy of ankle supports including restriction on range of motion, postural effects, neuromuscular control, and joint velocity.

The most commonly accepted mechanism for the effectiveness of bracing/taping is the apparent limitation of joint range of motion. Both taping and bracing reduce the range of motion up to 62% and dampen the inversion moment necessary to generate ligamentous inversion injury (5,11,13,14). In addition, both tape and lace-up bracing decrease the angle of supination at heel strike and increase the maximum pronation of the foot. Ultimately, the support devices serve to hold the foot farther from inversion.

Both bracing and taping seem to provide improved mechanical and functional stability. However, several studies provide differing explanations of this phenomenon. In addition to the restricted range of motion as discussed, many argue that ankle supports provide a proprioceptive benefit and augmented sensory input. Several electromyogram studies have noted a shortened reaction time of the peroneals with taping previously injured ankles as well as an increase in force production of 1.6 times (15). The most significant effect was seen in the most unstable ankles. Also, Robbins measured the accuracy of foot position awareness in the taped ankle before and after exercise (16). In spite of the loosening of the tape, there was clear improvement in proprioception both before and after exercise. This alteration of ankle-joint proprioception may have a greater effect on reduction of ankle injury than the restricted ROM. This is supported by the studies focusing on proprioceptive ankle training. Some argue against these beneficial effects of taping on ankle position awareness and conclude that only semi-rigid bracing significantly alters proprioception secondary to pressure from the support bars on cutaneous receptors as well as through a more rigid construct (17).

Multiple studies endorse the use of bracing/taping for the prevention of ankle sprains. A large study by Garrick used a combination of taping with high-top shoes. The athletes with the additional support of taping had an injury incidence of 6.5/1,000 games as compared to the control group with an injury incidence of 30.4/1,000 games without supportive tape (17). Another randomized trial of ankle bracing in soccer players by Tropp showed a 3% incidence of ankle sprains in the braced group as compared to 17% in the control group (4). Similar results were found in multiple other studies focusing on brace use in athletes with previous ankle injuries. In these athletes, ankle bracing can supplement the defective peroneal muscles and ultimately protect the ankle from common inversion injuries. Potentially this could be explained through a restriction of inversion velocity. In the uninjured, unsupported ankle, the peroneals fire too slowly to protect against a supination injury. However, bracing may slow this movement enough to allow the evertors to generate sufficient protective force. In addition, a randomized trial conducted by Surve et al. in soccer players with previous ankle sprains showed a significant decrease in recurrent ankle injury (18). Gross et al. also showed a beneficial effect of prophylactic bracing specifically for those high-risk athletes with previous ankle injury (1). Both of these studies utilized semi-rigid ankle stabilizers.

Unfortunately, this benefit is not maximally sustained throughout the period of activity (14). Ankle supports routinely have reduced efficacy in post-exercise testing secondary to loosening. Multiple studies have described loss of strength of tape support ranging from 20% to 50% following athletic activity from 10 to 60 minutes (1,14,19). This dramatic decrease in strength is seen most readily with the non-rigid supports, i.e., tape. Maximal protective effect occurs within the initial 20 minutes of activity at which point the tape has loosened to its residual restrictive capability, which is related to the type of exercise performed. Similarly, ankle braces have been shown to loosen, but allow for re-application/re-tensioning during the activity, hence reducing the duration of decreased efficacy during activity.

A wide variety of taping techniques offers different supports that may ultimately offer sports-specific protection. Nearly all taping techniques are a variation on the original basketweave pattern described by Gibney. One study by Rarick, focusing on the resistance to a plantarflexion and inversion motion, found that taping technique incorporating the basketweave with a stirrup and heel lock provided the highest resistance (20). In addition, Frankney showed taping the ankle with the Hinton–Boswell method (taping in a relaxed, plantarflexed position) provided the greatest resistance to an inversion force (21). Essentially, the taping technique needs to consistently lock the talus in neutral inversion–eversion with lateral support to resist the inversion moment. In addition to taping formation, it is critical to layer the tape. A single layer of tape fails at 10% the force required for ATFL injury. In addition, taping may be prohibitive to some athletic programs secondary to extreme costs. It has been estimated that taping costs $1.75 per ankle/per session (22). This may be difficult to justify when the use of reusable ankle braces provide equivalent or superior protection. In addition, braces often do not require skilled personnel for application and can be easily re-tensioned during athletic events.

Similarly to the variability in taping techniques and materials, multiple brace designs are currently available and offer differing benefits to athletes. Prophylactic ankle supports range from elastic/all cloth to lace-up and semi-rigid designs. The semi-rigid design withstands a longer duration of activity compared to the elastic/cloth version. This was demonstrated by Greene with a comparison between two semi-rigid brace designs and a non-rigid ankle support (23). Immediately post application, the semi-rigid designs resisted up to 48% ROM of the ankle. These resistive properties were maintained throughout a 90-minute workout for the ankle-ligament protector. This significantly outperformed the non-rigid brace that only maintained an 8% restriction to ankle ROM at 90 minutes (24). In other studies, the non-rigid supports rapidly lost resistance to a deforming force, similar to taping. Finally, Rovere found laced ankle stabilizers twice as effective as tape for reducing ankle instability in football players (13,25). This was primarily a result of the ability to retighten the stabilizer to maximal support. Overall, these studies support bracing as a more effective and cost-efficient mechanism to protect athletes from ankle injury.

ORTHOSES

In-shoe devices may also reduce the incidence of foot and ankle injury in the athlete. Foot orthoses are designed to either reduce the impact and cushion the foot or alter the foot position to a more biomechanically normal position during gait. Most studies supporting the use of in-shoe devices use military recruits as the subjects which limits the applicability in the normal population. Although limited, the information provided can certainly assist in the decision to prescribe orthotics as well as which type will be most beneficial to the patient.

Several varieties of orthotic devices are available. These vary both in the position the foot is placed in when molded as well as materials they are constructed from. Some orthoses serve to cushion the impact (soft/accommodating) while others serve to formally alter the foot position during activity (semi-rigid). Finestone found that semi-rigid orthoses are no better than soft-molded orthoses in prevention of over-use injury to the foot (26). A formal in vivo study demonstrated higher tibial strain during running with semi-rigid orthoses (27). In addition, there is no shown benefit for custom orthoses over the prefabricated type. This is important to recognize when prescribing orthotics for preventive measures. The most critical factor when discussing efficacy of orthoses is the usage rate. In the military population, Finestone reported 18% to 43% discontinuation of various orthotics secondary to discomfort (26). Patients have to be comfortable in the orthoses or they will discontinue use regardless of benefit to gait and foot position.

Foot orthoses are commonly utilized for the management of lower extremity over-use injury. Early use was prescribed for the over-pronated foot, which was thought to lead to stress injury and tendinopathies. When compared to a control population, studies demonstrate a significant decrease in overuse injury to the foot with use of foot orthoses (28,29). One study showed increased shock attenuation capability in footwear can reduce not only metatarsal stress fractures but also symptoms of metatarsalgia and arch pain (28). This was secondary to an increase in the viscoelastic properties of the footwear which reduced the vertical loads on the metatarsals.

In addition to a reduction to stress injuries to the foot, the use of orthotics may improve postural control and reduce recurrent injury in unstable ankles. Foot orthoses primarily impact subtalar motion. The athlete with lower extremity injury has been shown to have an increase in range of motion of the subtalar joint, specifically pronation (30). Biomechanical orthoses are formed with the subtalar joint in neutral alignment. Ultimately, this reduces maximum pronation to normal values and reorients the foot relative to the surface. In turn, these alterations optimize proprioceptive mechanisms and reduce surrounding muscular strain. Ultimately, the addition of molded foot orthoses in the injured athlete may prevent future injury if worn and tolerated by the athlete with specific lower extremity biomechanical abnormalities.

REFERENCES

1. Gross MT, Liu HY. The role of ankle bracing for prevention of ankle sprain injuries. *J Orthop Sports Phys Ther* 2003;33:572–577.
2. Osborne MD, Chou LS, Laskowski ER, et al. The effect of ankle disk training on muscle reaction time in subjects with a history of ankle sprain. *Am J Sports Med* 2001;29:627–632.
3. McGuine TA, Keene JS. The effect of a balance training program on the risk of ankle sprains in high school athletes. *Am J Sports Med* 2006;34:1103–1111.
4. Tropp H, Askling C, Gillquist J. Prevention of ankle sprains. *J Am J Sports Med* 1985;13: 259–262.
5. Verhagen E, van der Beek A, Twisk J, et al. The effect of a proprioceptive balance board training program for the prevention of ankle sprains: a prospective controlled trial. *Am J Sports Med* 2004;32:1385–1393.
6. McHugh MP, Tyler TF, Mirabella MR, et al. The effectiveness of a balance training intervention in reducing the incidence of noncontact ankle sprains in high school football players. *Am J Sports Med* 2007;35:1289–1294.
7. Engebretsen AH, Myklebust G, Holme I, et al. Prevention of injuries among male soccer players: a prospective, randomized intervention study targeting players with previous injuries or reduced function. *Am J Sports Med* 2008;36:1052–1060.
8. Wedderkopp N, Kaltoft M, Holm R, et al. Comparison of two intervention programmes in young female players in European handball–with and without ankle disc. *Scand J Med Sci Sports* 2003;13:371–375.
9. Bahr R, Lian O, Bahr IA. A twofold reduction in the incidence of acute ankle sprains in volleyball after the introduction of an injury prevention program: a prospective cohort study. *Scand J Med Sci Sports* 1997;7:172–177.
10. Pope RP, Herbert R, Kirwan J. Effects of ankle dorsiflexion range and pre-exercise calf muscle stretching on injury risk in Army recruits. *Aust J Physiother* 1998;44:165–172.
11. Park DY, Chou L. Stretching for prevention of Achilles tendon injuries: a review of the literature. *Foot Ankle Int* 2006;27:1086–1095.
12. Pope RP, Herbert RD, Kirwan JD, et al. A randomized trial of pre-exercise stretching for prevention of lower-limb injury. *Med Sci Sports Exerc* 2000;32:271–277.
13. Arnold BL, Docherty CL. Bracing and rehabilitation–what's new. *Clin Sports Med* 2004; 23:83–95.
14. Verhagen EA, van der Beek AJ, van Mechelen W. The effect of tape, braces and shoes on ankle range of motion. *Sports Med* 2001;31:667–677.
15. Lohrer H, Alt W, Gollhofer A. Neuromuscular properties and functional aspects of taped ankles. *Am J Sports Med* 1999;27:69–75.
16. Robbins S, Waked E. Factors associated with ankle injuries. Preventive measures. *Sports Med* 1998;25:63–72.
17. Callaghan MJ. Role of ankle taping and bracing in the athlete. *Br J Sports Med* 1997;31: 102–108.
18. Surve I, Schwellnus MP, Noakes T, et al. A fivefold reduction in the incidence of recurrent ankle sprains in soccer players using the Sport-Stirrup orthosis. *Am J Sports Med* 1994; 22:601–606.
19. Verhagen E, Van Mechelen W, De Vente W. The effect of preventative measures on the incidence of ankle sprains. *Clin J Sport Med* 2000;10:291–296.
20. Rarick GL, Bigley G, Karst P, et al. The measurable support of the ankle joint by conventional methods of taping. *J Bone Joint Surg Am* 1962;44:1183–1190.
21. Frankney JR, Jewett DL, Hanks GA, et al. A comparison of ankle tape methods. *Clin J Sport Med* 1999;3:20–25.
22. Mickel TJ, Bottoni CR, Tsuji G, et al. Prophylactic bracing versus taping for the prevention of ankle sprains in high school athletes: a prospective, randomized trial. *J Foot Ankle Surg* 2006;45:360–365.
23. Thacker SB, Stroup DF, Branche CM, et al. The prevention of ankle sprains in sports. A systematic review of the literature. *Am J Sports Med* 1999;27:753–760.
24. Hume PA, Gerrard DF. Effectiveness of external ankle support. Bracing and taping in rugby union. *Sports Med* 1998;25:285–312.
25. Rovere GD, Clarke TJ, Yates CS, et al. Retrospective comparison of taping and ankle stabilizers in preventing ankle injuries. *Am J Sports Med* 1988;16:228–233.
26. Finestone A, Novack V, Farfel A, et al. A prospective study of the effect of foot orthoses composition and fabrication on comfort and the incidence of overuse injuries. *Foot Ankle Int* 2004;25:462–466.
27. Ekenman I, Milgrom C, Finestone A, et al. The role of biomechanical shoe orthoses in tibial stress fracture prevention. *Am J Sports Med* 2002;30:866–870.
28. Finestone A, Giladi M, Elad H, et al. Prevention of stress fractures using custom biomechanical shoe orthoses. *Clin Orthop Relat Res* 1999;360:182–190.
29. Milgrom C, Finestone A, Shlamkovitch N, et al. Prevention of overuse injuries of the foot by improved shoe shock attenuation. A randomized prospective study. *Clin Orthop Relat Res* 1992;281:189–192.
30. Kilmartin TE, Wallace WA. The scientific basis for the use of biomechanical foot orthoses in the treatment of lower limb sports injuries–a review of the literature. *Br J Sports Med* 1994;28:180–184.

CHAPTER

28

Jordan Reichman
Jian-Ren Liu
Dexter Sun

Focal Nerve Injuries in the Foot and Ankle

OVERVIEW

Neurologic complications of athletic injuries to the ankle and foot are common (1) and may have a profound impact on morbidity. When nerve injury is correctly diagnosed, prognostic and treatment options are enhanced. Furthermore, the explosion of interest in neuroscience has led to a dramatic increase in the discovery of therapeutics for neurologic illnesses.

Diagnosis in clinical neurology is founded on accurate localization. Starting with the history, diagnostic maneuvers first aim to locate the area/areas of neuronal dysfunction. Efforts then focus on determining the pathophysiologic process responsible for signs and symptoms. This method will usually result in successful diagnosis and treatment of neurologic disorders. Hence, to develop clinical aptitude the relevant neuroanatomy is first reviewed. This review is followed by an outlined approach to the patient evaluation. Finally, specific nerve injuries and treatment are discussed.

NEUROANATOMY OF THE ANKLE AND FOOT

THE COMMON PERONEAL NERVE

The common peroneal nerve exits the popliteal fossa between the biceps femoris tendon and the lateral head of gastrocnemius, coursing anterolaterally across the fibular neck where it is palpable. It then gives off communicating branches to the sural nerve and the lateral cutaneous nerve of the calf. Subsequently, the nerve pierces the peroneus longus muscle and divides into deep and superficial branches.

The deep peroneal nerve runs between the extensor digitorum longus and the extensor hallucis longus 5 cm above the ankle mortise. At approximately 1 cm above the ankle joint, beneath the extensor retinaculum, the nerve divides into medial and lateral branches. The medial branch travels parallel to the dorsalis pedis artery. The lateral branch supplies proprioceptive fibers to the ankle joint and sensory fibers to the roof of the sinus tarsi, traveling in a fibrous tunnel beneath the extensor digitorum brevis. The deep peroneal nerve innervates the muscles of the anterior compartment, including tibialis anterior, extensor hallucis longus, extensor digitorum longus, peroneus tertius, and extensor digitorum brevis. It should be noted that the extensor digitorum brevis receives supplemental innervation from the superficial peroneal in roughly one-third of patients (2,3).

The superficial peroneal nerve innervates peroneus longus, peroneus brevis, and peroneus tertius. It exits the deep fascia of the leg 10 to 13 cm proximal to the tip of the lateral malleolus and remains subcutaneous. It then divides into the intermediate and medial dorsal cutaneous nerves (4). These divisions carry sensation from the anterior lower leg and dorsum of the foot. Anatomic variations of the superficial peroneal nerve are described in the reports of Kosinski and Horwitz (5,6).

THE TIBIAL NERVE

The tibial nerve passes through the popliteal fossa below the arch of the soleus muscle. Within the popliteal fossa, it gives off branches to the gastrocnemius, popliteus, soleus and plantaris muscles, as well as to the sural nerve. Distal to soleus, the tibial nerve innervates the tibialis posterior, flexor digitorum longus, and flexor hallucis longus muscles. It passes beneath the medial malleolus where it is bound by the flexor retinaculum in the "tarsal tunnel." Here it divides into medial and lateral plantar branches.

The medial plantar nerve passes beneath the insertion of the abductor hallucis and then travels within connective tissue attaching the flexor hallucis brevis to the tarsal bones. It innervates the abductor hallucis, flexor digitorum brevis, flexor hallucis brevis muscles, as well as the first lumbrical. Sensation is carried from the medial aspect of the sole, the medial three and one half digits, and the nail beds.

The lateral plantar nerve courses deep to the insertion of the abductor hallucis, passing between flexor digitorum brevis and quadratus plantae. It innervates quadratus plantae, flexor digiti minimi, adductor hallucis, all interossei, the three remaining lumbricals, and abductor digiti minimi muscles, and carries cutaneous sensation from the lateral sole and lateral one and one half digits.

Both the medial and lateral plantar nerves divide into interdigital nerves located beneath the transverse metatarsal ligament, terminating at the distal phalanges (7), and carry sensation from the plantar surfaces and web spaces between the toes. The medial plantar proper digital nerve supplies the skin on the medial aspect of the first digit.

THE SURAL NERVE

The sural nerve originates from the tibial and common peroneal nerves, carrying cutaneous sensation from the lateral aspect of the ankle, heel, and fourth and fifth digits. It also mediates foot proprioception, measures stretch in the Achilles tendon, and provides sensation from deeper tissues. Traditionally, the sural nerve is considered a purely sensory nerve, although electrophysiologic studies have demonstrated motor fibers. Kosinski, Tani, and Sekiya et al. have reported on variations of sural nerve anatomy (8–17).

DIAGNOSIS OF NERVE INJURY IN THE ANKLE AND FOOT

Evaluation of patients with athletic injury to the ankle and foot begins with a thorough history and physical examination. If nerve injury is suspected, electrodiagnostic and imaging studies may be indicated.

The history should include questions about the nature of the injury and any sensory change or muscle weakness. Complaints of burning pain, paresthesias, and numbness suggest injury to small diameter sensory fibers. Allodynia may be present. Dysfunction of large diameter sensory fibers can cause proprioceptive loss and lead to ataxia, tremor, or disequilibrium. High-functioning athletes may complain of subtle deficits in balance. Involvement of motor fibers is suggested by weakness. Complaints of difficulty walking or a change in appearance of gait not explained by pain or limited range of motion should raise suspicion for motor injury.

The neurologic examination typically follows the musculoskeletal examination and should include evaluation of sensation, motor function, reflexes, and gait. Abnormalities are more easily identified by comparison to the unaffected limb.

The sensory examination should include assessment of pain, temperature, light touch, vibratory sensation, and proprioception. Appropriate mapping of the affected areas localizes to the corresponding nerve. Nerves can also be palpated and percussed to ascertain the site of compression or entrapment.

Eliciting muscle weakness is a special challenge when examining athletes with acute injuries, as many suffer from severe pain. Analgesics may facilitate the examination. Care must be taken to accurately correlate the muscle with its corresponding joint movement. Certain joints must be properly positioned. For example, evaluating ankle inversion strength in patients with dorsiflexion weakness should begin with passive dorsiflexion by the examiner. Failure to do so gives the mistaken impression of tibialis posterior weakness (18).

In addition to strength, muscle bulk and tone are assessed. Chronic motor nerve injury leads to atrophy. Weak joints may assume an abnormal position. For example, the foot may assume an equinovarus position after peroneal nerve injury. The muscles should be closely inspected for signs of denervation, such as fasciculations or myokymia.

The gait is often revealing. Patients with ankle dorsiflexion weakness excessively flex the hip and knee when ambulating in order to raise the leg. This compensation allows passage of the paretic foot through the swing phase. Lack of a controlled descent of the foot causes a characteristic slapping noise. The resulting appearance of the patient attempting to step over an object has led to the term, "steppage gait."

ELECTRODIAGNOSTIC TESTING

Nerve conduction studies (NCS) and needle electromyography (EMG) add certainty to the location of nerve injury, and elucidate the nature and severity of impairment (19,20).

NCS measure the response of a nerve to a locally delivered electrical current, whereas needle EMG details the electrical properties of relaxing and contracting muscle by insertion of a needle electrode. The collective data from both NCS and EMG may help determine the temporal course of injury, differentiate neuropathy from myopathy, assess the severity of the axonal damage, and reveal signs of axonal regeneration. Also, the quantitative results of electrodiagnostic studies provide a measurement, which can be followed over time.

IMAGING STUDIES

Standard radiographs and computed tomography have little role in the characterization of neuropathies given an inability to directly visualize nerves. The modalities of interest to peripheral nerve injury are mainly ultrasound (US) and magnetic resonance imaging (MRI).

US

In recent years, US has gained wide acceptance as a useful tool in the evaluation of the musculoskeletal system (21–23). State of the art high-resolution transducers can depict individual nerve fascicles (24). The advantages of this technique include dynamic, real-time examination, and quick assessment of entire nerve segments; US is also non-invasive, well tolerated, and affordable, and can be performed in the office. Image quality is operator dependant (25).

Inflamed nerves can be identified by increased caliber or internal signal changes. Focal thinning with proximal fusiform swelling occurs with nerve compression (26). Analogous to electrodiagnostic testing, US can yield important information about muscle by differentiating phases of muscle contraction.

MRI

In 1996, Filler et al. reported on the use of MRI in peripheral neuropathy. Since then, there has been growing interest in MR neurography (27–33). As with US, MR provides resolution up to the level of the nerve fascicle.

The signal characteristics of peripheral nerves using traditional MR pulse sequences are well described. Relative to adjacent muscle tissue, T1 weighted images of normal nerve fascicles are hypointense, with hyperintense perineurial and epineurial fat surrounding them. Roughly the reverse is seen in T2 weighted images (27–29,32,34–37). Deviation from the normal signal characteristics of a nerve indicates pathology. T2 hyperintensity within the nerve is thought to reflect disruption of the blood–nerve barrier, leading to endoneurial or perineurial edema. However, the underlying pathogenesis remains uncertain (27,28,33,38). As with US, changes in nerve diameter should raise suspicion for pathology.

The fascicles in nerves distal to the common peroneal nerve are poorly visualized with MRI (33). Neuropathy in distal nerves is suggested by changes consistent with denervation myopathy (39–45). Denervated muscles are edematous in the subacute phase and atrophic in the chronic phase. T1 weighted images are useful for visualizing fatty deposits in chronically denervated muscle (44). Denervation myopathy is apparent on MRI up to 4 days after a traumatic nerve injury. The abnormal signal changes are reversible if there is reinnervation (45).

INDIVIDUAL NERVE INJURIES

THE COMMON PERONEAL NERVE

Table 28.1 lists common activities associated with injury of the peroneal nerve. Although frequently asymptomatic, peroneal neuropathy is a common complication of ankle injuries. Using electrodiagnostic studies, Nitz and co-workers found that 17% of patients with grade II ankle sprains and 86% with grade III sprains had evidence of subclinical motor impairment in the peroneal nerve (1). Symptomatic ankle dorsiflexion and eversion weakness result from plantarflexion and inversion injuries as seen in severe sprains or fractures of the distal tibia and fibula (47,48). The common peroneal nerve can be torn by sudden, extreme ankle inversion, leading to internal hemorrhage and ischemia (47–49).

After such injury, paralysis is usually immediate, but can be delayed for several days. Baccari et al. (49) reported six cases of delayed paralysis due to peroneal nerve injury following ankle sprain by up to 3 days. Patients with sensory injury to the common peroneal nerve may complain of numbness or burning pain from the knee to the top of the foot.

THE DEEP PERONEAL NERVE

Compression of the deep peroneal nerve may result from anterior compartment syndrome which is associated with a painful, tight, and swollen lower leg. Intramuscular pressure measurements facilitate diagnosis and electrodiagnostic studies may document the extent of involvement. Chronic compartment syndrome can occur in runners or other athletes experiencing repetitive lower extremity impact. Pain that increases on passive stretching and active contraction may be present. Generally, symptoms disappear once the offending activity is stopped.

The deep peroneal nerve can also be compressed against the talonavicular joint in crush injuries, post-surgical inflammation, and by tightly tied shoes (50,51). Compression occurs over the head of the talus when the ankle is plantarflexed and inverted (52). Chronic compression beneath the extensor retinaculum has been referred to as the "anterior tarsal tunnel syndrome." Kopell and Thompson first described this syndrome in 1963 (2,3,53). Patients with lateral branch compression typically complain of pain radiating to the lateral tarsometatarsal joints, whereas medial nerve compression causes symptoms within the first web space. The precise site of compression can be confirmed with a focal nerve block.

THE SUPERFICIAL PERONEAL NERVE

The superficial peroneal nerve can sustain traction injury during inversion ankle sprain (53) or become entrapped as it exits the deep fascia. Entrapment can be seen in dancers with a technique flaw referred to as "sickling" in which the foot is either inverted or everted during dancing. Hypertrophied peroneal muscles may also lead to entrapment by causing increased compartment pressure (54).

In dancers with lateral ligament deficiency or ankle instability, the superficial peroneal nerve may be tethered and stretched. Pain at the distal third of the lateral leg is precipitated by dancing and relieved by rest. The examiner may reproduce sensory symptoms over the dorsum and lateral aspect of the foot by dorsiflexing and everting the ankle. Nerve percussion can also reproduce symptoms.

THE TIBIAL NERVE

Table 28.2 lists common activities associated with injury of the tibial nerve. Entrapment of the tibial nerve within the tarsal tunnel has been frequently described in athletes. Any swelling of structures in or adjacent to the tunnel can lead to the so called "tarsal tunnel syndrome." Inflammatory tenosynovitis, edema related to trauma, and ganglia of adjacent joints or tendon sheaths are potential causes. The classic symptoms are pain in the heel and sole of the foot with accompanying sensory changes.

TABLE 28.1 Activities Associated with Injury to the Peroneal Nerve (46)

Running	Entrapment at the fibular neck; anterior tibial compartment syndrome; compression at the capitulum peronei by a mucous cyst
Dancing	Footwear compression
Martial arts	Impact nerve contusion
Football	Knee dislocation and/or ligamentous injury with subsequent nerve trauma (incidence of 24%)
Soccer	Entrapment at the fibular neck
Auto racing	Compression within small cockpit
Surfing	Chronic nerve trauma
Roller skating	Entrapment secondary to footwear

TABLE 28.2 Activities Associated with Injury to the Tibial Nerve (46)

Running	Chronic trauma within the tarsal tunnel caused by repetitive ankle dorsiflexion; Morton's neuroma; entrapment at the calcaneal nerve; injury of lateral and medial branches
Dancing	Morton's neuroma
Martial arts	Morton's neuroma
Hiking	Chronic trauma within the tarsal tunnel caused by repetitive ankle dorsiflexion
Hockey	Footwear compression at the tarsal tunnel

Morton's neuroma is a well-known cause of impingement of the interdigital nerves. Although the name implies a nerve tumor, histologic analysis reveals fibrosis and demyelination rather than hypertrophy or neoplasia (55). It is suspected that repetitive dorsiflexion of the toes against the transverse metatarsal ligament causes nerve trauma and subsequent fibrosis (56). Inflammation of the intermetatarsal bursa is another potential cause (57,58). Morton's neuroma can be found between any of the metatarsals, but most commonly occurs in the third followed by the second interdigital space (56,59–61). Although the exact incidence is unknown, it is considered to be a common cause of forefoot pain (59). Symptoms are exacerbated by running and tight fitted footwear (62). Female predominance may be due to footwear differences (63–65).

MRI is 90% sensitive and 100% specific for detecting Morton's neuroma (66) which is most easily detected in coronal view with an extremity coil. Patients should be positioned prone in the magnet, with the foot in plantarflexion (34,67). The diameter of the mass is usually 5 mm or larger with T1 and T2 hypointensity and occasional enhancement (66). A fluid collection may be seen within the intermetatarsal bursa. Greater than 3 mm of fluid is considered abnormal (68).

TREATMENT

Once the diagnosis is established, intervention should focus on minimizing further injury, treating symptoms, and accelerating recovery. Acute ankle and foot trauma may require surgery. Anti-inflammatory drugs can be used acutely as adjuvant or primary therapy to decrease edema and inflammation. The approach to chronic injuries is different, and likewise depends on the mechanism of injury. Interventions for compressive neuropathy may be as simple as apparel adjustment, as in deep peroneal nerve compression from tight footwear. In other cases, decompression may require surgery. Chronic repetitive trauma as occurs in dedicated athletes and performers may be difficult to prevent. Subtle improvements in technique may be necessary and are frequently painstaking. In less fortunate patients, the offending activity must be temporarily or permanently stopped.

Pain can be a disabling result of peripheral nerve injury. It is important to identify and treat neuropathic pain to prevent morbidity, given the high prevalence of comorbid depression in chronic pain patients (69,70). Among antidepressants, amitriptyline is most commonly used. Its efficacy has been demonstrated in diabetic neuropathy and post herpetic neuralgia (71,72). Another tricyclic antidepressant nortriptyline is better tolerated in the elderly. Duloxetine is a newer antidepressant that has proven effective in several randomized, double-blinded studies (73).

Gabapentin, carbamazepine, and pregabalin are anticonvulsants used to treat neuropathic pain. Gabapentin is used most frequently, and has proven efficacy (74,75). Carbamazepine is an older drug. It was the initial anticonvulsant investigated in the treatment of trigeminal neuralgia and is still considered first line therapy. N-methyl D-aspartate (NMDA) receptor antagonists, opioid analgesics, and topical agents are also useful treatment options. Combination therapy may be necessary to achieve adequate pain control. Recent efforts to better define drug interactions may lead to a more informed choice of drug combinations (76). The number of drugs available for neuropathic pain continues to grow.

Recovery from peripheral nerve injury is variable. Currently, physical medicine and rehabilitation offer the best options for injured athletes. Those who participate in rigorous rehabilitation programs have improved strength, agility, and balance. To add to this, growing interest in therapies to improve nerve regeneration has led to promising discoveries. Animal studies have identified several potentially effective pharmacologic compounds. FK506 is an immunosuppressive agent that increases the regeneration of sensory fibers in rats with sciatic nerve injury (77). Surgical treatment continues to be investigated. Neurotization is a technique by which an autologous nerve of little functional significance is transplanted to the site of disabling nerve injury. This technique has been used extensively in patients with brachial plexus injuries. In patients with tibialis anterior denervation, schwann cell transplant has been shown to enhance reinnervation after neurotization (46). There will continue to be development of novel therapies to improve peripheral nerve regeneration. However, these approaches are currently experimental and should only be considered on a case-to-case basis.

ACKNOWLEDGMENT

Michael Rubin, M.D.
Professor of Neurology
New York Presbyterian Hospital Cornell University Weill Medical College

REFERENCES

1. Nitz A, Dobner J, Kersey D. Nerve injury and grade II and III ankle sprains. *Am J Sports Med* 1985;13:177–182.
2. Akyuz G, Us O, Turan B, et al. Anterior tarsal tunnel syndrome. *Electromyogr Clin Neurophysiol* 2000;40:123–128.
3. Andresen BL, Wertsch JJ, Stewart WA. Anterior tarsal tunnel syndrome. *Arch Phys Med Rehabil* 1992;73:1112–1117.
4. Saraffian SK. *Anatomy of the Foot and Ankle: Descriptive, Topographic, Functional.* Philadelphia, PA: Lippincott; 1983.
5. Kosinski C. The course. Mutual relations and distribution of the leg and foot. *J Anal* 1926;60:274.
6. Horwitz MT. Normal anatomy and variations of the peripheral nerves of the leg and foot. *Arch Surg* 1938;36:626–636.
7. Sarrafian SK. *Anatomy of the Foot and Ankle: Descriptive Topographic, Functional.* 2nd ed. Philadelphia, PA: JB Lippincott; 1993.
8. Lippert H. Zur innervation der menschlichen fussgelenke. *Zeit Anat Entwick* 1962;123: 295–308.
9. Gardner E, Gray DJ. The innervation of the joints of the foot. *Anat Rec* 1968;161:141–148.
10. Stilwell DL. The innervation of tendons and aponeuroses. *Am J Anat* 1957;100:289–318.
11. Chang SC, Wei JY, Mao CP. Deep innervation of sural nerve. *Brain Res* 1983;279:262–265.
12. Kosinski C. The course, mutual relations and distribution of the cutaneous nerves of the metazonal region of leg and foot. *J Anat* 1926;60:274–297.
13. Tani J. Distribution of the sural nerve, as examined by fibre analysis. *J Juzen Med Soc* 1974;83:435–448.
14. Sekiya S, Kumaki K. Fiber analysis of sural–tibial communications in humans. *Acta Anat Nippon* 2000;75:69.
15. Liguori R, Trojaborg W. Are there motor fibers in the sural nerve? *Muscle Nerve* 1990;13: 12–15.
16. Ragno M, Santoro L. Motor fibers in human sural nerve. *Elec Clin Neurophysiol* 1995;35: 61–63.
17. Amoiridis G, Schöls L, Ameridis N, et al. Motor fibers in the sural nerve of humans. *Neurology* 1997;49:1725–1728.
18. Preston DC, Shapiro BE. Peroneal nerve palsy. In: Preston DC, Shapiro BE, eds. *Electromyography and Neuromuscular disorders: Clinical-Electrophysiologic Correlations.* 2nd ed. Philadelphia, PA: Elsevier; 2005:343–354.
19. Ma DM, Liveson JA. *Laboratory Reference for Clinical Neurophysiology.* Philadelphia, PA: FA Davis; 1992.

20. Johnson EW, Ortiz PR. Electrodiagnosis of tarsal tunnel syndrome. *Arch Phys Med Rehabil* 1966;47:776–780.
21. Tardieu M, Brasseur JL, eds. *Echographie de l'appareil locomoteur.* Paris: Masson; 2006.
22. Van Holsbeeck M, Introcaso JH, eds. *Musculoskeletal Ultrasound.* St. Louis, MO: Mosby; 2001.
23. Bianchi S, Martinoli C, eds. *Ultrasound of the Musculoskeletal System.* Berlin: Springer-Verlag; 2007.
24. Silvestri E, Martinoli C, Derchi LE, et al. Echotexture of peripheral nerves: correlation between US and histologic findings and criteria to differentiate tendons. *Radiology* 1995;197(1):291–296.
25. Martinoli C, Bianchi S, Gandolfo N, et al. US of nerve entrapments in osteofibrous tunnels of the upper and lower limbs. *Radiographics* 2000;20:199–213.
26. Stefano Bianchi. Ultrasound of the peripheral nerves. *Joint Bone Spine* 2008;75:643–649.
27. Spratt JD, Stanley AJ, Grainger AJ, et al. The role of diagnostic radiology in compressive and entrapment neuropathies. *Eur Radiol* 2002;12:2352–2364.
28. Grant GA, Britz GW, Goodkin R, et al. The utility of magnetic resonance imaging in evaluating peripheral nerve disorders. *Muscle Nerve* 2002;25:314–331.
29. Howe FA, Filler AG, Bell BA, et al. Magnetic resonance neurography. *Magn Reson Med* 1992;28:328–338.
30. Kuntz CT, Blake L, Britz G, et al. Magnetic resonance neurography of peripheral nerve lesions in the lower extremity. *Neurosurgery* 1996;39:750–756.
31. Cudlip SA, Howe FA, Griffiths JR, et al. Magnetic resonance neurography of peripheral nerve following experimental crush injury, and correlation with functional deficit. *J Neurosurg* 2002;96:755–759.
32. Filler AG, Kliot M, Howe FA, et al. Application of magnetic resonance neurography in the evaluation of patients with peripheral nerve pathology. *J Neurosurg* 1996;85:299–309.
33. Maravilla KR, Bowen BC. Imaging of the peripheral nervous system: evaluation of peripheral neuropathy and plexopathy. *Am J Neuroradiol* 1998;19:1011–1023.
34. Hochman MG, Zilberfarb JL. Nerves in a pinch: imaging of nerve compression syndromes. *Radiol Clin North Am* 2004;42:221–245.
35. Hormann M, Traxler H, Ba-Ssalamah A, et al. Correlative high-resolution MR-anatomic study of sciatic, ulnar, and proper palmar digital nerve. *Magn Reson Imaging* 2003;21: 879–885.
36. Filler AG, Howe FA, Hayes CE, et al. Magnetic resonance neurography. *Lancet* 1993;341: 659–661.
37. Jarvik JG, Kliot M, Maravilla KR. MR nerve imaging of the wrist and hand. *Hand Clin* 2000;16:13–24.
38. Gebarski SS, Telian SA, Niparko JK. Enhancement along the normal facial nerve in the facial canal: MR imaging and anatomic correlation. *Radiology* 1992;183:391–394.
39. Bendszus M, Koltzenburg M, Wessig C, et al. Sequential MR imaging of denervated muscle: experimental study. *Am J Neuroradiol* 2002;23:1427–1431.
40. Bendszus M, Wessig C, Reiners K, et al. MR imaging in the differential diagnosis of neurogenic foot drop. *Am J Neuroradiol* 2003;24:1283–1289.
41. Bredella MA, Tirman PF, Fritz RC, et al. Denervation syndromes of the shoulder girdle: MR imaging with electrophysiologic correlation. *Skeletal Radiol* 1999;28:567–572.
42. Inokuchi W, Ogawa K, Horiuchi Y. Magnetic resonance imaging of suprascapular nerve palsy. *J Shoulder Elbow Surg* 1998;7:223–227.
43. Linker CS, Helms CA, Fritz RC. Quadrilateral space syndrome: findings at MR imaging. *Radiology* 1993;188:675–676.
44. Sallomi D, Janzen DL, Munk PL, et al. Muscle denervation patterns in upper limb nerve injuries: MR imaging findings and anatomic basis. *Am J Roentgenol* 1998;171:779–784.
45. West GA, Haynor DR, Goodkin R, et al. Magnetic resonance imaging signal changes in denervated muscles after peripheral nerve injury. *Neurosurgery* 1994;35:1077–1085.
46. Polin R. Neurologic injuries associated with sporting activities. *MedLink Neurology.* San Diego: MedLink Corporation. Available at www.medlink.com. Accessed 8/26/2009.
47. Nobel W. Peroneal palsy due to hematoma in the common peroneal nerve sheath after distal torsional fractures and inversion ankle sprains. *J Bone Joint Surg Am* 1966;48:1484–1495.
48. Meals RA. Peroneal nerve palsy complicating ankle sprain: a report of two cases and review of the literature. *J Bone Joint Surg Am* 1977;59:966–968.
49. Baccari S, Turki M, Zinelabidine M, et al. Une etiologie rare de paralysie du nerf sciatique poplite' externe: l'entorse de la cheville. *J Traumatol Sport* 2000;17:208–212.
50. Kopell HP, Thompson WA. Peripheral entrapment neuropathies of the lower extremity. *N Engl J Med* 1960;262:56–60.
51. Mackey D, Colbert DS, Chater EH. Musculo-cutaneous nerve entrapment. *Ir J Med Sci* 1977;146:100–102.
52. Kennedy JG, Brunner JB, Bohne WH, et al. Clinical importance of the lateral branch of the deep peroneal nerve. *Clin Orthop Relat Res* 2007;459:222–228.
53. Kopell HP, Thompson WA. *Peripheral Entrapment Neuropathies.* Baltimore: Williams & Wilkins; 1963.
54. Styf J. Entrapment of the superficial peroneal nerve. Diagnosis and results of decompression. *J Bone Joint Surg Am* 1989;71B:131–135.
55. Graham CE, Graham DM. Morton's neuroma: a microscopic evaluation. *Foot Ankle* 1984; 5:150–153.
56. Lorei MP, Hershman EB. Peripheral nerve injuries in athletes. Treatment and prevention. *Sports Med* 1993;16:130–147.
57. Bossley CJ, Cairney PC. The intermetatarsophalangeal bursa and its significance in Morton's metatarsalgia. *J Bone Joint Surg Br* 1980;62:184–187.
58. Gauthier G. Thomas Morton's disease: a nerve entrapment syndrome. A new surgical technique. *Clin Orthop Relat Res* 1979;142:90–92.
59. Schon LC. Nerve entrapment, neuropathy, and nerve dysfunction in athletes. *Orthop Clin North Am* 1994;25:47–59.
60. Bencardino J, Rosenberg ZS, Beltran J, et al. Morton's neuroma: is it always symptomatic? *Am J Roentgenol* 2000;175:649–653.
61. Perini L, Del BM, Cipriano R, et al. Dynamic sonography of the forefoot in Morton's syndrome: correlation with magnetic resonance and surgery. *Radiol Med* 2006;111:897–905.
62. Hockenbury RT. Forefoot problems in athletes. *Med Sci Sports Exerc* 1999;31:448–458.
63. Bennett GL, Graham CE, Mauldin DM. Morton's interdigital neuroma: a comprehensive treatment protocol. *Foot Ankle Int* 1995;16:760–763.
64. Kilmartin TE, Wallace WA. Effect of pronation and supination orthosis on Morton's neuroma and lower extremity function. *Foot Ankle Int* 1994;15:256–262.
65. Greenfield J, Rea J Jr, Ilfeld FW. Morton's interdigital neuroma. Indications for treatment by local injections versus surgery. *Clin Orthop Relat Res* 1984;185:142–144.
66. Zanetti M, Ledermann T, Zollinger H, et al. Efficacy of MR imaging in patients suspected of having Morton's neuroma. *Am J Roentgenol* 1997;168:529–532.
67. Weishaupt D, Treiber K, Kundert HP, et al. Morton neuroma: MR imaging in prone, supine, and upright weight-bearing body positions. *Radiology* 2003;226:849–856.
68. Arnow B, Hunkeler E, Blasey C, et al. Comorbid depression, chronic pain, and disability in primary care. *Psychosom Med* 2006;68:262–268.
69. Mossey J, Gallagher R. The longitudinal occurrence and impact of comorbid chronic pain and chronic depression over two years in continuing care retirement community residents. *Pain Med* 2004;5:334–348.
70. Max MB, Culnane M, Schafer SC, et al. Amitriptyline relieves diabetic neuropathy pain in patients with normal or depressed mood. *Neurology* 1987;37:589–596.
71. Watson CP, Chipman M, Reed K, et al. Amitriptyline versus maprotiline in postherpetic neuralgia: a randomized, double-blind, crossover trial. *Pain* 1992;48:29–36.
72. Goldstein DJ, Lu Y, Detke MJ, et al. Duloxetine vs. placebo in patients with painful diabetic neuropathy. *Pain* 2005;116:109–118.
73. Dallocchio C, Buffa C, Mazzarello P, et al. Gabapentin vs. amitriptyline in painful diabetic neuropathy: an open-label pilot study. *J Pain Symptom Manage* 2000;20:280–285.
74. Yaksi A, Ozgonenel L, Ozgonenel B. The efficiency of gabapentin therapy in patients with lumbar spinal stenosis. *Spine* 2007;32:939–942.
75. Gilron I, Bailey JM, Tu D, et al. Morphine, gabapentin, or their combination for neuropathic pain. *N Engl J Med* 2005;352:1324–1334.
76. Steiner J, Connolly M, Valentine H, et al. Neurotrophic actions of nonimmunosuppressive analogues of immunosuppressive drugs FK506, rapamycin and cyclosporine A. *Nat Med* 1997;3(4):421–428.
77. Fukuda A, Hitoshi H, Koji A, et al. Enhanced reinnervation after neurotization with schwann cell transplantation. *Muscle Nerve* 2005;31:229–234.

CHAPTER

29

Robin Reiter

Rehabilitation of the Foot and Ankle

Optimal management of an injury to the lower leg is best achieved by a multidisciplinary team of medical professionals. When surgery or other invasive treatment methods are not advised, physical therapy is often recommended as a conservative option in the treatment of foot and ankle disorders. The goal of physical therapy is to decrease the athlete's pain and inflammation, while restoring range of motion, flexibility, and strength. Through a combination of passive modalities and therapeutic exercise, physical therapy helps the athlete return to full sport activity without limitations.

ASSESSMENT

Prior to developing a program for a patient, the physical therapist performs a thorough assessment of the individual's injury. The focus of initial evaluation is threefold: The injury is identified, the severity is graded, and a multidisciplinary plan is created to manage the patient and return the athlete to normal activity as soon as possible (1).

The initial evaluation begins with a complete patient history. This is especially useful when the practitioner is attempting to determine the mechanism of pain or injury, to identify any previous ankle dysfunction, and to establish the performance level of the individual (2). In order to identify the injury, the physical therapist obtains important information, including the patient's age, occupation, sports and hobbies. The patient reports the chief complaints of the injury, the date of onset, and the duration of pain. It is important to note previous treatment for the injury and results, if applicable.

The therapist carefully observes the patient in the weight-bearing (closed-chain) and non–weight-bearing (open-chain) positions. During open-chain motion, the talus is fixed, whereas during closed-chain motion, the talus moves. The weight-bearing stance of the foot shows how the body compensates for structural abnormalities. The non–weight-bearing posture shows functional and structural abilities without compensation (3).

Views from the anterior, posterior, medial, and lateral directions in both the standing and sitting positions should be included. This will provide information on the patient's bony and muscular symmetry as well as any obvious swelling or deformities in the lower leg.

A systematic palpation of the bony and soft tissue structures from the knee to the toes is performed to determine the presence of tenderness and/or structural deformity. Examination of the foot and proximal fibula also helps to rule out other injuries that occur simultaneously and may be disguised as ankle pain (4). The examiner palpates for any inflammation and notes the presence of pitting edema, which may suggest systemic disease or venous insufficiency. The skin's texture and temperature are also important components of the palpation. An ischemic foot with poor circulation will show loss of hair and inelasticity, and the foot will feel cold to the touch. It is important to palpate the pulse of the dorsalis pedis and tibialis posterior arteries, as absence of either of these pulses may suggest lower limb arterial disease (3). Dermatomes (L3–S2) and myotomes (L3–S3) are assessed, and the patient's patellar (L3–L4), Achilles (S1–S2), posterior tibialis (L5) and Babinski reflexes are tested.

Range of motion is evaluated with both active and passive movement assessment. Active movements are performed in weight bearing and non–weight-bearing, and passive movement is assessed by applying overpressure with specific movements. Table 29.1 depicts movements tested when determining range of motion limitations. Lower-leg strength is tested with resisted isometric movements in the sitting or supine position. The examiner evaluates knee flexion, ankle plantarflexion and dorsiflexion, ankle inversion and eversion, and toe flexion and extension. The peripheral joints of the knee and hip are assessed as well to rule out additional injury.

The examiner performs a variety of special tests on the lower leg, ankle, and foot. The neutral position of the talus is assessed in the weight-bearing (standing) position as well as the non–weight-bearing (supine and prone) positions. Alignment is measured between the leg and heel to determine heel inversion or eversion, and the forefoot and heel to show forefoot valgus or varus. The examiner may also test for tibial torsion, ligamentous instability, integrity of muscle attachments, and any leg-length discrepancy.

The last step of the evaluation is functional assessment. The patient is asked to perform a series of movements to determine how the joints and muscles of the lower leg interact. Squatting, standing on the toes, standing on one foot, single-leg heel raises, going up and down stairs, running, and jumping are examples of movements that help the therapist assess the patient's overall function.

TREATMENT

Once the assessment is completed, a rehabilitation plan is devised. In order to effectively treat foot and ankle problems,

TABLE 29.1 Assessment of Lower-leg Range of Motion

Active Weight-bearing Movements	Active Non–weight-bearing Movements	Passive Movements (with overpressure)
Ankle plantarflexion	Ankle plantarflexion	Ankle plantarflexion
Ankle dorsiflexion	Ankle dorsiflexion	Ankle dorsiflexion
Ankle inversion	Ankle inversion	Ankle inversion
Ankle eversion	Ankle eversion	Ankle eversion
Toe extension	Toe extension and flexion	Toe extension and flexion
Toe flexion	Toe abduction and adduction	Toe abduction and adduction

it is crucial to understand the biomechanics of both structures as they relate to sport activities. Studies show that the incidence of foot problems in the general population is as high as 80% (3). In athletes specifically, the prevalence of foot injuries is also high—in runners alone, 40% to 50% of all injuries occur below the knee (5).

During high-impact sports that involve running and jumping, there is great biomechanical stress placed on the foot. In running, the foot must withstand forces that are 3 to 4 times the normal body weight (6). The lack of muscle mass surrounding the bones, tendons, and ligaments in the foot decreases its ability to absorb shock and makes it vulnerable to overuse injuries.

Injuries in the foot that are commonly treated by physical therapists include ligamentous disorders, tendinopathies, injuries to the bone, and neural problems. Conservative treatment of these injuries involves a combination of modalities, soft tissue massage and stretching, and therapeutic exercise.

MODALITIES

Various modalities are effective in treating multiple aspects of foot and ankle disorders. According to Starkey, the definition of a modality is "the application of some form of stress to the body for the purpose of eliciting an adaptive response" (7). This includes thermal, mechanical, and electrical energy, and modalities play an important role in the treatment of injuries through the various stages of healing.

CRYOTHERAPY

Cryotherapy, or the application of cold to an injury, is an important component in the acute stages in reduction of inflammation. The local effects of applying cold include a decrease in metabolic rate, vasoconstriction, and decreased pain and swelling. The most beneficial effect of cold application during an acute injury is to decrease the need for oxygen in the area being treated (8). Applying cold decreases the metabolic rate of the cells, which in turn decreases the amount of oxygen needed by cells to survive. This limits the degree of secondary hypoxia by lessening the quantity of cells killed by a lack of oxygen. Since fewer cells are killed, smaller amounts of inflammatory substance are released into the injured area (7).

Muscle spasm is decreased by cold as well. Cryotherapy lowers the threshold of afferent nerve endings and lessens the sensitivity of muscle spindles. Combined, these decrease muscle spasm by inhibiting the stretch reflex mechanism (7,9,10). Pain transmission is inhibited by the application of cold. By stimulating the large-diameter neurons, cold acts as a counterirritant to inhibit transmission of pain. Cryotherapy reduces the speed of impulses by nerve fibers, thus inhibiting pain sensation.

Cold application is useful in the acute stages of inflammation and following physical activity. It may be applied in the form of an ice massage, an ice pack, or an ice bath. To perform an ice massage, the patient freezes a paper cup of water, and then peels down the cup to expose the ice. The cold is directly applied to the site of the injury using moderate pressure in a circular motion. The duration of this treatment is 5 to 10 minutes. An ice pack should be directly applied to the inflamed area for 10 to 15 minutes. An ice bath, which involves filling a shallow pan with water and ice and soaking the foot, should also be performed for 10 to 15 minutes.

HEAT THERAPY

Like cold application, the use of heat decreases pain and muscle spasm by altering the threshold of nerve endings. However, the application of heat accelerates inflammation by increasing blood flow to the injured area, and therefore is not recommended in the acute stages of injury.

Heat therapy is recommended in the subacute or chronic stages of inflammation, to encourage tissue healing, to reduce edema and ecchymosis, and to assist in range of motion prior to activity (7). It is generally applied via a heat pack, though more penetrating heat may be achieved with ultrasound (see below).

ULTRASOUND

Ultrasound is another frequently utilized modality in the treatment of injuries. Produced by means of a mechanical vibration of a crystal in the head of the ultrasound machine, this technique uses sound waves to penetrate the skin into the tissue below. This results in increased blood flow to the injured area, which promotes the healing process, breaks down scar tissue, and decreases swelling.

Ultrasound has both thermal and non-thermal effects on the area of injury (Table 29.2). These are dependent on the mode of application (pulsed or continuous), the frequency of the sound, the size of the treatment area and the type of tissue being treated.

Although it is widely used in the treatment of foot and ankle injuries, the efficacy of ultrasound remains questionable. Van der Windt et al. conducted a review of five trials involving 572

TABLE 29.2 Non-thermal and Thermal Effects of Ultrasound on Injured Tissue

Non-thermal Effects of Ultrasound	Thermal Effects of Ultrasound
Increased permeability of cell membrane and blood vessels	Pain reduction
Increased blood flow	Increased blood flow
Regeneration of tissue	Decreased muscle spasm
Decreased edema	Increased velocity of nerve conduction
Protein synthesis	Increased collage extensibility

patients, each trial having at least one study group treated with ultrasound for acute lateral ankle sprain. In all studies, the outcome measures included general improvement, functional disability, swelling, pain, or range of motion measures. They found that the use of ultrasound in the treatment of lateral ankle sprains was not supported by the trials (11). Brand et al. studied the effects of daily pulsed low intensity ultrasound on lower extremity stress fractures, and found that time off from normal activities was significantly minimized with the use of this modality (12).

IONTOPHORESIS

Iontophoresis is a therapeutic modality that uses a local electrical current to transdermally deliver medicine to an injured area. An electrode is placed over the inflamed tissue and the voltage is applied to drive the ionized medication into the injured tissue. Based on the ionic reaction between the machine's positive and negative poles, medication is delivered along the lines of force created by the current. Iontophoresis is particularly useful in treating injuries that present with localized pain and swelling, and has been shown to deliver medication to depths of 6 to 20 mm below the surface of the skin (7).

Iontophoresis has been proven effective in a variety of foot and ankle injuries. Japour et al. studied 35 patients with chronic heel pain who were treated with acetic acid iontophoresis over a 4-year period. At the conclusion of treatment, 94% of patients reported complete or substantial relief of heel pain after an average of 5.7 sessions over a period of 2.8 weeks (13). In a separate study by Neeter et al., the effects of iontophoresis using dexamethasone were assessed on 25 patients with acute Achilles tendonitis. At the end of the study, significant improvements were seen in the treatment group in areas of range of motion, pain, stiffness, and swelling (14).

NEUROMUSCULAR ELECTRICAL STIMULATION

Neuromuscular electrical stimulation (NMES) is a modality used for muscle strengthening and re-education and decreasing swelling post-injury or surgery. Electrodes attached to leads are placed on motor points of specific muscles, and an electrical stimulus is applied causing muscles to contract. Parameters such as current rate, amplitude, and waveform are adjusted to allow for a strong contraction while minimizing fatigue.

NMES has been proven an effective tool in the improvement of muscle strength. Delitto et al. found that when applied to a muscle, neuromuscular stimulation causes contraction that produces a torque equal to 90% of maximal voluntary training with electrical stimulation. They found an overall significant improvement in the muscle strength of subjects who trained with maximal voluntary isometric contractions induced by electrical stimulation versus those who did not use NMES to elicit contractions (15).

NMES also aids in the reduction of swelling and edema by enhancing venous and lymphatic return (7). Muscle contractions cause a pumping action in these vessels, allowing for the movement of fluids. In a study conducted by Man et al., subjects were studied to determine whether the increase in fluid volume of the foot and ankle after 30 minutes of motionless standing could be minimized by NMES. Researchers found significant differences in the mean volume of individuals who were treated with electrical stimulation after the 30 minutes versus those who were not (16).

The main role of therapeutic modalities in the rehabilitation of injury is to provide an optimal environment for healing to take place. When used properly and at the right stages of injury, modalities allow for a body segment to return to its normal function and recover fully.

COMMON FOOT AND ANKLE DISORDERS

Due to the constant stresses placed on the foot and ankle during daily life, injuries to these structures are frequent and varied. Below are some of the more common injuries and appropriate rehabilitation protocols for treatment. In all diagnoses, the use of the RICE method (rest, ice, compression, and elevation) is suggested in the acute stage to relieve pain, limit swelling, and protect the injured tissue. Once the injury becomes sub-acute or chronic, various manual and therapeutic exercise techniques help to speed up the healing process and return the athlete to sport. This section focuses on physical therapy treatment in the subacute and chronic phases of injury.

PLANTAR FASCIITIS

Plantar fasciitis, the most common ligamentous injury in the foot, is caused by repetitive microtears of the long fibrous plantar fascia ligament, resulting in pain and inflammation. Pain is most commonly reported along the medial tubercle of the calcaneus, where the plantar fascia originates. The classic sign of plantar fasciitis is report of increased pain in the plantar foot during the first few steps in the morning. Individuals may also report discomfort at the beginning of their sport activity that decreases as they warm up. Often pain is increased with prolonged standing, and may become worse at the end of the day.

Plantar fasciitis can often be a challenge to treat in the physical therapy clinic. Non-surgical management of plantar fascia pain can be grouped into three categories: Reducing pain and inflammation, reducing tissue stress to a tolerable level, and restoring flexibility and muscle strength in the foot (17). In addition to cryotherapy in the acute stages, the reduction of pain and swelling is achieved via the use of various modalities, including iontophoresis and NMES.

Due to its localized nature, plantar fasciitis is a condition that responds well to iontophoresis. Gudeman et al. conducted a study of 40 patients with the diagnosis to determine if iontophoresis of dexamethasone, when combined with other treatment modalities, provides more immediate pain relief than traditional modalities alone. They found that the combination of modalities and iontophoresis was superior to the use of modalities alone, and it provided immediate reduction of symptoms (18).

The efficacy of ultrasound in the treatment of plantar fasciitis, however, is questionable. Ultrasound has been shown to increase blood flow to the site of injury, which speeds up the healing process in the foot. In addition, it assists in decreasing swelling, which can cause much of the pain. However, Crawford and Snaith found that therapeutic ultrasound at a dosage of 0.5 w/cm^2 3 MHz, pulsed 1:4 for 8 minutes was no more effective in a group of patients with heel pain than a placebo treatment (19).

Manual techniques, including cross friction massage and passive stretching, are used to assist in breaking down scar tissue at the site of the injury and restoring proper range of motion. Cross friction massage applied over the medial calcaneus (i.e., the origin of the plantar fascia) breaks up scar tissue and promotes extensibility, and joint mobilizations of the first ray and subtalar joint improve mobility. Stretching of the foot and ankle is one of the most effective treatments in reducing tissue stress to a tolerable level. Pfeffer et al. studied the effects of Achilles and plantar fascia stretches in individuals with plantar fasciitis. Patients whose only treatment was to stretch the foot and ankle for 10 minutes, two times daily over an 8-week period still demonstrated decreases in pain and had a 71.8% response to treatment (20).

A passive and active stretching program is designed with the goal of decreasing tension put on the plantar fascia. This stress can be caused by tightness of the plantar fascia itself, and/or decreased flexibility of the Achilles tendon, which also causes stiffness of the fascia (20). Appropriate stretching includes stretch of the gastrocnemius–soleus complex on a slant board or wall, the dorsiflexion towel stretch, and the "stair-stretch" for the plantar fascia. Some studies suggest that a program of non–weight-bearing stretching exercise specific to the plantar fascia is superior to the commonly administered weight-bearing Achilles tendon stretches. DiGiovanni et al. studied 101 patients with chronic proximal plantar fasciitis, and divided them into two groups: Those who participated in a plantar fascia tissue-stretching program and those who performed an Achilles tendon stretching program. Follow-up analysis showed that the group managed with the plantar-fascia stretching program revealed greater improvements in pain, previous activity limitation, and overall patient satisfaction (21). However, the study did not have a long-term follow-up and nearly 20% of the participants dropped out before the end. Therefore, before definitive conclusions can be made, there must be improvements in study design (21,22).

To restore muscle strength into the foot, exercise programs should focus on the intrinsic muscles. Examples of non–weight-bearing exercises given to patients with plantar fasciitis are picking up marbles with the toes and towel curls (Fig. 29.1). To perform a towel curl, the patient sits with the heel flat on the floor and the foot flat on the end of a towel placed on the floor. While keeping the heel immobile, the patient curls the toes to move the towel toward the body (23). As the patient progresses and pain is decreased, weight-bearing exercises are introduced, including heel raises, single-leg stance, and heel/toe walks. These act to strengthen the muscles of the foot and lower leg, as well as improve balance and proprioception which are commonly affected with injury.

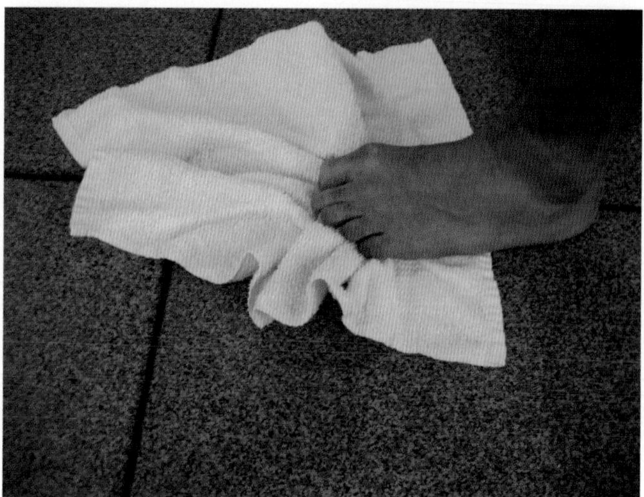

Figure 29.1. Towel scrunches.

LATERAL ANKLE SPRAIN

The two most commonly injured ligaments in the ankle are the anterior talofibular ligament and the calcaneofibular ligament. Together, they act to stabilize the lateral ankle and prevent excessive lateral movement. If these ligaments are loose, the ankle becomes unstable and an eversion sprain, or lateral ankle sprain, may occur. Common causes of this injury in sports include running on uneven ground, twisting the leg while the foot is planted, or unusual force or trauma applied to the joint.

Ankle sprains are classified by their severity into Grade I, II, or III (Table 29.3). They may also be grouped into either complicated or uncomplicated sprains. Complicated ankle sprains are more severe and often require surgical intervention, while uncomplicated sprains can usually be treated by conservative measures.

Lateral ankle sprains often do not present with gross deformity at the site of injury, though they may show marked swelling and discoloration. Special tests, such as the anterior drawer test, squeeze test, and external rotation test, are used to determine the location and severity of the injury (24).

Following initial management to decrease acute swelling and pain, the patient may begin progressive physical therapy with a goal of return to activity. It is extremely important to begin rehabilitation in a timely fashion, given that common post-injury problems include persistent pain, swelling, and joint laxity. In addition, by placing functional stress on the ankle, the body is stimulated to produce strong collagen to replace damaged tissue (25).

Initially, range of motion exercises are prescribed to restore movement in all directions. This includes stretching of the Achilles tendon, and gastrocnemius–soleus complex. In addition, the patient is encouraged to perform active range of

TABLE 29.3 Grades 1, 2, and 3 Ankle Sprains: Signs and Symptoms

Grade of Ankle Sprain	Signs and Symptoms
Grade 1	• Stretching of ligament without laxity • Pain and swelling • Able to ambulate without assistive device
Grade 2	• Severe partial tear of ligament with some laxity • Significant swelling or bruising • Pain with walking
Grade 3	• Complete tear of ligament with marked laxity • Severe pain and swelling • Unable to walk without assistive device • Complaints of instability in ankle joint

motion in plantarflexion, dorsiflexion, inversion, and eversion. Patients may also be instructed to perform clockwise and counterclockwise circles with the foot as well as ankle alphabet exercises.

Manual mobilizations are performed by the physical therapist to break down scar tissue and restore normal motion between the bones at the joint complex. One mobilization in particular, an anteroposterior glide on the talus at the talocrural joint, was shown to be effective in the treatment of ankle inversion sprains. Green et al. found that addition of this mobilization to the RICE protocol in the acute stage of injury necessitated fewer treatments to achieve pain-free dorsiflexion and improve speed of gait stride (26).

Once the patient has minimal swelling and pain, full range of motion, and normal gait, physical therapy focuses on pain-free strengthening. Four-way theraband is introduced in plantarflexion, dorsiflexion, inversion, and eversion, which helps to rebuild endurance in the injured ankle. The patient is instructed in balance and proprioception exercises, including single-leg stance and balancing on the rocker board, first bilaterally then unilaterally. The gastrocnemius–soleus complex is strengthened with bilateral heel raises, progressing to single-leg heel raises.

Advanced strengthening following a lateral ankle sprain is initiated once the patient demonstrates normal gait on all types of surfaces and good balance and proprioception. These exercises may include single-leg press, single-leg squats, and more advanced balance exercises, such as unilateral stance on a rubber disc or other soft surfaces. The patient may also be progressed to straight plane jogging and initiate controlled lateral agility work. The criteria to return the patient to sport is detailed below.

SYNDESMOSIS INJURY

Often referred to as a "high ankle sprain," this injury involves the ligaments above the ankle joint. In a syndesmosis injury, at least one of the ligaments connecting the distal ends of the tibia and fibula is sprained. These are the most severe types of ankle sprains and often take longer to heal. Patients with syndesmosis injuries present with complaints of pain and swelling on the lateral ankle. Reports of ankle instability are common in more chronic injuries, and weight-bearing movement of the ankle can cause radicular pain in the lateral leg.

Mild syndesmosis injuries are treated with the same protocol as lateral ankle sprains, and initial physical therapy treatment focuses on decreasing pain and swelling with modalities and cryotherapy. As the swelling subsides, stretching, strengthening, balance, and proprioception exercises are introduced. More severe syndesmosis sprains often require surgical intervention.

POSTERIOR TIBIAL TENDONITIS

The posterior tibial tendon passes behind the medial malleolus and has its insertion on the navicular bone. Injuries to the posterior tibial tendon can be traumatic, such as with a blow to the medial ankle or a twisting injury that may avulse the tendon, or chronic degeneration of the tendon. Individuals with posterior tibial tendonitis complain of pain in the midfoot and ankle. Physical examination reveals inflammation of the posterior tibial tendon and tightness in the posterior tibialis muscle (5).

Posterior tibial tendon injury is more prevalent in individuals with low medial longitudinal arches. Researchers have investigated correlations between arch structure and injury patterns in runners, and biomechanical analysis finds that runners with planus feet demonstrate increased eversion excursion and eversion velocity at the rear foot. This may require the medial foot structures, including the posterior tibialis, to exert more active and passive control to stabilize the foot. Runners with low arches reported three times as many incidences of posterior tibial tendonitis as high-arched participants (27).

While the most effective treatment of this disorder is orthotics, physical therapy can help to decrease inflammation, control pain, and strengthen the foot muscles. Rehabilitation for this injury includes a combination of stretching and eccentric and concentric progressive resistive exercises. The focus of strengthening is on plantarflexion and inversion aiming to decrease excessive pronation. Appropriate exercises include plantarflexion and inversion with resistance bands, heel raises, and heel/toe walks. When combined with custom-made orthotics to provide biomechanical correction, patients with posterior tibial tendonitis who engage in rehabilitation show a decrease in total pain and disability (28).

PERONEAL TENDONITIS

The peroneus longus and brevis muscles run behind the lateral malleolus and then diverge, with the brevis inserting into the base of the fifth metatarsal and the longus into the base of the first metatarsal and medial cuneiform. Acute tendonitis is caused by repetitive activity or trauma, and can become more chronic (tendonosis) if not treated effectively. Chronic peroneal injury is often seen in patients with excessive pronation, as this foot position places stress on the tendons and puts them at a mechanical disadvantage as they work to stabilize the foot. The overstretched tendon becomes easily fatigued and injury occurs. Peroneal tendonitis presents with pain and inflammation in the lateral ankle along either or both of the peroneal tendons (peroneus longus and peroneus brevis). Often the patient reports increased discomfort with weight bearing, stiffness after exercise, and inability to walk pain-free on uneven surfaces.

In the acute stages, physical therapy focuses on decreasing swelling and pain while maintaining normal range of motion. Peroneal tendonitis is associated with excessive pronation at toe off and weak plantarflexion, and these should be addressed in the strengthening phase of rehabilitation (29). The peroneal muscles are responsible for plantarflexion and eversion of the ankle, so appropriate strengthening exercises include standing heel raises, heel raise on the seated or incline leg press, and theraband eversion exercises. General exercises to improve balance and proprioception are also appropriate and include single-leg stance and balancing on the rocker board.

ANTERIOR TIBIAL TENDONITIS

Situated in the front of the lower leg, the anterior tibialis muscle assists with dorsiflexion of the ankle. Pain and inflammation of the tendon can result from activities that place excessive pressure on the tendon, such as repetitive high strain or force placed on the muscle. Over time, this leads to gradual degeneration of the tendon and swelling in the area, and shin splints may result. Activities that may lead to this injury include fast walking, sprinting up hills, and prolonged walking on uneven ground. Anterior tibial tendonitis is characterized by localized tenderness, crepitus, and pain with resisted dorsiflexion. Many individuals with this injury report pain increases with going down stairs or running downhill.

Rehabilitation of anterior tibial tendonitis begins with correction of gain mechanics. Two simple changes can be made to lessen the force on the tendon: (1) Decreasing the length of the stride, and (2) adding arch supports to decrease the functional length of the tibialis anterior. Both of these alterations will allow for less stress placed on the tendon of the muscle in gait. Stretching of the tibialis anterior muscle may be achieved by performing the "toe drag stretch" (Fig. 29.2). In addition, stretching the gastrocnemius and soleus is recommended, as tightness in these muscles causes biomechanical stress in walking by decreasing dorsiflexion. Strengthening of the tibialis anterior muscle through dorsiflexion and inversion exercises is introduced once pain is decreased and range of motion is normal. Theraband exercises are used to improve strength and endurance, and other exercises may focus on balance and proprioception.

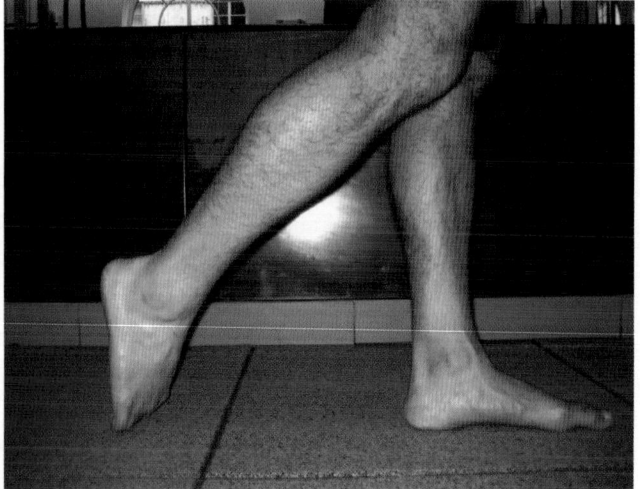

Figure 29.2. Toe drag stretch.

ACHILLES TENDONITIS

The etiology of Achilles tendonitis, while widely studied, is not fully clear. It is believed that overtraining, overpronation, and/or weakness of the gastrocnemius and soleus muscles all contribute to this disorder. Histologic studies of affected Achilles tendons show a fiber degeneration and collagen fiber derangement, suggesting it is a degenerative process (5). Individuals with a diagnosis of Achilles tendonitis present with tenderness 2 cm to 6 cm above the insertion into the calcaneus. Increased pain is elicited by stretching the ankle into dorsiflexion. Studies have shown that patients with Achilles tendonitis often present with biomechanical faults, including excessive pronation, limited mobility of the subtalar joint, and limited range of ankle dorsiflexion.

Physical therapy has been proven very effective in the treatment of Achilles tendonitis, and rehabilitation focuses on controlling pain and inflammation, correcting the aforementioned biomechanical deviations, and eccentrically strengthening the gastrocnemius–soleus complex. In a study by Clement et al., 109 runners diagnosed with Achilles tendonitis were treated conservatively without immobilization. Treatment consisted of pain and inflammation control, strengthening of the gastrocnemius–soleus muscle–tendon unit, and control of biomechanical parameters. At the end of treatment, one fair, 12 good, and 73 excellent results were reported with a mean recovery time of 5 weeks (30).

Eccentric strengthening of the calf has been proven very effective in the treatment of this injury. Alfredson et al. studied runners with chronic tendonitis to determine the efficacy of eccentric strengthening of the gastrocnemius–soleus complex. At the study's onset, all runners were found to have decreased calf-muscle strength in the involved leg when compared to the non-involved leg, and all had shown no improvement after being treated with rest from running, conventional physical therapy, non-steroidal anti-inflammatories and orthotics. Fifteen patients underwent surgery and fifteen were instructed to perform eccentric calf exercises twice daily for 12 weeks. At the end of 12 weeks, all patients who performed eccentric strengthening returned to running and felt they were at their pre-injury level. The surgical group also returned to running at their pre-injury level; however, their recovery took 6 months (31).

Achilles tendon rehabilitation begins with stretching of the gastrocnemius–soleus complex. The "runner's stretch" (Figs. 29.3 and 29.4) is performed against a wall, first with the posterior leg straight (to target the gastrocnemius) and then bent (to target the soleus). The foot should be positioned straight ahead to allow for linear stretching of the tissue. In addition to range of motion exercises, patients should engage in therapeutic exercises for calf strengthening, balance, and proprioception. To eccentrically strengthen the calf, the patient starts with a bilateral heel raise. At the top of the motion, the weight is shifted to the involved leg and the heel is slowly lowered down. To improve balance and proprioception, single-leg stance is performed, first

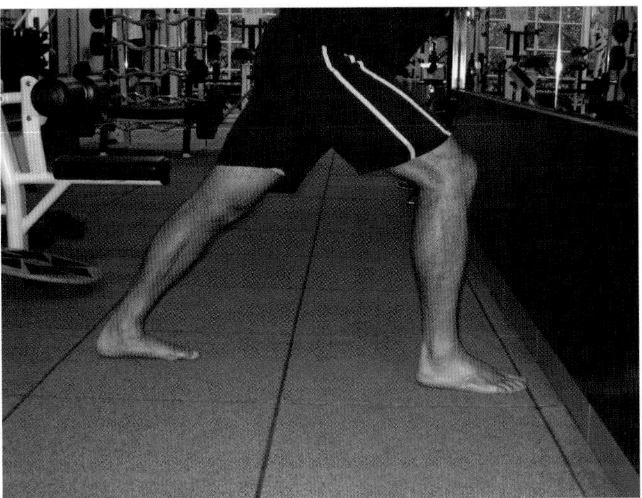

Figure 29.3. Runner's stretch with focus on gastrocnemius.

on a flat floor and later on unstable surfaces, such as cushions and wobble boards.

SHIN SPLINTS

Shin splints result from repetitive stress resulting in inflammation of the posterior peroneal tendon and adjacent tissues on the anterior lateral shin. One common cause of shin splints is increase in distance or intensity of a workout schedule, which may lead to overuse and inflammation in the anterior lower-leg muscles. Structural abnormalities in the foot and ankle may also p lay a role in shin splints. Individuals with pes planus (flat longitudinal arch) can develop shin splints due to over-stretching of the posterior tibialis and other muscles of the medial shin.

Vtsalo et al. studied 48 male athletes to determine biomechanical differences in the foot and ankle of those with and without shin splints. Each participant ran with bare feet on the treadmill and researchers noted: (1) The position of the lower leg and heel while standing, (2) the mobility of the subtalar joint, and (3) the Achilles tendon angle (the angular displacement between the calcaneus and midline of the lower leg).

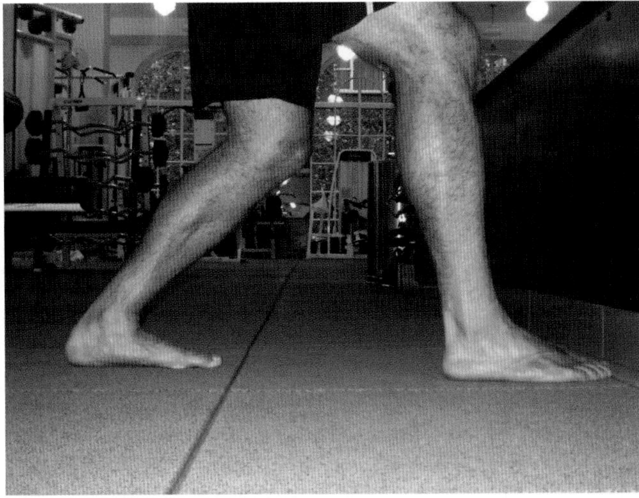

Figure 29.4. Runner's stretch with focus on soleus.

Those runners with shin splints presented with significantly greater Achilles tendon angles at heel strike, and greater mobility of the subtalar joint. In addition, the group with shin splints showed significantly greater angular displacement between the heel strike and the maximal everted position in running. Thus, results suggest that structural and functional differences are present in the feet and ankles between healthy athletes and those with shin splints (32).

Patients with shin splints present with dull, aching pain and tenderness over the anterior and lateral lower leg. Mild edema may also be present in more severe cases. These individual may report pain that is intermittent and only present with exercise, or constant pain that is present all the time.

Once pain and inflammation are controlled with modalities and/or anti-inflammatories, physical therapy focuses on stretching the posterior and anterior lower-leg muscles. Patients are then progressed to progressive resistive strengthening of the muscles of the anterior shin, and eventually return to limited running or other impact activity at a low speed.

METATARSALGIA

Metatarsalgia is a common condition that affects the bones and joints at the ball of the foot. It often presents under the second, third, and fourth metatarsal heads, or more isolated at the head of the first metatarsal. Its onset is due to excessive pressure over a long period of time, causing the heads of the metatarsals to become inflamed and painful. The use of shoes with high heels and the lack of proper footwear during high-impact activity can lead to metatarsalgia. Individuals present with pain over the metatarsal heads of the involved bones. Symptoms increase with standing and activity and decrease with rest. Mild metatarsalgia pain is localized; however, more severe cases may present with sharp, shooting pain that radiates into the toes.

The goal of rehabilitation for metatarsalgia is restoring full range of motion, strength, and foot function. Physical therapy in the acute stage is directed at decreasing pain and inflammation at the site of the injury with RICE and modalities. A metatarsal pad, which acts to alleviate pressure on the bone has also been shown effective in reducing symptoms (33). The pads are placed proximal to the affected metatarsal head and allow pressure on the plantar foot to be redistributed, thus relieving symptoms.

Once pain and inflammation are resolved, joint mobilization, stretching and strengthening exercises may be introduced. Mobilizing the metatarsophalangeal joint with long-axis distraction and dorsal/plantar glides helps to lubricate the articulation and improve movement. It is important to increase dorsiflexion range of motion, as this will permit improved forward progression of the tibia over the foot and decrease forefoot stress. Four-way theraband, marble pick-ups, and towel scrunches are good exercises to improve strength in the ankle and intrinsic foot muscles.

HALLUX RIGIDUS

Hallux rigidus, a form of degenerative arthritis, is a condition that presents at the base of the big toe. Patients with this condition initially report pain and stiffness in the joint, and as the problem becomes more chronic, limitations in range of motion can occur. The causes of hallux rigidus are often related to faulty biomechanics in the foot or structural abnormalities. Excessive pronators or those who have flat medial longitudinal arches are susceptible to this disorder. In this population, greater stress is placed on the joint of the great toe during the push-off phase of gait, which may, over time, lead to inflammation and chronic injury.

Physical therapy treatment of hallux rigidus focuses on decreasing pain and inflammation with modalities, as well as maintaining motion at the metatarsophalangeal and interphalangeal joints of the great toe. While they should be avoided in the acute stages, gentle mobilizations such as long-axis distraction at the great toe joints assist in pain reduction and joint lubrication in the subacute and chronic stages. Therapeutic exercises to strengthen the medial longitudinal arch without putting pressure on the great toe are recommended, such as theraband plantarflexion, seated towel scrunches, and marble pick-ups.

HALLUX VALGUS (BUNION)

Hallux valgus, also known as bunion deformity, occurs when there is a medial deviation of the first metatarsal and a lateral deviation of the hallux. The cause of hallux valgus is frequently improper footwear, specifically shoes with a narrow toe box and high heels. Use of these shoes causes the front of the foot to be pushed forward into the narrow box, and the toes become squeezed together. Over time, this may lead to the bunion deformity. In addition, genetics play a role and those who have a family history of bunions are more likely to develop them. Patients with hallux valgus present with complaints of pain with walking, redness and inflammation at the joint, as well as a visible prominence on the medial aspect of the foot.

In more severe cases of hallux valgus, a surgical osteotomy has been proven very effective in treating pain and dysfunction (34). However, if the patient opts for physical therapy, treatment begins with education. The patient is advised to change footwear to alleviate symptoms and prevent progression of the bunion. Appropriate shoes have a wide toe box, low heel, and good arch support. Rehabilitation focuses on pain reduction and stretching. In addition to ultrasound and moist heat application, gentle massage of the affected area helps to break up scar tissue and increase blood flow. Slowly and gently stretching the great toe into flexion and extension prevents loss of motion.

STRESS FRACTURES

Due to the repetitive stress on the foot and ankle during sports activities, stress fractures are common injuries to the tarsal, metatarsal, phalangeal, and ankle bones. Most stress fractures are seen in the weight-bearing portions of the lower leg, and result from repetitive striking of the foot on the ground. Factors such as overtraining, poor equipment, faulty technique, and bone insufficiency contribute to the development of stress fractures.

Often, stress fractures are the result of muscle insufficiency, such as when the muscles become overtired and are no longer able to absorb the shock of the repeated impact. Stresses are then transferred to the bones, causing them to develop cracks. Common sites of stress fractures in the lower leg are the second and third metatarsals, calcaneus, fibula, and navicular bones. Patients present with complaints of localized foot and ankle pain and swelling that increase with weight-bearing activity and decrease with rest. There may be point tenderness over the site of the injury, and some discoloration may be noted.

The most important treatment for stress fractures is to stop the activity that caused the injury. Stress fractures generally heal in 6 to 8 weeks, and during that time, patients are advised to engage in low-impact activities that do not place stress on the injury. Physical therapy focuses on decreasing the pain and swelling at the site of the injury using modalities, heat and cold therapy, and gentle massage. In addition, stretching is recommended to maintain muscle flexibility. Muscle re-education is crucial to prevent further injury, as stronger intrinsic foot muscles allow for better shock absorption during activity. This is best achieved through stabilization exercises such as single-leg stance on various surfaces (including flat ground, the BAPS board, and the rubber disc). Intrinsic muscle strengthening is achieved through towel scrunches and marble pick-ups, and four-way theraband exercises help to improve ankle muscle endurance.

MORTON'S NEUROMA

Morton's neuroma is an enlarged nerve that most frequently occurs between the third and fourth toes, in the third interspace. A neuroma results from thickening of the nerve resulting from constant compression or irritation, which causes enlargement. Frequently, forcing the foot into a shoe with a narrow toe box causes this type of injury. In addition, acute or chronic hyperextension of the metatarsophalangeal joints, which may be incurred in activities like walking in high-heel shoes, can cause this disorder (35). Sports such as running or jumping that involve repetitive impact on the ball of the foot can lead to Morton's neuroma.

Patients with this type of injury present with complaints of pain, numbness, and tingling in the third interspace. They often report feeling as though there is an object stuck inside the ball of the foot. Initially, the patient reports symptoms only during walking; however, as the disorder progresses, pain is felt at rest and may be worse at night.

Biomechanical foot correction is the best treatment for Morton's neuroma, consisting of a supportive pad under the heads of the metatarsals and improving foot position with orthotics (35). Physical therapy can be useful to decrease symptoms of swelling with cryotherapy and modalities, as well as stretching and soft tissue massage. When conservative measures are not successful in treating the symptoms of a Morton's neuroma, surgical excision of the fibrotic area is recommended.

RETURN TO ACTIVITY FOLLOWING INJURY

The final phase of physical therapy is preparing the athlete to return to sport. During this time, rehabilitation should focus equally on increasing strength and improving endurance, as muscle fatigue predisposes athletes to recurrent injury (36). Because the lower leg absorbs much of the shock of repetitive impact, it is imperative to reach pre-set goals for muscle strength, endurance, and neuromuscular performance that should be met prior to release. Returning to sport too quickly may lead to further injury, while prolonged inactivity can cause unnecessary deconditioning.

General guidelines can help to determine if it is safe for an athlete to return to sport. These include full and pain-free range of motion, strength returns of at least 90% (37), a pre-injury level of balance and proprioception, and a thorough understanding of the risk of re-injury and how to prevent it. The decision to return an athlete to sport should involve many people, including the coach, the physical therapist, the doctor, and the team's athletic trainer. Sporting activities should be resumed at a sub-maximal intensity, and the athlete should be progressed to higher intensities as strength gains are made.

The final phase of physical therapy treatment focuses on activities and drills geared toward ensuring that all goals have been met and the patient is ready for return to sport. Exercises performed in this phase of rehabilitation include advanced balance and proprioception activities, intense agility drills, and plyometrics. Balance and proprioception exercises include single-leg stance using unstable surfaces such as wobble boards and cushions. Athletes may combine balancing on one leg with other activities, such as tossing a ball on a rebounding trampoline or bending down to pick up weights. Agility drills, which focus on complexity and speed, are performed in forward, backward, and side-to-side directions. Examples include running sprints, lateral shuffles, and cariocas. Plyometric exercises geared toward increasing power include hopping, skipping, and bounding, and progress to more intense activities such as box jumps.

Physical therapy is an invaluable tool in the treatment of lower-leg injuries. A successful rehabilitation program addresses all aspects of an athlete's lower-leg injury—from treating the acute stages of pain and inflammation to preparing the patient for full return to sport. The right combination of modalities, stretching, and therapeutic exercise often allows a patient to avoid more invasive measures of treatment, which ultimately may decrease the time away from sport.

REFERENCES

1. Geffen SJ. Rehabilitation principles for treating chronic musculoskeletal injuries. *Med J Aust* 2003;178:238–242.
2. Marder RM. Current methods for the evaluation of ankle ligament injuries. *J Bone Joint Surg Am* 1994;76:1103–1111.
3. Magee DJ. *Orthopedic Physical Assessment.* 4th ed. Philadelphia, PA: W.B. Saunders Company; 2002.
4. Baumhauer JF, Nawoczenski DA, DiGiovanni BF, et al. Ankle pain and peroneal tendon pathology. *Clin Sports Med* 2004;23:21–34.
5. Barr KP, Harrast MA. Evidence-based treatment of foot and ankle injuries in runners. *Phys Med Rehabil Clin N Am* 2005;16:779–799.
6. Birrer RB, Buzermanis S, DellaCorte MP, et al. Biomechanics of running. In: O'Connor BL, Wilder RP, Nirschl R, eds. *Textbook of Running Medicine.* New York, NY: McGraw Hill; 2001:11–19.
7. Starkey C. *Therapeutic Modalities for Athletic Trainers.* Philadelphia, PA: F.A. Davis Company; 1993.
8. Knight KL. *Cryotherapy: Theory, Technique, and Physiology.* Chattanooga, TN: Chattanooga Corporation; 1985.
9. Grana WA, Walton WL, Reider B. Cold modalities. In: Drez D, ed. *Therapeutic Modalities for Sports Injuries.* Chicago, IL: Year Book Medical Publishers; 1989:25–32.
10. Halvorson GA. Therapeutic heat and cold for athletic injuries. *Physician Sportsmed* 1990;18:87.
11. Van Der Windt DA, Van Der Heijden GJ, Van Den Berg SG, et al. Ultrasound therapy for acute ankle sprains. *Cochrane Database Syst Rev* 2002;1:CD001250.
12. Brand JC, Brindle T, Nyland J. Does pulsed low intensity ultrasound allow early return to normal activities when treating stress fractures?: a review of one tarsal navicular and eight tibial stress fractures. *Iowa Orthop J* 199;19:26–30.
13. Japour CJ, Vohra R, Vohra PK, et al. Management of heel pain syndrome with acetic acid iontophoresis. *JAPMA* 1999;89(5):251–257.
14. Neeter C, Thomeé R, Silbernagel KG, et al. Iontophoresis with or without dexamethasone in the treatment of acute Achilles tendon pain. *Scand J Med Sci Sports* 2003;13(6): 376–382.
15. Delitto A, Rose SJ. Comparative comfort of three wave forms used in electrically eliciting quadriceps femoris muscle contractions. *Phys Ther* 1986;66:1704–1707.
16. W Man IO, Lepar GS, Morrissey MC, et al. Effects of neuromuscular stimulation on foot/ankle volume during standing. *Med Sci Sports Exer* 2003;35(4):630–634.
17. Cornwall MW, McPoil TG. Plantar fasciitis: etiology and treatment. *J Orthop Sports Phys Ther* 1999;29(12):756–760.
18. Gudeman SD, Eisele SA, Heidt RS Jr, et al. Treatment of plantar fasciitis by iontophoresis of 0.4% dexamethasone. *Am J Sports Med* 1997;25(3):312–316.
19. Crawford F, Snaith M. How effective is therapeutic ultrasound in the treatment of heel pain? *Ann Rheum Dis* 1996;55:265–267.
20. Pfeffer G, Bacchetti P, Deland J, et al. Comparison of custom and prefabricated orthoses in the initial treatment of proximal plantar fasciitis. *Foot Ankle Int* 1999;20(4):214–221.
21. Digiovanni BF, Nawoczenski DA, Lintal ME, et al. Tissue-specific plantar fascia-stretching exercise enhances outcomes in patients with chronic heel pain. *J Bone Joint Surg Am* 2003;85:1270–1277.
22. Stuber K, Kristmanson K. Conservative therapy for plantar fasciitis: a narrative review of randomized controlled trials. *J Can Chiropr Assoc* 2006;50(2):118–133.
23. Young CC, Rutherford DS, Niedfeldt MW. Treatment of plantar fasciitis. *Am Fam Physician* 2001;63(3):467–475.
24. Wolfe MW, Uhl TL, Mattacola CG, et al. Plantar fasciitis: etiology and treatment. *J Orthop Sports Phys Ther* 1999;29(12):756–760.
25. Karlsson J, Lundin O, Lind K, et al. Early mobilization versus immobilization after ankle ligament stabilization. *Scand J Med Sci Sports* 1999;9:299–303.
26. Green T, Refshauge K, Crosbie J, et al. A randomized controlled trial of a passive accessory joint mobilization on acute ankle inversion sprains. *Phys Ther* 2001;81(4):984–994.
27. Williams DS III, McClay IS, Hamill J. Arch structure and injury patterns in runners. *Clin Biomech (Bristol, Avon)* 2001;16:341–347.
28. Kulig K, Reischl SF, Pomrantz AB, et al. Nonsurgical management of posterior tibial tendon dysfunction with orthoses and resistive exercise: a randomized control. *Phys Ther* 2009;89(1):26–37.
29. Simons SM. Foot injuries in the runner. In: O'Connor FG, Wilder RP, Nirschl R, eds. *Textbook of Running Medicine.* New York, NY: McGraw-Hill; 2001:213–216.
30. Clement DB, Taunton JE, Smart GW. Achilles tendinitis and peritendinitis: etiology and treatment. *Am J Sports Med* 1983;12(3):179–184.
31. Alfredson H, Pietila T, Jonsson P, et al. Heavy-load eccentric calf muscle training for the treatment of chronic Achilles tendinosis. *Am J Sports Med* 1998;26(3):360–366.
32. Vtasalo JT, Kvist M. Some biomechanical aspects of the foot and ankle in athletes with and without shin splints. *Am J Sports Med* 1983;11(3):125–130.
33. Kang J, Chen M, Chen S, et al. Correlations between subjective treatment responses and plantar pressure parameters of metatarsal pad treatment in metatarsalgia patients: a prospective study. *BMC Musculoskelet Disord* 2006;7:95–102.
34. Torkki M, Malmivaara A, Seitsalo S, et al. Surgery vs. orthosis vs. watchful waiting for hallux valgus: a randomized controlled trial. *JAMA* 2001;285:2474–2480.
35. Winkel D, Matthijs O, Phelps V. *Diagnosis and Treatment of the Lower Extremities.* Maryland, MD: Aspen Publishers; 1997.
36. Zöch C, Fialka-Moser V, Quittan M. Rehabilitation of ligamentous ankle injuries: a review of recent studies. *Br J Sports Med* 2003;37:291–295.
37. Sundberg S. Returning to sports after an ankle injury. Gillette Children's Specialty Healthcare: A Pediatric Perspective 2003;12(5):1–4.

CHAPTER

30

Mark A. Caselli
Rock G. Positano
Meaghan M. Colletti
Rock CJ. Positano

Sport Specific Prescription Foot Orthoses

INTRODUCTION

Today's age of sports medicine, with its focus on the prevention and treatment of foot and ankle injuries, has led to an increase in the use of foot orthoses. Both competitive and recreational athletes frequently utilize foot orthoses to promote pain free activity. Orthoses and insoles are the mainstay of mechanical foot therapy as it has developed over the last century. Over the past two decades, tremendous advances have been made in the diagnosis and treatment of mechanical problems pertaining to gait, and thus the design and use of foot orthoses and insoles. Computer technology, new materials, and advances from orthotic laboratories have played a significant role in patient care.

FOOT ORTHOSES AND INSOLES

By definition, an orthosis is a device that is used to protect, support, or improve function of parts of the body that move (1). The terms orthoses and orthotics are used to describe a wide range of devices that are placed inside the shoe. Other terms used for orthoses include inserts, insoles, inlays, supports, and cushions.

The three basic types of foot orthoses are prefabricated, customized, and custom molded. A prefabricated orthosis is one that is mass produced and is intended to be dispensed to the user without modification. Prefabricated orthoses are usually designed to provide either increased support or shock absorption for a specific area of the foot, such as an arch support or heel cushion. They may also provide cushioning to the entire foot as is the case with the use of a full insole. A customized orthosis usually consists of a prefabricated base component that is modified in some way, such as adding a metatarsal pad or heel lift. A custom-molded orthosis is one made from a model of the patient's foot that was crafted using some form of three-dimensional impression taking procedure. These devices are used for patients with more severe or complicated foot problems. They are commonly composed of a shell, the layer of material next to and in total contact with the foot, and posting material, filling the space between the shell and the shoe. Custom orthoses can be further modified by adding materials to the top of the shell to either redistribute pressure or provide cushioning.

Foot orthoses are often described as being either accommodative or functional. An accommodative orthosis is designed primarily to accommodate a rigid or deformed foot, or one that is at risk. A functional orthosis is designed to realign a more flexible foot by providing joint stability and support. In reality, most orthoses offer some degree of both accommodative and functional properties. In general, foot orthoses are designed to accomplish one or more of the following: (1) reduce shock, (2) reduce shear, (3) relieve areas of excessive plantar pressure, (4) stabilize and support the joints of the foot, (5) limit motion of joints (2).

ORTHOTIC MATERIALS

These materials are commonly divided into three basic types: soft, semiflexible, and rigid. Examples of soft materials include polyethylene foams such as Plastazote (Bakalite Xylonite LTD, {BXL} UK), closed-cell neoprene impregnated with nitrogen bubbles such as Spenco (Spenco Medical Corporation, Waco, TX), open-cell foams such as Poron (Rogers Corporation, Rogers, CT), and gel-like viscoelastic polymers such as silicone. Leather and cork materials are usually considered to be semi-flexible. Semiflexible materials are somewhat accommodative but provide more functional support than the soft type and do not "bottom out" as quickly. Rigid materials include acrylic plastics and thermoplastic polymers. They are moldable at high temperatures and are primarily functional in nature. These are the most durable and supportive of the three types. This method of classifying materials provides a good general guideline for selecting materials either alone or in combination for the fabrication of a foot orthosis. The problem with this classification system is that it could be misleading without a thorough knowledge of the properties of each of the materials. Many of the materials can range from being soft to rigid, depending on the thickness, number of layers, or form of the material used. A good example of this is an orthotic made from Plastizote, which can range from soft (a single layer of medium grade) to rigid (laminated layers of rigid grade). A better method is categorizing the materials as either being natural or synthetic with specific properties assigned to each material.

NATURAL MATERIALS

Natural materials used for the fabrication of orthoses are those found in nature and include leather, rubber butter, and cork.

LEATHER

Leather orthoses can be either functional or accommodative depending on material combinations and casting techniques. Leather devices may include various materials from firm to soft depending on the needs of the patient. The basic shell of a leather orthosis consists of adding layers of leather to one another to form a lamination that can be shaped to a positive cast of the patient's foot or molded to the foot or to the inside of a shoe directly.

The benefits of leather as an orthotic material are a direct result of its intrinsic natural characteristics. The collagen fibers that make up leather are woven in a three-dimensional pattern. Collagen's chemical properties give leather its distinctive porosity or breathability. As a result, leather can absorb up to 30% of its weight in water vapor without feeling wet. Tanning also gives leather the ability to retain its shape and resist the aging process. The refinement of high performance leather has resulted in features that include improved water repellency, low water absorption, fast and soft drying, and durability. Other advantages of leather orthoses include the fact that leather conforms to foot contours and deformities and can be easily modified to disperse pressure from bony prominences. They are also well tolerated by patients of all ages. In order to give leather orthoses more shock attenuation properties, the underside of a leather shell is often filled with other softer materials. Leather devices can be readily reshaped, remodeled, and adjusted in the office. The disadvantages of leather orthoses are that they tend to be more bulky than those made from the thermoplastics for a given degree of motion control. They also tend to breakdown when worn by very active or obese individuals. While they can withstand a limited amount of moisture, they do not hold up well under repetitive soaking (3).

RUBBER BUTTER

Rubber butter is a generic substance formulated by mixing liquid latex with either cork, wood, or leather shavings, each producing a slightly different material. The rubber butter which is composed of latex and leather grindings has more shock attenuation than the latex cork mixtures. Rubber butter–like materials are manufactured by several companies and are available under various trade names. Cushion Cork (JMS Plastics, Neptune, NJ) is a latex and cork combination available in sheets that are supplied in thicknesses measuring 1/6 to 1/2 in., and is commonly used for fabricating wedges and lifts. Korex is a cork latex mixture manufactured by Armstrong. Thermocork (Apex Foot Health Industries, Teaneck, NJ) is the only heat-molded product in this group and is available in thicknesses measuring 1/8 to 3/8 in. Rubber butter which is composed of latex and leather grindings has more shock attenuating properties than the latex and cork mixtures, however, because of its leather content, it is susceptible to a greater degree of breakdown over time (4). These materials are also effective when used specifically as accommodations, either in conjunction with a standard-length foot orthosis or alone.

SYNTHETIC MATERIALS

The synthetic materials used in the fabrication of foot orthoses were developed to possess desired properties not found in naturally occurring materials.

POLYETHYLENE AND POLYPROPYLENE THERMOPLASTICS

Polyethylene is a polyolefin which is synthesized from the monomer ethylene oxide. Polyethylene thermoplastics possess the properties of toughness and flexibility with good dimensional stability, are heat moldable, lightweight, and possess favorable weight/strength ratios. They are generally classified as being low, medium, high, or ultrahigh density. They are available for orthosis fabrication primarily as Ortholen and Sub-Ortholen (Teufel, Stuttgart, Germany).

Ortholen is an extremely high-density thermoforming polyethylene with a molecular weight of 1 million. It is a very tough material which is resistant to chemical erosion and is nonbrittle at low temperatures. Ortholen is available in thicknesses of 3 to 6 mm and is heat molded by heating to 350°F for 10 to 15 minutes. Orthoses fabricated from Ortholen are indicated when a functional or semi-functional device is desired as it provides efficient pronation control in situations where a moderately flexible orthosis is required. Sub-Ortholen is an ultrahigh-density thermoforming polyethylene with a molecular weight of 500,000. Although related to Ortholen, it has less toughness and strength but is easier to mold by heating to 300°F. Sub-Ortholen is available in thicknesses of 1 to 6 mm (4).

Polypropylene is also a polyolefin synthesized from the monomer ethylene oxide. As with polyethylene, polypropylene is a thermoplastic that is heat-formable and heat-adjustable at approximately 360 to 390°F. Polypropylene differs from polyethylene in that it is a polymer of greater density and molecular weight, causing it to have a higher stiffness-to-thickness ratio. This results in polypropylene having generally less rapid and less severe plastic, or shape deformation than the polyethylenes (5).

ROHADUR

Rohadur nylon acrylic is a copolymer consisting of methylmethacrylate and acrylonitrile. It was first developed for orthopedic use by the Rohm Haas Company of Germany in 1951 as Thermolast-1. Sheets of this material were marketed by various companies under such trade names as Plexidur, Nyloplex, Sadur, and Cyrodur (all JMS Plastics, Neptune, NJ). In 1976, Thermolast-1 was found to be possibly carcinogenic in its manufacturing process and was therefore reformulated and a new Rohadur resin was introduced as Thermolast-II. Rohadur thermoplastic is heat moldable and indicated for orthotic devices in which functional control is desired. In addition to its use in fabricating orthoses to control pronation, Rohadur is commonly used in the fabrication of gait plates which are used in the treatment of in-toe gait. Rohadur is available in sheets measuring 2, 2.5, 3, 3.5, 4, 5, and 6 mm in thickness, with the 3 to 4 mm thickness most frequently used (4).

CARBON GRAPHITE

Carbon graphite orthotic devices are fabricated by laminating very thin sheets of carbon graphite fiber cloths using a liquid resin. The number of laminations varies depending on the strength desired, but for most foot orthosis applications, the shell is approximately 2 mm in thickness. This produces a thin rigid shell that is appreciably thinner than other thermoplastic orthoses.

TL-2100 (Performance Materials Corp., Camarillo, California) is manufactured with an acrylic-based thermoplastic resin system reinforced with carbon fiber and combined in a sandwich configuration. This allows thermoformability and heat adjustability similar to that of polypropylene. The graphite reinforcement provides stiffness for support and strength for durability. There are four versions of TL-2100 available: ultrastrength, so named because it is manufactured with approximately 50% more graphite than the other versions, rigid, semi-rigid, and semiflexible. Thicknesses range from 1.8 to 2.8 mm (5).

POLYETHYLENE FOAMS

Polyethylene foams make up the most common group of materials used in the fabrication of pressure reducing insoles and orthoses. Polyethylene foams are synthetic materials also classified as polyolefins. These foams are closed-cell foams that are nontoxic, resistant to chemicals and fluids, light, and when heated to suitable temperatures, are moldable. They are readily washable and discourage bacteria growth. Orthotic shells may be fabricated using one type of polyethylene foam or by laminating different foams together. A variety of polyethylene foams are available in assorted durometers or hardnesses. Polyethylene foams are manufactured under different trade names, with each company implementing its own system to name the materials' various durometers. Some of the more commonly encountered trade names of polyethylene foams are Plastizote, Evazote, Pelite (all Bakalite Xylonite LTD, {BXL}, UK), and Aliplast (Alimed, Needham, MA) (6).

Plastizote is the most commonly used and well known of the polyethylene foams; it originally received fairly extensive clinical use in the 1960s by Dr. Paul Brand for the treatment of the insensate foot of leprosy patients. It was used as a shoe insert, or, more frequently, constructed into a shoe or sandal. It offered protection by eliminating high pressure points to feet which had lost all sensation, as well as to feet which had actually undergone ulcerations. Plastizote foams are known for their memory or ability to retain moldable shape, as well as their smooth feel.

Plastizote is heat moldable at 140°F and is self-accommodating to lesions and bony prominences as well as being very lightweight. Plastizote is available in thicknesses of 1/16 to 1 in. It is also available in three durometers: medium, firm, and rigid. The medium and firm durometers are commonly used in the fabrication of accommodative and dynamic insoles, while the rigid durometer is used in the fabrication of semi-functional orthotic devices. Evazote is available in only one durometer which is very self-accommodating and lightweight. Pelite is available in four durometers and is commonly used as a liner for prosthetics. Aliplast is comparable to Plastizote and is supplied in four durometers (4).

Applications of polyethylene foams include the fabrication of orthoses for the relief of pain associated with burns, plantar fascial strain, synovitis, hyperesthesia, and high pressure points of the deformed foot. While these polyethylene foams are excellent materials for orthotic fabrication, they are poor shock attenuators. After a period of time, they will experience a loss of thickness due to both compression and shear-compression stress and must be replaced. The clinical lifetime of these foams is affected by their ability to dissipate the force of walking through their compression rather than breakdown of the plantar skin. For this reason, these foams are often combined with other materials such as Poron, Spenco, and leather.

POLYURETHANE FOAMS

Polyurethane foam is a thermosetting, non-heat moldable foam that is manufactured either as an opened- or closed-cell foam. The opened-cell type is the most commonly used. Poron, an opened-cell polyurethane foam made from a combination of polyether and polyester resins was developed by the Rogers Company of Connecticut utilizing a patented process. It is used wherever the reduction of pressure from static or dynamic forces is to be achieved, as in the production of foot orthoses or shoe inlays. This polyurethane foam is stable in form, elastic, shock-absorbing, odorless, and washable. As an opened-cell foam, medical grade Poron dissipates heat well and, by allowing water vapor transmission, enables perspiration to be transmitted away from the foot. This opened-cell nature also allows the air to circulate according to the weight lying on the material.

Poron retains its form stability and always returns to its original position, even after permanent load, while polyethylene foams such as Plastizote tend to permanently compress or "bottom out." When used as a shock attenuating soft tissue supplement for the plantar aspect of the foot, it is available in thicknesses ranging from 1/16 to 1/2 in. in a single durometer. The material is manufactured both perforated and non-perforated with a variety of surfaces and topcovers including smooth, abraded, felt, and multistretch nylon. Poron was once marketed by Langer Inc. of Deer Park NY under the name PPT. Today, however, PPT is no longer made of Poron, though it has similar properties (6).

RUBBER FOAMS

The term *rubber* refers to a group of compounds (both natural and synthetic) with elastic properties. The chemical industry classifies this group as elastomers. In the mid-1930s, Dupont invented the synthetic rubber neoprene, a polychloroprene. Once a Dupont trademark, neoprene is now used extensively industry-wide in the manufacture of foot orthoses, usually on the undersurface of a rigid or semi-rigid plastic shell. It is used as a balancing or posting material and is also used for providing some degree of cushioning and shock absorption.

In an attempt to produce an insole that would better absorb lateral and oblique forces and decrease the problem of blisters, Wayman Spence, MD and Marlin Shields, PT, in 1966, developed Spenco (Spenco Medical Corp., Waco, TX). Spenco is neoprene closed-cell foam with entrapped nitrogen bubbles and a nylon (polyamide) topcover. Spenco insoles are currently available in 3/32, 1/8, and 1/4 in. thicknesses. They are indicated for absorbing vertical forces, torque, and fore, aft, and lateral sheer, thus preventing blisters in athletes. Spenco insoles are also used to help prevent neuropathic and rheumatoid ulcerations by reducing the increased plantar foot pressure responsible for skin breakdown. Spenco does, however, retain heat and moisture due to its closed-cell nature (6).

Lynco (Apex Foot Health Industries, Teaneck, NJ), an open-cell neoprene foam insole with a nylon topcover better dissipates heat than Spenco, but due to its open-cell nature, it is felt not to be as good a shock attenuator.

SILICONE

Silicones are entirely synthetic polymers containing repeating silicon and oxygen atoms with organic groups directly attached to the silicon atom. Depending on the length of its polymer chain and the degree of cross-linking, silicone can be present in many different types of commercial products ranging from fluids to rubbers. Silicone rubbers are compositions containing a high molecular weight dimethyl silicone linear polymer and are commonly used in the fabrication of foot orthoses. Products containing silicone polymers tend to be relatively expensive. In the case of orthotic devices, those made of true silicone tend to be more costly than similar products made from other materials such as polyurethane foams. Silicone, however, has many properties that make it highly desirable for use in the manufacture of orthoses.

Silicone rubber offers excellent viscoelastic properties capable of providing shock absorption by dissipating the energy evading the body during ambulation. It accomplishes this task without bottoming out as quickly as other materials used for the same purpose, thus making it an excellent substitute for the natural viscoelastic body tissues. Silicone rubber has the ability of remaining flexible at very low temperatures and is not distorted by heat up to 400°C (752°F). Orthoses made from silicone can be heated and cooled without drying or cracking. Other important characteristics include a high degree of chemical inertness which allows the silicone devices to be soaked in many types of solutions for both cleaning and disinfecting without loss of any function. This chemical inertness also reduces the chance of allergies upon contact with the skin and does not support bacterial growth or odor. Disadvantages include a tendency to retain heat and an inability to be ground for adjustment (7).

A variety of both heel and full foot orthoses fabricated from silicone are currently available on the market. Although they differ somewhat in appearance, they are all designed primarily for both shock attenuation and weight dispersion. Several of the silicone orthoses incorporate precisely positioned softer padding, targeting the metatarsal and heel regions of the foot where shock load is highest. Some full-length insoles also include contouring that provides both heel and arch support, as well as shock absorption.

EVALUATING THE EFFECTS OF ORTHOSES AND INSOLES ON FOOT FUNCTION

Technologic advancements have provided objective methods of accurately determining the effects of orthoses and insoles on specific features of foot function, specifically pedal plantar pressure. In order for a device to be of value in assessing pedal plantar pressure, it must be capable of measuring the pressure at the shoe–foot interface or the orthotic/insole–foot interface during ambulation. There are currently a number of systems on the market that are capable of accomplishing this task. One of the commonly used systems is the F-Scan In-Shoe System (Tekscan, Inc., Boston, MA). This system utilizes an ultrathin (7/1,000 in.) pressure sensitive insole sensor containing 960 individual pressure sensing points. The F-Scan software records and calculates stance times and pressures at the shoe–foot interface. Increasing pressure is depicted by color changes ranging from violet (lowest pressure) to red (highest pressure) along the standard color spectrum. In-shoe plantar pressure can thus be a valuable tool in detecting both areas of increased plantar pressure and the ability of shoegear, insoles, and orthoses to offload these high pressure areas (8).

The plantar surface of the lesser metatarsals is the area of the foot most commonly associated with pathology due to excessive pressure (especially during the push-off phase of gait). Conditions such as metatarsalgia, hyperkeratosis, and stress fractures have been attributed to excessive pressure in this area.

Metatarsalgia is described as a localized or generalized pain in the region of the distal aspect of one or more of the metatarsals during weight bearing. Pain may be the result of either positional or functional malalignment of the metatarsals. The most common type of metatarsalgia involves a long lesser metatarsal bone (typically second or third) that projects past the theoretically perfect curve. The increased pressure and friction from this long metatarsal occurs during the push-off phase of gait, when the foot is fully loaded. Metatarsalgia may also be caused by a plantarflexed lesser metatarsal resulting from a contracted hammertoe condition. The plantar weight-bearing area under the metatarsal often begins to form a protective callus, and eventually a deep, painful plantar keratoma may develop (9,10). Metatarsal stress fractures (or march fractures) are also the result of increased repetitive pressure on the sub-metatarsal area of the foot. Once the most commonly diagnosed stress fractures, occurring often in military training during prolonged marches, these fractures affect a significant number of athletes (11).

THE EFFECT OF ORTHOSES AND INSOLES ON EXCESSIVE LESSER METATARSAL PLANTAR PRESSURE

The following figures demonstrate the effects of various foot orthoses and insoles on the plantar pedal pressure of a patient exhibiting excessive sub-lesser metatarsal plantar pressure. F-Scan readings were taken at the push-off phase of gait when the sub-lesser metatarsal pressure was at its peak. The measurements were recorded using the F-Scan In-shoe sensor with the patient wearing an all-purpose type athletic shoe. The readings were taken first with the shoe alone containing the manufacturer supplied shoe sockliner, then with various types of foot orthoses and insoles replacing the sockliner. The orthoses were custom made from an impression cast of the patient's feet and fabricated from a variety of both natural and synthetic materials as described. They represent what would be considered either functional, semi-functional, or accommodative devices. The insoles are made of some of the various types of biomaterials described in this paper (Figs. 30.1–30.8).

USE OF ORTHOSES IN THE TREATMENT OF OTHER COMMON SPORTS RELATED PROBLEMS

Sport-specific foot orthoses are designed to both improve athletic performance and reduce sports-related injury. They are prescribed for running, tennis, squash, golf, basketball, baseball, volleyball, football, dance, alpine and cross-country skiing, cycling, soccer, lacrosse, hockey, figure skating, walking, and hiking. Each activity applies different mechanical stresses on the lower extremities,

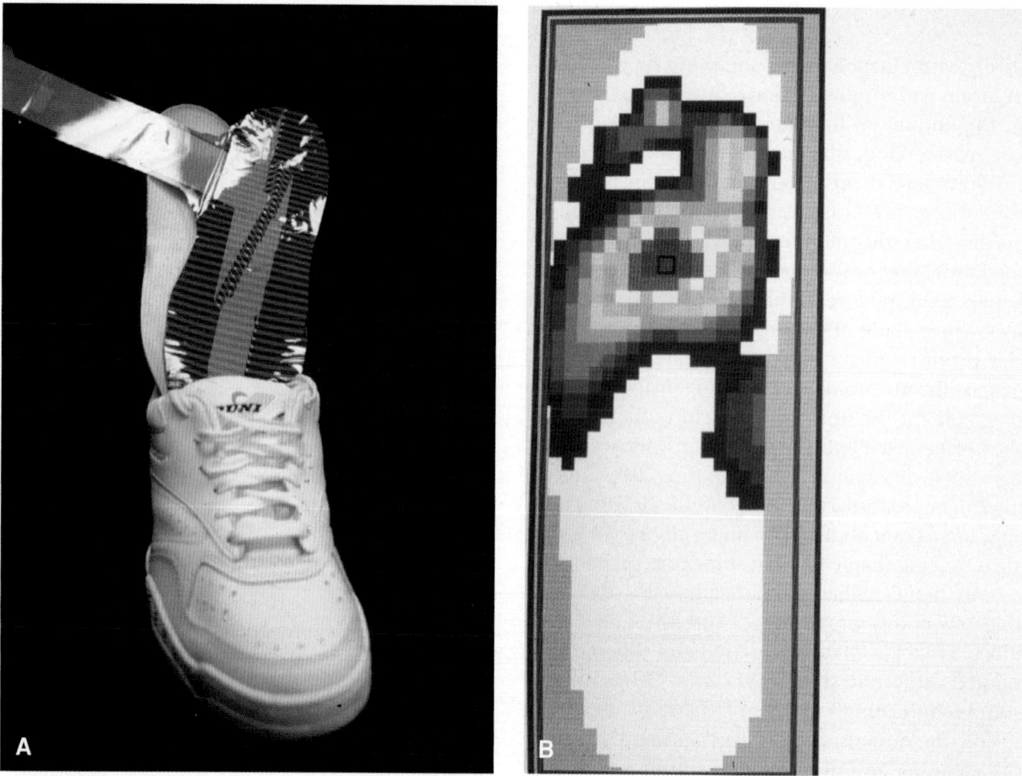

Figure 30.1. **A:** F-Scan insole sensor being placed in an athletic shoe with the manufacturer's supplied shoe sock liner. **B:** F-Scan recording using the shoe alone demonstrating high pressure areas under metatarsal heads.

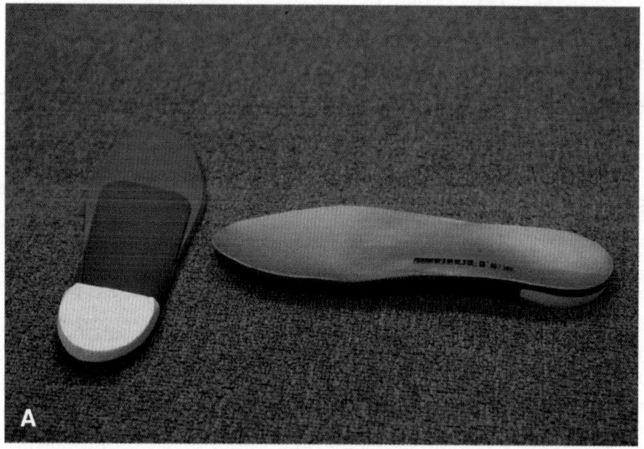

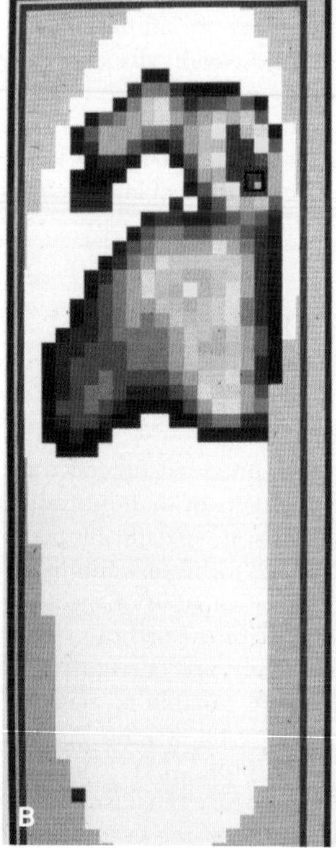

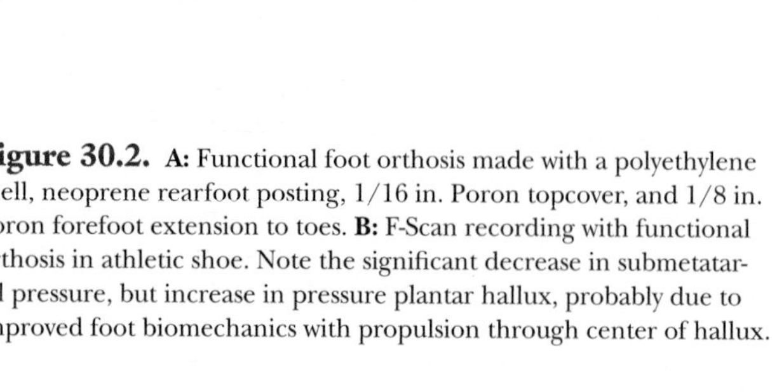

Figure 30.2. **A:** Functional foot orthosis made with a polyethylene shell, neoprene rearfoot posting, 1/16 in. Poron topcover, and 1/8 in. Poron forefoot extension to toes. **B:** F-Scan recording with functional orthosis in athletic shoe. Note the significant decrease in submetatarsal pressure, but increase in pressure plantar hallux, probably due to improved foot biomechanics with propulsion through center of hallux.

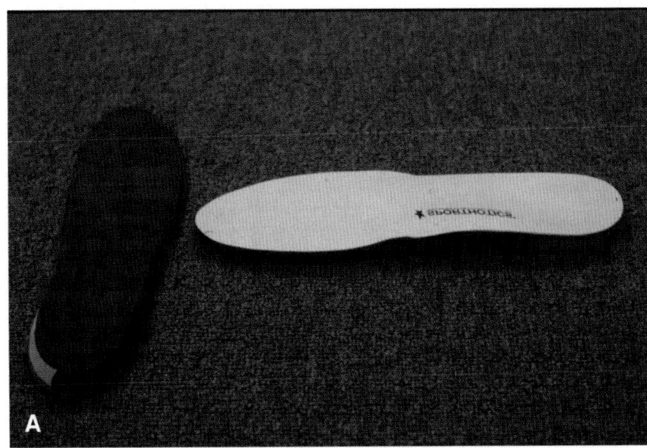

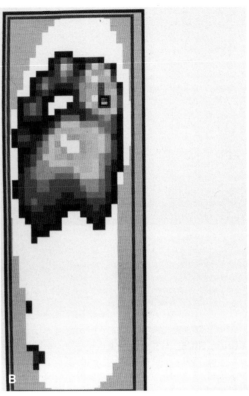

Figure 30.3. **A:** Semi-functional foot orthosis made with thinner polyethylene shell, Poron longitudinal arch reinforcement, lower durometer neoprene rearfoot posting, 1/16 in. Poron topcover, and 1/8 in. Poron forefoot extension to toes. **B:** F-Scan recording with semi-functional orthosis in athletic shoe. Note slightly less decrease in submetatarsal pressure than with the functional orthosis, but also the decrease in pressure plantar hallux probably due to its less functional design.

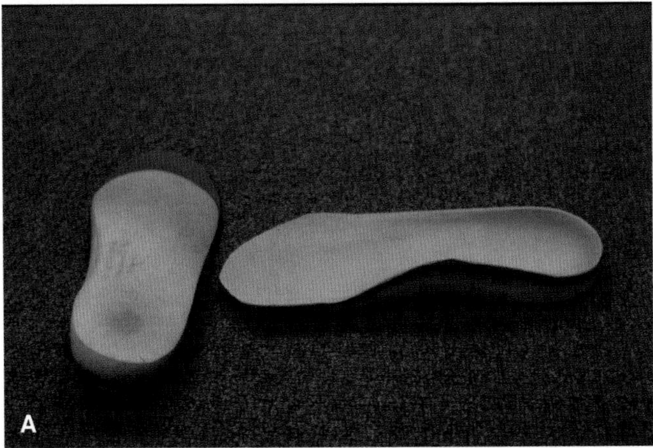

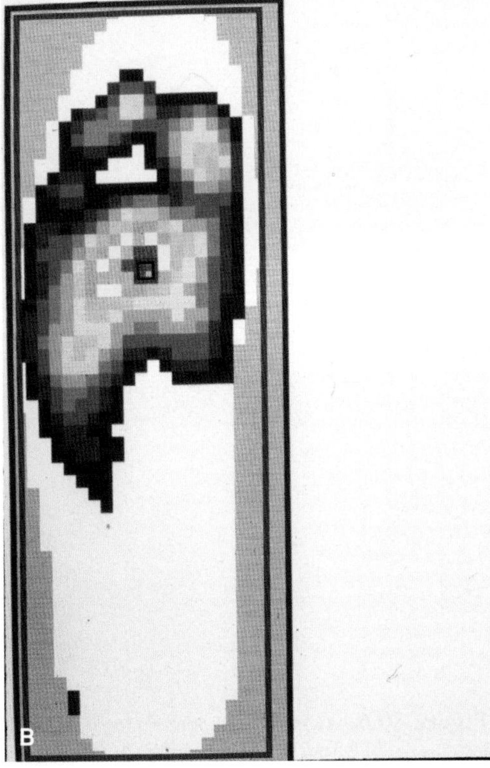

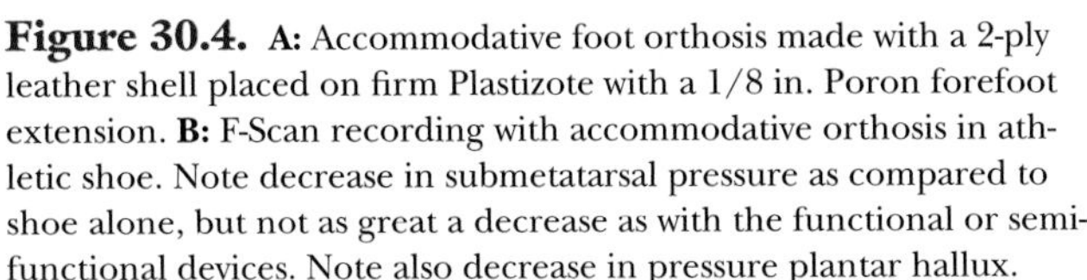

Figure 30.4. **A:** Accommodative foot orthosis made with a 2-ply leather shell placed on firm Plastizote with a 1/8 in. Poron forefoot extension. **B:** F-Scan recording with accommodative orthosis in athletic shoe. Note decrease in submetatarsal pressure as compared to shoe alone, but not as great a decrease as with the functional or semi-functional devices. Note also decrease in pressure plantar hallux.

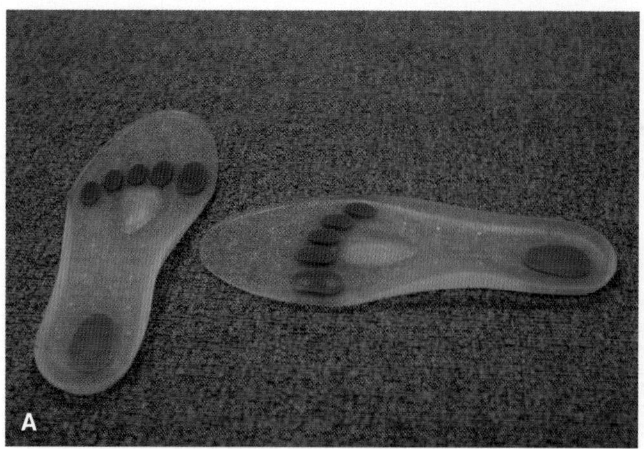

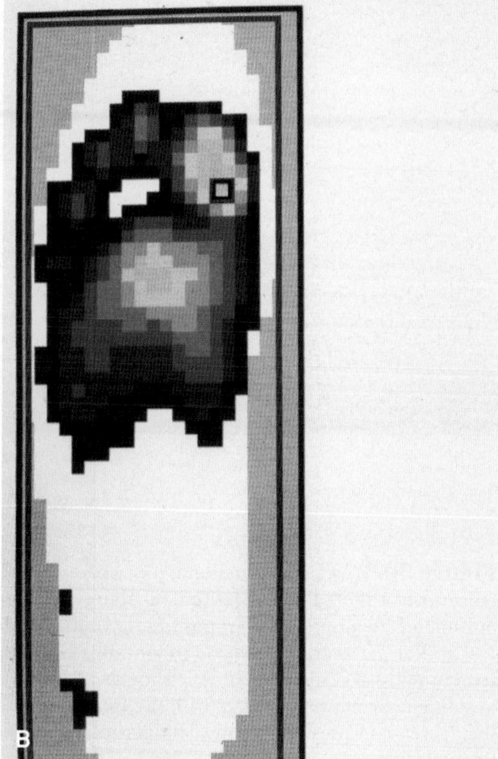

Figure 30.5. **A:** Silicone full-length insole with heel and arch support contouring, metatarsal pad, and softer padding at the metatarsal and heel areas. **B:** F-Scan recording with silicone insole in athletic shoe.

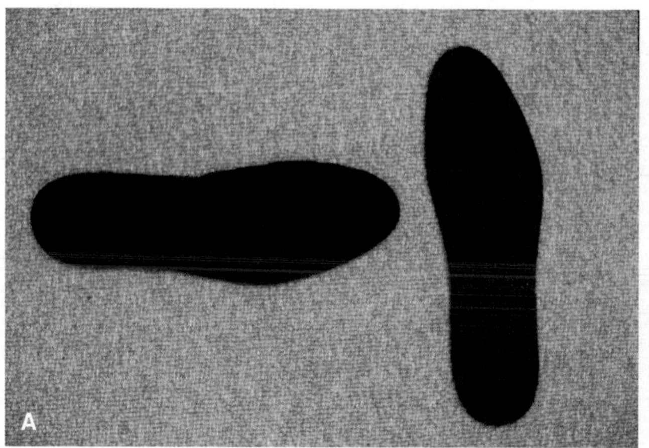

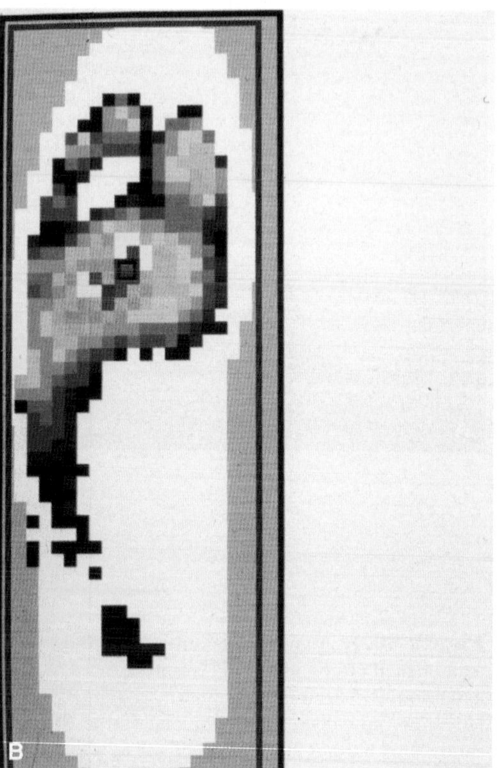

Figure 30.6. **A:** Spenco (neoprene closed-cell foam) 1/8 in. full foot insole. **B:** F-Scan recording with Spenco insole in athletic shoe.

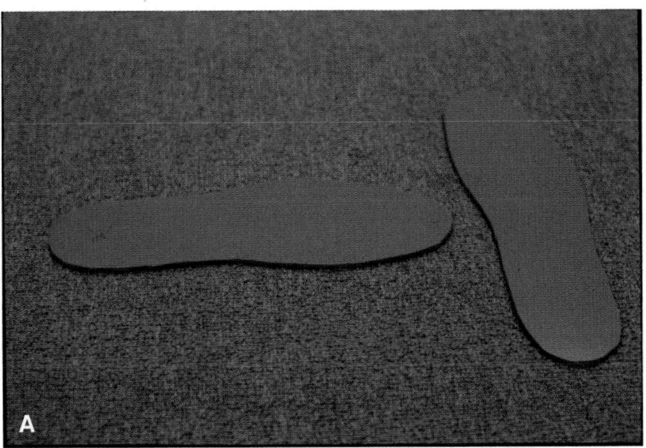

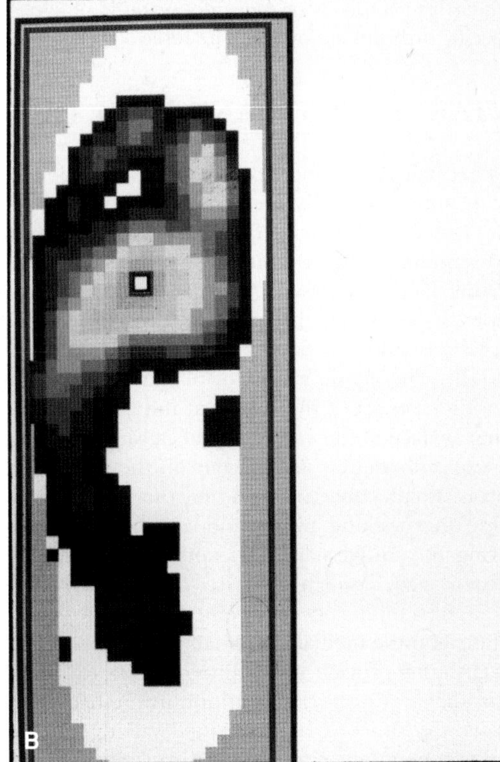

Figure 30.7. **A:** Poron (opened-cell polyurethane foam) 1/8 in. full foot insole. **B:** F-Scan recording with Poron 1/8 in. insole in athletic shoe.

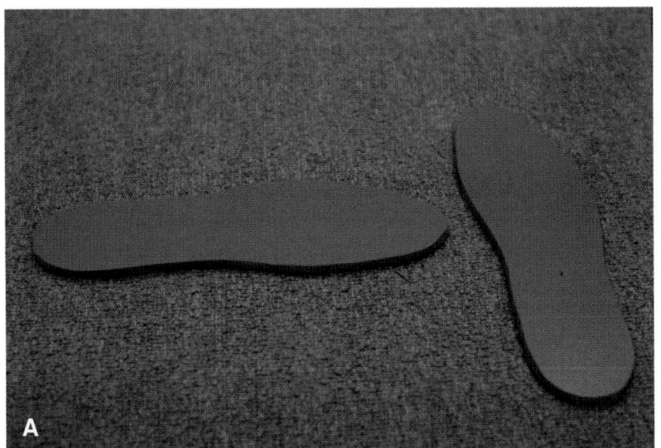

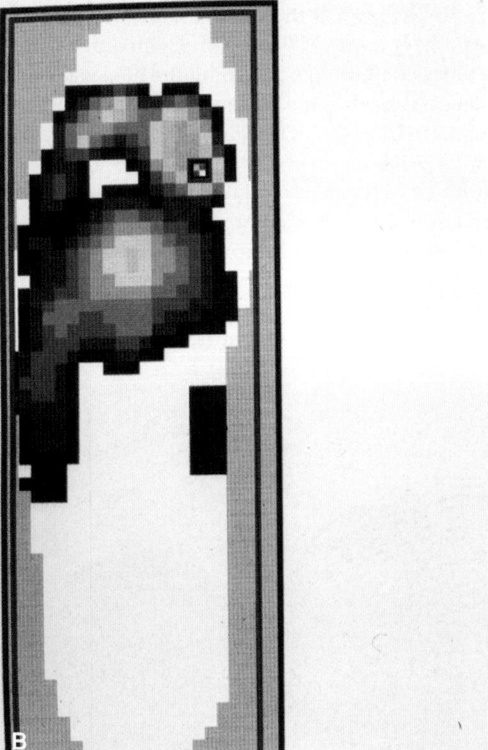

Figure 30.8. **A:** Poron (opened-cell polyurethane foam) 1/4 in. full foot insole. **B:** F-Scan recording with Poron 1/4 in. insole in athletic shoe.

therefore each warrants its own distinct orthotic design. Various sports-specific orthoses are outlined in Table 30.1.

PLANTAR FASCIITIS AND HEEL PAIN

Plantar heel pain is the most common foot problem seen in athletes; plantar fasciitis is the most common cause of this problem (12–17). The plantar fascia supports the longitudinal arch and is under constant strain during walking and running. Precipitating factors leading to plantar fasciitis include overuse injuries, hyperpronated foot, cavus foot, aging with degenerative changes, and systemic disorders such as inflammatory arthritis (18). The classic history of plantar fasciitis is marked by the insidious onset of sharp pain at the fascial insertion on the plantar surface of the anteromedial calcaneus. Arch fatigue and generalized soreness are present on the sole of the foot. The pain is usually more severe when the patient first arises, eases some after walking awhile, and returns at the end of the day. During the initial stages of exercise, the symptoms are more pronounced, easing as exercise continues. Palpation typically reveals heel tenderness anteromedially at the origin of the plantar fascia on the medial calcaneal tubercle.

Heel cushions provide a first line of relief for plantar fasciitis, providing extra shock absorption in the heel area. They help absorb the shock of heel strike in walking and running. Heel pads are generally constructed of polyvinyl chloride, silicone, leather, polyethylene foam–like Plastizote, and thermoplastics. Soft heel cups cushion and contain the fat pad and are effective for a plantar calcaneal bursitis or plantar heel spur syndrome. In patients with heel pain from fat pad atrophy, hard plastic heel cups (M-F Athletic Company, Cranston, RI) are sometimes effective in positioning the heel pad underneath the calcaneus, restoring the natural cushioning and compressibility (Fig. 30.9) (19,20). The SofSpot Viscoheel (Bauerfeind, Germany) is a silicone heel cushion that has a built-in area of softer durometer especially designed to disperse weight around the plantar medial tubercle of the calcaneus (Fig. 30.10). Sometimes a heel lift is helpful to shift pressure to the forefoot. A heel lift in the shoe should be no thicker than 1/4 in.

Excessive pronation lowers the arch and puts tensile strain on the plantar fascia. Similarly, weight bearing on the high arched

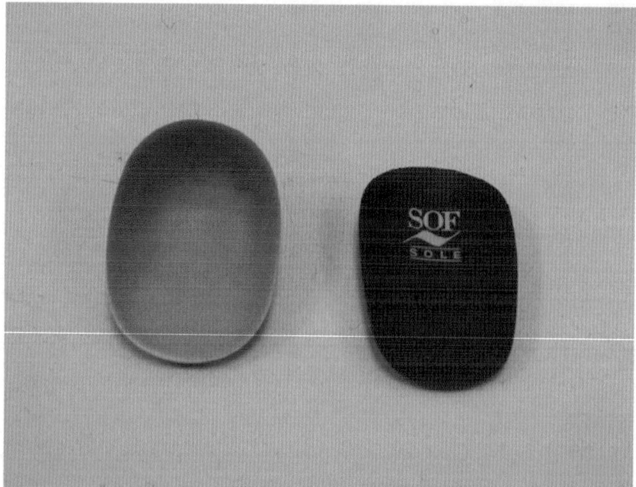

Figure 30.9. Hard plastic heel cup left and soft heel cushion right.

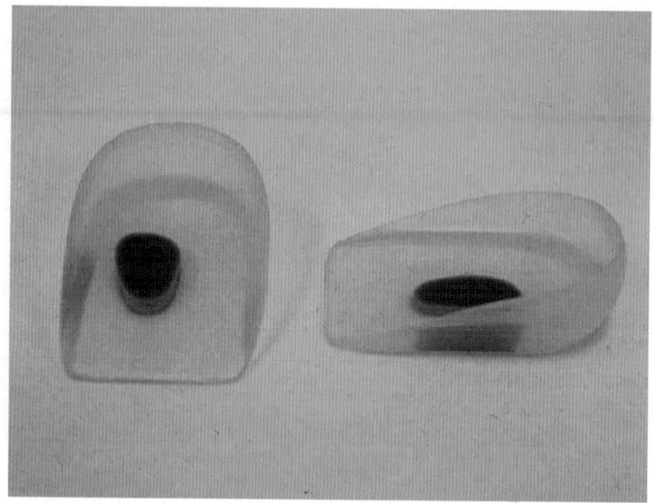

Figure 30.10. Silicone dual durometer heel cushion.

foot places the plantar fascia under tension. A foot orthosis with a raised medial arch can be used to reduce arch strain associated with plantar fasciitis. Prefabricated foot orthoses are commercially available in a wide variety of styles. Premade orthoses are adequate for many athletes with plantar fasciitis and are significantly less expensive than custom-made orthoses (Fig. 30.11).

A custom-made foot orthosis may be required for the more severe athletic foot injury. Custom foot orthoses can be made of leather or plastic. Leather has the advantage of comfort and ease of orthotic adjustments (Fig. 30.12). A whale pad design and deep heel seat leather orthosis is well suited for the treatment of heel pain as a result of plantar fasciitis. A custom device is more important for the cavus foot type than for the hyperpronated foot, which will often improve with a well-constructed prefabricated orthosis.

POSTERIOR TIBIAL TENDINITIS

The causes of posterior tibial tendinitis include overuse of the pronated foot, trauma, and degeneration as a result of rheumatic diseases. There is an association between posterior tibial tendinitis and the pes planovalgus foot type (21). Insertional posterior tibial tendinitis is associated with an accessory navicular bone, which clinically can be detected as a bony promi-

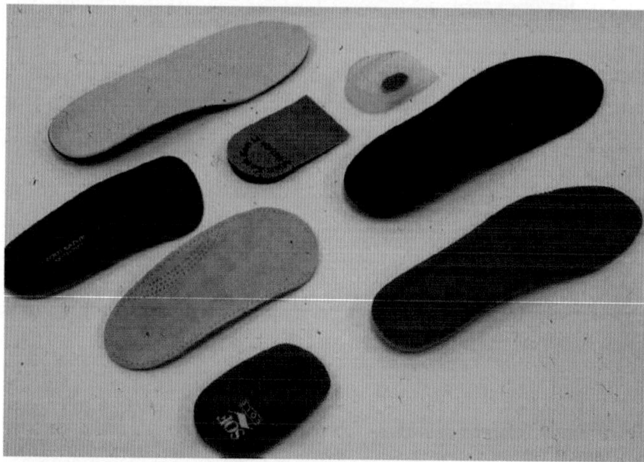

Figure 30.11. Various types of prefabricated foot orthoses.

TABLE 30.1 Sport Specific Prescription Foot Orthoses Design

Running—Running orthoses provides shock absorption (cushioning), stability (control), and durability. It stabilizes stride, reduces muscle fatigue, and improves peak performance. These orthoses are full length and semi-rigid to allow the foot to function as normally as possible. The foot must be able to pronate sufficiently to dissipate shock without causing excessive knee motion. Common adjustments made to running orthoses include: metatarsal raise pads, metatarsal bars, neuroma pads, longitudinal arch pads, Morton's extensions, heel lifts, heel cushions, heel spur pads, extrinsic heel posts, and forefoot post to sulcus.

Hiking boot—Hiking boot orthoses are both durable and flexible. They provide for increased support of the heel and back of the foot to protect against ankle sprains, shin splints, and Achilles tendonitis. Their biomechanical construction yields greater control to maximize both foot and leg function while reducing foot fatigue and medial longitudinal arch strain.

Ski—A ski boot orthoses enables effective transfer of foot movement to the edges of the skis improving skiing style, edge control, reduction of excessive pronation, and other foot imbalances. Since there is no heel-toe dynamic in skiing, this device is more rigid than an orthosis designed for use in everyday footwear, the rigidity of the orthosis is used to lock the foot in a neutral position thereby reducing pronation. With less pronation, there is a more direct and efficient transfer of pressure from the lower leg to the ski edge. Without an orthosis in place, as the knee passes over the mid-line of the foot, leverage to the edge of the ski is not maintained because there is no support of the foot and energy is lost to the flattening of the foot. This flattening of the foot translates to a loss of the effective lever arm of the lower leg to the ski edge. Overall performance and efficiency are enhanced by further adjustment of the devices based upon skiing ability, style (GS turns vs. fall line, competitive downhill and super G), and terrain (powder, hard pack, and ice surfaces).

XC Ski—This ski orthotic is thinner, lighter, and more flexible than the ski boot orthosis. Increased flexibility enables a skier to push off from side to side providing optimal medial and lateral loading while decreased volume affords the foot and toes more room to function during the step and glide motion of the sport. The rear foot is stabilized with a deep heel pocket, supplying improved power and more stable glide. These devices are regularly used to alleviate arch strain, heel pain, knee discomfort, and lower back ache.

Cycling—Cycling orthoses are designed to accommodate both recreational and professional cyclists. These orthoses improve foot mechanics, distribute plantar pressures, increase comfort, and improve cycling efficiency. The majority of cycling shoes are made without arch support. This lack of support allows unwarranted motion of the feet, ankles, and knees; thus an inefficient pedal stroke. This uncontrolled motion over-stresses the muscles and can lead to overuse injuries. The orthoses serve to position and support the feet in the most neutral position to provide for better energy transfer between the foot and pedal.

Figure skating—Figure skating orthoses are used to correct for biomechanical deficiencies thereby eliminating the need for a skaters muscles to compensate for faint imbalances; this reduces fatigue and promotes muscle function allowing for enhanced performance. Once the foot is properly aligned, skating becomes more mechanically efficient effecting quicker starts and stops, faster spins, and higher more explosive jumps. These orthoses are flexible enough to allow for the freedom of motion needed in jumping, but rigid enough to control the pronatory motion of the foot improving balance, edge control, and power in the skating stroke.

Hockey—This orthoses is manufactured with the same biomechanical advantages and features as the figure skating orthotic; however, it uses a much more rigid orthotic shell designed to handle the loads that a much larger and more aggressive skater produces. It provides support for the proper foot mechanics needed to distribute force more evenly during skating thereby increasing edge control and overall performance while decreasing fatigue in musculature throughout the body. Recreational skaters can employ these orthoses to improve the interface between the foot and the blade while satisfying individual clinical needs.

Speed skating—This skating orthoses is similar in design to the cross country ski orthotic. It differs in the types of material used and the amount of flexibility in the shell. The speed skating devices are composed of a neutral orthotic shell made out of graphite and other composites, intrinsically posted in the rear foot to provide increased stability. These devices improve a skater's mechanics increasing both speed and efficiency.

Tennis—These orthoses are composed of a thermoplastic orthotic shell with a full foot extension to the toes. The selected materials are designed to address the increased shear forces endured by the foot in this multidirectional sport. The rear foot is neutrally posted with an extrinsic heel to provide maximum biomechanics control. The forefoot is fully balanced to help redistribute the increased pressure, placed on the balls of the feet, across the entire foot reducing foot fatigue and lateral overload. This orthotic design reduces the occurrence of ankle sprains, shin splints, and knee injuries.

Squash—A specialized squash orthotic can be either three-quarters to the metatarsals or full-length. It provides more efficient lateral movement, facilitates quick changes in direction, and reduces the risk of peroneal tendon overload. This low profile device is composed of high impact flexible shells that are both durable and supportive. Common foot problems treated with this orthosis include: ankle instability, metatarsalgia, arch strain, plantar fasciitis, and Jones fracture.

Basketball—Basketball orthoses are thin, light, and durable. These semi-rigid devices provide increased shock absorption to deal with the increased forces placed on the ankles and feet, thereby protecting against chronic injuries such as stress fractures of the shins and metatarsals. Rear foot posting improves rear foot and subtalar joint control allowing for more effective control of knee tracking.

Baseball cleat—The baseball orthosis is made from high-density thermoplastic and is manufactured with an extrinsic rear foot post and a full foot extension to provide increased stability and control in both running and pivoting. Specialized modifications are made to accommodate the differing requirements of each position. A more rigid orthosis is used to provide better support during push off in pitching, while an orthosis with more flexion in the ball of the foot is used to accommodate the squatting position of the catcher.

Fishing wader—This device is made of a thermoplastic, which is durable enough to withstand constant immersion in water while maintaining the same biomechanical control of a regular orthosis. It provides increased stability to allow balance on uneven surfaces in 2–4 feet of water.

Golf—The golf specific orthosis retains the same attributes of both the tennis and basketball orthotic; however, it has an extrinsic forefoot post extension to the sulcus. This additional adjustment properly aligns stance and decreases force in the heel and Achilles region. Stance alignment results in a straighter drive of the golf ball due to increased stability through the golf swing. The forefoot posting also opens up the hips thereby improving the mechanics of the tee shot.

Dance shoe—These orthoses are made of thin flexible graphite and are designed to redistribute the large forces applied to the balls of the feet, toes, arches, and ankles during all types of dance. Dependent on the dance style and shoe type, metatarsal pads are discretely placed across the second, third, and fourth met heads to balance the forefoot area distributing body weight more evenly across the foot. Overall the dance specific orthotic provides for less stress on the forefoot, mid-tarsal, and heel.

(*continued*)

TABLE 30.1 Sport Specific Prescription Foot Orthoses Design (*continued*)

Soccer/lacrosse/rugby cleat—These orthoses are manufactured from graphite and other composite shells. The device increases contact surface area under the foot, stabilizing the rear-foot and mid-foot; thereby influencing knee alignment during rapid deceleration and protecting the foot through sudden changes of direction. The increased contact area provides a more stable plant foot when kicking resulting in increased balance, stability, power, and accuracy.

Football cleat—The football device is a fully reinforced orthotic with increased stabilization for running, jumping, pivoting, sprinting, cutting, backpedaling, and kicking. The device reduces the stress incurred by the foot when generating the large amount of torque required in sudden impacts from blocking, tackling, and quick pivoting. The orthosis also helps absorb high impact forces and reduce the occurrence of injuries such as turf toe and metatarsalgia.

Volleyball—This device is both lightweight and flexible. It is fully posted in the rearfoot to provide increased stabilization and control. A soft lined topcover cushions the foot and ankle against the repetitive stresses inherent in volleyball.

Walking—The walking specific orthosis is a semi flexible device. It is biomechanically balanced from rearfoot to forefoot providing increased support and thereby reducing the occurrence of shin splints, ankle pains, Achillies tendonitis, and calluses.

NB: These are general descriptions. Devices are prescribed and made to meet the specific clinical parameters of the patient in addition to meeting the sports and performance needs of the activity (i.e., novice skier does not have the same skills and abilities and may not have the same pathologic foot type as a pro skier and therefore may require variations of these devices).

Acknowledgements: Gregory Sands, C.O. at Ortho-Rite Laboratory for assistance with table design and creation.

nence anterior and inferior to the medial malleolus (22). Symptoms of posterior tibial tendinitis include pain in the medial aspect of the hindfoot aggravated by weight bearing. There is tenderness, thickening, and swelling from the navicular to the medial malleolus and along the course of the tendon. The pain is aggravated by active inversion and passive dorsiflexion and eversion, which stretches the tendon.

During the acute period of posterior tibial tenosynovitis, there is acute medial pain and swelling. Mechanical therapy at this time might include immobilization for 6 to 8 weeks and an ankle stirrup brace (23). During the more chronic phases of the condition, while the foot is still flexible, a foot orthosis may be appropriate. The purpose of the foot orthosis for posterior tibial tendinitis is support of the flattened arch (24). Prefabricated or custom-made orthoses may be effective. A rearfoot varus heel post added to the orthosis will also supinate the foot.

PERONEAL TENDINITIS

Peroneal tendinitis results in pain in the lateral aspect of the rearfoot and ankle. Tenderness is present along the course of the peroneal tendon from the base of the fifth metatarsal where the peroneus brevis inserts into the posterior aspect of the lateral malleolus. Active eversion and passive inversion stretching of the tendon will elicit pain. The foot orthosis used to treat peroneal tendinitis must reduce the pressure on the peroneal tendon and decrease excessive supination (25). Lateral support in the midfoot and hindfoot will perform this function. This may consist of a valgus post on the forefoot and rearfoot of the foot orthosis (Fig. 30.13).

HALLUX RIGIDUS

Hallux rigidus is a painful condition involving the metatarsophalangeal joint of the great toe. It represents an insidious and annoying condition in the athlete which can lead to significant limitations in the athlete's ability to perform. Hallux rigidus is characterized by a limitation of motion in this joint, chiefly in the direction of dorsiflexion. This limitation of motion results from a reactive proliferation of bone along the dorsal aspect of the joint and is associated with painful, degenerative arthrosis of the first metatarsophalangeal joint. Hallux rigidus is a local arthritic process, typically without accompanying arthritic degeneration of other joints of the foot and ankle.

Hallux rigidus generally presents as an isolated arthritis in the young adult without a systemic arthritic condition. This

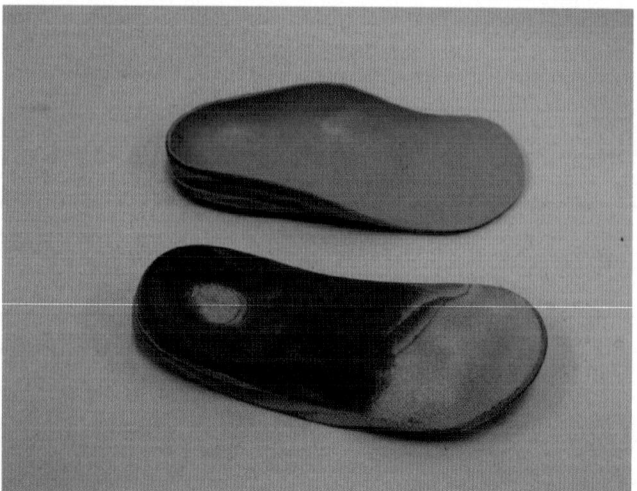

Figure 30.12. Custom-made leather foot orthosis with deep heel seat and high medial and lateral flange.

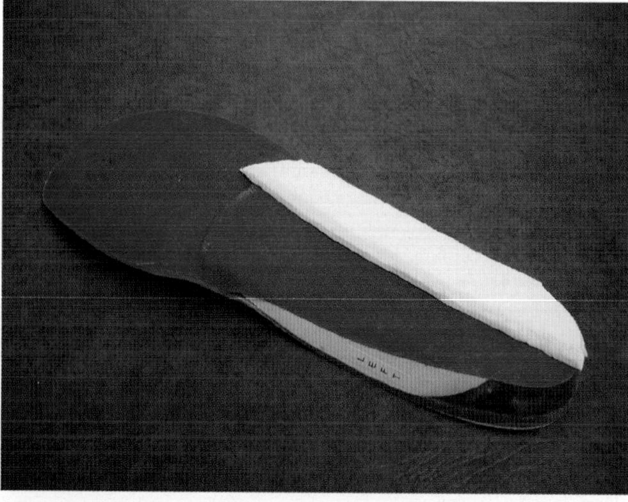

Figure 30.13. Valgus posted foot orthotic used in the treatment of peroneal tendinitis.

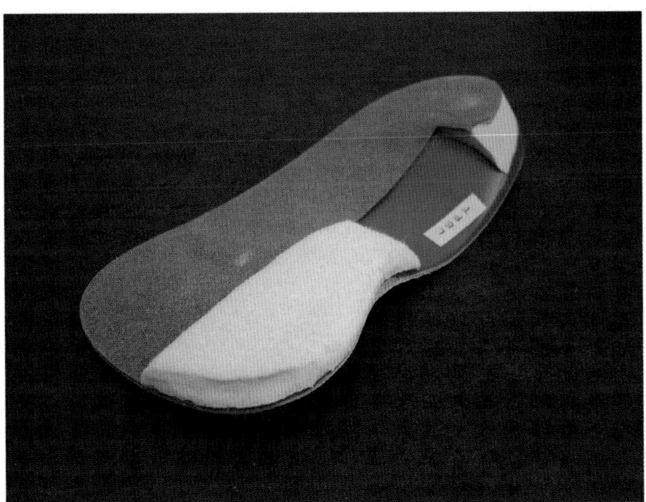

Figure 30.14. Foot orthotic with extrinsic forefoot posting used in the management of hallux rigidus.

suggests that the degenerative process is caused by some local pathologic alteration in the first metatarsophalangeal joint. Secondary joint degeneration may occur after a recognized traumatic event (26). Other theories suggest that hallux rigidus is caused by extra strain on the first metatarsophalangeal joint in a pronated foot or by an elevated first metatarsal resulting in a limitation of hallux dorsiflexion (27,28). In any case, the condition tends to be progressive.

Pain about the first metatarsophalangeal joint is the presenting symptom of patients with hallux rigidus. The patient may or may not be aware of the limitation of joint motion. Because of the limitation of dorsiflexion, patients may complain of increased difficulty with activities that place greater dorsiflexion demands such as walking up an incline, squatting, or running. Any activity that requires significant dorsiflexion of the first metatarsophalangeal joint results in impingement or jamming, which is painful. Swelling may be present around the joint, and a dorsal bony proliferation may be palpated.

Hallux rigidus presents several problems to a runner. The size of the exostosis can result in shoe rubbing and irritation from the toe box of the shoe. Stiffness of the first metatarsophalangeal joint may result in abnormal biomechanics which cause the runner to compensate by running on the lateral border of the foot or abducting the foot to roll over the medial aspect of the hallux. These forms of compensation, if left uncorrected, often lead to both foot and proximal leg pain.

It is not uncommon to observe a hyperextension deformity of the hallux interphalangeal joint as a result of hallux rigidus. This hyperextension deformity develops as a result of compensation for lack of motion in the first metatarsophalangeal joint. The interphalangeal joint may experience increased stress as dorsiflexion of the metatarsophalangeal joint becomes more limited. Palpable thickening and enlargement of the joint are also present owing to osteophyte formation. An associated plantar callosity beneath the interphalangeal joint may also result.

Shoe gear plays an important role in the management of hallux rigidus. Initial steps are aimed at relieving pressure placed on the enlarged joint by poorly fitting athletic shoes. This may be accomplished by wearing shoes with soft uppers or shoes with adequate depth and width of the toe box to accommodate the enlarged joint. The use of a stiff-soled shoe can help to decrease the dorsiflexion force. Shoe modifications can include an extended steel shank or a rocker bottom sole. However, an excessively stiff-soled shoe should be used with caution since it may promote conditions such as Achilles tendinitis and shin splints or interfere with motion, and for example, impair the delivery of the high performance pitcher.

A foot orthosis can also be a valuable tool in the management of hallux rigidus. It should be fabricated to hold the longitudinal arch in a corrected position while incorporating a sufficient (at least 5 degree) "extrinsic" forefoot varus posting to raise the head of the first metatarsal bone (Fig. 30.14). This modification allows the limited amount of dorsiflexion present to be used to the best mechanical advantage.

LEG-LENGTH DISCREPANCY

Chronic overuse problems that persist despite appropriate care are the hallmarks of the presence of a leg-length difference. The symptoms associated with leg-length discrepancies are diverse and at times vague and confusing. The incidence of lower extremity asymmetry varies from 60% to 95% in the general population (29–31). A high index of suspicion to the presence of leg-length asymmetry should always be considered in the athlete with back or lower extremity complaints.

There are three categories in the classification of limb-length asymmetry. The two major categories are structural and functional. The one minor category is environmental. It is important to be able to differentiate between structural, functional, and environmental leg-length asymmetry because the treatment for each is different. Structural discrepancies result from an actual anatomic shortening of one or more of the bones of the lower extremity. Structural leg-length differences can also result from spinal abnormalities such as scoliosis or surgical procedures such as total hip or knee replacements. Functional leg-length differences are far more common than structural pathologies. Conditions that result in functional leg-length differences include pelvic obliquity, adduction or flexion contractures of the hip, genu varum, valgum or recurvatum, calcaneovalgus, equinovarus, and rearfoot pronation. Environmental factors such as drainage crowns built into roadways, banked running surfaces, and excessive wear of shoes can create a situation mimicking a leg-length difference. These environmental factors can also either accentuate or correct structural and functional length differences depending how the athlete is running on a given surface (32).

The most common symptom associated with leg-length asymmetry is backache. Other symptoms affecting the lower extremity with a structural discrepancy usually appear first on the long leg side and include flank pain, arthritis of the knee, psoasitis, arthritis of the hip, patellar tendinitis, patellofemoral pain syndrome, plantar fasciitis, medial tibial stress syndrome, and metatarsalgia. Symptoms affecting the short extremity include iliotibial band syndrome with lateral knee pain, trochanteric bursitis, sacroiliac discomfort, Achilles tendinitis, and cuboid syndrome.

The treatment for leg-length differences often depends on whether or not symptoms are present. If the body is compensating for a length difference without causing biomechanical stress in other areas, correcting the difference may alter the body mechanics in such a way as to cause an injury. If the

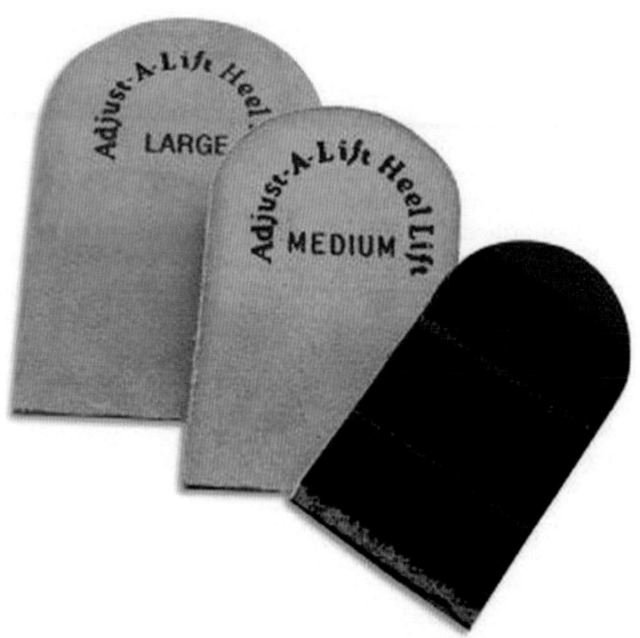

Figure 30.15. Example of adjustable heel lift.

discrepancy is causing symptoms, it must be addressed in order for the full recovery to take place.

Treatment depends on the classification of the asymmetry. Functional asymmetry due to unilateral foot pronation is corrected with the use of properly posted foot orthoses. Environmental asymmetry secondary to improper foot gear of canted running surfaces is easily treated with the use of new or appropriate foot wear or a change in the running surface. Structural limb asymmetry is treated with a heel lift (Fig. 30.15).

The purpose of the heel lift is to level off the sacral base and correct compensatory scoliosis caused by the short leg. Typically, several different types of heel lifts are used for different shoes and activities. Lifts used for sports activities require firm support to retain control and prevent injuries. A well-designed heel lift should be long enough to extend well forward under the arch to avoid "bridging" between the heel and the ball of the foot. If the lift is too short along the length of the foot or has a "slope" that is too steep, it can cause the foot to slip forward in the shoe, especially when running. The longer the heel lifts, the better it functions. A shoe lift should add elevation with minimal compressibility to avoid creating vertical heel motion and rubbing in the shoe. Firm shoe lifts are mandatory for active sports to avoid loss of control through excess motion in the shoe which can result in injuries, many of which are ankle sprains.

Most heel lifts are made of cork, foam rubbers, or various plastics. Adjustable heel lifts are available which allow for the changing of the height of the lift by removing and replacing layers of materials (15). Adjustable heel lifts are available in two varieties: Those composed of three layers of rubber or plastic foam, and a multi-layered lift, which is made of many thin layers of firm plastic. The amount of heel lift needed is determined by the indirect method of evaluating a structural shortage. This is accomplished by having the patient stand with their subtalar joint in neutral position. Then a material of known thickness is placed under the short limb until the iliac crests are level. The thickness of the heel lift under the short leg is the amount of limb-length inequality present. When using a heel lift, the heel lift height should be measured at the point where the calcaneus rests upon it, not at the back end of the lift.

The amount of heel lift that is used initially is about half of the anatomic discrepancy. This amount is used to realign the superstructure in a gradual manner. Using patient feedback, the clinician determines the final amount of lift that will produce the best results in regards to the underlying symptoms. Approximately 1/4 to 3/8 in. heel lift can fit into the average adult shoe. If more correction is required, an addition may need to be added to the outside of the shoe.

ACKNOWLEDGMENT

The authors wish to thank *Podiatry Management* for permission to use material from the article *Orthoses, Materials, and Foot Function* by Mark A Caselli.

REFERENCES

1. Pedorthic Footwear Association. *Pedorthic Definitions*. Columbia, MD: Pedorthic Footwear Association; 1996.
2. Janisse DJ. Orthoses, shoewear, and shoe modifications. In: Myerson MS, ed. *Foot and Ankle Disorders*. Philadelphia, PA: WB Saunders Co.; 2000:195–212.
3. Pribut S. Leather as an orthotic material. *Biomechanics* 1997;4(4):61–65.
4. Levitz SJ, Whiteside LS, Fitzgerald TA. Biomechanical foot therapy. *Clin Podiatr Med Surg* 1988;5(3):721–736.
5. Olson WR. Orthotic materials. In: Valmassy RL, ed. *Clinical Biomechanics of the Lower Extremities*. St. Louis, MO: Mosby; 1996:307–326.
6. Jones LS, Caselli M. Foam zone. *Biomechanics* 1996;3(1):73–77.
7. Caselli M. Silicone. *Biomechanics* 1995;2(1):55–58.
8. Caselli MA. Foot management guidelines for the diabetic athlete. *Podiatr Manag* 1998; 17(9):45–58.
9. Caselli MA, George DH. Foot deformities: biomechanical and pathomechanical changes associated with aging, part 1. *Clin Podiatr Med Surg* 2003;20(3):487–509.
10. Caselli MA, Levitz SJ, Clark N, et al. Comparison of Viscoped and Poron for painful submetatarsal hyperkeratotic lesions. *J Am Podiatr Med Assoc* 1997;87(1) 6–10.
11. Leach RE, Zecher SB. Stress fractures. In: Guten GN, ed. *Running Injuries*. Philadelphia, PA: WB Saunders Co.; 1997:30–46.
12. Dale SJ, David DJ, Sykes TF. Effective approaches to common foot complaints. *Patient Care* 1997;31:158.
13. Pfeffer GB, Baxter DE, Graves S, et al. Symposium: the management of plantar heel pain. *Contemp Orthop* 1996;32:357.
14. Duddy RK, Duggan RJ, Visser HJ, et al. Diagnosis, treatment, and rehabilitation of injuries to the lower leg and foot. *Clin Sport Med* 1989;8:861.
15. Mitchetti ML, Jacobs SA. Calcaneal heel spurs: etiology, treatment and a new surgical approach. *J Foot Surg* 1983;22:234.
16. Graham CE. Painful heel syndrome: rationale of diagnosis and treatment. *Foot Ankle* 1983;3:261.
17. LaMelle DP, Kisilewicz P, Janis LR. Chronic plantar fascial inflammation and fibrosis. *Clin Podiatr Med Surg* 1990;7:385.
18. Batt ME, Tanji JL. Management options for plantar fasciitis. *Phys Sport Med* 1995;23:77.
19. Snook GA, Christman OD. The management of subcalcaneal pain. *Clin Orthop* 1972;82:163.
20. Jorgensen U, Bojsen-Moller F. Shock absorbency of factors in the shoe-heel with special focus on role of the heel pad. *Foot Ankle* 1989;9:294.
21. Williams R. Chronic Non-Specific Tendovaginitis of Tibialis Posterior. *J Bone Joint Surg Br* 1963;45:542.
22. Gellman R, Burns S. Walking aches and running pains. *Prim Care* 1996;23:263.
23. Myerson M. Adult acquired flatfoot deformity: treatment of dysfunction of the posterior tibial tendon. *J Bone Joint Surg Am* 1996;78:780.
24. Lin SS, Lee TH, Chao W, et al. Nonoperative treatment of patients with posterior tibial tendinitis. *Foot Ankle Clin* 1996;1:261.
25. Janisse DJ. Indications and prescriptions for orthoses in sports. *Orthop Clin North Am* 1994;25:95–107.
26. Clanton TO, Ford JJ. Turf toe injury. *Clin Sports Med* 1994;13:771.
27. Jensen M. Hallux valgus, rigidus, and malleus. *J Orthop Surg* 1921;3:87.
28. Lambrinudi C. Metatarsus primus elevatus. *Proc R Soc Med* 1938;31:1273.
29. Klein KK, Buckley JC. Asymmetries of growth in the pelvis and legs of growing children. *J Am Correct Ther* 1968;22:53.
30. Pappas AM, Nehme AME. Leg length discrepancy associated with hypertrophy. *Clin Orthop* 1979;144:198.
31. Pearson WM. A progressive structural study of school children. An eight year study of children in the rural areas of Adair County, Missouri. *J Am Osteop Assoc* 1934;33:286.
32. Baylis WJ, Rzonca EC. Functional and structural limb-length discrepancies: evaluation and treatment. *Clin Podiatr Med Surg* 1988;5(3):509–520.

Amol Saxena
Brian Fullem

CHAPTER

31

Plantar Fascia Injuries

Disclosures: Drs. Saxena and Fullem have performed funded research for Storz Medical AG and received something of value. Dr. Saxena receives royalties from Mondeal NA/Tekartis, holds stock in Alter-G, Inc and serves on their advisory board.

Plantar fascia pathology, aka plantar fasciopathy, is one of the most common entities encountered by musculoskeletal specialists. It is estimated that 20% of the general population will experience some type of plantar heel pain at some point in their lives and 2 million are treated annually in the United States alone (1–6). The condition plantar fasciitis, aka "heel-spur syndrome" (which is also now coined "fasciosis" due to histopathologic findings) is common with many types of sports participants (7). It is one of the most common complaints in running athletes. Classic symptoms include pain with the first steps in the morning and after rest (post-static dyskinesia). It typically feels better with activity, though over-zealous exercise can exacerbate symptoms during activity. Chronic plantar fasciitis/fasciosis can be debilitating and may last 12 or more months but it does not have to be as we will discuss below. It has been reported that over 90% of these types of cases resolve by 12 months; this is difficult to accurately report due to the fact that patients may seek treatment from many providers (1,3,5,6,8–11). Unless follow-up assessments occur at 12 or more months after onset by the same provider, this may only be conjecture. Most studies on non-operative treatments only evaluate patients for symptoms up to 1 year or less, and do not report on the activity level (or the need for cessation). We believe most plantar fasciitis is controlled, but not necessarily cured. In addition to "classic" plantar fasciitis, other conditions such as calcaneal stress fractures and periostitis, plantar fascia and muscle ruptures, and local nerve entrapment can occur (12). Table 31.1 shows common differential diagnoses for plantar fasciopathy. The current evidence-based treatment options of these conditions will be discussed, with a focus on athletically active individuals.

FUNCTIONAL ANATOMY

The plantar fascia is an aponeurosis that covers the plantar structures of the foot, deep to the subcutaneous tissue and heel fat pad. The central portion of the plantar fascia courses from the medial process of the calcaneal tuberosity distally to blend with the flexor tendon sheaths. There are three distinct bands: Medial, central and lateral. The lateral band attaches to the lateral process of the calcaneal tuberosity proximally. The proximal fibers blend with the periosteum of the calcaneus which also blends with the distal Achilles expansion (13–15). "Classic," aka "proximal plantar fasciitis," is located in the region of the medial process of the calcaneal tuberosity where the medial and central bands attach (Fig. 31.1). The plantar aponeurosis has been described to act like a "windlass" mechanism. Clinically, this is demonstrated by dorsiflexion of the digits which causes retrograde increase in arch height due to the windlass mechanism (13–15). This is also known as the "Hubscher maneuver" or the "test of Jack" (Fig. 31.2). Inferiorly, the plantar fascia is covered by the calcaneal fat pad which consists of columns of fibrous septae containing adipose tissue. More distal, the fascia is covered by a thin layer of subcutaneous tissue. Deep (superior) to the plantar fascia is the first plantar muscular layer which includes the abductor hallucis, flexor digitorum brevis and abductor digiti minimi (13–15).

The so-called infra-calcaneal spur if present is located within the first plantar muscular layer or the deeper intrinsic muscle layers (such as the quadratus plantae) that originate from the plantar aspect of the calcaneus. (One should note that an infra-calcaneal spur is essentially a component of myositis ossificans of the plantar muscles, not the fascia. This calcification is present in approximately 40% of asymptomatic individuals, therefore the "heel spur" is generally of inconsequence.) The innervation to the region primarily occurs from the medial and lateral plantar nerves off of the tibial nerve. The muscular branch from the lateral plantar nerve to the abductor digiti minimi can become entrapped, causing symptoms such as neuritis and heel pain (12). The vascular supply to this region occurs from the posterior tibial artery which also has medial and lateral plantar branches. The venae comitantes (paired veins) course within the neurovascular bundle in the posterior medial ankle and have branches that course deeply to the fascia and muscular layers. Engorgement of these veins can cause "pseudo-tarsal tunnel" syndrome (12,16).

CLINICAL EXAMINATION AND DIAGNOSTIC CONSIDERATIONS

A typical history is obtained. Given that many patients have symmetric foot type and range of motion (ROM), there should be an attempt to find the causative agent such as erroneous

TABLE 31.1 Differential Diagnoses for Plantar Fasciitis

Local etiology:
1. Plantar fascia rupture
2. Plantar muscular strain/rupture
3. Infra-calcaneal bursitis
4. Calcaneal stress fracture/periostitis
5. Plantar nerve entrapment
6. Tarsal tunnel syndrome
7. Flexor tenosynovitis
8. Posterior tibial dysfunction
9. Spring ligament sprain/tear
10. Midfoot stress fracture
11. Plantar fibroma
12. Fat-pad atrophy
13. Chronic compartment syndrome
14. Achilles tendofasciitis
15. Calcaneal apophysitis
16. Tumor or cyst

Systemic:

17. Enthesopathy/inflammatory arthropathy
18. Spondyloarthropathy
19. Peripheral neuropathy
20. Paget's disease

Referred:

21. Radiculopathy
22. Spinal stenosis

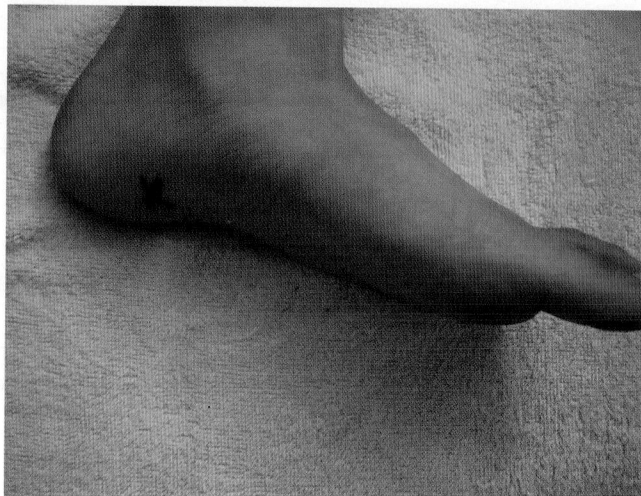

Figure 31.1. Typical plantar fasciitis location.

shoe gear or training error. This is substantiated by the observation that many athletes already have inserts or orthoses when they develop plantar fasciopathy. Patients often relate with plantar fasciitis that their symptoms began the morning after extended activity or use of atypical shoe gear. Their symptoms typically are worst with the "first morning steps," after prolonged sitting, and gets better with activity unless they over-extend themselves; then the pain can get worse, causing them to limp. Typical pain is at the medial tubercle of the calcaneus, though gait modification can cause symptoms laterally as well (Fig. 31.3). Repetitive activity, over-working one limb, such as practising a tennis serve or running on a track in one direction can be causative factors. Patients usually can bear weight with plantar fasciitis. Burning maybe present with typical plantar fasciitis but numbness and tingling should not be, nor should swelling, throbbing or bruising. Evaluation of lower-extremity ROM and foot type is performed (neutral, planus, or cavus). Asymmetry in ROM or limb length is assessed. Increased BMI has been associated but most athletes, other than American football players, have normal BMI (17). In fact, most runners who usually have lower BMI are commonly afflicted (11).

History is, however, the most important for differential diagnosis. If patients felt a sudden "pop," suspicion should be for a plantar fascia rupture. Previous localized corticosteroid injection, oral steroid and quinolone use may have occurred prior to onset of rupture. Patients with ruptures often cannot bear weight easily, and relate that they felt as if their "arch met the shoe" or their arch suddenly collapsed. Their posterior

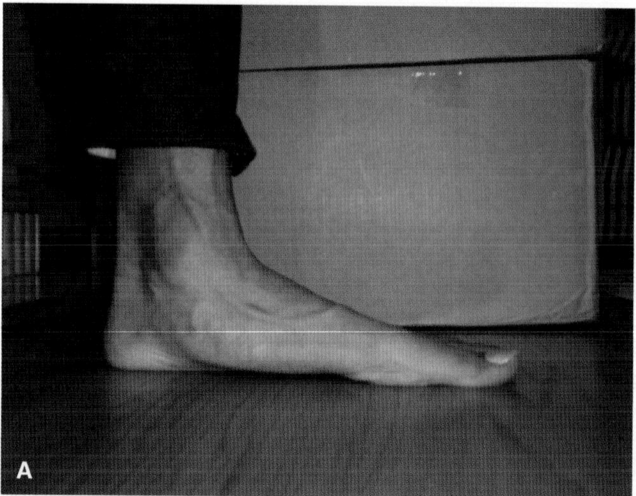

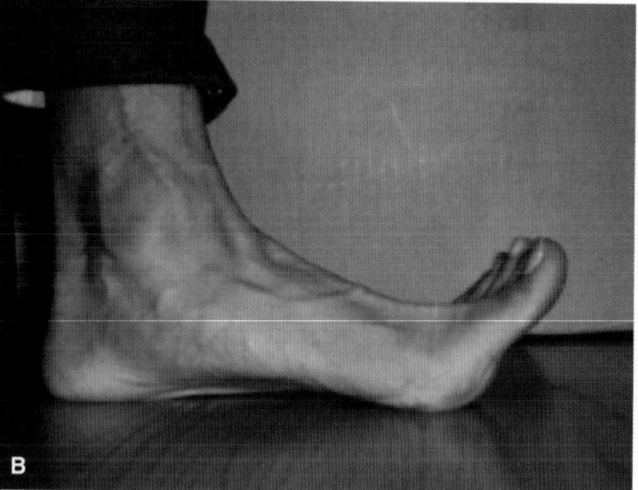

Figure 31.2. **A:** Hubscher maneuver will increase arch height **B:** dorsiflexion of the hallux.

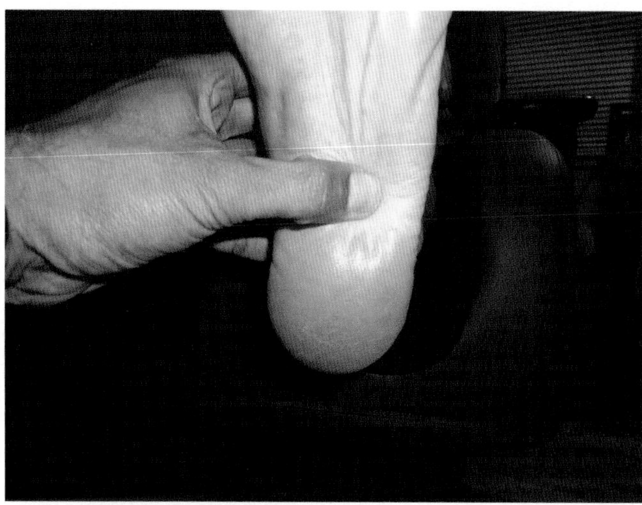

Figure 31.3. The location of lateral column pain.

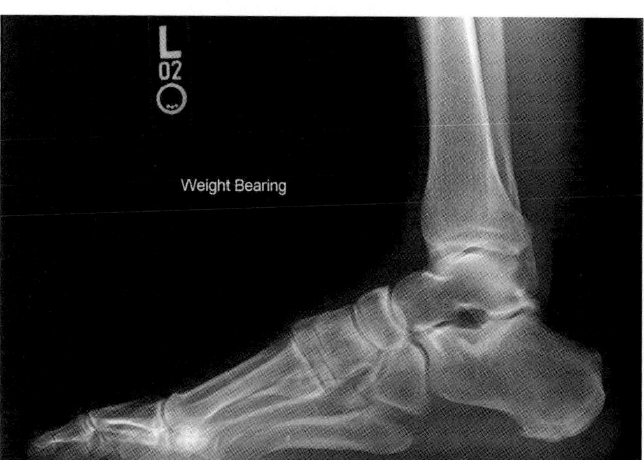

Figure 31.5. Infra-calcaneal spur in a patient with inflammatory arthropathy.

tibial and flexors will be intact. In addition, passive extension of the toes causes pain as it stretches the ruptured ligament and possibly associated intrinsic plantar muscles such as the abductor hallucis. Bruising and swelling are present with ruptures of both the fascia and the muscles (17–21) (Fig. 31.4).

Patients with stress fractures and periostitis often complain of pain that increases with activity, along with the presence of throbbing. If there is pain with squeezing the calcaneus (positive "squeeze test") then suspicion should be high for at least periostitis if not stress fracture (17). Radiographs such as plain x-ray are often *not* helpful in early cases of plantar fasciitis; however, when patients complain of "bony" symptoms, x-rays are typically performed. A large calcaneal spur or inferior erosions are associated with inflammatory arthropathy (16) (Fig. 31.5). Appropriate lab tests for gout, rheumatoid arthritis, and seronegative arthropathies such as Reiter's, psoriatic or ankylosing spondylitis via an HLA B27 marker can be ordered

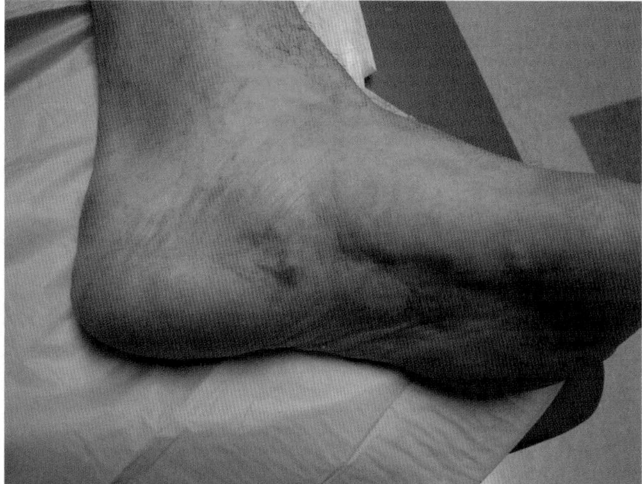

Figure 31.4. Patient with plantar fascia rupture. From Fullem B, Saxena A. Plantar Fasciitis. In: Saxena A, ed. *International Advances in Foot and Ankle Surgery.* London: Springer;2012:253–260.

in these situations. A clinical pearl is that anti-inflammatories (NSAIDs) typically do not help much in most cases of plantar fasciitis/fasciosis, since most often no inflammation may be present; however, when NSAIDs do help, there may be one of these underlying conditions. Referral to a rheumatologist should be considered in this situation and when labs are "positive." As mentioned earlier, many asymptomatic patients have a "spur" present, whereas many symptomatic patients have no spur. This is one reason why x-rays are not often requested initially. Our practice is to take initial x-rays (lateral, axial and often oblique views) when patients complain of "bony" symptoms, if bruising and swelling are present, and if there is a positive "squeeze" test. Calcaneal stress fractures can be seen on plain film, as well as technetium bone scans and MRI scans. Diagnostic ultrasound is useful to determine ruptures as is MRI. The thickness of the plantar fascia has been utilized to determine if cases will become chronic or require surgery (22,23). However, caution should be taken on judging the severity of plantar fasciitis by its thickness alone. Some ethnic groups and athletes have thicker plantar fascia with no symptoms (24). We prefer MRI over ultrasound, as other entities such as stress fracture, tenosynovitis of the deeper flexor tendons, plantar fibromas, dilatation of veins and space-occupying lesions can be evident.

Nerve symptoms manifest by numbness and tingling in the arch and/or heel. These symptoms will be present despite rest and activity. Local nerve entrapment can be aggravated by increased activity level, such as in tarsal tunnel syndrome; this can be caused by traction of the tibial nerve from excessive pronation for instance, or increased venous dilatation from prolonged standing can occur. Lateral plantar nerve entrapment usually occurs on the plantar lateral aspect of the heel (as opposed to typical plantar fasciitis and ruptures in which symptoms occur primarily medially). Note should be taken that not all lateral symptoms are due to nerve conditions; lateral compensation from medial heel pain can overload the ligaments and tendons on this side of the foot as well. Electro-diagnostics tests such as EMG/NCV can help delineate local versus more proximal nerve entrapment (such as radiculopathy and spinal stenosis) (12,16,22).

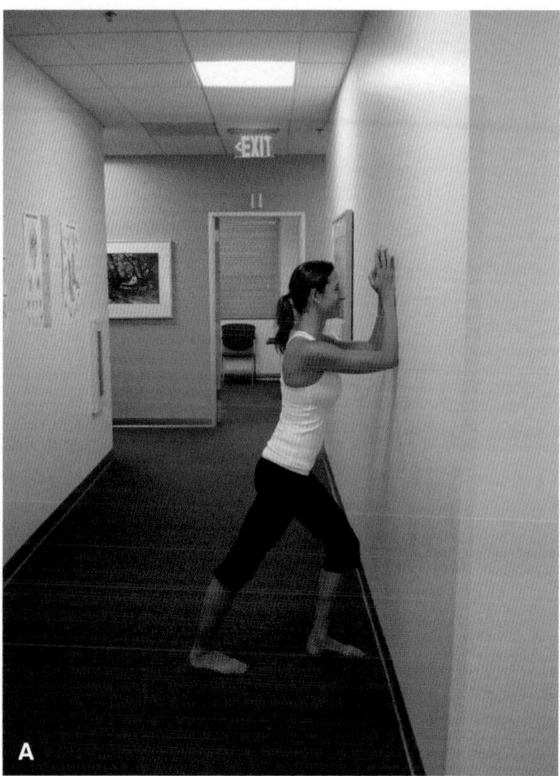

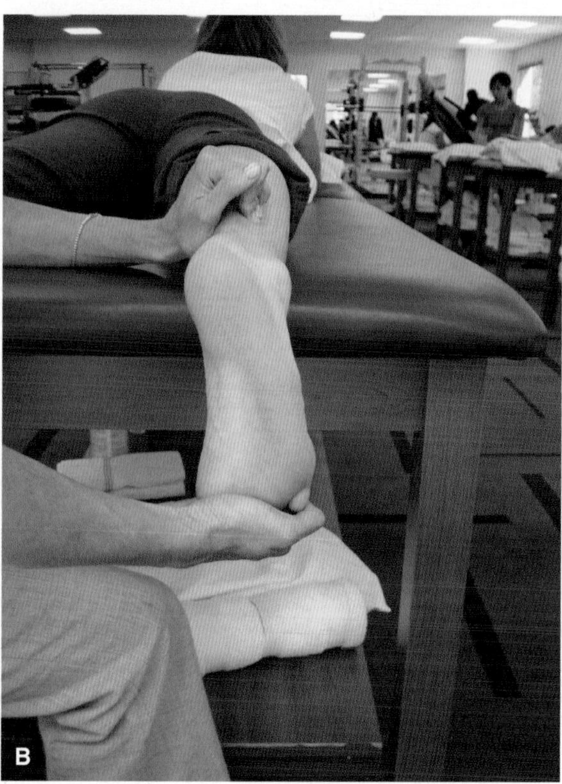

Figure 31.6. **A:** Calf stretch. **B:** Arch stretch. With permission from Saxena A, Granot A. Post-operative physical therapy for foot and ankle surgery. In: Saxena A, ed. *International Advances in Foot and Ankle Surgery.* London: Springer;2012:509–534.

THERAPEUTIC OPTIONS FOR PLANTAR FASCIITIS

Plantar fasciitis is a frustrating condition to providers and patients alike in that there are so many causative agents and therefore many therapies that seemingly "work" and it is difficult to predict "healing time." For athletes, return to activity (RTA) and return to competition can be critical (17). Recently, more evidence-based treatment approach has been adopted. We recommend an initial "three-pronged" approach: Stretching, support, and icing, along with activity modification as needed.

PHASE 1 (0 TO 3 MONTHS FROM ONSET)

The first line of treatment for plantar fasciitis is calf and arch stretching. Contracture of the gastrocnemius–soleus complex has been shown to be associated with plantar fasciitis. Caution should be taken when dealing with athletic patients as many of them have symmetric contracture (aka "equinus") and are often only symptomatic on one side. Stretching the arch and plantar fascia seems to have more of an impact (25–29) (Fig. 31.6). We have our patients hold these stretches for 15 to 30 seconds and perform them twice daily.

The next line of treatment for plantar fasciitis is appropriate shoe gear and inserts. A stiff-shanked athletic-type shoe is recommended. A shoe that flexes in the arch can cause and exacerbate symptoms (30) (Fig. 31.7). Current basketball and soccer shoe designs incorporate these "cut-out" features in order to make the shoe more light and flexible, but have been associated with an increased incidence of plantar fasciopathy in our practice. In addition, there is a current phenomenon of "barefoot running" and "minimalist shoes."

Current scientific evidence shows that when running "less protected," there is an increase in stride cadence, and subsequent decrease in contact time. While there may be less impact on the heel since the gastrocnemius–soleus complex needs to contract sooner, there is more force taken up elsewhere in the

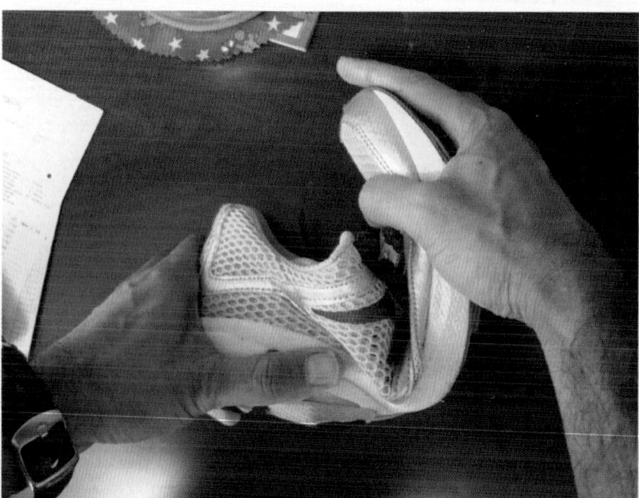

Figure 31.7. Inappropriate shoe flexibility. With permission from Fullem B, Saxena A. Plantar Fasciitis. In: Saxena A, ed. *International Advances in Foot and Ankle Surgery.* London: Springer; 2012:253–260.

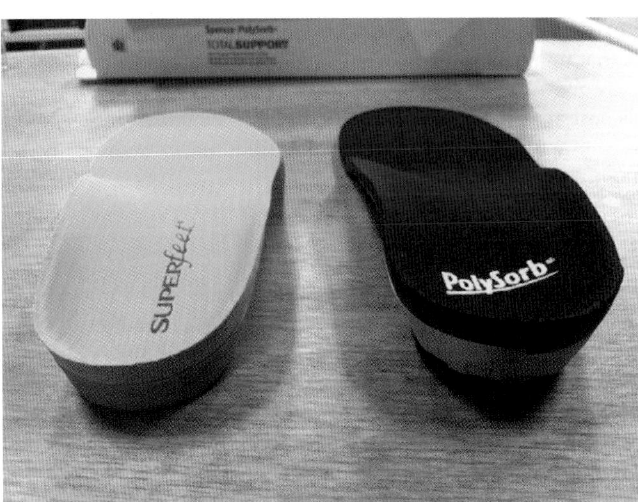

Figure 31.8. Sample over-the-counter arch supports with built-in heel cup.

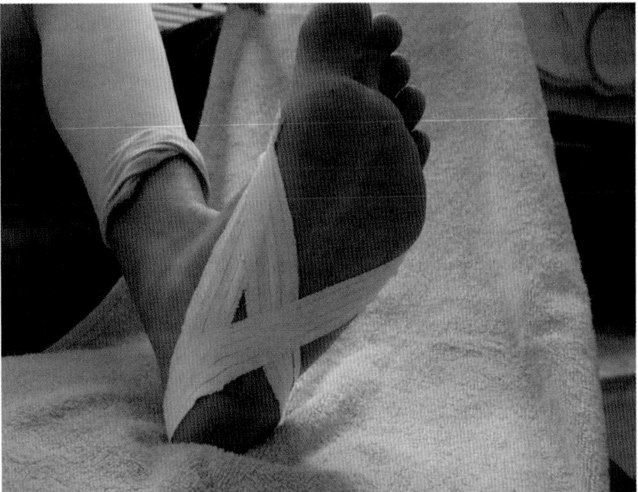

Figure 31.9. Figure of 8 arch tape as alternative to "Low-Dye" tape. With permission from Fullem B, Saxena A. Plantar Fasciitis. In: Saxena A, ed. *International Advances in Foot and Ankle Surgery.* London: Springer; 2012:253–260.

foot. Lower–heel-height shoes (and barefoot) do increase the strain on the Achilles complex, but decrease the force on the patellofemoral joint (31–35). More research needs to be done to see which type of athletes will benefit from minimalistic shoe gear, but we caution asymptomatic runners to only try barefoot running in limited amounts on safe surfaces such as grass or a cushioned track. More study needs to be done to evaluate the effects of strengthening barefoot as well, especially in regards to prevention of foot injury such as plantar fasciopathy.

Research has shown that an over-the-counter arch support with a heel cup can be helpful (8,31) (Fig. 31.8). Some patients try a heel cup or heel cushion, or even a higher-heeled shoe, but biomechanical studies show that this can increase the tension on the plantar fascia distally. Similarly, an insert with too high an arch can actually increase the tension on the medial fascia or aggravate the flexor tendons. We recommend that patients try an arch support which feels comfortable immediately, rather than have them try to "break it in." Taping is an option particularly for athletes who do not use supportive shoe gear or need to be barefoot during their sport (36,37) (Fig. 31.9). We try to have patients avoid walking barefoot during this phase. Finally, the third line of treatment is to reduce pain and inflammation if present. This is where patients can try NSAIDs but we also have them massage their arch and heel for 5 minutes by rolling their heel to the arch on a frozen water bottle, twice daily (Fig. 31.10). The primary benefit of cryotherapy for plantar fasciitis appears to be analgesia. The added benefit of massage concomitant with cryotherapy is unknown.

Physical therapy is often prescribed for plantar fasciitis and modalities such as ultrasound and iontophoresis. In studies comparing both ultrasound and iontophoresis, no significant long-term benefit has been documented. Iontophoresis using 5% acetic acid was found to be more beneficial than 0.4% dexamethasone, though both were only evaluated in the short term (6 weeks post-treatment) (37,38). We find that the benefit of physical therapy is for the evaluation of gait and functional weaknesses, limb-length inequality and to establish core strengthening which has been associated with many lower-extremity pathologies. One randomized study showed that mechanical exercise was more beneficial than utilizing electrophysiologic agents such as ultrasound followed by iontophoresis with dexamethasone in physical therapy. Patients in the mechanical-exercise group had several mobilization and stretching maneuvers performed on them for their entire lower extremity by a licensed physical therapist, twice weekly for 2 weeks, then once a week for another 2 weeks (six visits total). The patients in both groups had BMIs greater than 30, so unlikely they were athletic and no mention was made of activity level. Though this study had power, the end point was 6 months post-treatment so it is difficult to know the lasting effects of the interventions (28). As of now, based on the current literature, iontophoresis and ultrasound benefits appear short term and minimal significance for plantar fasciitis (28,37,38).

If patients are having plantar fascia symptoms during or immediately after their activity, we have them decrease or even discontinue the offending activity. Cross-training with non-impact sports or running on an Alter-G™ (Alter-G, Inc.,

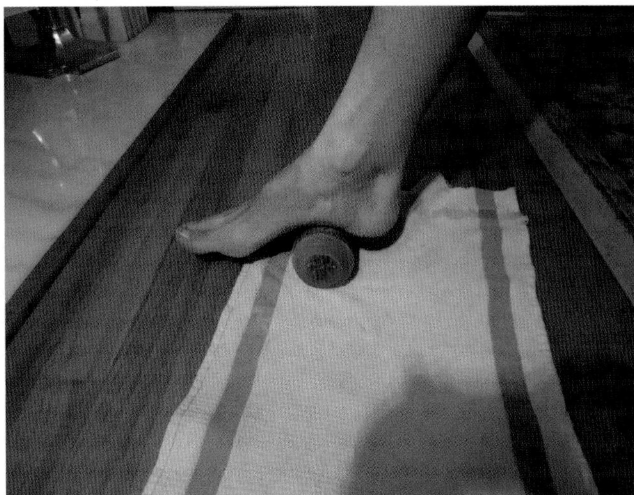

Figure 31.10. Rolling on frozen water bottle for massage and cryotherapy.

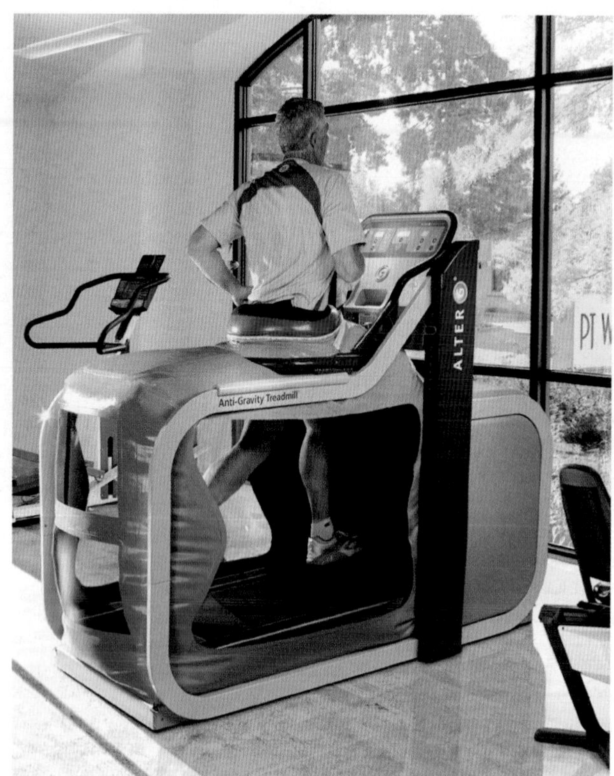

Figure 31.11. Alter-G Treadmill (courtesy Alter-G, Inc., Milpitas, CA, USA). With permission from Saxena A, Granot A. Post-operative physical therapy for foot and ankle surgery. In: Saxena A, ed. *International Advances in Foot and Ankle Surgery.* London: Springer; 2012:509–534.

Milpitas, CA, USA) treadmill may be allowed (Fig. 31.11). This treadmill allows weight-bearing activity at reduced bodyweight. Air is pumped in a chamber over the treadmill such that bodyweight can be reduced as low as 20%. We typically allow running at 60% and progress them to higher values, all the way up to 100% (full) bodyweight. We also try to have patients decrease the amount they are standing during the day.

Night splints have been found to be of value for patients complaining of morning pain (39,40). Because most patients find difficulty sleeping with them through the night and most athletes are not as concerned with the "first-step" pain, we recommend them as an adjunct, but not a primary treatment. Some athletes erroneously adopt the "more is better" approach and apply the night splint too aggressively; traction neuritis of the tibial and sural nerves has been anecdotally noted from excessive ankle dorsiflexion.

PHASE 2

If patients have been compliant with the stretching, OTC supports, icing and activity modification, and are still limited by their plantar fasciitis symptoms, then we consider three other options: Injections, custom orthoses and radial pulsed pressure wave therapy, aka "sound waves," such as D-Actor EPAT™ (Storz Medical AG, Tägerwilen, Switzerland) or SwissDolorclast™ (EMS Medical Systems, Switzerland). Unfortunately, in the United States, patients (and oftentimes providers) will only recommend therapies that are covered by indemnity insurance. On the other end of the spectrum and equally unfortunate, is that financial incentives such as "cash" for uncovered services may motivate recommendations as well. These factors such as cost and financial incentives, need to be taken into account as therapeutic guidelines are established in an evidence-based manner.

INJECTION THERAPY

Corticosteroid injections are generally covered by insurances. Therefore this is a common practice. We recommend these injections if the patient is unable to do their daily activities ("adls") and sport. The theory behind these injections is that they break down the degenerated tissue, decrease pain and provoke a healing response (31). Risks include rupture of the plantar fascia and plantar fat-pad atrophy. Anecdotally, the two authors of this chapter have experienced less than 10 possible steroid-injection-induced ruptures that they are aware of in over 40+ years of clinical practice between them. Generally 1 to 1.5 cc of medium-term–acting steroid (such as betamethasone 6mg/mL or a mixture of dexamethasone 4mg/mL and depo-medrol acetate 40 mg/mL) is deposited in the fascia space inferiorly and superiorly to the fascia origin, generally from a medial or plantar medial approach (Fig. 31.12 A–C). Ultrasonic-guided injections have been anecdotally reported to be more accurate; however, the familiarity of the anatomy of the provider rendering the injection has not been studied (41). An experienced provider (i.e., musculoskeletal specialist) should be able to render a corticosteroid injection without ultrasonic guidance, thereby saving additional medical costs. If a palpable inferior mass is felt (so-called "infra-calcaneal bursa"), this can be injected. Tumors in this region are rare; however, if there is suspicion, MRI should be performed prior to injection. Plantar fibromas have been noted in approximately 25% of surgical cases of plantar fasciitis; it may be difficult to differentiate between the two pathologies in this location (23).

Patients are advised to refrain from running and jumping for 1 week post-corticosteroid injection and must maintain their regimen from Phase 1. If the first injection was significantly helpful, a second injection can be rendered 1 or more months later. We rarely give more than three injections to one area; however, if there is a long time span, it may be considered safe. The number of injections to this area over a certain timeframe has not been thoroughly studied.

Platelet-rich plasma (PRP) and autologous blood injections (ABI) have been rendered for plantar fasciitis. These injections have not been critically studied (Level III or higher) in regards to this condition. However, when compared to placebo for Achilles tendinopathy, no significant difference has been found with PRP/ABI. There are several confounding factors with PRP such as an individual's platelet count, preparation technique, and post-injection protocols (42–45). Also, as noted above, finances play a factor. Because PRP injections are not covered by insurance, they are often not recommended early in the treatment phase. Though PRP injections appear safe, and in other applications may have a role in stimulating healing, a recent meta-analysis determined there is insufficient beneficial evidence for tendinopathy and plantar fasciopathy (45). Given the fact that there is only anecdotal evidence at this time, we generally do not recommend these based on the current literature for plantar fasciopathy (42–45).

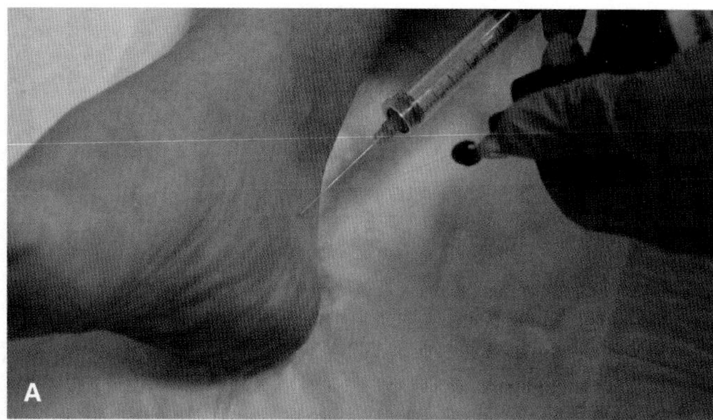

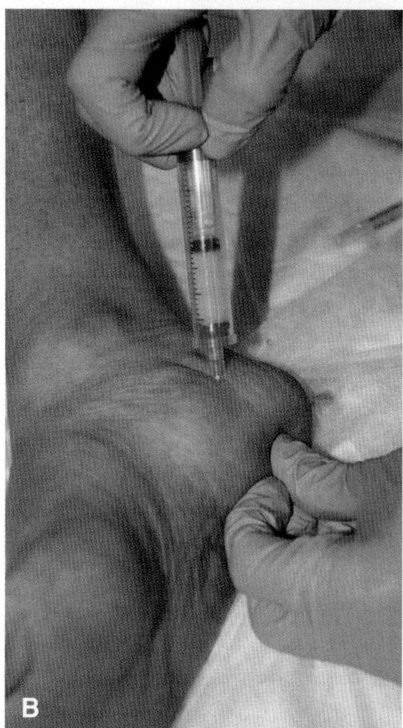

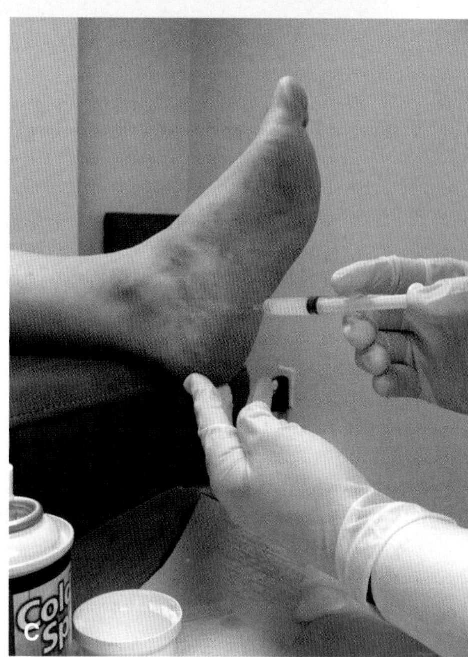

Figure 31.12. Injection techniques. **A:** Medial approach with anesthesia first being injected. **B:** Injection with corticosteroid after medial heel is numb, slightly inferior to plantar fascia origin. **C:** Plantar medial approach.

FOOT ORTHOSES

If over-the-counter arch supports have provided some degree of relief, and patients have been compliant with the other "Phase 1" components of plantar fascia "therapy," we will recommend custom devices to be considered. In the United States, there is a large variability on insurance coverage of these devices. Unfortunately, there are no definitive theories on the types of devices based on foot morphology, as there is much variability with this issue as well. Plantar fasciitis occurs in all foot types. One study found no difference with heel valgus but a higher medial arch was noted (46). It has been postulated that cavus feet benefit from softer, more accommodative inserts, whereas planus foot types benefit from firmer and more supportive inserts (46,47).

"Functional" (often thermoplastic) devices that are constructed by molds or scans of a patient's foot that take into account the foot type, lower-extremity ROM or restrictions, activity level, body habitus and shoe gear; these would be considered custom devices. These devices are typically "posted" or canted in varus to reduce excessive pronation or valgus to reduce excessive supination. Kogler et al. showed on a cadaver model that there is less tension on the plantar fascia medially when the forefoot is placed on a forefoot valgus wedge (48). A plantar fascia "groove" can be incorporated into the foot orthosis to decrease pressure on the tender fascia band or prominent tendons. This is an orthotic modification in which there is an accommodation several millimeters deep that transverses the long axis of the orthoses (Fig. 31.13A and B). Scherer relates that though many orthosis manufacturers have this as an option, there are no published data on the effectiveness of this accommodation (47). Studies show effectiveness of custom foot orthoses for plantar fasciitis to be as high as 91%, though at best, only Level III evidence exists (5,31,48,49,50). Uden et al. found several high level studies supporting the use of orthoses, but admittedly, it is difficult to conduct a Level II or higher study (31).

While it is generally acknowledged that patients should utilize their foot orthoses with ambulation while they are symptomatic with their lower-extremity condition, it is unknown for how long they should maintain them (46,47,51). We generally see if patients can "wean" themselves off their devices as their condition becomes under control. An analogous

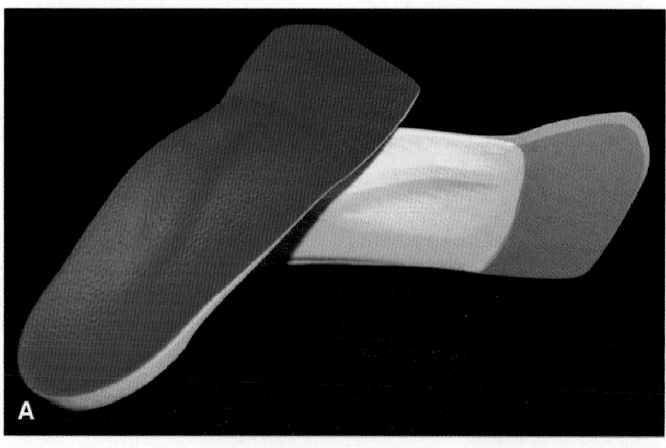

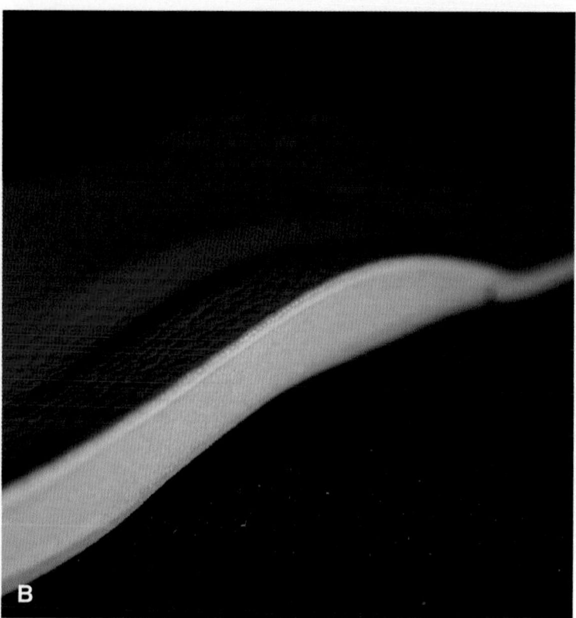

Figure 31.13. **A:** Semi-rigid thermoplastic custom device with plantar fascia groove. **B:** Cavus foot type of flexible device with plastic foam and poly-shell. (Photos courtesy of Plus Labs, Rancho Santa Fe Springs, CA, USA.)

situation is a cervical collar after whiplash; as patients recover, they no longer need their splint. Conversely, when patients necessitate eyeglasses, they only receive benefit when they use them. If patients do seem to have significant structural malalignment, we recommend them to continue with their foot orthoses. This needs to be studied further. It may be unrealistic to consider plantar fasciitis "cured" if patients need to continue with their devices; a better term would be "controlled."

PLANTAR FASCIA RUPTURES

Plantar fascia ruptures are increasingly common and should be included in the spectrum of plantar fasciopathy (17–21). This may be due to more awareness of the condition and also the increased use of MRI/ultrasound to evaluate plantar fascia conditions. Patients with ruptures notice an acute onset of intense symptoms in the arch or heel, and may even relate a "pop" sensation. Ecchymosis is common as seen in Figure 31.4. There is difficulty with weight bearing and pain with passive extension of the toes. There may be a history of prior plantar fasciitis symptoms and even prior injections. Differential diagnosis includes heel contusion, calcaneal fracture/stress fracture, pathologic fracture and heel fat-pad rupture (Fig. 31.14). Athletes in lateral motion sports such as basketball and soccer are increasingly using lighter shoe gear with less arch support. The stress of lateral sports places more torque on the arch structures making plantar fascia common with these sports. MRI examination is helpful in certain situations, particularly when "downtime" assessment is needed (Fig. 31.15). Generally, plantar fascia ruptures take longer to heal than plantar "muscle" ruptures. In our study, using our treatment protocol, athletes were able to return to their sport on an average of 9 weeks after plantar fascia rupture (17). Treatment for plantar fascia rupture includes cast-boot immobilization, with non—weight-bearing the first three weeks. Weight bearing is allowed when edema and pain have subsided. Often, an arch support is placed within the boot when weight bearing is commenced. Patients maintain their boot until they are pain-free, which is generally 3 to 6 weeks post-rupture. Cross-training is allowed on a stationary bike with the boot on, as well as swimming with the boot off (but no "flip turns"). Physical therapy is initiated at 3 to 6 weeks which included gradual stretching and strengthening, along with modalities such as electrical stimulation and cryotherapy as needed. Gradual return to sport with an arch support or custom orthosis generally occurs around 9 or more weeks post-rupture. In our study on 18 athletes, using this protocol with an average follow-up of 4 or more years, none of the patients in our series necessitated surgery, had chronic

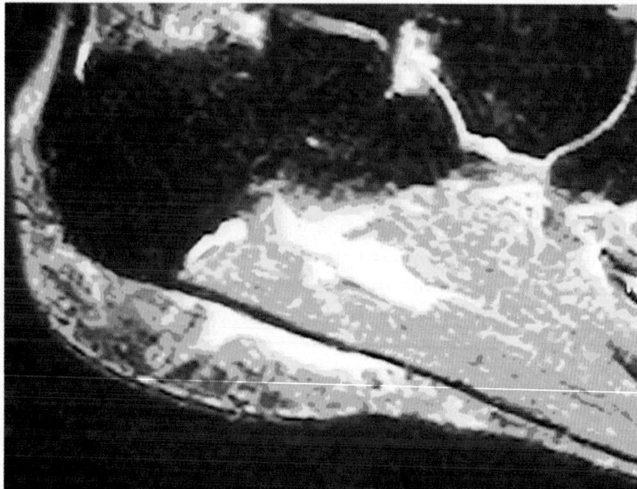

Figure 31.14. MRI of a fat-pad rupture in an elite triple jumper. Note the intact fascia and musculature, and disruption of the fat pad.

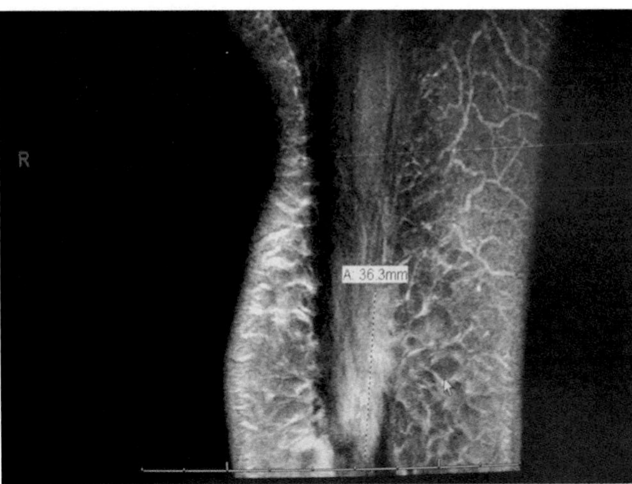

Figure 31.15. MRI of plantar fascia rupture. Longitudinal rupture in a basketball player who was able to return to play in 2 weeks. With permission from Fullem B, Saxena A. Plantar Fasciitis. In: Saxena A, ed. *International Advances in Foot and Ankle Surgery.* London: Springer; 2012:253–260.

plantar fasciitis, nor sustained a re-rupture with an average follow-up range of 2 to 10 years. We surmise that a plantar fascia rupture essentially releases the tension on the fascia and is essentially a "self-performed" surgery, with seemingly excellent results.

CALCANEAL STRESS FRACTURES/ PERIOSTITIS

Some patients with chronic plantar fasciitis can develop periostitis and stress fractures at the proximal attachment. This appears to be more common in osteopenic females. With plantar fascia ruptures, the weak point is the degenerated fascia attachment. When there is osteopenia or osteoporosis, the calcaneus is the weak point and it fatigues. These patients relate that their pain gets worse with activity, has a throbbing or deep ache quality, usually exhibit swelling and have difficulty weight bearing. They have a positive "squeeze test"; compression of the calcaneus from medial to lateral creates significant pain (Fig. 31.16). X-rays may show sclerosis in the calcaneal tuberosity often perpendicular to the plantar fascia pull (30) (Fig. 31.17 A and B). Bone scans and MRI are diagnostic (Fig. 31.18 A and B). The stress fractures associated with plantar fasciitis are different from other overuse stress fractures of the calcaneus which show sclerosis more superior and parallel to the subtalar joint (30). Metabolic assessment for calcaneal stress fractures and endocrine consult can be helpful. The treatment for calcaneal stress fractures/periostitis is cast boot immobilization for 4 to 6 weeks. As with plantar fascia ruptures, cross-training in a boot on a stationary bike or swimming is allowed. Normalization of endocrine or metabolic abnormality such as diabetes, anorexia, hyperthyroidism should be achieved before the athlete is allowed to return to weight-bearing sport. The use of an Alter-G™ (Milpitas, CA, USA) treadmill may be allowed during the healing phase. Generally patients return to their sport after 6 to 12 weeks.

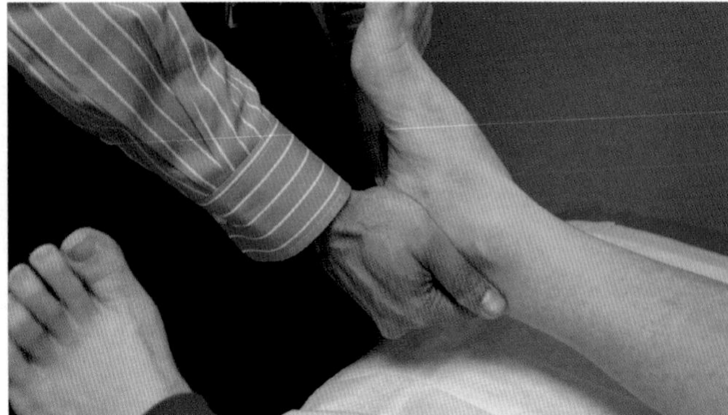

Figure 31.16. Squeeze test to determine calcaneal stress fracture and periostitis.

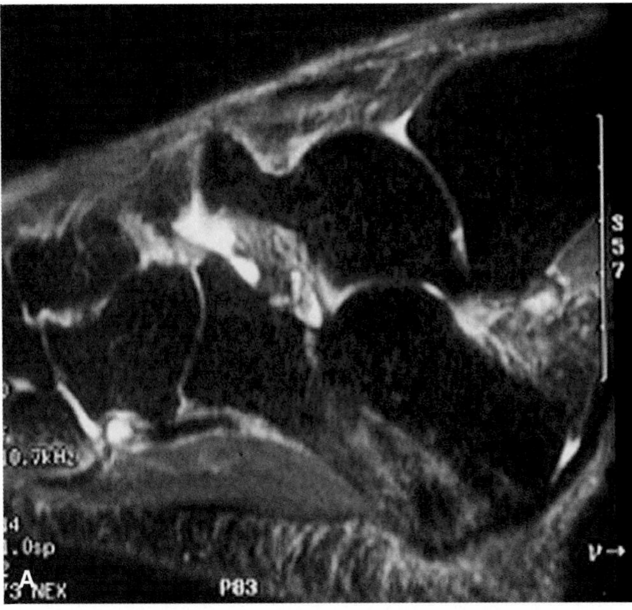

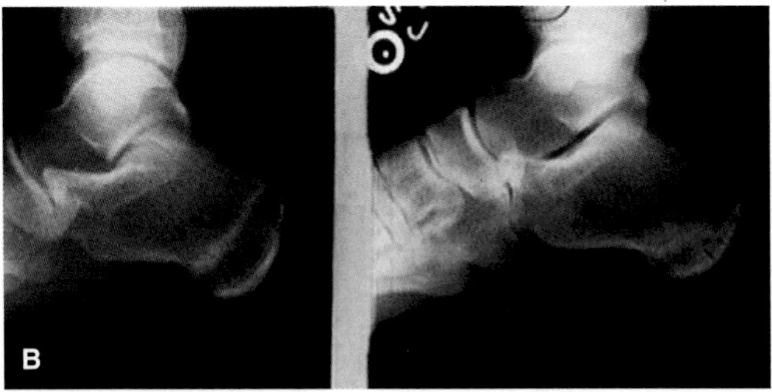

Figure 31.17. **A:** MRI showing stress fracture from plantar fasciitis. **B:** X-ray showing bilateral stress fractures from osteoporosis. Note the difference in fracture orientation.

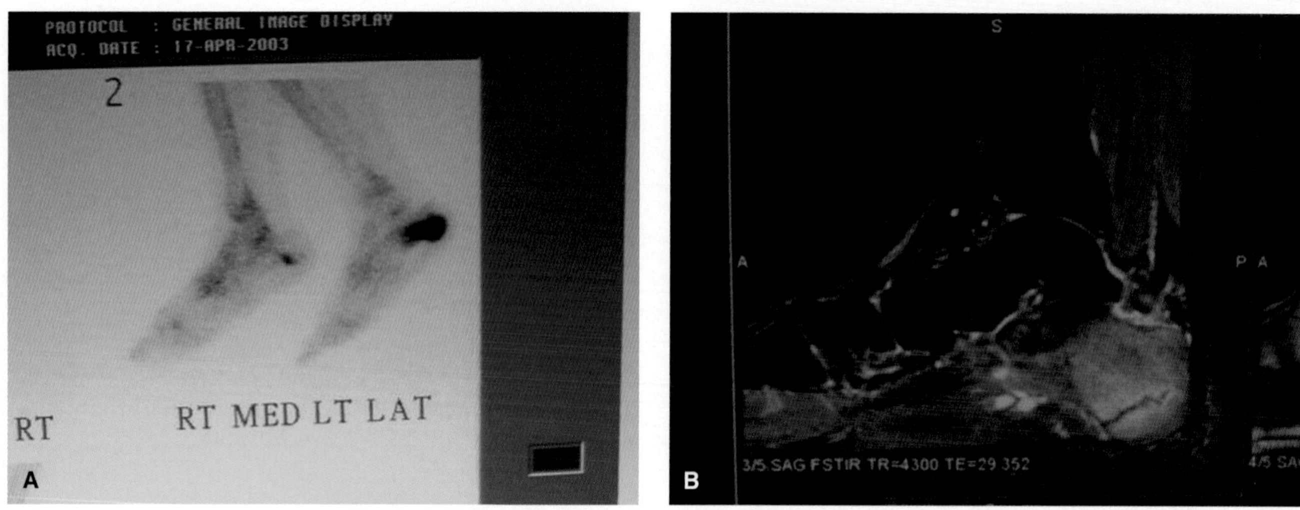

Figure 31.18. **A:** Bone scan for stress fracture. **B:** MRI for stress fracture.

EXTRACORPOREAL SHOCK WAVE THERAPY/SOUND WAVE

Extracorporeal shock wave therapy (ESWT) was first described for the treatment of plantar fasciitis by Rompe in 1996 (52). Since then, many authors have studied different forms of ESWT or orthotripsy for plantar fasciitis (9,10,52–61). The term "shock wave" is not accurate for many of the current effective devices available in the United States (56). In fact, two of the most readily available devices in the United States, D-Actor EPAT™ (Storz Medical AG, Tägerwilen, Switzerland) and SwissDolorclast™ (EMS Medical Systems, Switzerland) emit radial pressure waves, not shock waves (56). Furthermore, the terminology "high energy" and "low energy" is outdated and inaccurate.

While it has been found that "low-energy" devices produce more favorable results for plantar fasciitis and Achilles tendinopathy, many machines including radial devices can generate "high energy" (defined as ≥0.25 mJ/mm^2). The current differentiation between "sound-wave" devices are the radial pressure devices such as the ones noted above, and pulsed ultrasonic devices such as the Duolith™ (Storz Medical AG, Tägerwilen, Switzerland). The radial pressure devices are generally less costly, but both technologies can be administered without anesthesia. In fact, local anesthesia has been shown to decrease efficacy (58,59). The pulsed ultrasonic devices have broader applications beyond enthesopathies such as treatment for non-unions, avascular necrosis and wound healing. We collectively term both technologies, radial and ultrasonic, as "sound wave."

The actual sound-wave treatment involves introducing sound waves to the injured area to help regenerate the damaged tissue with local hyperemia, inhibition of pain fibers possibly through denervation and provide for growth of new blood vessels (neovascularization). The application had historically been divided into ultrasonic, aka "high energy," via one treatment, and radial, aka "low energy," using three to four treatments with weekly intervals. Early reports on the efficacy of ESWT showed a wide range of effectiveness from 40% to 70% and in some cases it was less effective than placebo. However, Rompe et al. reported that the use of local anesthesia, which was required for high-energy applications, lowered the effectiveness of the treatment. They stress the importance of being able to perform the ESWT/sound wave without anesthesia at the point of maximal tenderness for the best results; this is termed "patient focused" (58). Recently Klonschinski et al. concluded that ESWT dose-dependently activates and sensitizes primary afferent nociceptive C-fibers, and that both activation and sensitization were prevented if local anesthesia (LA) was applied in the treatment area. These results suggest that LA substantially alters the biologic responses of ESWT (59). Similar to other studies of the effectiveness of treatments for plantar fasciopathy, the follow-up and outcome-evaluation period is at the most, 1 year post-treatment. It is important to decipher the literature based on the energy level, blind versus unblinded, placebo-controlled, whether local anesthesia was utilized and post-treatment follow-up.

More recent Level I and II studies of sound wave, in particular with radial devices, show very favorable results. In many randomized, placebo-controlled studies, significant differences in outcomes between actual therapy and placebo have been documented. In one recent Level I study presented at both the American Academy of Orthopedic Surgeons Annual and American Orthopedic Society for Sports Medicine meetings showed 69% reduction in pain for plantar fasciitis with a focused pulsed ultrasonic device as compared to 34.5% for placebo after 1 year post-treatment. In this study of 246 patients, no other intervention was allowed, including refraining from NSAIDs, and a 6-week "wash-out" period from prior corticosteroid injections. Athletic patients were allowed to continue to exercise and no ruptures of the plantar fascia occurred post-treatment. Patients in this study were followed up to 2 years post-treatment (57).

Our current protocol for sound wave is to treat patients who are unresponsive to other treatments such as the ones described above in Phase 1. If patients have a relatively neutral foot type and appropriate shoe gear, and are limited in their

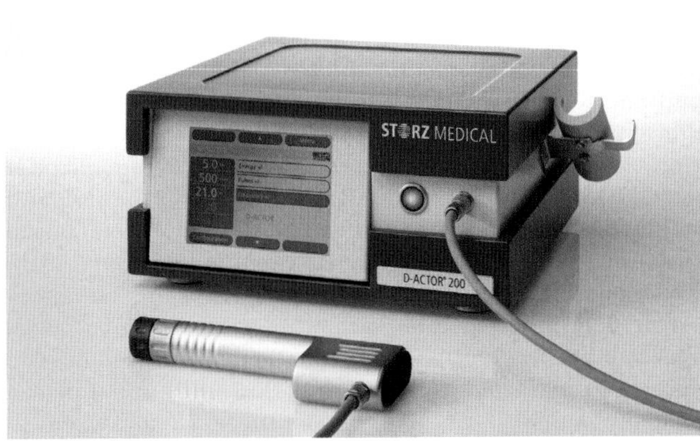

Figure 31.19. "EPAT/D-Actor" sound-wave machine. (Storz Medical AG, Tägerwilen, Switzerland). With permission from Fullem B, Saxena A. Plantar Fasciitis. In: Saxena A, ed. *International Advances in Foot and Ankle Surgery*. London: Springer; 2012: 253–260.

activity level by their plantar fasciitis, then we will offer them sound wave. Some patients may choose a corticosteroid injection first, realizing that there is a small chance of rupture with the injection and that they must restrict running and jumping activity for at least a week. Sound-wave treatment should ideally be delayed for 6 weeks after a corticosteroid injection as this may blunt the desired response. Sound-wave treatments are typically rendered three times, at weekly intervals for 2,500 pulses at 11 Hz, and 4.0 Bar with radial devices (Fig. 31.19). Patients are advised to avoid NSAIDs, and ideally ice, as both of these may decrease the body's response. Treating the calf trigger point has been anecdotally advocated. If athletic patients are sore after activity, we let them use ice and acetaminophen if needed (9,10,57). Maximum effectiveness is typically seen at 12 to 20 weeks following treatment with very few side effects being reported (9,10,55,57–59). Objective findings such as decreased plantar fascia thickness noted on ultrasound, has been shown to correlate with decreased symptoms (22,60). Consistent with other high-level studies using these types of devices, we are able to relieve approximately 70% of our patients' symptoms (9,10,55,57–59).

Cost-effectiveness is becoming critical in the treatment of many chronic medical conditions. When figuring costs associated for the typical treatment paradigm for plantar fasciopathy, on average over US $2,500 (excluding radiologic examinations) is incurred prior to the decision to consider sound wave (Table 31.2). Other than cost of treatment, there is little to no downside to the use of sound-wave technology. An argument could be made to consider sound wave earlier in the treatment algorithm, as it is perhaps the most rigorously studied therapy for treatment of plantar fasciopathy. A randomized study showed that stretching is more effective for initial treatment of plantar fasciitis than sound wave, so we recommend a trial of Phase-1 treatments first (61). However, when dealing with athletes, given the relative safety of sound-wave devices, early intervention may prevent chronic fasciitis and allow faster RTA. Sound wave should be strongly considered as treatment option before considering surgical management for plantar fasciopathy.

TABLE 31.2 Sample Charges in US$ From 12 Orthopedic and Podiatric offices for the Treatment of Plantar Fasciopathy Nationwide (Excluding Radiologic Examinations) Before Considering Sound Wave, Surgery, etc.

Doctor's office visits (initial and 2+ follow-up)	$700+
Physical therapy (minimum 6 visits)	$1,200+
Over-the-counter inserts and night splint	$60+
NSAIDs (OTC and Rx)	$15+
Custom orthoses	$350+
Corticosteroid injection	$250+
TOTAL	**$2,560+**

SURGERY FOR PLANTAR FASCIITIS

Surgery for plantar fasciitis is generally reserved for the less than 10% of the patients who are unresponsive to non-surgical treatment. Saxena reported results of a prospective Level III study on endoscopic plantar fasciotomy. His cohort comprised of 29 patients who underwent surgery for isolated plantar fasciitis, out of 866 patients seen for plantar fasciitis during the 5-year study period (11). Mean pre-operative treatment prior to surgery was 19.6 months and minimum post-operative follow-up was 2 years. This underscores the number of patients who may necessitate surgical intervention is low and that the duration of pre-operative symptoms prior to considering surgery is much more than a year.

One of the most difficult and essentially undocumented aspects of treating patients with plantar fasciopathy is how to determine if surgery is indicated. We generally do not operate on patients unless they have had symptoms and treatment for a minimum of 12 months. However, if athletic patients have had all the appropriate non-surgical treatments mentioned above, and have been unable to return to sport to their desired activity level for 6 months, we may recommend surgery for these individuals. In some unusual cases with elite runners, if there is no improvement after 3 months, because the findings show return to running is often 2 to 3 months, and even sooner with an Alter-G™, we rarely may consider surgery at this point, particularly if the Olympics or major championships are looming within a year (11). Two things to keep in mind are that for many individual sports such running and tennis, there is often no "down season" and the athletes have a very defined way of measuring their recovery (i.e., maintaining their speed or ranking). Patients may not want to rest for fear of losing fitness. We do not recommend operating on these individuals unless they have refrained from the offending activity for at least 2 months.

In general, there are relatively few studies on foot and ankle surgery on athletes. Two studies from the 1980s described an open approach, with good results (62,63). Interestingly, most studies on athletic patients who had good outcomes are on runners (11,62,63). Saxena's study was prospective, used an endoscopic approach and is the largest on athletic patients. All the athletic patients returned to their sports on average 2.7 months post-surgery with a minimum 2-year follow-up with only one patient with transient lateral symptoms. Even patients with BMI over 27 had good outcomes if they were motivated to exercise (11).

Plantar fascia surgery can be performed in three basic ways: Open, percutaneous, and endoscopic. It is generally accepted that partial plantar fascia release is the critical portion of the procedure and that a spur, if present, does not need to be removed. This is substantiated by the finding that many *asymptomatic* individuals have an infra-calcaneal spur (64). The open technique is performed from a medial approach, with an oblique incision, with the release of the abductor hallucis, and transection of the medial portion of the central plantar fascia. With this approach, nerve decompression for nerve entrapment can be performed, though different incisional approaches may be needed if nerve pathology is the primary problem (65–68). Studies comparing the open to the endoscopic approach, show a longer RTA, higher wound complications and nerve entrapment along with longer healing time with the open technique (11,12). One thing that all approaches have in common, including nerve release, is that they all include partial plantar fascia release and have protection post-operatively.

A percutaneous "instep" plantar fasciotomy can be performed for plantar fasciitis. The incision is made transversely, within the skin lines, distal to the plantar fascia origin (Fig. 31.20). The medial and lateral margins of the central plantar fascia band are indentified; the medial 50% is transected (69,70). There are no studies reporting the activity level of patients with this technique but it does appear that it is analogous to creating a plantar fascia rupture.

The senior author's preferred technique for plantar fasciotomy is the endoscopic approach. The patient is placed supine. A 4.0 30 degree endoscope is utilized. A medial incision within the skin lines is made distal to the plantar fascia origin. A fascial elevator is used to create a pathway inferior to the plantar fascia. An obturator/cannula assembly is placed in the medial incision and advanced laterally along the pathway, tenting the skin laterally. The endoscope is introduced medially; the plantar fascia should be visualized superiorly. Transillumination is used laterally to create a lateral portal; the cannula is then advanced through the skin and stabilized. The endoscope is then placed in the lateral portal to confirm tissue planes, again showing the fascia superiorly. The camera is then temporarily rotated 180 degrees inferiorly to determine the mid-point of the central plantar fascia. This will be the "end point" of the medial transection. The endoscope is rotated back and an endoscopic knife is placed medially (Mondeal NA/Tekartis, San Diego, CA and Mondeal Gmbh, Mülheim, Germany). As the blade is advanced from medial to the lateral end point, the endoscope is kept stationary so that inadvertent lateral transection does not occur. The toes are dorsiflexed to aid in transection. Sterile cotton swabs or suction can be used to aid in visualization. The ends of the transected plantar fascia should be visible (Fig. 31.21A–H). After irrigation, and instrument removal, 1cc of dexamethasone phosphate is injected in the region of the transection. Any remaining medial fibers are transected under direct visualization. The skin is re-approximated. Post-operatively, patients are placed in a short walker boot for 4 weeks; the first 2 weeks non—weight-bearing. Sutures are removed at 2 weeks. Physical therapy is begun at 4 weeks. The post-operative non—weight-bearing phase is critical in avoiding post-operative lateral column pain. Runners can RTA as soon as 4 weeks on an Alter-G treadmill and 7 weeks on regular running surfaces (11,71–74).

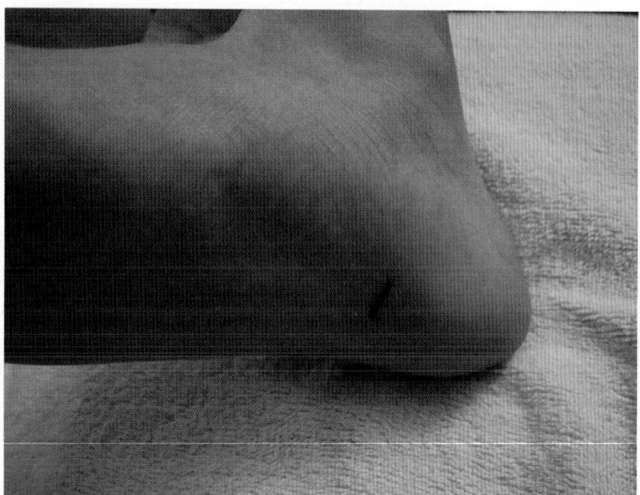

Figure 31.20. Instep plantar fasciotomy incision. With permission from Fullem B, Saxena A. Plantar Fasciitis. In: Saxena A, ed. *International Advances in Foot and Ankle Surgery*. London: Springer; 2012:253–260.

Other researchers have studied "indirect" surgery for plantar fasciopathy. Because ankle equinus has been correlated with plantar fasciitis, surgery to reduce the contracture has been studied. A recent Level IV study showed reasonable results from a proximal medial gastrocnemius tenotomy in relieving patients' symptoms. Abbassian et al. reported on 21 patients who had this procedure, with no weakness noted post-surgery, no brace was needed and 81% had good to excellent results (75). Surgery for gastrocnemius equinus may address the etiology of plantar fasciopathy but keep in mind that athletic patients may have symmetric equinus bilaterally and symptoms only unilaterally. Many asymptomatic individuals may have equinus, particularly athletes (76).

Another technique that has gained interest for the treatment of plantar fasciitis is the "TOPAZ" technique (Arthrocare, San Diego, CA). The technique uses radiofrequency in the region of the plantar fascia symptoms. To date, only Level IV studies have been reported with follow-up of 6 to 12 months (77,78). Epidermal cyst formation has been noted from this modality (79). Another radiofrequency technique is utilized for nerve ablation to the plantar fascia region. Significant reduction of the patients' pain using the VAS in this retrospective study was found. Similar to gastrocnemius recession and TOPAZ™, nerve ablation is somewhat novel as the plantar fascia integrity is maintained (80). As with most surgical results being reported, activity levels such as return to sports have not been reported by these "alternative" techniques.

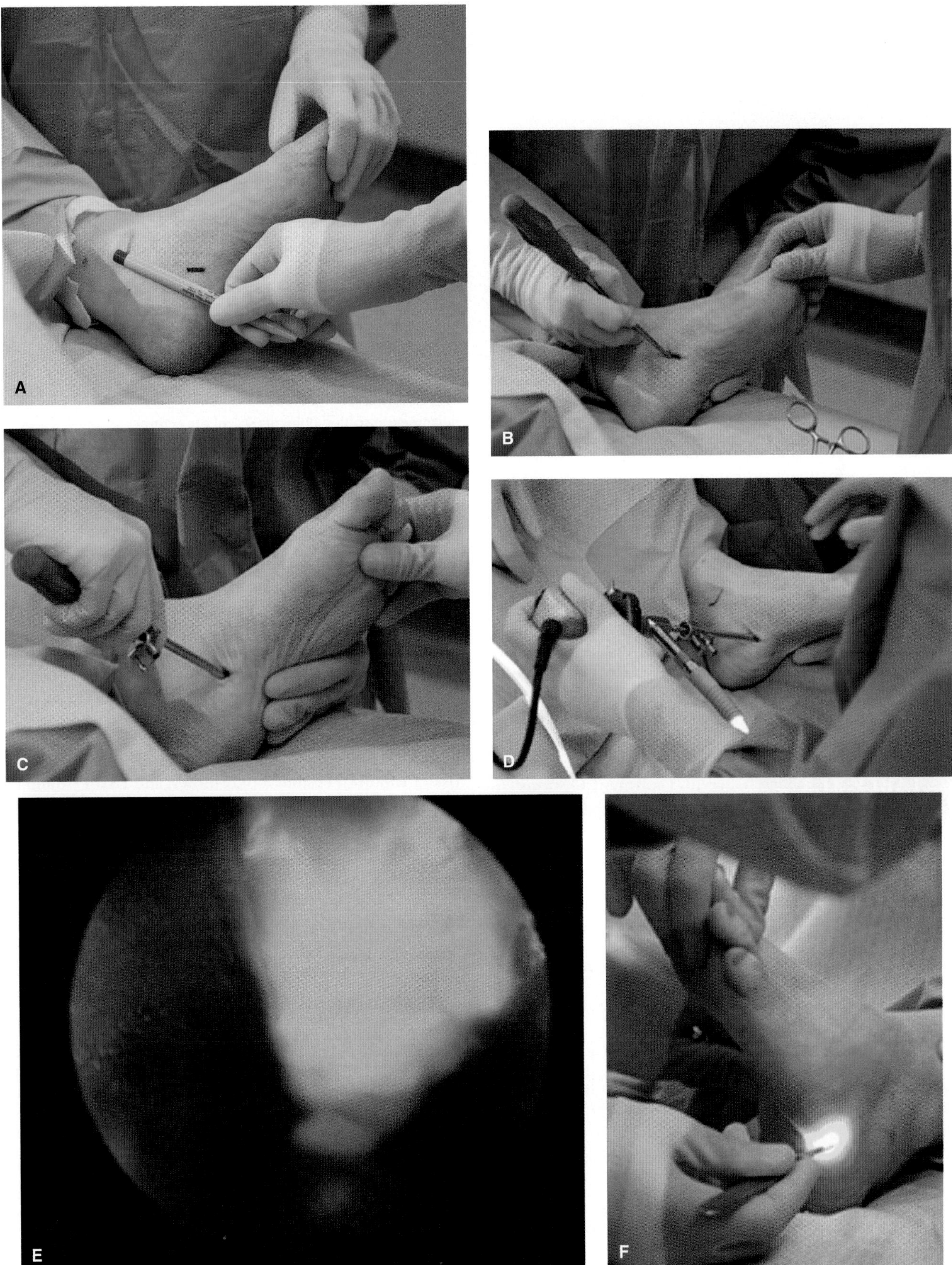

Figure 31.21. **A:** Medial incision from endoscopic plantar fasciotomy. **B:** Insertion of fascial elevator. **C:** Insertion of obturator cannula. **D:** Insertion of endoscope. **E:** View of plantar fascia superiorly. **F:** Lateral portal. **Note:** incision should be horizontal. (*continued*)

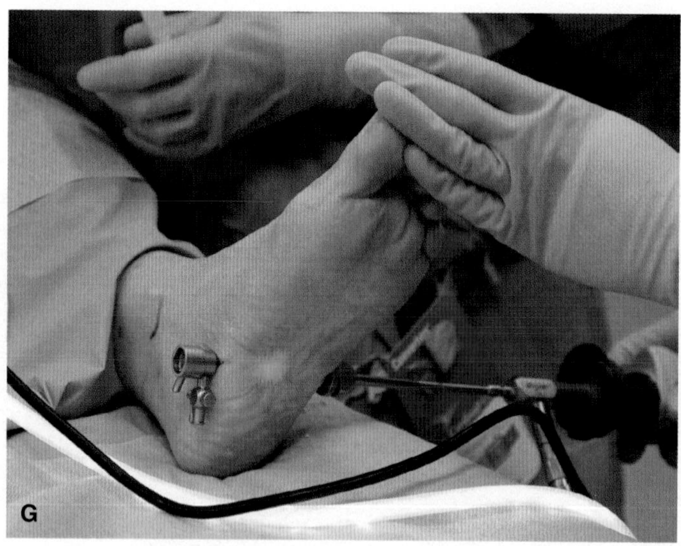

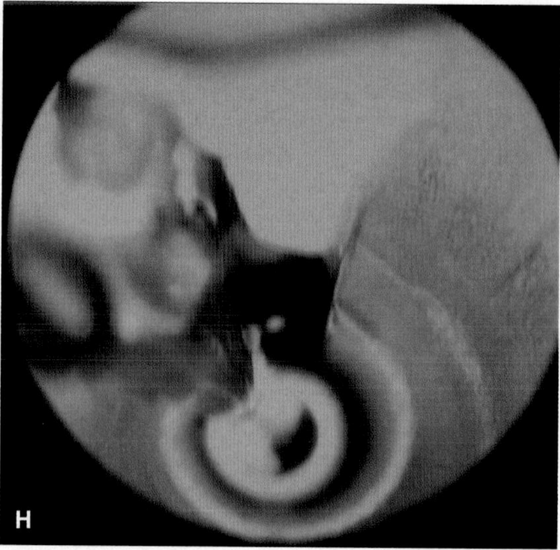

Figure 31.21. (*continued*) **G:** Transillumination to determine transection point at 50% of the central band's width. **H:** View of endoscopic blade (Mondeal Gmbh, Mühleim, Germany). With permission from Fullem B, Saxena A. Plantar Fasciitis. In: Saxena A, ed. *International Advances in Foot and Ankle Surgery.* London: Springer; 2012:253–260.

SUMMARY

Plantar fasciitis is a condition that has multiple etiologies and often lasts 12 months. Definitive diagnosis to rule out other entities such as rupture, stress fracture, and nerve entrapment is crucial. It is reported that 90% of cases "resolve" by a year, though this is difficult to determine for certain. Further study is needed to understand how some therapeutic options such as cryotherapy work and when to employ certain diagnostics such as x-ray (81,82). Plantar fasciitis is a condition that is controlled, but not necessarily cured. Table 31.3 summarizes recent research findings. Current evidence-based literature recommendations for initial ("Phase 1") treatment include stretching the calf and arch, pain control with cryotherapy and possible NSAIDs, and the use of an arch support or tape, along with appropriate shoe gear and activity modification. In unresponsive cases to these measures, the next level of treatment ("Phase 2") options such as corticosteroid injection (though athletes have to refrain from running and jumping for a week due to risk of rupture), custom foot orthoses, and ESWT/sound-wave therapy can be commenced. Recalcitrant cases, particularly runners, benefit from surgical partial plantar fasciotomy.

TABLE 31.3 Summary of Benefits of Current Treatment Options for Plantar Fasciopathy

PHASE 1:	
Stretching of calf and arch	High-level evidence
Over-the-counter arch supports	Medium-level evidence
Cryotherapy	Medium-level evidence
Night splints	High- and medium-level evidence
NSAIDs	Low level (unless inflammatory arthropathy)
Physical therapy (US and Ionto)	Low level
PHASE 2:	
ESWT/sound wave	High-level evidence
Custom orthoses	Medium-level evidence
Corticosteroid injection	Medium-level evidence
PRP/ABI	Low level
SURGERY:	
Endoscopic plantar fasciotomy	High- and medium-level evidence
Open and percutaneous fasciotomy	Low level
Gastrocnemius recession	Low level
TOPAZ	Low level

Experimental/Under-reported therapies: LASER, acupuncture, needling, massage.
Note: High = Level I and II, Medium = Level III, Low = Level IV and V.

REFERENCES

1. Taunton JE, Ryan MB, Clement DB, et al. A retrospective case-control analysis of 2002 running injuries. *Br J Sports Med* 2002;36(2):95–101.
2. Riddle DL, Schappert SM. Volume of ambulatory care visits and patterns of care for patients diagnosed with plantar fasciitis: a national study of medical doctors. *Foot Ankle Int* 2004;25:303–310.
3. Wolgin M, Cook C, Graham C, et al. Conservative treatment of plantar heel pain: long-term follow-up. *Foot Ankle Int* 1994;15:97–102.
4. O'Brien D, Martin WJ. A retrospective analysis of heel pain. *J Am Podiatr Med Assoc* 1985; 75:416–418.
5. Scherer PR. Biomechanics Graduate Research Group for 1988: Heel spur syndrome: pathomechanics and nonsurgical treatment. *J Am Podiatr Med Assoc* 1991;81:68–72.
6. Lynch DM, Goforth WP, Martin JE, et al. Conservative treatment of plantar fasciitis: a prospective study. *J Am Podiatr Med Assoc* 1998;88:375–380.
7. Lemont H, Ammirati KM, Usen N. Plantar fasciitis: a degenerative process (fasciosis) without inflammation. *J Am Podiar Med Assoc* 2003;93(3):234–237.
8. Pfeffer G, Bacchetti P, Deland J, et al. Comparison of custom and prefabricated orthoses in the initial treatment of proximal plantar fasciitis. *Foot Ankle Int* 1999;20(4):214–221.
9. Gerdesmeyer L, Frey C, Vester J, et al. Radial extracorporeal shock wave therapy is safe and effective in the treatment of chronic recalcitrant plantar fasciitis: results of a confirmatory randomized placebo-controlled multicenter study. *Am J Sports Med* 2008;36(11): 2100–2109.
10. Gollwitzer H, Diehl P, von Korff A, et al. Extracorporeal shock wave therapy for chronic painful heel syndrome: a prospective, double blind, randomized trial assessing the efficacy of a new electromagnetic shock wave device. *J Foot Ankle Surg* 2007;46(5):348–357.
11. Saxena A. Uniportal endoscopic plantar fasciotomy: a prospective study on athletic patients. *Foot Ankle Int* 2004;25(12):882–889.

12. Wapner KL, Puri RD. Heel and subcalcaneal pain. In: Thordarson DB, ed. *Orthopaedic Surgical Essentials: Foot & Ankle.* Philadelphia, PA: Lippincott Williams & Wilkins; 2004:182–194.
13. Bøjsen-Möller F, Flagstad KE. Plantar aponeurosis and internal architecture of the ball of the foot. *J Anat* 1976;121:599–611.
14. Pontious J, Flanigan KP, Hillstrom HJ. Role of the plantar fascia in digital stabilization. A case report. *J Am Podiatr Med Assoc* 1996;86:43–47.
15. Sarrafian S. *Anatomy of the Foot and Ankle: Descriptive, Topographic, Functional.* Philadelphia, PA: Lippincott; 1993:591–602.
16. Gould JS. Tarsal tunnel syndrome. *Foot Ankle Clin* 2011;16(2):275–286.
17. Saxena A, Fullem B. Plantar fascia ruptures in athletes. *Am J Sports Med* 2004;32(3):662–665.
18. Acevedo JI, Beskin JL. Complications of plantar fascia rupture associated with corticosteroid injection. *Foot Ankle Int* 1998;19(2):91–97.
19. Sellman JR. Plantar fascia rupture associated with corticosteroid injection. *Foot Ankle Int* 1994;15:376–381.
20. Leach R, Jones R, Silva T. Rupture of the plantar fascia in athletes. *J Bone Joint Surg Am* 1978;60:537–539.
21. Kim C, Cashdollar MR, Mendicino RW, et al. Incidence of plantar fascia ruptures following corticosteroid injection. *Foot Ankle Spec* 2010;3(6):335–337.
22. Mahowald S, Legge BS, Grady JF. The correlation between plantar fascia thickness and symptoms of plantar fasciitis. *J Am Podiatr Med Assoc* 2011;101(5):385–389.
23. Hafner S, Han N, Pressman M, et al. Proximal plantar fibroma as an etiology for recalcitrant plantar heel pain. *J Foot Ankle Surg* 2011;50(2):153-157.
24. Uzel M, Cetinus E, Ekerbicer HC, et al. The influence of athletic activity on the plantar fascia in healthy young adults. *J Clin Ultrasound* 2006;34(1):17–21.
25. Digiovanni BF, Nawoczenski DA, Lintal ME, et al. Tissue-specific plantar fascia-stretching exercise enhances outcomes in patients with chronic heel pain: a prospective, randomized study. *J Bone Joint Surg Am* 2003;85:1270–1277.
26. Patel A, Digiovanni B. Association between plantar fasciitis and isolated contracture of the gastrocnemius. *Foot Ankle Int* 2011;32:5–8.
27. Sweeting D, Parish B, Hooper L, et al. The effectiveness of manual stretching in the treatment of plantar heel pain: a systematic review. *J Foot Ankle Res* 2011;4:19.
28. Cleland JA, Abbott JH, Kidd MO, et al. Manual physical therapy and exercise versus electrophysical agents and exercise in the management of plantar heel pain: a multicenter randomized clinical trial. *J Orthop Sports Phys Ther* 2009;39(8):573–585.
29. Digiovanni BF, Nawoczenski DA, Malay DP, et al. Plantar fascia-specific stretching exercise improves outcomes in patients with chronic plantar fasciitis. A prospective clinical trial with two-year follow-up. *J Bone Joint Surg Am* 2006;88(8):1775–1781.
30. Fullem B, Saxena A. Plantar Fasciitis. In: Saxena A, ed. *International Advances in Foot and Ankle Surgery.* London: Springer; 2012:253–260.
31. Uden H, Boesch E, Kumar S. Plantar fasciitis - to jab or to support? A systematic review of the current best evidence. *J Multidiscip Healthc* 2011;4:155–164.
32. Squadrone R, Gallozzi C. Biomechanical and physiological comparison of barefoot and two shod conditions in experienced barefoot runners. *J Sports Med Phys Fit* 2009;49:6–13.
33. Smith GA, Bressel E, Branscomb J. Impact acceleration of the leg: comparison of shod and barefoot treadmill running. *Med Sci Sports Exer* 2010;42:133–134.
34. Divert C, Mornieux G, Freychat P, et al. Barefoot-shod running differences: shoe or mass effect. *Int J Sports Med* 2008;29:512–518.
35. Squadrone R, Gallozzi C. Biomechanical and physiological comparison of barefoot and two shod conditions in experienced barefoot runners. *J Sports Med Phys Fitness* 2009;49:6–13.
36. van de Water AT, Speksnijder CM. Efficacy of taping for the treatment of plantar fasciosis: a systematic review of controlled trials. *J Am Podiatr Med Assoc* 2010;100(1):41–51.
37. Osborne HR, Allison GT. Treatment of plantar fasciitis by LowDye taping and iontophoresis: short term results of a double blinded, randomised, placebo controlled clinical trial of dexamethasone and acetic acid. *Br J Sports Med* 2006;40(6):545–549.
38. Gudeman SD, Eisele SA, Heidt RS Jr, et al. Treatment of plantar fasciitis by iontophoresis of 0.4% dexamethasone. A randomized, double-blind, placebo-controlled study. *Am J Sports Med* 1997;25(3):312–316.
39. Berlet GC, Anderson RB, Davis H, et al. A prospective trial of night splinting in the treatment of recalcitrant plantar fasciitis: the ankle dorsiflexion dynasplint. *Orthopedics* 2002;25(11):1273–1275.
40. Al-Bluwi MT, Sadat-Ali M, Al-Habdan IM, et al. Efficacy of EZStep in the management of plantar fasciitis: a prospective, randomized study. *Foot Ankle Spec* 2011;4(4):218–221.
41. Louwers MJ, Sabb B, Pangilinan PH. Ultrasound evaluation of a spontaneous plantar fascia rupture. *Am J Phys Med Rehabil* 2010;89(11):941–944.
42. Taylor DW, Petrera M, Hendry M, et al. A systematic review of the use of platelet-rich plasma in sports medicine as a new treatment for tendon and ligament injuries. *Clin J Sport Med* 2011;21(4):344–352.
43. Andia I, Sánchez M, Maffulli N. Platelet rich plasma therapies for sports muscle injuries: any evidence behind clinical practice? *Expert Opin Biol Ther* 2011;11(4):509–518.
44. Paoloni J, De Vos RJ, Hamilton B, et al. Platelet-rich plasma treatment for ligament and tendon injuries. *Clin J Sport Med* 2011;21(1):37–45.
45. Sheth U, Simunovic N, Klein G, et al. Efficacy of Autologous Platelet-rich plasma use for orthopedic indications: a meta-analysis. *J Bone Joint Surg Am* 2012;94:298–307.
46. Ribeiro AP, Trombini-Souza F, Tessutti V, et al. Rearfoot alignment and medial longitudinal arch configurations of runners with symptoms and histories of plantar fasciitis. *Clinics (Sao Paulo)* 2011;66(6):1027–1033.
47. Scherer P. Chapter 3: Mechanically Induced Plantar Fasciitis and Subcalcaneal Pain in Recent Advances. In: Scherer P, ed. *Orthotic Therapy: Improving Clinical Outcomes with a Pathology-Specific Approach.* Albany, NY: Lower Extremity Publishing LLC; 2011:43–55.
48. Kogler G, Veer FB, Solomonidis SE. The influence of medial and lateral placement of orthotic wedges on loading of the plantar aponeurosis. *J Bone Joint Surg Am* 1999;81A:1403–1413.
49. Landorf KB, Keenan AM, Herbert RD. Effectiveness of foot orthoses to treat plantar fasciitis. *Arch Intern Med* 2006;166(6):1305–1310.
50. Baldassin V, Gomes CR, Beraldo PS. Effectiveness of prefabricated and customized foot orthoses made from low-cost foam for non-complicated plantar fasciitis: a randomized controlled trial. *Arch Phys Med Rehab.* 2009;90(4):701–706.
51. Roos E, Engstrom M, Soderberg B. Foot orthoses for the treatment of plantar fasciitis. *Foot Ankle Int.* 2006;27(8):606–611.
52. Rompe JD, Hopf C, Nafe B, et al. Low-energy extracorporeal shock wave therapy for painful heel: a prospective controlled single-blind study. *Arch Orthop Trauma Surg* 1996;115(2):75–79.
53. Ho C. Extracorporeal shock wave treatment for chronic plantar fasciitis (heel pain). *Issues Emerg Health Technol* 2007;96(1):1–4.
54. Chuckpaiwong B, Berkson EM, Theodore GH. Extracorporeal shock wave for chronic proximal plantar fasciitis: 225 patients with results and outcome predictors. *J Foot Ankle Surg* 2009;48(2):148–155.
55. Marks W, Jackiewicz A, Witkowski Z, et al. Extracorporeal shock-wave therapy (ESWT) with a new-generation pneumatic device in the treatment of heel pain. A double blind randomised controlled trial. *Acta Orthop Belg* 2008;74(1):98–101.
56. Saxena A, Ramdath S, O'Halloran P, et al. Letter to the editor. *J Foot Ankle Surg* 2011; 50(6):753–754.
57. Gollwitzer H, Saxena A, Didomenico L, et al. Focus ESWT for chronic plantar fasciitis. *J Bone Joint Surg* 2012 (in press)
58. Rompe JD, Meurer A, Nafe B, et al. Repetitive low-energy shock wave application without local anesthesia is more efficient than repetitive low-energy shock wave application with local anesthesia in the treatment of chronic plantar fasciitis. *J Orthop Res* 2005;23(4): 931–941.
59. Klonschinski T, Ament SJ, Schlereth T, et al. Application of local anesthesia inhibits effects of low-energy extracorporeal shock wave treatment (ESWT) on nociceptors. *Pain Med* 2011;12(10):1532–1537.
60. Hammer DS, Adam F, Kreutz A, et al. Ultrasonographic evaluation at 6-month follow-up of plantar fasciitis after extracorporeal shock wave therapy. *Arch Orthop Trauma Surg* 2005;125(1):6–9.
61. Rompe JD, Cacchio A, Weil L Jr, et al. Plantar fascia-specific stretching versus radial shock-wave therapy as initial treatment of plantar fasciopathy. *J Bone Joint Surg Am* 2010; 92(15):2514–2522.
62. Snider MP, Clancy WG, McBeath AA. Plantar fascia release for chronic plantar fasciitis in runners. *Am J Sports Med* 1983;11:215–219.
63. Leach RE, Seavey MS, Salter DK. Results in surgery in athletes with plantar fasciitis. *Foot Ankle Int* 1986;7:156–161.
64. Shama SS, Kominsky SJ, Lemont H. Prevalence of non-painful heel spur and its relation to postural foot position. *J Am Podiar Med Assoc* 1983;73(3):122–123.
65. Sinnaeve F, Vandeputte G. Clinical outcome of surgical intervention for recalcitrant infero-medial heel pain. *Acta Orthop Belg* 2008;74:483–488.
66. Hendrix CL, Jolly GP, Garbalosa JC, et al. Entrapment neuropathy: the etiology of intractable chronic heel pain syndrome. *J Foot Ankle Surg* 1998;37:273–279.
67. Dellon AL. Technique for determining when plantar heel pain can be neural in origin. *Microsurgery* 2008;28:403–406.
68. Baxter DE. Release of the nerve to the abductor digiti minimi In: Kitaoka HB, ed. *Master Techniques in Orthopaedic Surgery of The Foot and Ankle.* Philadelphia, PA: Lippincott Williams and Wilkins; 2002:359.
69. Woelffer KE, Figura MA, Sandberg NS, et al. Five-year follow-up results of instep plantar fasciotomy for chronic heel pain. *J Foot Ankle Surg* 2000;39(4):218–223.
70. Boberg J. Plantar fascia surgery in master techniques. In: Chang T, ed. *Podiatric Surgery: The Foot and Ankle.* Lippincott: Philadelphia, PA; 2005:222–224.
71. Bazazz R, Ferkel R. Results of endoscopic plantar fascia release. *Foot Ankle Int* 2007;28: 549–556.
72. Shapiro S. Endoscopic plantar fasciotomy. In: Scuderi G, Tria A, eds. *Minimally Invasive Surgery in Orthopedics.* New York, NY: Springer; 2009:427–436.
73. Bader L, Park K, Gu Y, et al. Functional outcome of endoscopic plantar fasciotomy. *Foot Ankle Int* 2012;33(1):37–43.
74. Saxena A. Endoscopic plantar fasciotomy versus pulsed ultrasonic soundwave in runners. *J Musc Lig Tend* (in press)
75. Abbassian A, Kohls-Gatzoulis J, Solan MC. Proximal medial gastrocnemius release in the treatment of recalcitrant plantar fasciitis. *Foot Ankle Int* 2012;33(1):14–19.
76. Saxena A, Kim W. Ankle dorsiflexion in adolescent athletes. *J Am Podiatr Med Assoc* 2003;93(4):312–314.
77. Weil L Jr, Glover JP, Weil LS Sr. A new minimally invasive technique for treating plantar fasciosis using bipolar radiofrequency: a prospective analysis. *Foot Ankle Spec* 2008;1(1): 13–18.
78. Sean NY, Singh I, Wai CK. Radiofrequency microtenotomy for the treatment of plantar fasciitis shows good early results. *Foot Ankle Surg* 2010;16(4):174–177.
79. Ferguson K, Thomson AG, Moir JS. Case study: Epidermoid cyst following percutaneous Topaz coblation for plantar fasciitis. *Foot (Edinb)* 2012;22(1):46–47.
80. Liden B, Simmons M, Landsman AS. A retrospective analysis of 22 patients treated with percutaneous radiofrequency nerve ablation for prolonged moderate to severe heel pain associated with plantar fasciitis. *J Foot Ankle Surg* 2009;48(6):642–647.
81. Bizzini M. Ice and modern sports physiotherapy: still cool? *Br J Sports Med* 2012;46: 219.
82. Levy JC, Mizel MS, Clifford PD, et al. Value of radiographs in the initial evaluation of non-traumatic adult heel pain. *Foot Ankle Int* 2006;27(6):427–430.

CHAPTER

32

Stephen L. Comite
Natalia Mozol
Melanie Ng
Ashley Mehl
Jessica Siegelheim
Carmen Alcala

Sports Dermatology of the Foot and Ankle

INTRODUCTION

The skin is our largest organ and, of course, the most visible. Nearly everyone has some dermatology problem some time during one's lifetime. Indeed for Olympic athletes, dermatologic issues were the most common complaint (1).

This chapter will focus on skin problems, both common and uncommon, that can affect the feet of athletes. The chapter is divided and grouped arbitrarily into infectious, mechanical, environmental, papulosquamous, nail, and miscellaneous topics. For further details on any particular subject, the references should help guide the way. Now, it is our best feet forward.

VERRUCA PLANTARIS, VERRUCA VULGARIS

Verruca vulgaris, commonly known as warts, are termed verruca plantaris or plantar verruca when located on the foot (Fig. 32.1). They often are hyperkeratotic and occur in areas of pressure such as the heel and ball of the foot (2). Periungual warts are especially difficult to treat. Multiple warts that fuse together are known as mosaic warts.

Foot warts are a common problem and may be painful and spread to other locations on the feet, often causing morbidity in athletes. In one report, a college tennis player experienced weeks of pain causing her to discontinue playing; imaging studies including an x-ray and a bone scan to rule out a stress fracture were performed (3).

When these tests were negative, the athlete was advised to rest. After 2 weeks, the symptoms recurred during her next tennis match. She again went to the emergency room, where it was finally determined that she had a verruca vulgaris within her calluses. Indeed, two teammates had been treated for plantar verrucas, and had used the same shower facilities.

Plantar warts are caused by the human papillomavirus (HPV) and affect approximately 7% to 10% of the population. HPV is divided into several subtypes, dependent on its tendency to affect a specific body part. Verruca plantaris, for instance, affecting plantar feet, is mainly caused by subtypes 1, 2, 4, 27, and 57 (4,5).

Warts are generally transmitted through contact between hosts, through a cut or abrasion in the skin. In one study of participants who used a public bath, plantar warts were found in about 5% of the boys and 10% of the girls (6).

The virus most commonly manifests in children, adolescents, and those who are immunocompromised; warts are more common in females than in males (7). Although the virus proliferates in warmer environments, it can also survive in cooler settings, even without a host. Therefore, athletes and those using public showers while barefoot are at risk for developing warts (8).

A study done in a public school in Nashville, Tennessee compared the incidence of plantar warts in swimmers; those who use public shower rooms versus those who only use public locker rooms were evaluated. It was found that the affected number of individuals with warts who used public shower rooms (27%) was much greater than those non-users (1%) (9). Along with swimming pool decks, locker rooms, and showers, plantar warts can also be spread in changing rooms (7). In another study, swimmers were 1.81 times more likely to have warts than non-swimmers, though the results were not statistically significant (10). Participants in the Special Olympics had a rate of verruca similar to that of the general population although this was an observational survey without further laboratory or other evaluation (11).

While warts elsewhere on the body are usually exophytic, because of pressure from ambulation, plantar warts are generally endophytic. Individuals affected by the virus may have pain in the affected foot, as well as leg or back pain.

Physicians diagnose the plantar warts clinically; if in doubt as to the diagnosis, the affected foot can be soaked in water for 5 to 10 minutes followed by debridement of the lesion. The clinician should note the absence of the usual dermatoglyphic lines and the presence of black dots due to bleeding within the verruca. Dermatoscopy may be of assistance as well (12).

The warts can also be analyzed histopathologically showing acanthosis and hyperkeratosis, increased mitotic activity, and elongated rete ridges arranged in a centripetal manner (13). Additional characteristic features of verruca vulgaris are foci of vacuolated cells, vertical tiers of parakeratotic cells, and foci of clumped keratohyalin granules (14). These changes are pronounced in young verruca vulgaris, but less so in older ones (15).

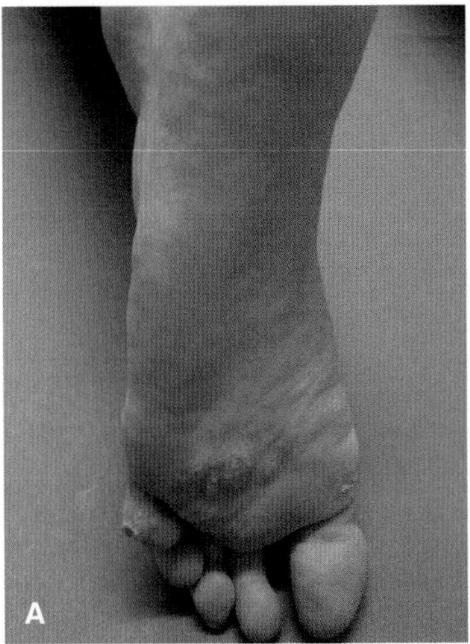

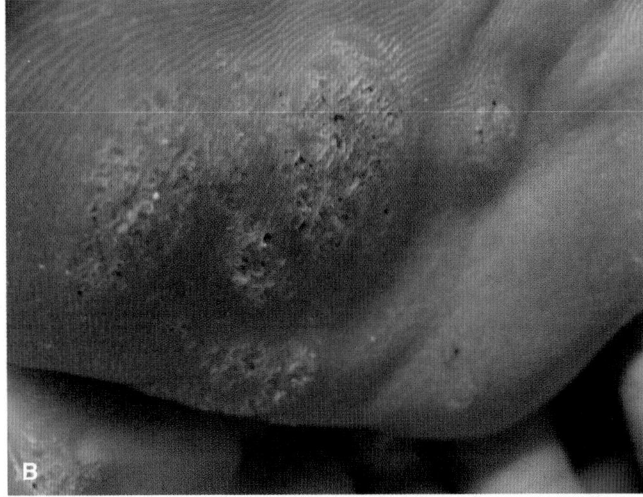

Figure 32.1. Verruca vulgaris foot. **A:** Foot with mosaic warts. **B:** Close-up of mosaic warts. Note the black dots from thrombosed blood vessels.

In most athletes, plantar warts need to be treated because of the pain, the risk of spreading, and the possibility of limitation upon one's sport (9). In healthy individuals, warts may resolve by themselves in months to years (13). Today there is a wide array of treatments available for the treatment of verruca plantaris. Treating warts can be a challenge as warts may be resistant to many therapies and therefore a patient may have variable responses. Often treatments have to be used in combination with one another for optimal results. While not always possible, one main objective is to avoid scarring.

We recommend a biopsy in all cases of suspicious, long-term, or recalcitrant warts. Occasionally what has been treated as a wart is actually a verrucous carcinoma or even a melanoma (16,17). Other diagnoses that should be considered include calluses, corns, keratoacanthomas, non-healing ulcers, foreign bodies, and nevi.

Before seeking professional help for plantar warts, often patients resort to over-the-counter salicylic acid medications, which may or may not be strong enough for resolution (18). In order to use most of these products properly, one should soak the wart for a few minutes to soften it and scrape off the excess debris with either a pumice stone or an emery board.

Topical treatments for warts are myriad but data is severely lacking as to efficaciousness. According to a Cochrane review, simple treatments including salicylic acid are more effective than placebo, but studies have been inadequate overall (19).

Physicians commonly use cryotherapy as a first line of therapy, whereby liquid nitrogen at a temperature of −196°C is used to freeze the lesions and repeated every 2 to 3 weeks for variable lengths of time. This treatment can cause pain, though it is generally minimal and temporary, and may occasionally cause blisters (4). Blisters tend to be less common on the feet as they often go unnoticed since they may be removed by ambulation. One study showed that of the 34 patients treated with cryotherapy, 14 (41%) experienced complete resolution (20). Cryotherapy alone is, in many cases, insufficient; other topical treatments are often necessary. Some patients ask about freeze products that are over-the-counter such as Verruca-Freeze®. This product freezes tissue only to −70°C compared to cryotherapy, which as stated above, gets much colder (4).

Duct tape is another easy-to-use approach for the treatment of warts, but the results are variable (21). In one study, duct tape was more successful than cryotherapy, but few of the patients in the study had plantar warts (22). The method of action for duct tape is unclear; it works perhaps by occlusion or heat. Since occasionally warts not under duct tape occlusion also resolve, perhaps there is an immune system effect as well. Irritation and maintaining placement are typical problems associated with duct tape use. The recommended technique is to leave the duct tape on for 6 days, and then remove on the 7th day. On the day the tape is removed, the wart can be soaked and gently scraped with a pumice stone or an emery board. In one double-blind controlled study, the researchers found no statistically significant difference between moleskin and duct tape for the treatment of warts in adults (7); however, they used transparent, acrylic-based duct tape rather than silver, rubber-based duct tape (23). Many of the patients had difficulty maintaining the pads, and the size of the duct tape was smaller than the wart. The study did not differentiate between types of warts and their location on the body. In another study, while 60% of the patients had resolution of their warts using cryotherapy, 85% had resolution using duct tape (24). However, in this paper it was unclear if the study participants were completely blinded and if the follow-up was complete.

Though cantharone or 0.07% cantharadin, derived from the blister beetle, is no longer FDA-approved in the United States, it can be used as part of a compound and remains a safe and effective treatment, with a success rate of up to 80%. This treatment should be repeated every 2 to 3 weeks and can cause blisters, so it should be used with care in athletes (18). In one retrospective study of 144 patients, 95% showed clearance after a compounded solution of cantharadin 1%, podophyllotoxin 5%, and salicylic acid 30% was used. Only 9% of patients required a second application (25). There is a similar commercial preparation available outside of the United States containing cantharadin 1%, podophyllin 2%, and salicylic acid 30% in an acetone, ether, and alcohol solution.

One combination that appears promising is the twice-daily application of topical salicylic acid with fluorouracil (26). In a study of 20 patients, all achieved full resolution though two patients temporarily developed local dermatitis.

Other destructive modalities include intralesional bleomycin (27–32). Bleomycin sulfate's mode of action is that it inhibits both DNA and RNA synthesis and consequently protein synthesis, processes required for a wart's survival. Injection of bleomycin into the wart causes vascular microthrombosis and hemorrhagic necrosis, which result in the wart decreasing in size and subsequent destruction. In one study, all patients treated with bleomycin experienced a decrease in the size of the plantar wart, and 54 of 62 (87%) patients experienced complete resolution after 6 months (32). Recently, however, supplies of bleomycin have been limited. Many patients who have been treated with bleomycin experience pain, inflammation, and eschar formation, so the clinician should be aware of these side effects when treating the athlete (33). Rare complications include flagellate hyperpigmentation (34), localized urticaria in hand warts (35), Raynaud's phenomenon (36) and nail loss if bleomycin has been used for periungual verruca (31,37,38).

Another destructive modality is the injection of fluorouracil. It is thought to be effective as it replaces a component of the viral DNA, thereby eliminating the proliferation ability of the wart. It was shown that 70% of verrucas treated by injections with 5-FU plus lidocaine with epinephrine showed complete response (100% decrease), while 18% showed partial response (50% to 100% decrease), and 12% showed no response (less than 50% decrease) (39). Another paper also discussed the use of intralesional 5-FU, lidocaine, and epinephrine (40). Complete resolution was observed in 64% of warts treated with this mixture, while in the placebo group there was only a 34% response. The injections were given weekly for 4 weeks. However, besides noting that the warts were symmetrical, there was no discussion as to where the warts were located, and the participants found the injections very painful.

Another option a physician may opt to use is immunotherapy with medications such as imiquimod, candida, and cimetidine; these are thought to be effective in treating viral-induced diseases because they activate the immune system and prevent the propagation of HPV (5). Imiquimod cream 5% was shown to resolve warts in 50% of 109 patients treated, with 13% experiencing recurrence (41). In a case report of two patients, imiquimod combined with paring was helpful for resistant plantar warts (42).

Intralesional candida has been used with success in the treatment of warts (41). In a retrospective review of 149 adult and pediatric patients, of which 104 participated in the study, 75 out of 104 (72%) experienced complete resolution within 8 weeks of their last injection, which were spaced in 4-week intervals (43). Another study reported 87% resolution with weekly injections of candida to plantar verrucas. However, there were many dropouts in the study, and many patients were treated concurrently with other treatments. In another study of 223 patients with warts, intralesional immunotherapy using candida, mumps, or trichophyton skin tests were found to be an effective treatment for warts and better than interferon alpha-2B alone (44).

Interferon (IFN) has been tried in the treatment of plantar warts. In one study of 53 patients with resistant warts, one wart was treated with a single injection of 4.5 million units of IFN-α2a in 24 of the patients with single warts, while 8 control patients were treated with intralesional saline (45). Twenty-one patients had multiple warts, both palmar and plantar. Cryosurgery was used as local anesthesia and paracetamol (acetaminophen) was used to prevent flu-like symptoms. The patients were followed for a year. In patients with single warts, 19 of the 24 had complete resolution (79%), while none of those injected with saline had resolution. The treatment was not as effective for patients with multiple warts. Interferon was fairly well tolerated although a few patients had headaches and 32 had flu-like symptoms. However, the IFN dose used was high, and was used in combination with cryosurgery.

Oral cimetidine has been used with variable results in the treatment of plantar verrucas. This treatment can be successful and can be used in children as well but requires long-term therapy and compliance can be an issue (46).

Surgical treatments include curettage, dissection, and electrodessication (47). While there have been many successful reports, scarring is commonly a problem as with any surgical treatment (4). In addition, scars on the feet can be painful, persistent, and difficult to treat.

Various other methods have been tried such as chemical cautery with silver nitrate, hypnosis, and hyperthermia hot water, but compelling evidence as to their effectiveness is lacking (4). In one single-blinded, randomized, placebo-controlled study from China, using a patented hyperthermic device, heat for 3 consecutive days, then 2 additional days 2 weeks later resulted in a 53% cure rate after three months (48).

A study from India studied autoimplantation of a wart into the flexor forearm and reported an 80% cure rate in 20 patients with palmoplantar warts (49).

Laser surgery is another option to be considered. Among the lasers used are the carbon dioxide and the pulsed dye lasers. The carbon dioxide (CO_2) laser has a reported clearance rate of 52% (50), and the pulsed dye laser seems to be no more effective than cantharadin or cryotherapy (51). Another option is photodynamic therapy using a photosensitizer (52). In one study using PDT with a 4 to 8 hours incubation time after paring the wart and applying ALA in a cream, the warts were incubated for 15 to 20 minutes using an incoherent multiple-band light source. Patients were treated an average of 2.3 times. There was clearance in 42 of the 48 patients. About 18% of patients complained of stinging pain and 16% of itching and tingling. There was one patient with hyperpigmentation. A study comparing three treatments of paring alone versus paring with intense pulsed light (IPL) showed no difference in the clearance rate of plantar warts. A Japanese study used the carbon dioxide laser to the lipid layer followed by nylon suturing with artificial dermis. Of 35 patients, 31 or 88.6% achieved clearance. Local anesthetic was required. Interestingly, there were no instances of severe hypertrophic scars or pain (42). These lasers all require additional and expensive instrumentation.

Oral zinc sulfate has been tried with some success. In one study, common and plane warts resolved successfully with this treatment. The dose used was 10 mg/kg daily up to 600 mg. All the patients experienced nausea, vomiting, epigastric pain, and were found to have low zinc levels. When the warts responded, they often itched and increased in size initially.

It is important to note that the treatment of warts varies from individual to individual. Frequently therapies have to be personalized accordingly with a combination of one to several treatment modalities.

Prevention is the mainstay of treatment. Measures can be taken to prevent infection of both warts and other communicable skin infections common to athletes (9). Sandals or flip-flops should be worn in locker rooms or showers. Towels and equipment should be cleansed regularly. Protective gloves should be used with weightlifting equipment. Clothing towels, razors, and protective equipment should not be shared. Showers should be taken immediately after practices or competitions.

TINEA PEDIS

Tinea pedis, also known as athlete's foot, is a broad term used for various cutaneous mycoses or fungal infections caused by dermatophytes (53) (Fig. 32.2). According to numerous studies, there is an increased prevalence of tinea pedis in athletes as compared to the general population (54). In one epidemiologic study of over 100,000 people, athletes were found to have 1.6 to 2.3 times as many occurrences of tinea pedis as compared to non-athletes (55).

There have also been various studies that have looked at the prevalence of tinea pedis among athletes of different sports. Runners have an increased tendency to have tinea pedis: in two studies, 22% and 31% respectively of the runners tested were infected (56,57). Soccer players also have a high prevalence as compared to the general population (58). Athletes who participate in sports in which there were shared shower facilities and/or swimming pools are at greater risk (54).

Other sports studied for the prevalence of athlete's foot include, basketball, swimming, judo, water polo, and hockey (54). Interestingly, one study looking at a professional ice hockey team found no increased incidence of tinea (59). Another study of professional Brazilian and Chinese soccer players also showed no increased prevalence of tinea pedis (60). Although the reasons are not completely clear, the authors hypothesized that the good health of the athletes as well as "institutional provisions" on hygiene may account for the surprising results (59).

According to a study performed by Pickup and Adams, there was no significant difference between the prevalence of tinea in college male and college female soccer players versus non-athletes (61). However, numerous studies have shown that there is higher prevalence of tinea in males over females (62). This study also noted a significant difference in the prevalence between athletes and non-athletes (61). Some studies have shown a positive correlation between prevalence of tinea pedis and age; this may be a result of changes in immunity as people age (62). Participants in the Special Olympics had a rate of tinea higher than that of the general population although this was an observational survey without further laboratory or other confirmation (11).

The skin of the foot provides favorable conditions for dermatophyte infection (58). The foot lacks sebaceous glands and inhibitory fungistatic lipids, therefore decreasing the defenses against infection (58). Athletes often tend to wear synthetic and occlusive clothing and footwear, which increases sweating (60). Sweating consequently softens the stratum corneum and increases maceration of the skin, allowing for easier dermatophyte entry (58). The stratum corneum is the top layer of skin and made up of keratin, which is what the dermatophytes survive on (53). Athletes are at an even greater risk of infection because of an increased chance of trauma, which also facilitates mycoses (61). Often, symptoms are first noticed between the fourth and fifth toes.

Fungal infections can be spread by person-to-person contact, animal contact, and contact with inanimate objects, as the spores shed can sometimes live for months outside the host (53,63). Some studies sampling community baths, pools, and dressing rooms have revealed *Trichophyton mentagrophytes* present on various surfaces (64,65).

There are numerous dermatophyte and non-dermatophyte causes of tinea pedis, although the two most common types are *T. rubrum* and *T. mentagrophytes* (58). The majority of studies show that *T. rubrum* accounts for the highest percent of tinea pedis in the general population, while *T. mentagrophytes* causes the highest percent of tinea pedis amongst athletes (58). Other less common causes include *Epidermophyton floccosum* and non-dermatophyte molds such as *Candida, Scopulariopsis, Scytalidium, Acremonium,* and *Fusarium* (58).

When the body is infected by a dermatophyte, it protects itself by increasing growth of the basal cell layer, causing the skin to thicken which leads to the scaling that is often symptomatic of athlete's foot (66). Increased hyperkeratosis can occasionally occur, which will require additional treatments (67).

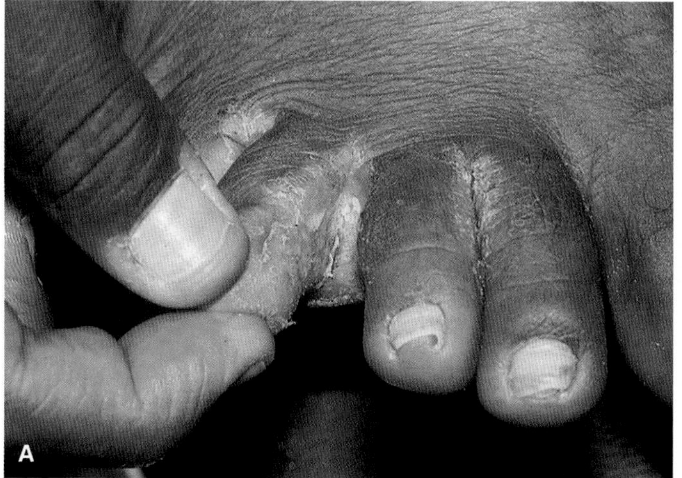

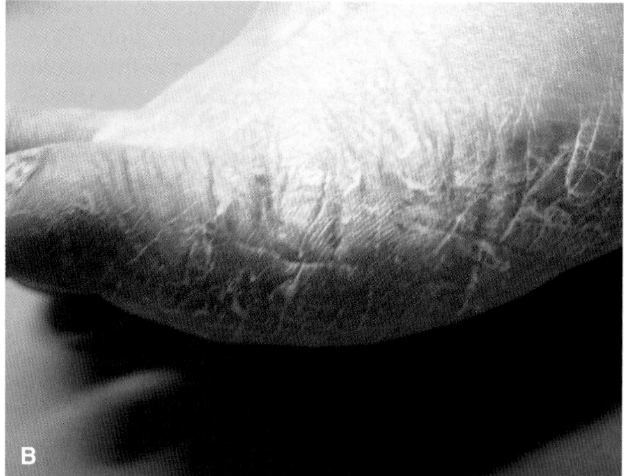

Figure 32.2. Tinea pedis. **A:** Interdigital. **B:** Moccasin type.

Secondary to the fungal infection, the skin can also become infected with *Staphylococcus* or *Pseudomonas* (54). Viewed under a Wood's lamp, the plaques may appear greenish in color, which is indicative of *Pseudomonas* superinfection (54). Other complications include onychomycosis and cellulitis (58).

Frequently, clinical examination of patients is sufficient to make the diagnosis. Tinea pedis has three main presentations: interdigital, moccasin (Fig. 32.2B), and vesicular (66,67). The interdigital type, generally presents with maceration, scaling, and erythema between the toes, usually between the fourth and fifth toes (54). The moccasin-like pattern presents as ill-defined and scaly, often with erythematous plaques (54). These two types are caused by the *T. rubrum* dermatophyte. The third vesiculobullous variant is caused by *T. mentagrophytes* and clinically presents with intense pruritus, scaling, erythema, papules, and vesicles on the instep (67).

The differential diagnoses to tinea pedis include psoriasis, dyshidrotic eczema, xerosis, contact dermatitis, candida, erythrasma, and pitted keratolysis. If the clinician is in doubt, potassium hydroxide (KOH)-treated scrapings can be examined under the microscope, which will reveal multiple, septate hyphae, and spores. The clinician can also perform a fungal culture. According to numerous studies, the KOH-stain is often a more accurate diagnosis than a culture because of the risk of co-infection of agars by other bacterium (58). While KOH stain is more sensitive than fungal culture, the latter is more specific (68).

Co-infection with bacteria may make a culture less sensitive (69). The diagnosis can be confirmed by culturing on a Sabouraud's peptone–glucose agar; however, this may take 1 to 4 weeks to confirm.

Occult tinea pedis is also common to athletes, which may increase transmission (56–58,62,64,70). In one study looking at swimmers, a significant amount of subjects (36%) infections that were occult, which allows for unintentional spreading (62). Also, many athletes often mistake the scaly plaques for dry skin or calluses (67).

The primary course of treatment for tinea pedis is topical antifungal creams. The two main classes of antifungal agents include the allylamines and the imidazoles. Allylamines, such as topical terbinafine and naftifine, have been preferred since they are fungicidal, while imidazoles, such as ketoconazole, miconazole, and clotrimazole are fungistatic (53,71–74). Ciclopiroxamine is a separate class of antifungal topical medication. One recent meta-analysis showed no differences in any of these classes of antifungal topical medications (75).

Sometimes the skin may become hyperkeratotic and require keratolytic agents, including salicylic acid or urea (58,67). A complementary medical alternative, Ageratina pichinchensis worked as well as 2% ketoconazole in a randomized, double-blinded, placebo-controlled 160 patient Mexican study, with therapeutic cures of 34 to 42% (76).

Co-infection of gram-negative bacteria can also occur, and thus antibacterial treatments are often needed as well (58). Many feel gram-negative toe web infection is a separate entity and this condition will be reviewed elsewhere in this chapter. Topical steroids are often used to relieve the uncomfortable itching (58). If a topical cortisone cream is used alone, however, the fungal infection will frequently worsen.

If topical treatments fail, which is common when the fungal infection involves the nail, termed onychomycosis, systemic antifungal medications are the next step. This will be further elaborated upon in this chapter's section on onychomycosis. Oral medications for tinea pedis include itraconazole, fluconazole, and terbinafine. A Cochrane review noted that terbinafine was more efficacious than griseofulvin, and that terbinafine and itraconazole were more effective than placebo (77). Recurrence rates for tinea pedis are as high as 70% (78).

Prevention is necessary in order to reduce the number of athletes infected. Athletes should wear sandals in the locker room, shower, and pool decks. The use of antifungals as well as routine, consistent screenings for possible signs of infection may decrease the incidence of tinea pedis (61,67). Adams and others advocate antifungal drying powders, and moisture-wicking socks as preventatives. Other recommendations include keeping nails short, discarding shoes after 500 miles of training, and having an adequate size toe box in shoes (58,79,80). Frequent cleaning and hosing of shower room, pools, and locker rooms may help to decrease the incidence of tinea pedis (58). Compliance with treatment regimens is often poor (62). Because of the high incidence of occult disease and recurrence, trainers and physicians need to be vigilant in examining, diagnosing, and treating tinea pedis.

While there are specific NCAA rules regarding an athlete's return to play after being infected with tinea capitis and tinea corporis, there are no NCAA rules regarding tinea pedis.

GRAM-NEGATIVE TOE INFECTION

Gram-negative toe web infections are a little known cause of infection that can easily be confused with tinea pedis or fungal infections (Fig. 32.3). This condition has sometimes been termed foot intertrigo (81). Patients frequently complain of a burning sensation and pain (82). The pain may become so severe as to impede walking (83). Sometimes the condition may be malodorous. It can be difficult to determine the origin of toe web infections. The condition may be characterized by erythema, vesicopustules, erosions, and marked macerations. Lesions are found in the interdigital web and inflammation can extend toward the digitoplantar sulcus, the sole, and the back of the foot (82).

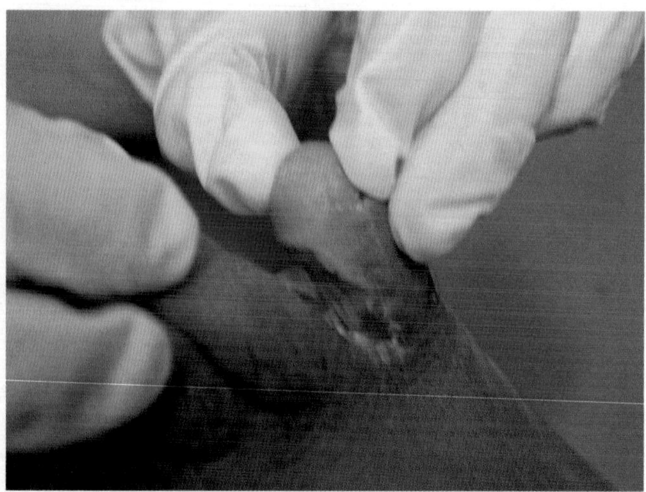

Figure 32.3. Gram-negative toe web infection.

Some cases have noted the development of a hyperkeratotic rim (84). Patients often complain of thick toes and tight interdigital spaces (85). Hyperhidrosis is often noted among patients who are active but it is unclear whether it is a result or a cause of gram-negative toe web infection (83).

Gram-negative toe web infections may also be mistaken for candidiasis, erythrasma, tinea pedis, intertrigo, and hyperhidrosis (83). Often patients are incorrectly treated for tinea, and as the condition is often recalcitrant to fungal treatment, it will not be responsive. Gram-negative infections are often caused by *Pseudomonas aeruginosa* alone or in combination with other gram-negative bacteria such as *Moraxella, Alcaligenes, Acinetobacter,* and *Erwinia* (81).

Despite the name of the condition, there are other organisms besides gram-negative bacteria that can cause it. Other organisms that may be involved in this infection include dermatophytes, yeasts, *Corynebacterium minutissimum,* and *Staphylococcus aureus* (81). These infections are often polymicrobial (82). In one study, 84 patients (28 females and 56 males ages 16 to 89 years) with foot intertrigo underwent KOH prep and Wood's light exams of the affected areas. After isolating the pathogens on culture mediums, 17.9% were infected by coagulase-negative staphylococci, 11.9% were infected by dermatophytes, 16.7% were infected by *P. aeruginosa,* 2.4% were infected by a beta-hemolytic streptococcus, 11.9% were infected by *C minutissimum,* 11.9% were infected by *S aureus,* and 1.2% were infected by *P. mirabilis* (81).

According to a study conducted at Cagliari University, males are more commonly affected by toe web infections caused by gram-negative bacteria than females, with a male/female ratio of 4 to 1 (82). Overgrowth of gram-negative bacteria may cause the infection but the moist environment caused by excessive sweating of the feet may also play a role (83). This particular infection can also be associated with tight-fitting shoes and among those who physically exert themselves during athletic, recreational, and or occupational activities (83). Infections from gram-negative bacteria in many cases start at the stratum corneum, where dermatophytes destroy the composition of the bacterial flora and develop antibiotic-resistant strains responsible for lesions (82). The infections can be a result of exposure to bacteria in spa pools (81).

Diagnostic tests that may be indicated include Wood's light examination to rule out Corynebacterium, as well as KOH preps, fungal, and bacterial cultures.

Topical therapy is often the first course of treatment, often econazole nitrate topicals. This has been shown to decrease aerobic flora, large-colony diphtheroids, lipophilic diphtheroids, and gram-negative bacteria (83). In addition to econazole nitrate, Castellani's paint, a fungicidal and bactericidal liquid, is another option that has both anesthetic and antiseptic effects (83). Gentamicin sulfate is an antifungal topical that helps to fight gram-negative infections and can be useful (83).

While initially many clinicians try to use topical medications to treat gram-negative toe web infection, these often fail; systemic therapy is frequently necessary for resolution. Oral ciprofloxacin is frequently a part of the treatment regimen as it inhibits bacterial DNA synthesis and consequently, growth (83).

In order to prevent relapses in the most severe cases where yeasts or dermatophytes are still observed in the microbial flora after the beginning of treatment, antifungal drugs are added in order to ensure complete recovery (82). In the cases where a hyperkeratotic rim develops interdigitally, a curettage may be needed to debride the surface. Most often the rim must surgically be removed so that the infecting agent no longer has a protected environment in which to grow; moreover, the rim can serve as a hindrance in the healing of the wound that lies underneath (84). In addition, this will remove the nidus of infection so that the skin in the area becomes less dense and therefore the topical treatments can be more effective (86).

It can be helpful to change or clean the patient's athletic footwear in order to be rid of the causative bacteria (54). Drying the interdigital web areas is a crucial part of treatment (83). In order to prevent this gram-negative infection, those who are physically active may apply 20% aluminum chloride to their feet in order to decrease plantar hyperhidrosis. Plantar hyperhidrosis often makes footwear wet which is an environment conducive to *Pseudomonas* colonies (54). Plantar hyperhidrosis is discussed in another part of this chapter. Plantar hyperhidrosis can also be treated with iontophoresis as well as botulinum toxin type A injections.

PSEUDOMONAS/HOT-FOOT SYNDROME

Pseudomonas hot-foot syndrome, also known as hot hand–foot syndrome, is a very rare condition that has been noted in an outbreak at a community swimming pool as well as in a hot tub. Two outbreaks have been reported in children (87,88). Ten patients, 9 children and 1 adult, were affected by a recent outbreak in Germany. One required hospitalization and intravenous antibiotics (89).

Although not necessarily restricted to children, it is possible that children are more susceptible because children have a thinner stratum corneum than adults, which could lead to easier entry of microorganisms (87).

Overlap of hot tub folliculitis and pseudomonas hot foot may have occurred in other case reports as well (90,91).

Patients typically present with a significant amount of pain in the soles of both feet. In one case study of 40 patients, the mean age of presentation was 6 (87).

The outbreak can occur 6 to 48 hours after exposure (88). Other symptoms commonly experienced include lethargy, malaise, nausea, swelling, redness, and a sensation of heat (87,88). On physical examination, this condition can present with diffuse, dusky erythema of the soles, and deep, exquisitely tender, red-to-purple, 0.5- to 2-cm nodules on the weight-bearing surfaces of the foot (87,88). Most commonly affected areas on the feet were the plantar toes, metatarsal heads, heels, and lateral surfaces of the feet (87). Foot pain was associated with erythema and nodules (87).

Ambulation and weight bearing may be exquisitely painful (88). Three patients showed lymphangiitis of the instep though no inguinal or popliteal lymphadenopathy. Patients may be febrile (87,88).

Although the cause of pseudomonas hot-foot syndrome is not completely clear, it is believed that it may be caused by the namesake microorganism, *P. aeruginosa,* the gram-negative bacterium more commonly responsible for outbreaks of hot tub folliculitis, contracted from pools and hot tubs (54). Hot tub folliculitis is not usually seen on the palms or soles (54). These two entities, hot tub folliculitis and pseudomonas hot hand–foot syndrome, have generally been reported separately. In one recent outbreak, however, there was overlap in two patients in that both types of lesions were reported in the same patients (88). *P. aeruginosa,* identical to that found in the pool, was recovered from a pustule in some affected children both with pseudomonas hot foot and the overlap condition (87,88). Besides the pool, in one study, inlets, floors, and drains yielded *Pseudomonas* (87).

Blood work can show leukocytosis, neutrophils, and elevated sedimentation rate and elevated C-reactive protein (87,88).

Among the differential diagnoses are idiopathic palmoplantar hidradenitis, suppurative panniculitis, erythema nodosum, traumatic-pressure urticaria, meningococcemia, and Rocky Mountain spotted fever (87,88). Palmoplantar hidradenitis is inconsistent with the symptoms because although the etiology is unknown, trauma-induced destruction of the eccrine glands and excessive moisture are often cited as the main causes (87). Suppurative panniculitis, which can also be caused by *P. aeruginosa,* differs from past cases of hot-foot syndrome because there is no history of a communal cause; all cases have been completely random (87).

If the condition is clinically recognized, then biopsy may be unnecessary. Histology performed in two patients showed a perivascular and perieccrine neutrophilic infiltrate; one biopsy showed a dermal microabscess and a focal area of vasculitis with fresh thrombin in the blood vessel (87).

The majority of the patients were treated symptomatically with analgesic agents, cold compresses, and elevation of the feet (87). In all patients, the symptoms completely resolved within 1 to 14 days and generally within 7 days (87). Some patients required a course of ciprofloxacin, usually 500 mg twice daily; however this is only necessary in patients with recurring infections or those that are immunosuppressed (92). Quinolones should be used cautiously in children. In one study, three patients had recurrent lesions when they again went in the pool (87).

Besides quinolones, antibiotics used include cephalosporins and aminoglycosides. Adjunctive treatment include amikacin 5% gel topical and hot compresses with 2% to 5% solutions of acetic acid for 15 days. In more severe cases, along with ciprofloxacin, intramuscular injections of ceftazidime or cefotaxime for 10 days may be needed.

Green foot, a specific type of gram-negative infection, may particularly affect those who are involved in athletic activities. The infection can develop due to the occlusive, sweaty nature of athletic shoes (54).

In the cases when *Pseudomonas* is the bacteria causing the infection, the feet and toenails may appear green and the color does not scrape or wipe off. *Pseudomonas* can be ruled in or out as the causative organism with a culture. While cultures of the skin may be negative, cultures should be taken of the patient's athletic shoes as well in order to rule out other bacteria (54).

The best way to prevent the spread of pseudomonas hot-foot syndrome according to the reports and the Centers for Disease Control is to superchlorinate pool water, maintaining a free chlorine or bromine concentration of 3 to 6 ppm, and the pH between 7.6 and 7.8, reduce abrasion of pool floors, and scrub floors, water pipes, and inlets of pools with quaternium ammonium compounds, followed by treatment with ozone to disrupt the contaminated biofilm (87,88,93).

In order to prevent this condition; those who are physically active may apply 20% aluminum chloride to their feet in order to decrease plantar hyperhidrosis. Other alternative treatments for plantar hyperhidrosis include iontophoresis and botulinum toxin injections—see our section elsewhere in this chapter for further elaboration. Plantar hyperhidrosis often makes footwear wet which enables growth of *Pseudomonas* colonies (54).

PITTED KERATOLYSIS

Pitted keratolysis is also known as sweaty sock syndrome, keratolysis sulcata, and keratolysis plantare sulcatum (Fig. 32.4). This condition is most commonly seen among barefooted individuals or individuals using occluded shoes living in warm, humid environments. Pitted keratolysis is seen worldwide and there is no racial predilection (94). Pitted keratolysis is frequently seen in patients who wear occlusive or protective shoes (95), which include many athletes, such as basketball players, tennis players, and runners (7,54,96). In one study of 184 athletes, 26 were affected (97). Males have been reported to be 97% of affected individuals in case studies performed. Children and adults can be infected.

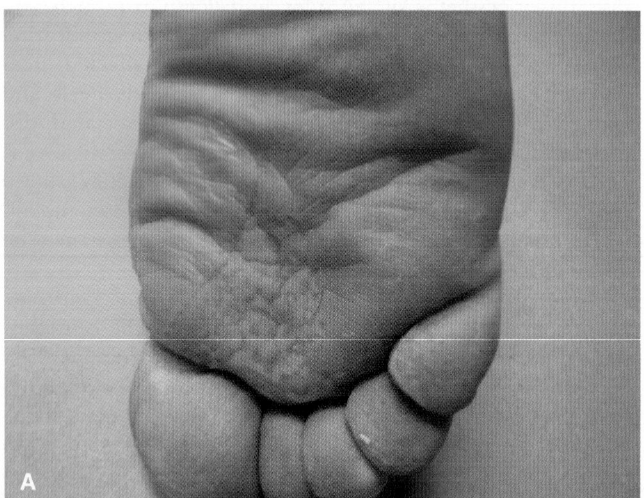

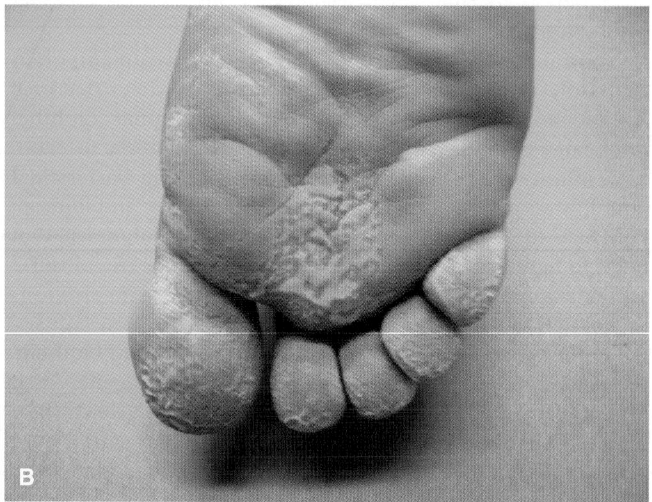

Figure 32.4. Pitted keratolysis. **A:** Before soaking in water. **B:** After soaking in water for 5 minutes.

These pits are less than 7 mm in diameter and are found where the foot experiences the greatest force, such as the soles, heels, and toe pads (96). Pitted keratolysis is almost always bilateral (95). For those wearing occluded shoes, a warm and humid environment may be provided by hyperhidrosis of the feet. A study showed that 96% of individuals with pitted keratolysis experienced hyperhidrosis. Many patients also complain of hyperhidrosis (68%) and smelly feet (66%) (95,98). Although pitted keratolysis has been reported to be generally painless, in one study 47% of patients complained of pain (95).

Pitted keratolysis is a cutaneous infection caused by one of three gram-positive bacteria: Usually *Corynebacterium,* but also *Kytococcus sedentarius* (previously *Micrococcus sedentarius*) and *Dermatophilus congolensis* (99). Under ideal conditions, such as warm, humid environments, these bacteria can grow and reproduce producing enzymes that will eat the stratum corneum, therefore creating small holes on the feet. The malodor and pits in the keratin have been attributed to the production of sulfides, thiols, and thioesters as well as two extracellular enzymes by *K. sedentarius* (99,100).

Many physicians can identify the condition by clinical observation and its distinctive malodor. Most patients present with pits on the feet but a few have erythematous coalescent lesions (95). If the diagnosis is in doubt, the feet can be soaked in water for a few minutes which allows the pits to become clinically much more obvious (Fig. 32.4). Dermatoscopy may be helpful (101).

Biopsies are sometimes performed to confirm the presence of bacteria (98). On histology, gram stain, periodic acid–Schiff (PAS), and methanamine silver can reveal the bacteria (95). The bacteria are coccoid forms generally found between and within the keratinocytes in the upper stratum granulosum as well as in corneocytes (95).

Included in the differential diagnosis for pitted keratolysis are common infections such as tinea pedis, plantar warts, and eczema (99,102). Less common differential diagnoses include punctate hyperkeratosis, porokeratosis, basal cell nevus syndrome, arsenic keratosis, tungiasis, yaws, and keratolysis exfoliativa (99).

The mainstay of treatments is a topical antibiotic, such as erythromycin, clindamycin solution, fusidic acid cream, and mupirocin (103). Domeboro soaks can be helpful (102). While benzoyl peroxide should be helpful, as it is both antimicrobial and drying, it is often painful (54). One study involving four patients utilized a clindamycin (1%)–benzoyl peroxide (5%) topical gel (duac) with good results (94). Similar combination topical antibiotics plus benzoyl peroxide would likely be similarly efficacious. Deeper infections may require oral antibiotics. With appropriate treatment, pitted keratolysis resolves within 3 to 4 weeks.

Since hyperhidrosis is thought to be one of the main etiologic factors of pitted keratolysis since it provides optimal environment for bacteria proliferation, treatment for reduction of sweating was tried as treatment of pitted keratolysis. Two case studies involved individuals who were diagnosed with hyperhidrosis of the feet and pitted keratolysis. When both individuals were treated for hyperhidrosis with botulinum toxin type A, their excessive sweating was minimized and the pitted keratolysis resolved within 30 days (102).

As prevention, moisture-wicking socks and open footwear can be helpful (54). In addition, topical antisweating agents such as aluminum chloride can be efficacious in prevention (54).

CUTANEOUS LARVA MIGRANS

Cutaneous larva migrans (CLM) is mainly seen in tropical, developing countries in warmer and humid areas, as the worm responsible for the condition is found in these areas of the world (104). There is one report of a volleyball player developing CLM; volleyball players are particularly at risk of exposure to the larva that live in the sand (105). There is no sexual or racial affinity of the affecting larva. However, it is commonly seen in children and younger adults, as this group is more likely to be in exposed areas, such as the beach (106).

Lee first described CLM as a "creeping eruption" over 100 years ago. Cutaneous larva migrans is usually diagnosed clinically by its appearance and the patient's travel history. Because of the migratory nature of CLM, it gives rise to a linear pruritic, serpiginous plaque (Fig. 32.5). Patients usually experience itchiness and tingling upon infection. The itching can be severe enough to disturb sleep (107).

On the foot, CLM is usually seen on the dorsa or between the toes, though it can be seen elsewhere in the body as well. There may be bulla formation in the tracts (108).

If the diagnosis is in doubt, a biopsy of the area can reveal the existence of larva in the skin (104,109). Confocal microscopy was used in one patient to locate the larva (110).

The nematodes typically migrate 1 to 2 cm daily. The differential includes other types of dermatitis. CLM may also cause Loeffler's syndrome, resulting in increased IgE levels. If there is suspicion of migratory pulmonary infiltrate, imaging studies may be indicated (54).

This creeping eruption is caused by infection of a person's skin with animal larvae, *Ancylostoma braziliense* in the Western hemisphere, but other species worldwide, most commonly, *Ancylostoma caninum* and *Uncinaria stenocephala* (109). Since humans are unintended hosts, these larvae are unable to penetrate beyond the cutaneous layer of the skin and thus remain superficially, which facilitates its diagnosis (111).

Cutaneous larva migrans is mainly seen in low-income countries because of the prevalence of stray dogs and cats affected with the hookworm but can be seen in more developed countries

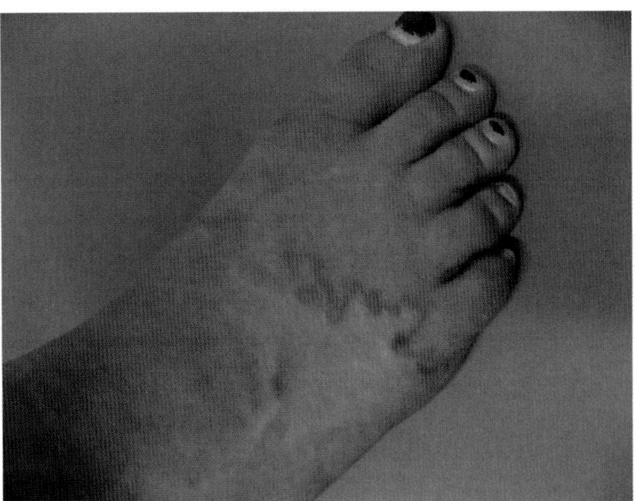

Figure 32.5. Cutaneous larva migrans infection after playing beach volleyball in Puerto Rico.

because of travel and tourism. An increase in CLM is seen during the rainy season, as the larvae eggs in the sand have a higher survival rate in these conditions; this increase is also due to the fact that the hosts of this nematode, cats and dogs, are more vulnerable during wet and humid weather (109).

There are several methods of treatment, both oral and topical. Topical treatments include application of albendazole ointment, twice a day for about 10 days, or similarly application of topical thiobendazole (104,109). These medications are often difficult to obtain in the United States. Oral treatments include anthelmintics, namely ivermectin, thiobendazole, and albendazole (110).

Ivermectin is prescribed as a single dose of 12 to 18 mg daily, an off-label usage, depending upon a patient's weight. A single dose of ivermectin has a higher efficacy rate than one single dose of albendazole, which is prescribed as 1 to 3 doses of 400 mg daily. Both medications are usually well tolerated (109).

Cutaneous larva migrans is easily prevented by wearing occlusive footwear while visiting areas that are likely to be infested with the larva (104). On a larger scale, stray dogs and cats should not be allowed in public areas where there is a tendency for visitors to be barefoot, and/or the strays should be given anthelmintic drugs (109). The condition is self-limiting and does not need to be treated, but we generally do treat because it may take weeks to resolve, frequently causes intense pruritus, and may upset the patient emotionally.

FRICTION BLISTERS

Friction blisters are likely the most common injury affecting athletes. Frictional forces between the skin and some object, usually footwear, cause these blisters (Fig. 32.6).

Major tennis players such as Pete Sampras, Roger Federer, and Maria Sharapova have been adversely affected by blisters in Grand Slam events (112). Consequently, any sport involving walking or running can cause the formation of foot blisters (113,114). The most common dermatologic complaint among marathon runners is blisters (115). Indeed, the incidence of blisters in marathon runners is up to 42% (112).

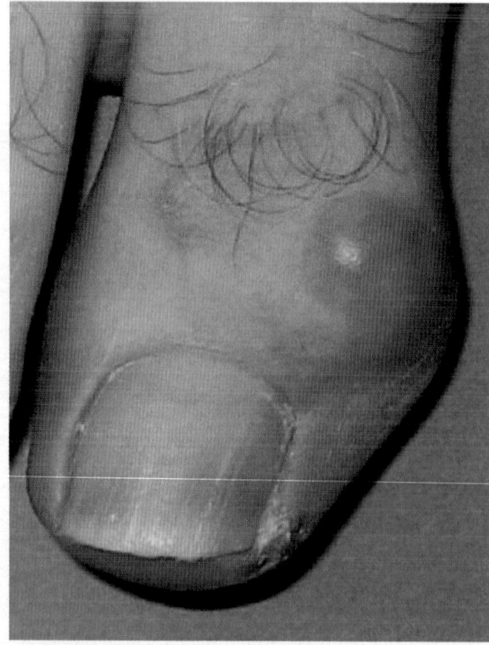

Figure 32.6. Blister from new shoe.

Blisters tend to form in areas where the skin has a thicker stratum corneum, such as the soles and palms (116). The locations that are the most common for friction blisters on the feet are the balls of the feet, the tips of the toes, and the posterior heel (117). The frictional forces due to shearing can cause a separation between the stratum spinosum and the layers above within the epidermis (116).

Generally, a blister begins with mild erythema often following slight exfoliation. There may be stinging or burning. After pallor develops around the erythematous area, the pallor can extend into the region of erythema and cause a blister (83).

The formation of a blister is dependent on numerous factors. In regards to the external force, however, the magnitude of the frictional force and the number of times the surface moves across the skin are most important in determining whether a friction blister is likely to occur (83). Rubbing moist skin produces a greater frictional force than rubbing extremely dry or wet skin (118). Dampness and temperature greater than 104 degrees have been implicated in blister formation; feet that are very wet or very dry are less likely to form blisters (119). Interestingly, athletes have often used emollients including petroleum jelly, which actually decrease the formation of blisters for up to an hour of activity. However, after that first hour of activity, the friction ratio begins to increase and consequently, so does the risk of blister formation (116). Increasing skin hydration seems to cause gender-specific changes in the mechanical properties and possibly the surface topography of human skin, leading to skin softening and increased real contact area and adhesion, at least in the upper arm (120).

The use of tobacco products may also be a risk factor for blister formation (119). Increased loads and heavy backpacks are additional risk factors for blisters (116). Historically, athletes and the military have been most greatly affected by blisters because of the activities in which they are involved (119). Although there have been no studies that have found a higher incidence of friction blisters based on race, age, or sex, a higher risk factor has been found in people who are more active (83,118).

Ill-fitting and worn out shoes are the most common cause of blisters but heat, maceration, and sweating may be causal factors as well (83). Plantar shear stress may be elevated in athletes prone to blisters (112).

Although typically the most common complications due to blisters are localized pain and delayed ability to return to the relative sport, there have been instances when secondary impetigo, cellulitis, sepsis, and rarely toxic shock syndrome occur as complications (83,121).

Blisters are diagnosed via clinical examination. If the etiology is unclear or related to a systemic disease, a biopsy for histopathology as well as for immunofluorescence can be indicated to rule out such conditions as bites, epidermolysis bullosa acquisita, and other bullous and cutaneous diseases.

Blisters less than 5 mm in size can be treated with protective donuts such as moleskin. Although there is limited evidence that moleskin, and hydrogel or hydrocolloid products such as duoderm are helpful, they seem to be helpful anecdotally (116).

If a blister is greater than 5 mm, the fluid that forms between the skin layers of the blisters should be drained with a sterile needle so as to prevent pain. The roof of the blisters should be left intact. If the blister appears infected, systemic antibiotic therapy should be initiated (116). If the roof of the blister tears or comes off completely, then the blister should be treated as an open wound. Hydrocolloid dressings have also been proven to decrease discomfort and encourage healing (83).

Prevention is the best method for treating blisters. In one double-blind placebo-controlled study of U.S. military cadets, it was found that those who used antiperspirant at least three nights before a hike were significantly less likely to form a blister. While the cadets were not especially compliant, results indicated that the incidence of skin irritation and dryness increased dramatically in those who used the antiperspirant consistently. This often led to discontinuation of the product (118). Lowering the percentage of antiperspirant used might prove equally or even more efficacious since there would likely be less irritation, but additional studies need to be performed.

Insoles and orthotics for significantly flat or high-arched feet may be helpful in preventing blisters (116,122,123). In addition, stopping tobacco products may also help prevent friction blisters (116). The evidence for the use of tincture of benzoin and foot powders to prevent blisters is lacking (116).

Advancements in fabric development have led to the use of several fabrics that have been found to significantly reduce the likelihood of blister formation. Runners who wore acrylic woven socks had less prevalence of friction blisters than those runners who wore socks of other materials (124); but acrylic was not better than wool socks (124). Cotton and wool socks tend to absorb moisture therefore increasing blister formation (116). A thin polyester sock under a standard thick military sock may be useful in minimizing blisters as well (125).

NODULES AND PADS

Athletes develop many nodules and pads generally as a result of repeated trauma in a sport. Another name for this condition is "Nike nodules," but an overall and inclusive term is "athlete's nodules" (126).

Athlete's nodules are not limited to a specific sport or activity, although they often affect surfers, boxers, and football players (127). Surfer's nodules most commonly develop on the dorsal aspect of the foot, while football players often develop such dermal nodules on the ankles (127). One female athlete acquired pads over both ankles because of the repetitive use of shin guards and athletic shoes used for soccer and softball (128). Athletes sometimes experience these conditions as a result of chronic rubbing from tight or ill-fitting shoes (54).

The nodules that form on ice skaters can also be called "double ankle bones"; they can be seen over the lateral malleoli, the skin overlying the Achilles tendons, the lateral sides of the feet or some combination thereof (129).

Skater's pads are more superficial than skater's nodules. Ice skaters may also suffer from pump bumps, caused by Haglund's deformity of the calcaneal tuberosity. These are bony enlargements on the back of the heel overlying the Achilles tendon; a painful bursitis may occur as well (129).

Other case reports have illustrated athlete's nodules on the lateral side of both feet and lateral malleoli of 1 year's duration in a soccer player who wore tight shoes; with nodules on the side of the feet and right lateral malleoli of 10 years duration in a karate and track and field athlete; and a nodule on the right lateral malleolus for 4 years in a skier (129).

Athlete's nodules often present as asymptomatic, symmetrical and flesh-colored nodules ranging in size from 5 to 40 mm (127). If the diagnosis is in doubt, a punch or excisional biopsy can confirm the diagnosis. The differential diagnosis includes ganglion cysts, granuloma annulare, rheumatoid nodules, gout, foreign body reactions, and elastomas (127).

Upon histopathology, a biopsy will likely reveal the presence of a collagenoma (54). In addition, an excess of dermal collagen and an acanthotic, hyperkeratotic epidermis is often indicative of the condition (127). Nodules specific to surfers, called surfer's nodules, are often composed of soft tissue swellings. The lesions eventually become firm, fibrous and less painful (54). Ganglion-like cysts on the dorsal feet of surfers are common. Athlete's nodules can be differentiated from dermatofibromas histologically by the dermal tumorous proliferation of fibroblasts and epidermal reactive hypertrophy (129).

Differentiating between surfer's nodules, athlete's nodules, and pads is not necessarily clear. All three conditions are caused by trauma and occur in similar anatomic areas. The conditions are histologically similar as well. The most significant difference is their appearance as either a nodule or in the case of pads as a plaque (126).

Often these nodules do not need to be treated, as to many athletes they are a "badge of honor" indicating history and proficiency at a sport. Consequently, these lesions will often go untreated. If an athlete does wish for the lesions to be treated or if they become symptomatic, the clinician can try topical keratolytics such as salicylic acid, urea, and lactic acid (54). If topical treatments are not effective, intralesional steroids such as triamcinolone may be used at a concentration of 5 or 10 mgs/cc, titrating higher if not successful (54). If intralesional cortisone is not successful, lesions can be excised but the risk of keloids, severe scarring, and recurrence make this treatment less desirable (54). As a preventative method, protective padding can be worn in areas of known friction (54). The risks of leaving these often benign nodules untreated, especially in the case of surfer's nodules, include secondary infection and cellulitis (54).

Cessation of the sport may help lessen the nodule but often they can persist. Minimizing friction, tight athletic shoes, and shin guards can be helpful as well (126).

Unlike nodules, sports-related pads that can also occur as a result of chronic friction in the ankle and foot region are more likely to resolve as a direct outcome of the cessation of activity, while nodules often need more direct and aggressive treatment (54), so here may be one way to differentiate nodules and pads. Skaters may require heel pads, high arches, and custom orthotics (129). Like nodules, sports-related pads may be prevented through the use of extra padding (54).

CALLUSES

Calluses or callosities are hyperkeratotic well-defined plaques on the foot, usually as a result of rubbing and friction. No prevalence studies exist, however, calluses occur commonly in athletes because of the constant friction and pressure due to certain equipment.

Callosities frequently develop on the balls of the foot, as well as the medial aspect of the first toe (54). They are generally due to repeated friction, irritation, or pressure (54,130). The margins of calluses are not well demarcated, like corns (130). It is thought that abnormal mechanical stress on the skin helps form several layers of the horny layer of the epithelium (130). While calluses are quite common on the hands, generally from athletic equipment, dancers usually present with them on the toes. Skaters such as hockey players and figure dancers often prefer to maintain their calluses to provide additional protection and prevent blistering (131).

In addition, ice hockey players and figure skaters can develop from "skate bite" or "lace bite": calluses along the midline anterior tibialis or inflammatory pseudonodules along the hallucis longus tendon from poorly fitting ice skates (132). Bunga pads and specially fitted ice skates can help in testament (131,133).

Calluses can often be confused with verruca vulgaris. In order to differentiate the two, the clinician should pare the lesion, preferably after soaking the area. If black dots are visualized, then the lesion is likely a verruca, as these dots represent thrombosed capillaries. If there are no black dots, and no central core (which would indicate a corn), then the lesion is likely a callus.

Calluses can be left alone unless they become symptomatic (132). Regular paring of the lesion is often done to prevent the calluses from becoming too large, which may cause fissures (130). Additional measures to control calluses by minimizing friction include: Synthetic socks, extra toe box room, shoe inserts and orthotics, and evenly placed padding (117).

Soaking the calluses in water for 20 to 30 minutes each night, and then rubbing them with a pumice stone can be very helpful (54,129). Other instruments commonly used include foot files, rotary tools, or scalpels (134).

CORNS

A corn is a well-circumscribed, well-demarcated hyperkeratotic lesion with a central, conical core of keratin. The conical core is formed by the thickening of the stratum corneum due to physical pressure (130). Hyperkeratosis is a normal response of the skin to chronic pressure or friction, as a protection of the bone (130). Corns and calluses occur more frequently in athletes from faulty mechanics including irregular distribution pressure and repetitive motion injury (135).

Corns are divided into two main categories: The hard corn and the soft corn. The most common, the hard corn, has a hard central core and are mostly found on the top of the fifth toe (130). The soft corn results from excessive moisture and has a macerated appearance (130). Paring must be done with care, especially in patients with impaired circulation such as diabetics.

Corns need to be differentiated from both verruca and callosities. Warts are generally more painful with lateral pressure, while callosities are more painful with direct pressure (135). After palpation, one can pare the lesion, preferably after soaking. In a wart, one notes the absence of dermatoglyphics, otherwise known as skin markings and the presence of black dots representing the hemorrhage in a verruca. In a callosity, the dermatoglyphics are maintained. In a corn, one sees smooth skin.

Biopsy, and subsequent histopathology, can be helpful in ruling out such conditions like lichen simplex chronicus (LSC), porokeratosis, plantaris discreta, porokeratosis plantaris disseminatum, palmoplantar keratoderma, and warts (135).

Radiologic studies may be helpful in discerning underlying causes. MRI of the foot may help in defining any diabetic foot disease (135). One common source of hard and soft corns is the hammertoe deformity (130). Typically, this type of corn can be painful and can develop between any of the toes (54). Podiatric or orthopedic referral, orthotics, and conservative footwear with extra foot space can be beneficial (130,135).

The first step in treatment is to provide pain relief, which is commonly done by removing the hyperkeratotic tissue with a scalpel (130). If the lesion is not painful, then a pumice stone can be used. Repetitive paring can be counter-productive (131).

Protective pads may also be used in order to reduce the pressure and friction on the foot by the footwear (130). It is best to use salicylic acid compounds with percentages between 10% to 17% because higher concentrations can cause problems for those with impaired circulation. Secondly, the cause of the pressure should be determined (i.e., non-fitting footwear or foot deformities). If proper footwear and padding can relieve symptoms and prevent further corns from forming then the treatment will be successful. There is little evidence to support corticosteroid injections or silver nitrate. If this treatment is not successful, then surgery may be needed in order to correct deformities that are causing the corns to form (130,132). Surgery is indicated only if conservative procedures fail.

MOUNTAINEER'S HEEL

The blisters and erosions that are caused from activities such as mountain climbing are common to those who participate in activities that involve repetitive movements and friction, like running and hiking (136). For mountaineers, the effect of low oxygen partial pressure and low temperatures at high altitudes can create conditions in which the skin's defense mechanisms are limited (136). For these reasons, mountaineer's heel is clinically distinct from regular blisters (136). The blisters associated with mountaineer's heels in this one case were large and deeply ulcerated and were located on the medial aspects of the heels (136).

In this case, a patient presented with severe erosions on both heels after a prolonged climb. He had been rock climbing for two-and-a-half days with crampons at the Matterhorn. The mountaineer reported pain in the area and stated that he was unable to remove his boots during the climb for 60 straight hours (136).

Prevention of mountaineer's heel is often more effective than treatment. Prevention includes ensuring that climbers are able to get adequate rest and remove their feet from their boots, and the boots must be broken in before extended trips. Adequate rest and broken in boots will allow for callus formation during climbing, which help to prevent blistering (136).

In the event that blisters form, they should be drained via a relatively small puncture wound (136). After the blisters are drained, potassium permanganate ($KMnO_4$) (1:10,000 dilution) baths as well as hydrocolloid dressings can be used and applied (136).

One case study reports a 35-year-old mountaineer with large ulcerated lesions on his heels. The lesions fully resolved after $KMnO_4$ treatment baths and rest for four weeks (136).

BLACK HEEL/TALON NOIR

Black heel, otherwise known as talon noir or calcaneal petechiae, are generally black lesions found mainly on the heels of athletes. This condition has been reported frequently in patients performing sports which generally require quick turns and stops such as tennis, basketball, lacrosse, gymnastics, running, soccer, ice hockey, and football, (117,131,137–145). Black heel has been known by many other names including basketball heel, tennis heel, post-traumatic punctate hemorrhage of the skin, and purpura traumatica pedis (146,147). In one study of 596 young, healthy athletes, 2.85% were found to have black heel (148).

Talon noir is due to the presence of blood in the stratum corneum. The presence of blood occurs from hemorrhage in the papillary dermis, caused by repeated lateral force of the epidermis sliding over the papillary dermis, which is where the blood vessels may have less protection (141). Despite the word 'black' in black heel, some lesions may also appear blue or reddish brown. And despite the word 'heel' in black heel, lesions may be present on the soles or on the toes (149). In fact, there are a variety of conditions, which are due to hemorrhage into the skin, not necessarily black and not necessarily on the heel (146,150). These lesions are also found on the palms of many athletes as well and are then known as "tache noire." Since there are a variety of ways that bleeding into the skin can present, Urbina et al. have proposed this condition to be called "post-traumatic, cutaneous, intracorneal blood" (146). Another proposed name for this entity is "post-traumatic punctate hemorrhage of the skin" (147,150).

Talon noir is generally diagnosed clinically by physicians who are familiar with the condition. It is asymptomatic. Lesions may be individual and isolated or multiple and punctiform or affecting large areas (146). Dermatoscopy, which may help in the diagnosis of certain skin lesions, especially pigmented ones, has been reported to be helpful in the diagnosis of these kinds of subcorneal hematomas (151). Forty percent of lesions had a red-black hue, the most common color. The most common pattern of pigmentation seen was homogenous (151).

Due to the need to rule out atypical pigmented lesions such as melanoma, the condition can be diagnosed by paring the horny layer with a no. 15-scalpel blade. Pre-soaking the foot in lukewarm water for 10 minutes may facilitate this paring down. Generally, layers of the skin can be removed without bleeding, or can be sent for histologic evaluation (146). Often removal of the lesion for histopathology will show small lakes of coagulated blood under the surface keratin (140). In one review of two histologic specimens, upon serial sections it was noted that the blood was squeezed out from the tips of normal-appearing papillae (140). In addition, there was loss of the granular layer and parakeratosis in several areas of the suprapapillary dermis (140). Coagulated blood can sometimes be found within the lumina of the eccrine sweat ducts, in the intrakeratinous portion (140). Unlike a verruca, there was no abnormal keratin or bleeding tips (140). The shavings can then be tested using a benzidine or other stains, which would show the presence of hemoglobin (149). Histology may also show hyperkeratosis with pigment within the stratum corneum (152). Focal deposits of coagulated blood can be seen in the horny layer, shown as eosinophilic amorphous material, and scattered hemosiderophages may be found in the papillary dermis (147,153).

Talon noir is generally asymptomatic, and if so, only reassurance is necessary. Lesions generally disappear with time, as well as when the particular sport is discontinued at the end of the season (145).

SUNBURN AND SKIN CANCER

In general, athletes are at a high risk for sunburn and other sun-related conditions. Cyclists, triathletes, tennis players, and sailors have all been shown to be exposed to high levels of ultraviolet exposure (117,154,155).

Athletes whose sport requires them to be barefooted, such as swimmers and others involved in outdoor aquatic sports, occasionally will experience sunburn on the foot. Sunburn is associated with increased risk of precancerous solar (actinic) keratoses as well as skin cancer, especially basal cell cancer, as has been seen in athletes who are involved with water sports (156). In addition, athletes often practice during the peak hours of UV radiation (157). It has been found that excessive exercise may lead to suppressed immune function, which may assist in the formation and growth of tumors (156). Increased physical activity does seem to be associated with a higher incidence of sunburn (158).

Sunburn, as defined by Han and Maibach, ". . . is the acute reaction of the skin to damage by ultraviolet light exposure, [which] can range from painless erythema to edema to vesicle and bullae formation (159)." The actual cause of sunburn is believed to be due to vasodilatation of blood vessels in the upper dermis and increased vascular permeability leading to edema (159). The cause of skin cancer is likely due to long-term exposure to UV radiation, which causes mutations in a person's DNA leading to pyrimidine dimer formation in the dermal and epidermal tissue (156). According to Hachman et al., pyrimidine dimer formation is positively correlated with the extent of erythema. In addition, "UV radiation may causes unique mutations in the p53 tumor suppressor gene; these mutations are found in more than 90% of squamous cell carcinomas and in most basal cell carcinomas (160)."

Sunburn is usually straightforward to diagnose upon clinical examination and history. The patient usually has a well-demarcated area of erythema occurring within a day following excessive sun exposure. Sunburn can occur quicker if a patient is on a phototoxic or photosensitizing medication such as doxycycline, commonly used for acne.

Although the recommendations for the treatment of sunburns vary, prevention is the best method. Mechanisms of prevention include avoiding the sun during peak ultraviolet radiation hours and wearing sun-protective clothing including hats (156). Wearing a high-numbered sunscreen is critical. While most sunscreens protect against UV-B rays, sunscreens should protect against UV-A rays as well. Water-resistant sunscreens containing at least one or more of the following ingredients are recommended: avobenzone, parsol-1789, mexoryl, zinc oxide, or titanium dioxide. Sunscreens, even those labeled water-resistant, need to be reapplied frequently, and more often on hot days, especially if the athlete swims or sweats during sports participation.

Treatments for sunburns include symptom reduction, which helps to reduce healing time. Systemic cortisone has not been shown to reduce healing time (159). NSAIDs, however, may reduce erythema, but need to be taken immediately after sun exposure (54). Various studies have shown that the use of topical corticosteroids applied after the skin is burned reduced recovery time, and this reduction was correlated with the vasoconstriction of the individual corticosteroids (159).

Antihistamines have not been found to be helpful in the treatment of sunburns (159).

The study of antioxidants in the prevention/treatment of sunburns has yielded conflicting results. Taking antioxidants as supplements prior to ultraviolet exposure appears to have no effect in preventing erythema (159). However, several studies done by Bangha et al. found that when melatonin was applied 15 minutes prior to UV irradiation, this was able to almost completely suppress the development of erythema 24 hours later (161). In addition, when 0.5% melatonin was applied immediately after exposure to UV radiation, it was shown that erythema was significantly reduced 8 hours after the exposure (159).

According to a study performed by Schleider et al. assessing the effectiveness in treating sunburns with emollients applied prior to sun exposure, peanut and corn oil have no effect; bath and baby oils helped slightly; while petroleum jelly, petrolatum, and hydrophilic ointment were significantly helpful in reducing erythema (159).

Different sports will lead to different probabilities of an athlete's development of skin cancers. However, there is a lack of data related to skin cancers of the foot. Marathon runners had more atypical nevi, solar lentigines, and lesions suggestive of non-melanoma skin cancer (162). Mountaineers were also found to be at higher risk for developing precancerous and cancerous skin lesions (156). In order to diagnose skin cancers, a biopsy should be performed and confirmed upon histopathology.

In a study done by Hamant et al., sunscreen use among college athletes was assessed (157). The participants in the study were both male and female college athletes on either soccer or cross-country teams. Each of the students was given an anonymous survey that inquired about the physical characteristics including skin type, gender, sport, age, school year, college, and sunscreen use. Forty-eight percent of the participants were female, and the mean age was 20 years. The results showed that 85% of participants had not used sunscreen in the past week. Although there were no significant differences between most of the factors, those who were fair-skinned did tend to wear sunscreen more often than those who were darker skinned. In addition, not one athlete reapplied sunscreen during practice (157).

Clearly, there is a need for greater education by parents, teachers, trainers, and team physicians regarding the important use of sunscreens, and especially those which are water resistant. If possible, athletic training should take place during hours of low sun exposure and a dermatologist should regularly examine athletes.

PERNIO

Pernio is also known as chilblains, comes from the Anglo-Saxon term "chill" meaning cold and "blain" meaning sore or blotch (163). While anyone is susceptible to developing this condition, numerous studies have found that it is more common in populations living in wet and cool climates. It is also more common in young children, women, the elderly, African Americans, and smokers (163–165). In addition, other populations that are often affected include those of low socioeconomic status and the military (163,166). Athletes who participate in outdoor sports in both cold and wet environments, such as fishing and tobogganing, are also at risk (167).

The direct cause of chilblains is overexposure to non-freezing cold, damp temperatures (163,166,168). In order to combat cold temperatures, the extremities have a cold-induced vasodilatory reflex (CIVDR) that is stimulated by cold weather (163). The reflex is triggered when the skin's temperature drops below 50°F (163). The reflex allows momentary bursts of blood flow into the skin, allowing the skin to warm up (163). However, problems with an individual's CIVDR have been found in certain populations, which correlate with the populations with a higher prevalence of chilblains: African Americans, women, and nicotine users (163). This leads to excessive vasoconstriction, which then causes hypoxia and inflammation of the vessel wall (164).

Initially the extremities become hyperemic and then appear cyanotic, which results in swelling (169).

Pernio may be either primary or secondary, as it can occur in association with numerous systemic diseases. Diseases associated with pernio, or secondary pernio, can be syndromes of neuromuscular instability, chronic tissue hypoxia, hyperviscosity syndromes, abnormal subcutaneous fatty tissue distribution, and medication related (163). The neurovascular instability syndrome diseases associated with pernio include Raynaud's phenomenon, acrocyanosis, complex regional pain syndrome, and livedoid vasculopathy. Diseases of chronic tissue hypoxia include erythromelalgia and peripheral arterial occlusive disease. Hyperviscosity syndromes include systemic lupus erythematosus (SLE), cryoproteinemia, and pre-leukemic or leukemic syndromes. Abnormal lipid distribution can be seen in obese individuals and those with anorexia nervosa. Sulindac is a medication which is associated with secondary pernio.

Pernio may either be acute or chronic (163) and can occur within several hours of exposure. Chronic pernio is seen with repeated exposure to the elements over the same season or over different years (163).

In acute pernio lesions, there is usually a history of exposure to wet or humid but non-freezing conditions. There may be single or multiple violaceous, brown, yellow or erythematous patches, or plaques on exposed areas (163,170–172). Lesions are most commonly seen on the toes and fingers, although the cheeks, ears, nose, shins, thighs, hips, and heels may be involved as well. On the feet, the plantar surfaces of the toe and the dorsal parts of the proximal digits of the toes are most at risk (54). Blisters can occur (164). Diagnosis is typically based on both physical examination and the patient's history; usually some prolonged exposure to the cold will be mentioned (163). In acute pernio the lesions resolve over several days to weeks as long as there is no cold exposure. The lesions are usually intensely painful, pruritic, or burning (163,164).

In chronic pernio, complications include ulceration, permanent discoloration likely from hyperpigmentation, skin laceration, and scarring (163). Heat, rubbing, and scratching may worsen the condition.

Depending upon the clinical presentation, among the differential diagnoses associated with blue toes, the clinician should consider including emboli, either atheromatous or thrombotic, and peripheral arterial disease (163).

Biopsy can be helpful to rule out conditions besides pernio or rule out secondary causes of pernio. Many believe that there is no specific histology for chilblains, though some disagree (163,173). Other studies may include blood work such as CBC, ANA, metabolic panel, rheumatoid factor, cryofibrinogen, cold agglutinins, cryoglobulins, and vascular laboratory studies.

It is important to discuss prevention with patients as well as treatment methods (164). Repeated cold-exposure can lead to a chronic form of chilblains that occurs more frequently and may persist into periods of warm weather (166). Patients should wear temperature-appropriate clothing, avoid exposure to the cold, especially when wet, maintain hydration, and avoid nicotine (166). Nicotine use increases the vasospastic responses to cold and lessens the rescue CIVDR (163). In addition, it is recommended to avoid alcoholic beverages because although alcohol has vasodilatory effects allowing the blood to flow to the extremities, alcohol actually leads to a loss of heat despite the temporary feelings of warmth (163).

Once chilblains has developed, it is important to avoid overheating, rubbing, or scratching the lesions (163). The most common form of treatment involves the use of the dihydropyridine calcium channel blockers, such as nifedipine at a dose of 20 mg, three times daily (163,164,174). Treatment can be continued until warm weather resumes, even if the lesions have resolved (163). In many cases in order to prevent recurrence, the medication is resumed when the weather starts to get cold (163). According to various studies, this dose reduces the duration, severity, and recurrence of chilblains (163). No topical creams are currently recommended, but extremity elevation is helpful in decreasing swelling (169). The skin should be kept both warm and dry (54).

While it is unlikely for athletes to suffer from trench foot, those in long endurance events may be at risk; it is more common in the military. After long exposure, the feet become hyperemic and eventually discolored, edematous and painful. Exposed patients must be returned to dry ground and not return to their sport until 6 to 9 months after this problem has resolved (175).

Raynaud's phenomenon, a vasculopathy that is related to cold, can affect the fingers and the toes, is common among figure skaters (176).

Raynaud's may be primary or secondary to numerous other conditions. Primary Raynaud's is more common in athletes and can generally be managed conservatively with warm clothing and maneuvers to increase circulation to extremities. If these measures are not adequate, then calcium channel blockers can be utilized.

FROSTBITE

Any athlete participating in cold and wet conditions is susceptible to frostbite, as heat conservation in cold weather leads to peripheral vasoconstriction (177). While joggers are most commonly affected by frostbite (169), incidence is increasing in athletes participating in winter sports such as skiing, high-altitude climbing, and hiking (178). Both alpine and Nordic skiers as well as cyclists, speed skaters, luge, and football players can be affected as well (54,169,178).

There are a number of other factors that appear to play a role in the increased incidence of frostbite: Alcohol abuse, mental illness, peripheral vascular disease, peripheral neuropathy, malnutrition, chronic illness, tobacco use, and race, especially blacks (178). Other conditions such as Raynaud's disease, erythroderma, hyperhidrosis, hypotension, shock, vasoconstrictor drugs, stress, and diabetes mellitus also increase the risk of frostbite (177,179). Environmental risk factors include increased humidity, low ambient temperatures, high wind-chill factor, high altitude, and prolonged exposure (169). Improper clothing such as tight boots, constrictive clothing, inadequate clothing and shelter as well as cramped positioning can cause frostbite (179). Skin sensitivity to cold in the toes may be blunted and can lead to poor decision making at high altitudes (180).

Other ways to develop frostbite include overexposure to cold compresses placed against the skin, which can cause cold-induced injury (181). Similarly, ethyl chloride spray can produce frostbite (54) and lead to a vasoconstrictor response which helps retard heat loss and defend core temperature, but at the expense of a decline in skin and muscle temperatures (179).

Besides the feet, frostbite can also affect the nose, hands, face, ears, and even the penis (182).

Contact frostbite can occur when bare skin comes into contact with an extremely cold object. When this occurs, heat is lost at a much faster rate via conduction (179). Certain liquids such as petroleum products, fuel, oil, antifreeze, and alcohol can remain liquid at −40°C and touching these objects or highly conductive metal or stone with bare skin can cause instantaneous contact frostbite (179).

The temperature of the limbs will decrease until it reaches the freezing point of tissues, 28°F (−2°C); slightly lower than the freezing point of water because of the increased molecular content (179). Extracellular ice crystals form in the plasma, causing changes in the osmotic gradient, subsequently leading to cellular dehydration. This cellular dehydration will eventually lead to a loss of overall cell structure, and at the same time, the sizable amount of fluid emptying into the vessels can lead to vessel damage as well as vascular thrombosis (177). As the temperature decreases, the ice forming within the cells begins to increase leading to physical destruction of the cell membranes (178).

As the body becomes dehydrated, the vessels constrict, and body temperature decreases. The circulation is further retarded because the blood viscosity increases (183). Without adequate circulation the tissues become hypoxic and will inevitably die if continually deprived of oxygen (183). After the tissues become hypoxic, inflammatory mediators are released (184). Repetitive freeze–thaw cycles are responsible for much of the damage seen in frostbite (177).

Frostbite may be straightforward to diagnose as it is often connected to outdoor athletics. Early signs of frostbite include localized cold, pain, and numbness. The absence of sensation in the affected tissue signals deep-tissue involvement (184). Frostnip can often appear to be frostbite; however, it does not result in irreversible tissue damage (183). According to Patel and Patel, clinically there are two types: "Superficial frostbite manifests as erythema and bulla formation; and deep frostbite, involves subcutaneous tissue and usually leads to tissue loss" (184). Symptoms of deep frostbite may include hemorrhagic blisters, ulcerations, gangrene, anesthesia, or hyperesthesia (184). Deep frostbite can damage the cartilage, bone, and even nerves (183). Signs of a poor prognosis include non-blanching cyanosis, firm skin, and dark, cloudy, fluid-filled blisters (184).

The differential diagnosis of frostbite includes burns, insect bites, pemphigus vulgaris, bullous pemphigoid, staphylococcal skin infections, and herpes simplex (184).

Frostbite is categorized into four degrees of tissue damage, similar to the classification of burns. One can also categorize the first two stages as superficial and the latter two as deep (177).

First degree: This is partial skin freezing and only the epidermis is involved. There is erythema, edema, and hyperemia but no blisters (177). A central whitish area surrounded by erythema characterizes lesions (178,184). Symptoms can include throbbing, aching, transient stinging and burning, and hyperhidrosis (177).

Second degree: This is a full-thickness injury (177). Both the dermis and the epidermis are involved; a blister forms, often filled with clear or cloudy fluids (178,184). There can be erythema and edema. The blisters can desquamate and form blackened eschars (177). Symptoms can include numbness, and if severe, vasomotor disturbance (177).

Third degree: This is full-thickness skin injury and subcutaneous freezing. The subdermal tissue is damaged and a hemorrhagic bulla forms which may progress to hard black eschars (178,184). There can be skin necrosis and blue-gray discoloration (177). Symptoms include possible joint pain (177).

Fourth degree: Along with full skin thickness and subcutaneous tissue, this may involve tendons, muscle and bone and may result in gangrene (177,178,184). There is little edema. While the skin is initially cyanotic, mottled, and deep red, but eventually the skin appears dry, black, and mummified (177).

Treatment should begin immediately, no matter what the severity of damage has been. Preventing further cold exposure and mechanical injury are the primary goals (178). Re-warming should only begin once it is determined that the individual can be maintained at a constant warm temperature; however, it is important that treatment of frostbite should not occur until the patient's core body temperature is greater than 95°F (178). Warming and then re-freezing can result in even greater tissue damage (183). Consequently it is better to keep an area frozen than to thaw and risk refreezing prematurely (175).

The affected area is then rapidly heated by placing it in a water bath containing a mild antibacterial at 104°F to 107.6°F, for 15 to 30 minutes (178). Rubbing and mechanical pressure should be avoided to the affected areas as they can result in even greater tissue damage (183). During rewarming, sensation will often return and in many cases can be very painful. Narcotics and non-steroidal antiinflammatory drugs (NSAIDs) can be indicated and helpful (177).

If the skin remains cold, black, and numb, then gangrene is likely and the patient should be given IV antibiotics and tetanus prophylaxis (178). Clear blisters should be drained and open wounds should be treated with antimicrobial agents (178), but this is controversial as some say blisters should not be drained (169). Patients should not be allowed to bear weight on the extremity (177). Smoking should be prohibited (178). Whirlpool, physical therapy, and occupational therapy are frequently indicated (178). In the most severe of cases, amputation is often necessary. Since demarcation of the affected areas can be difficult, however, amputation should not be performed until at least several weeks to 90 days after the initial injury (177,178,183).

Prevention is critical in frostbite. Athletes should wear the proper warm equipment (177,179). Change of clothing is often needed. Athletic events in cold and windy weather that can induce injury should be postponed (177). When the wind chill falls below −27°C (−18°F), increased surveillance of athletes is warranted (177). In one study, the authors looked at a large group of mountaineers in order to find the incidence and possible preventions of frostbite. Of the 637 mountaineers studied, 467 reported frostbite in some part of their body. It was found that the main factor contributing to the likelihood of frostbite was lack of proper equipment (185). In addition to deficient equipment, athlete-induced wind such as what runners and skiers produce can help bring about frostbite (179). Layering clothes and wearing non-constrictive clothing as well as proper footwear can be helpful (179,185). Athletes, especially mountaineers, should not remain in one location for too long so as to help minimize the risk of frostbite (185). Foot warmers can be useful as well, as long as they do not burn the skin (54). Those athletes with recent frostbite are contraindicated from having additional cold exposure for 6 to 12 months (175).

Late sequelae of frostbite include persistent symptoms and impaired function including hypersensitivity to cold, decreased sensation, hyperhidrosis, and general autonomic dysfunction in affected extremities, nail deformities, and growth plate disturbances (169,178,183).

SEA-URCHIN ENVENOMATION

Sea-urchin envenomation commonly affects the feet of swimmers, divers, snorkelers, and surfers in both tropical and subtropical areas (186–188) (Fig. 32.7). Since the creatures tend to be nocturnal, divers are most commonly injured in dark waters during night-diving activities, particularly in small caves or in shallow turbulent waters (189).

Sea urchins are small, spherical and slow-moving marine animals belonging to the class of *Echinoidea,* phylum *Echinodermata* (186). They are the most significant echinoderm in United States waters (189). Most sea urchins live between corals or below rocks, but some live in the sea-world soil (190). They live

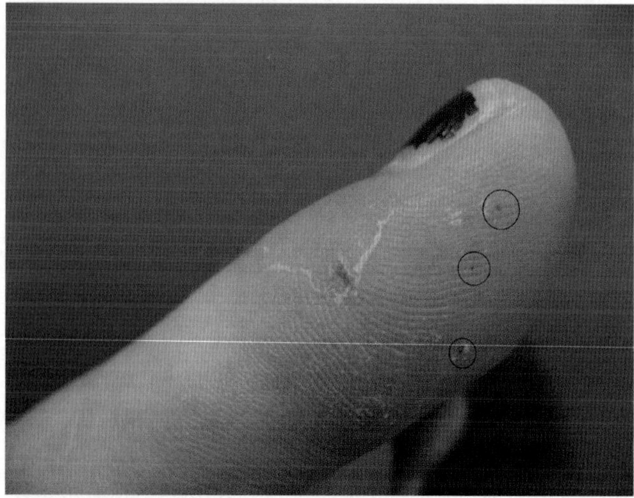

Figure 32.7. Sea urchin envenomation with circles around barbs.

both in deep water as well as along the continental shelf. The animal may be globular or flat and is covered with spines. The spines are permanently attached to the base by muscles and ball-and-socket joints, allowing the animal to wave its spines at intruders. The long, sharp spines are made of calcium carbonate and coated with a layer of epithelium. It is unclear if the spines are truly venomous. It may be the case, as it is with other aquatic tropical species, that the urchins possess pedicellariae, triple-jawed, pincer-like structures that are intermingled with the spines that function to inject venom. Sea-urchin venom is poorly characterized, but similar to other marine venoms. It contains heat labile, high-molecular-weight toxins, including steroid glycosides, hemolysins, proteases, serotonin, and cholinergic substances.

Members of the *Diadematidae* and *Echinothuridae* families possess long hollow spines, which can be dangerous to touch (190). Some spines have reverse hooks, which can increase the possibility of injury (190). Of the 600 species of sea urchins, approximately 28 to 80 may be venomous to humans (190,191). The spines can easily penetrate flesh, rubber-soled shoes, or wet suits, and because they are brittle and break off easily, they can leave calcareous material deep in the wound.

Human envenomations often occur after handling, stepping, or falling on an urchin. Forceful contact results in numerous puncture wounds. The brittle spines often break off in the wounds and dark color pigment is visible in the surrounding tissues (186). The discoloration is thought to be a temporary tattooing of the skin resulting from dye in the spines. Absence of a spine in the skin is indicated by the discoloration spontaneously resolving within 48 hours (192). Injuries result from a combination of factors: (1) reactions to foreign proteins caused by the epithelial covering, (2) reactions to foreign bodies as the spines are retained in the skin, and (3) bacterial infections resulting from puncture wounds (193).

Sea-urchin spine injury can result in local irritation, infection, granuloma formation, or a systemic illness. Following injury, burning or local pain of varying degrees may occur. Discomfort is typically at its most severe minutes to 24 hours after the initial insult (186). Envenomation leads to an immediate local reaction with erythema and edema. Secondary infections and indolent ulcerations are common. Patients may have problems bearing weight (186).

Sea-urchin injuries are known to cause both acute and delayed hypersensitivity reactions. A pruritic eruption due to a delayed hypersensitivity reaction may occur (190). Most often, these are local granulomatous nodules or rashes (194,195). Uncommon delayed reactions such as the appearance of 2 to 5 mm pink to cyanotic non-painful and possibly keratotic nodules have been reported 2 to 12 months after injury. Biopsy of such nodules shows histiocytic–epithelioid granulomas rarely containing crystalline material (193,196). Cystic lesions have also been described (196). Excision of these nodules and cysts is recommended since they rarely heal spontaneously (196).

Optimal treatment for sea-urchin envenomenation is unclear and recommendations vary considerably. Many topical remedies are anecdotal and vary according to local custom. Proper wound care and analgesics are the mainstays of treatment. A commonly recommended treatment is the use of non-scalding hot water soaks for 30 to 90 minutes in an attempt to relieve pain and theoretically inactivate any toxins (189). However, there is no evidence that this treatment is effective in humans as some toxins are heat resistant (189,190,192). Any pedicellariae still attached to the skin should be removed or envenomation will continue. Applying shaving foam and gently scraping with a razor may accomplish this (189). If easily accessible, spines can be removed with forceps or fingers (192). Although removing any pedicellariae is an important part of treatment, attempting to remove the spine may also cause it to break off at the skin and cause further injury or infection. Some authorities recommend not removing the spines if they are asymptomatic (196). Therefore, unless spines are easily accessible, it may be best to avoid removal but this approach is controversial and many recommend removal (196). Since granuloma formations are uncommon, surgical removal of all spines is not routinely indicated. Once granulomas form, they rarely heal and can cause significant disability, making surgical removal advisable (193,196). The erbium-doped yttrium aluminum garnet (Er:YAG) laser has been used successfully, without local or general anesthetic, for removal of sea-urchin spines on the foot (197).

For spines that are close to a joint or a neurovascular structure, surgical extraction may be necessary, preferably using an operative microscope (186,192,193). If the presence of a spine is in question, soft-tissue density radiographs, ultrasound, or MRI may locate spine fragments (189).

Wounds should be irrigated copiously, and tetanus prophylaxis should be administered when indicated. Antibiotics are indicated if signs of infection develop (196). Intralesional injection with a corticosteroid (triamcinolone acetonide, 5 mg/mL) is less efficacious, but can sometimes be successful (189).

Multiple wounds of venomous species may result in systemic symptoms, including nausea, vomiting, paresthesias, numbness, muscular paralysis, abdominal pain, syncope, hypotension, cranial nerve dysfunction, hepatitis, and respiratory distress (186,196). Retained spines without symptoms can be absorbed or extruded through the skin (196).

The proteinaceous covering of sea urchins tends to cause immune reactions of variable presentation. A case report of hypersensitivity reaction to black sea-urchin exposure resulted in eosinophilic pneumonitis requiring mechanical ventilation and prolonged hospitalization but the patient ultimately did recover (198). Osteoarticular symptoms may include bursitis, arthritis, tenosynovitis, and fasciitis (191,199). When implantation occurs near a joint, synovitis followed by arthritis may be an unusual, but not rare sequelae. A plain x-ray may not show the subtle soft tissue and osseous changes associated with such injury; the use of MRI was be beneficial in one case 30 months after penetration (191). Serum examination may be necessary if systemic symptoms are present (190).

One should try to prevent sea-urchin injuries by not stepping where they are located. The spines can penetrate protective gear including diving fins, so care should be taken to avoid them if possible.

TRAUMATIC PLANTAR URTICARIA

Traumatic plantar urticaria is also known as plantar hidradenitis, neutrophilic eccrine hidradenitis, and plantar erythema nodosum (200). All of these reported conditions appear to be relatively similar and possibly identical.

Most involve painful red papules and nodules on the plantar feet, and are typically found in children. These lesions are usually tender to both touch and pressure (201). The development of this condition has been linked to wearing wet sneakers (200). According to one paper, healthy, active individuals seem to be very susceptible (201). Adams notes that basketball players and runners seem to have a higher rate of traumatic plantar urticaria than the general public (54). Ice hockey participants and figure skaters who have prolonged exposure to damp skates may be affected by palmoplantar eccrine hidradenitis as well (176).

Generally, the diagnosis is made by clinical examination. The condition has an acute onset and ambulation can be painful (176).

The differential includes bites, chilblains, panniculitis, vasculitis, embolism, and migratory angioedema (200). A biopsy can be helpful as it often shows the presence of perivascular neutrophilic infiltration in both the superficial and deep dermis, which is seen in the acute stage of neutrophilic eccrine hidradenitis (54).

While a variety of treatments have been suggested including NSAIDs, antibiotics, systemic steroids, potassium iodide, and soaks, there are no controlled studies. Generally, the condition resolves upon discontinuing the physical activity and bed rest (200). The pain typically ceases within 24 hours of bed rest and the lesions typically resolve within a few days to a few weeks (176,201).

POISON IVY

Poison ivy, also known as rhus dermatitis, most often affects athletes whose activities bring them near or into wooded areas (202). This includes cross-country runners and golfers (54). Urushiol is the oil of the plant that causes contact dermatitis (54).

The most important member of the Anacardiaceae family, *Toxicodendron,* which includes common or northern poison ivy (*Toxicodendron radicans*), western poison ivy (*T. rydbergii*), eastern poison oak (*T. toxicarium*), western poison oak (*T. diversilobum*), and poison sumac (*T. vernix*) (203).

Clinically, poison ivy appears as linear, erythematous, vesicular papules, and plaques, but can frequently present atypically (Fig. 32.8). The rash is not limited to the areas of the body that were exposed to the plant, as athletes and others who are affected have a tendency to spread the causative protein to other parts of the body (54). The resin can remain on clothing or pets and be allergenic. It has been reported that the pruritic blisters and dermatitis may cover more than 50% of one's body (204).

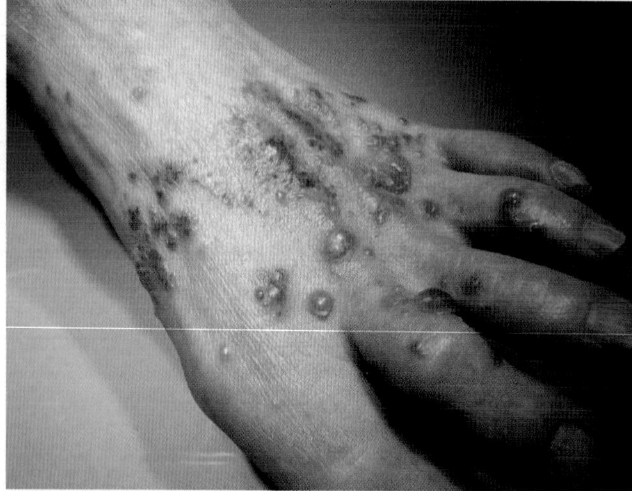

Figure 32.8. Poison ivy.

While the foot alone is rarely the only area of the dermatitis, the linear pattern is a key indicator in the diagnosis. The differential diagnosis includes atopic dermatitis, eczematous drug eruptions, and viral exanthems. Patch testing and biopsy can be performed if the rash cannot be confidently confirmed on a clinical basis (54).

The rash can be treated with medium to high potency (class I–II) topical steroids especially before vesicles have arisen. In severe cases, a rapid burst of oral steroids for 2 to 3 weeks or intramuscular (IM) injection of triamcinolone may be needed. If the clinical decision is made to use IM cortisone, the patient must be warned of the numerous potential side effects associated with parenteral corticosteroids including mental status changes and osteonecrosis of the femoral head (204). Cool compresses, calamine lotion, antipruritic lotions containing menthol and phenol, and oatmeal baths can be soothing. In milder cases, topical immunomodulators may be sufficient (54). Sedating antihistamines can be helpful if patients have difficulty sleeping. The condition can last for up to 2 months; therefore in order to continue sports comfortably, it is necessary to have the condition treated (204).

Barrier creams such as bentoquatam (Ivy Block) may be helpful in preventing dermatitis but can leave a clay-like residue (205).

As it is such a prevalent myth, it is important to note that the blisters do not contain urushiol so they are not contagious. In addition, washing should be performed immediately; if it is delayed by as little as 10 minutes, only 50% of the urushiol will be removed; by 60 minutes washing is ineffective (206).

DERMATITIS

Both allergic contact and irritant dermatitis occur commonly on the feet. They are often triggered by heat, sweating, and occlusion (207,208). They can present from acute to subacute and can also be chronic (208). Atopic dermatitis has been observed to be more common among elite athletes, but does not usually present on the feet (209).

Irritant or primary dermatitis presents similarly to allergic contact dermatitis; however, the former is due to an irritant effect and is not allergic in nature.

Contact dermatitis is allergic in nature and also known as contact allergic dermatitis. These are Type IV allergic reactions that are cell mediated and usually result in local reactions (210). This is in contrast to a Type I mediated allergic reaction, which can cause anaphylaxis; this can occur rarely from running shoes (211). Virtually any type of sports equipment including footwear and medications can cause a contact allergic dermatitis rash on the feet.

Among the common contactants on the foot are shoes, athletic tape, jogging cream, and swimming fins (54,207, 208,212,213). Any athlete who uses athletic tape can develop contact dermatitis (54). Jogging cream, used by runners to prevent blisters, can occasionally cause contact dermatitis (54). Contact dermatitis from fins can affect scuba divers and snorkelers (54). The common allergens in fins include dibutylthiourea, diethylthiourea, and isopropylaminodiphenylamine (214).

Shoe dermatitis is a result of different chemicals in combination with heat and humidity within the shoe, and can be experienced by runners and joggers (207,208). Among the possible contactants are rubber and neoprene innersoles (208,215,216). In some foam rubber, the offending agent is ethylbutylthiourea (217); polyurethane insoles are an alternative material. In addition, other compounds found in shoes, including leather, dyes, and glues have also been implicated in allergic contact dermatitis (7,208,215).

In a study performed among student athletes, many allergens, most notably benzocaine and lanolin were thought to be causative factors of contact dermatitis; it was concluded that benzocaine and epoxy resin were among the allergens that cause dermatitis on the feet (218). Many ingredients in analgesic sprays can cause contact dermatitis. In one case, a runner using jogging cream was allergic to four different components of the cream (208,219).

A 59-year-old woman detailed her 5-year history of a rash on her lower legs and feet during and after playing golf. The patient applied peppermint foot spray in order to cool the irritation she felt while playing golf. The patient was diagnosed with golfer's vasculitis. Patch testing was performed on clippings of grass and the patient's foot spray as well as the standard medicament series, facial series, fragrances series, and plant series. Positive reactions were reported to amerchol and the peppermint foot spray. The foot spray's purpose is to provide a cooling sensation for the irritation on the lower extremities that accompany golfing activities. In the case of this patient, she developed an allergic contact dermatitis to her foot spray as a secondary event to her golfer's vasculitis (220).

Walkers became sensitized from components of shoes including nickel, cobalt, and paraphenylenediamine (221). Ice hockey players and figure skaters can become sensitized to a wide variety of materials (176). One figure skater had foot contact dermatitis from a Bunga Pad; it was tested and due to lanolin (222).

Generally, contact dermatitis appears as symmetrical lesions. The clinician will usually see focal pruritic erythematous patches. The rash, however, can be vesicular and asymmetrical, and usually occurs from a few hours to a few days after the allergen is in contact with the patient. Allergic contact dermatitis never occurs the first time the skin is in contact with the allergen, as sensitivity must develop. Among the differential diagnosis are non-contact dermatitis, pressure urticaria, psoriasis, dyshidrosis (pompholyx), atopic dermatitis, and dermatophyte infection. KOH tests can rule out fungus; biopsies and allergy testing can often confirm contact dermatitis (54).

In order to prevent this rash, the clinician should attempt to find the offending chemical(s) if possible. They can sometimes be determined by the patient's history. Generally, however, the athlete should be referred to a dermatologist who can patch test the patient. Patch testing for contact dermatitis involves testing the athlete with a number of different potentially contributing factors to the condition. The patch test is generally placed on the back and is left on for 2 days; the area is then evaluated twice over the following 2 to 5 days. The second reading is necessary to rule out sensitivity to the tape or to all of the allergens known as "angry back syndrome." Patch testing during the athlete's sport season is frequently not practical because the area needs to remain dry for 2 days and then left alone by avoiding sweating and showering until the final reading is done. Consequently, patch test evaluations often need to be delayed until a break or after the sports season is over.

Dermatologists as well as allergists can both perform patch testing. Often, allergists depend on dermatologists for more comprehensive patch testing, but allergists generally have access to rapid epicutaneous tests that can be used as a primary method of evaluation for some products (223). Once the offending agent is recognized, the clinician should hopefully be able to provide non-allergic alternatives directly to the patient. Once the chemical is removed from the athlete's environment the dermatitis should resolve and not recur.

High-strength corticosteroids are the best way to treat most forms of primary and allergic contact dermatitis. However, if the allergic reaction is severe, or if symptoms and outbreaks have not resolved after the traditional course of topical steroids, a short period of oral steroids and/or an intramuscular cortisone injection may be added to the treatment regimen (54). For mild or chronic conditions, topical immunomodulators such as pimecrolimus may be administered to lessen the symptoms (54). Barrier creams may be helpful. Allergen-proof barrier socks can be helpful, but may be difficult to wear (224).

If it is possible to continue sports participation without the use of the equipment causing the allergic contact dermatitis, then the irritation can be decreased in this way.

PLANTAR PSORIASIS

Plantar psoriasis refers to psoriasis on the plantar surfaces of the feet. While there are no prevalence studies in athletes, this condition can potentially be confused with a variety of other papulosquamous dermatologic conditions, and can affect athletic performance.

Psoriasis is a genetic disease whose mechanism of inheritance is not fully elucidated. It is immune mediated. Clinical observation is the most common means of diagnosis of plantar psoriasis. Fissures within elevated lesions and plaques are often present when affecting the feet. Such plaques are usually well-defined and are typically a very red color. The plaques also often have a dry, thin, silvery-white or micaceous scale (225).

Local factors that contribute to the development of psoriasis include various kinds of trauma including infections, cold, and trauma (225). Excessive scratching can trigger the condition, as well as excessive exposure to sunlight. Psoriasis can improve with moderate sun exposure. Systemic factors that may contribute to the development of psoriasis include HIV infection, pharyngeal streptococcal infections, and certain drugs such as beta-blockers, NSAIDs and antimalarials. The likelihood of developing psoriasis has also been noted to increase with certain hormonal changes, as well as smoking and alcohol use. Some have reported an increase in the severity of symptoms with psychological stress, but this has yet to be proven.

Mild or high potency topical cortisones can be helpful, and are often combined with calcipotriene. Both psoralen plus ultraviolet A (PUVA) and Oral PUVA are treatments that have been shown to significantly decrease the severity of psoriasis symptoms (226,227). Topical 0.1% tazarotene cream can be efficacious (227). If severe, additional treatments include methotrexate, cyclosporine, ultraviolet light therapy, and biologics such as etanercept.

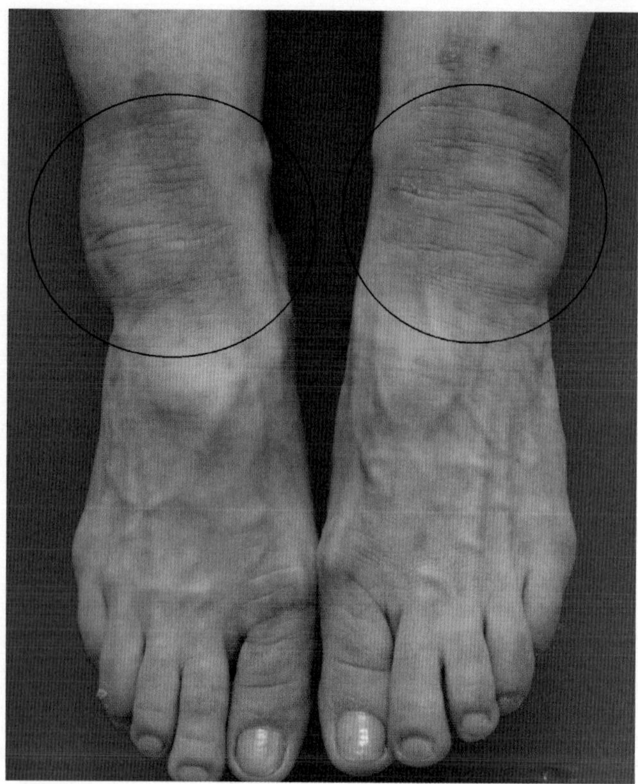

Figure 32.9. Lichen simplex chronicus (LSC) ankles.

LICHEN SIMPLEX CHRONICUS

Lichen simplex chronicus frequently occurs on the ankles, but can occur anywhere there is unrestrained rubbing and scratching (Fig. 32.9). Because of chronic rubbing, the skin becomes thickened and toughened. The need to scratch may be due to a number of factors such as infection, local trauma, depression, stress, anxiety, a history of atopic dermatitis, insect bites, scars, or a history of allergic contact dermatitis (228). Some studies have shown that LSC is more common in Asians and African Americans (184). Those who are most often affected by the condition are between the ages of 35 and 50 (229). Women are also more often affected than men (229).

Generally, the diagnosis is made clinically. If asked by the clinician, often a patient will demonstrate how they scratch. Physical indicators include thickening of the skin, hyperpigmentation, scaling, and itchy plaques (230). The condition is easily identified by such erythematous, well-defined plaques with excoriations due to scratching (228). The primary symptom is itch, which can usually be resolved after excessive scratching. The relief is usually then followed by another attack of pruritus, which is again resolved by scratching, in turn perpetuating the itch-scratch cycle. The ankles are a common site for this condition as well as the neck, scalp, vulva, pubis, scrotum, and extensor forearms. The differential diagnosis for LSC includes psoriasis, tinea, mycosis fungoides, lichen planus, and lichen amyloidosis (229).

Lichen simplex chronicus can be confirmed, if necessary, by biopsy. KOH preparation can be helpful in ruling out tinea. Clinical features are usually enough to diagnose the condition; however, biopsies and radiologic imaging studies can be performed in order to rule out any suspicion of lymphoma.

LSC is usually treated by high-strength topical cortisone, which has shown to resolve the lesions within 1 month of treatment (230). Topical cortisone in the form of a tape, cordran, which can be applied to the affected area for 24 hours at a time, can be helpful as this prevents the athlete from rubbing the area. Yet another effective treatment is the placement of an Unna boot, which not only has medicated bandages to treat the area but also prevents the patient from further scratching. When the lesions are smaller, another treatment option is to inject the lesions with intralesional cortisone, rather than using topical cortisone. Antihistamines and anxiolytics can be used occasionally as well.

It is important to emphasize other means of relief from the symptoms of the condition aside from scratching. For example, ice pack application may cause itching to subside and will not produce the negative side effects associated with scratching (228).

This condition is also often associated with depression and dissociative experiences. As a result of this connection, the field of psychodermatology has developed out of concern and interest in the relationship between skin diseases and the psyche (229).

ONYCHOMYCOSIS

Onychomycosis, otherwise known as tinea unguium, is infection of the toenails with tinea or fungus (Fig. 32.10B). Onychomycosis is more common in those who are active in sports (55). It is also four times more likely in toenails than in fingernails. This condition often affects those who visit swimming pools (231,232). Onychomycosis is associated with tinea pedis in 1/3rd of patients (232).

Other factors that have been associated with onychomycosis include being male, nail trauma, peripheral vascular disease, smoking, history of diabetes, immunosuppression, history of tinea pedis, and a family history of onychomycosis (79,233).

Onychomycosis is caused by fungi that flourish in moist and warm environments, such as the inside of a shoe (55). Since runners, cyclists, and other athletes use airtight and sweaty shoes, they are more at risk for developing onychomycosis. For these same reasons, the occlusive skates of professional ice hockey players, which are often saturated with sweat for several hours at a time, represent a typical environment in which fungus can grow (59). Athletes who use a swimming pool floor are also at greater risk for developing onychomycosis (231). Other areas similar or adjacent to swimming pool floors, which may be infected with tinea include public showers, health-club bathing facilities, and changing rooms (55). These locations tend to be common places for such fungal infections to reside; the fungi reproduce spores that then scatter throughout floor surfaces and thereby spreading to footwear and making it easier to transmit and/or re-infect an individual's feet (55). Participation in contact sports may compromise the patient's ability to defend against infections by reducing physical barriers as well as by impairing immune defenses (55).

The Achilles Project surveyed 100,000 subjects from 18 European countries for relevance between sports participation and the prevalence of foot diseases; 70% of those screened were active in sports (55). Among those who were active, 56.6% had clinically infected feet as a result of their respective sports. Among children, the odds were 1.7 times higher for finding a fungal infection of the foot and/or nail among those that were active compared to those that were not. For young adults, the odds were 1.4 times higher. For middle-aged adults, the effects of sports participation was not significant in fungal infection rates. For the elderly, the odds were 1.4 times higher (55). In a review from Brazil, while athletes, mostly soccer players, had additional onychomycosis, tinea pedis, and combined disease, the numbers apparently did not reach statistical significance (234).

Participants in the Special Olympics had a rate of onychomycosis similar to that of the general population although this was an observational survey without further laboratory or other confirmation (11).

The three main types of dermatophytes to cause nail infection are *Trichophyton, Epidermophyton,* and *Microsporum* (54). *Trichophyton,* mostly *T. rubrum* and *T. mentagrophytes,* are the primary causative species of most onychomycosis, with the ratio in a normal population of *T. rubrum* to *T. mentagrophytes* being greater than 9:1 (235).

The various subtypes of onychomycosis present differently but often overlap (236).

The subtypes include: distal lateral subungual onychomycosis (DLSO), white superficial onychomycosis (WSO), proximal subungual onychomycosis (PSO), endonyx onychomycosis (EO) and total dystrophic onychomycosis (OM). DLSO's clinical presentation manifests in the nail plate with a thickened and opacified appearance. In addition, subungual hyperkeratosis, onycholysis, and discoloration from white to brown may be present. EO presents as a milky white color; however, there is no clinical presentation of subungual hyperkeratosis or onycholysis. WSO is typically isolated to the toenails and presents as small, white-speckled or powdery areas on the nail plate. The nail is rough and often falls apart with ease. PSO presents with leukonychia in the proximal nail fold. The nail plate is normal distally, while it is white proximally (237). Lastly, total dystrophic onychomycosis can be recognized by its presentation of the nail as thickened, opaque, and yellow/brown. It involves both the nail plate in its entirety as well as the nail matrix (237).

When onychomycosis is diagnosed, the entire foot must be examined as all toes have the potential to be affected (54). Any one part of the nail unit, the nail matrix, nail bed, or nail plate may be all or partially affected (237). In addition, the hands should be examined as well. It can be helpful to examine the entire skin because certain rashes can occur as a result of tinea.

Onychomycosis may cause altered negative self-image as well as pain (238). It is also a risk factor for increased soft tissue infections of the leg and cellulitis (239).

Onychomycosis should be confirmed with laboratory testing. Periodic acid–Schiff (PAS) examination of the material under the nail by histology laboratory is the most sensitive test to determine dermatophyte infection (240). The condition can also be diagnosed via KOH mount and fungal culture examination of a sample specimen (241). A curette can be used to scrape the subungual debris. Vertical drilling of any proximal affected nail may allow more sensitive diagnosis but can leave a temporary nail deformity (242).

The differential diagnosis of onychomycosis includes onycholysis from a variety of causes, trauma, lichen planus, paronychia (55), psoriasis (59), dystrophic nail, and subungual hematoma such as tennis toe and jogger's toes (54) (see related section in this chapter).

After laboratory testing confirms a fungal etiology, but before treatment is initiated, the athlete's concurrent medications should be reviewed, as there may be interactions with the oral antifungal drugs (240). Typically, liver function tests and complete blood counts should be monitored while on oral antifungals (240).

Onychomycosis can be treated with either oral or topical medications. Nail lacquer, including ciclopirox and amorolfine, may also be beneficial but the cure rate is low (79). An alternative treatment includes cutting back the nail and treating the exposed skin with topical nystatin or an antifungal cream in hopes of enabling a healthy nail to grow back (241). If the nail is thickened, application of urea and 40% cream twice a day may be needed to thin the nail so that the topical antifungal can better penetrate the nail (54).

Systemic antifungal medications are much more effective than topical medications in treating onychomycosis. Terbinafine, itraconazole, griseofulvin, and fluconazole are all tested oral medications to treat the fungus. Terbinafine is clinically the most effective compared to the other treatments.

Cochrane meta-analysis revealed the superiority of terbinafine relative to alternative oral treatments such as itraconazole, griseofulvin, and fluconazole (233,243). For each agent, terbinafine and itraconazole, randomized controlled trials are compared to open studies via overall meta-analytical averages of both of the treatments' mycologic and clinical response rates (243). A cumulative meta-analysis of systemic antifungal agents for the treatment of onychomycosis suggests that over time, even as new randomized controlled trials have been observed, efficacy rates remain constant (243).

While common side effects of systemic therapy include gastrointestinal distress and headaches, serious side effects can occur in less than 1% of patients, most notably liver toxicity and even death (244).

The FDA recommends monitoring liver function tests. Systemic therapy should not be given to patients with active or chronic liver disease (245). Moreover, an additional side effect in patients treated with itraconazole can be congestive heart failure.

In one study published in 2002, 46% of the subjects who took systemic daily terbinafine for 12 to 16 weeks were cured, while only 13% of the subjects who took itraconazole were cured. Six months after treatment had ceased 9% of the terbinafine-treated patients and 22% of the itraconazole-treated patients experienced mycologic relapse (246). Seventy-two patients underwent a second intervention of terbinafine; 88% of those patients obtained mycologic cure (246). After 31 to 36 months, very few relapses were observed in either group (246).

Oral terbinafine taken for 12 weeks was also more effective than pulse dosing of itraconazole. Here pulse dosing means taking itraconazole twice daily for 1 week, then no medication for 3 weeks, then repeating the cycle two times.

Onychomycosis frequently recurs, with percentages ranging from 10% to 53%; patients who took terbinafine had lower recurrence rates than those who took itraconazole (247).

Debridement of infected nails has not been well studied nor has chemical or surgical avulsion of the nail, but they may have a therapeutic role especially in patients in whom drug therapy has failed (236).

Onychomycosis often goes undiagnosed and untreated. Although this infection can be relatively minor, it is important to treat onychomycosis in athletes so as to prevent spreading of the disease to other athletes (55).

It is better for athletes to prevent onychomycosis because toenails can be difficult to treat due to the length of time it takes for them to grow out (240). Synthetic moisture-wicking socks should be used and then immediately removed after athletic activity. After the removal of socks, the feet should immediately be washed. If public showers are used, the athlete should be encourage to wear sandals or some other sort of protective footwear such as flip-flops while walking on public floors (240). Athletes should be educated in proper nail care, including keeping nails clean and cut short. They should not share nail clippers or footwear (236).

Antifungal foot powders should be applied to shoes and proper footwear should be worn daily as well as when in communal areas. It is unclear whether athletes who have previously suffered from onychomycosis should apply prophylactic topical antifungal medications. It may also be important to treat family members and close friends of athletes who are diagnosed with onychomycosis (79).

Since facilities such as locker room floors, showers, and pool decks can be infected with dermatophytes, it is critical that the cleaning staff of facilities clean those areas thoroughly and confirm periodically that the surface area is negative for the fungus (54).

While there are no specific guidelines from the NCAA regarding onychomycosis, according to the NCAA guidelines on skin infections, athletes with tinea pedis who have exposed feet during competition should receive prompt therapy for their tinea. In general, "infectious skin conditions that cannot be adequately protected should be considered cause for medical disqualification from practice and competition (67)."

SUBUNGUAL HEMATOMA

Forces upon the toenail in many athletic endeavors can cause changes to the toenail. Frequently, these changes result in bleeding beneath the nail known as subungual hematomas. Other nail changes can be seen as well, such as nail dystrophy and subungual hyperkeratosis (141). In addition, onycholysis, edema, and erythema can be noted (248). Splinter hemorrhages may also be caused by trauma to the nail unit (249). Onycholysis can be seen in football players as well as ballet dancers who dance on *en pointe* (250). Leukonychia, generally seen as transverse white bands, can occur in athletes who do karate as well as other martial arts that involve a significant amount of force to their toenails (249). White nail beds can occur as well (249). If karate is discontinued, these nail changes will often normalize within 3 to 6 months (249). Occasionally, the nail may be partially or fully lost temporarily if enough nail separation has taken place (251,252). Often black-blue discoloration is observed under the distal nail-plate, not the proximal nail plate (78) (Fig. 32.10). Sometimes the discoloration affects the tip of the toe and spares the toenail (253).

These related conditions, however, if common to specific sports, may also be expressed according to the affected individual's sport, such as jogger's toe, skier's toe, climber's toe, hiker's toe, tennis toe, and sportsman's toe (7,54,249,252,254–261). Specific sports commonly have specific co-morbidities, which are dependent on the type of trauma to the nail bed. Football toe, for example, is sometimes accompanied by the complete loss of the toenail, also known as onychoptosis defluvium, even in the absence of subungual hematoma (252,262). Professional skaters, whether in hockey, figure-skating, or entertainment commonly have onychauxis, splinter hemorrhages, subungual hyperkeratosis, leukonychia, onycholysis, and pincer nail in addition to the subungual hematoma (54,249).

The affected digit is generally determined by the sport. The abrupt stops and quick starts in certain sports such as tennis, squash, basketball, and racquetball can affect either the first or second toe depending upon which is longer. In these sports, the force exerted on the toe into the front of the shoe is more common laterally than medially (7,139,259,262,263). Tennis toes can be involved bilaterally (264,265). The third, fourth and fifth toes of runners and joggers are generally affected, while the second and third toes are more likely to be involved in soccer and football kickers (127,252,257,263,266–268). The medical records of 635 marathon runners were reviewed

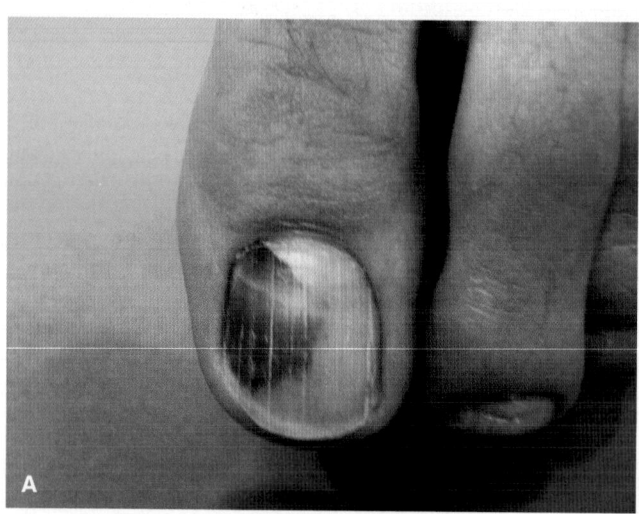

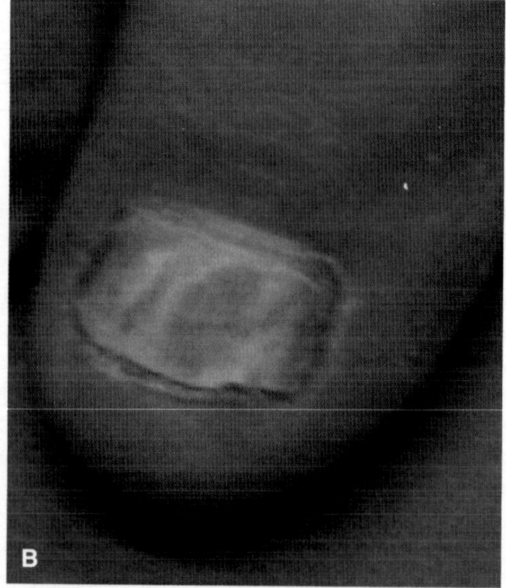

Figure 32.10. **A:** Subungual hematoma from skiing. **B:** Onychomycosis.

showing an incidence of 2.5% of subungual hematomas (269). Crush injuries can also cause subungual hematomas as in the case report of a gymnast dropping a 100-pound pommel horse on her foot (270). Windsurfers' toe or "toe jam" usually affects the big toe because of the pressure caused by planting toes tightly on the surfboard (54). Skiers' and skaters' toes are a result of ill-fitting boots or skates, which allow for excessive movement within the toe box (54,249,260,271). In skiers, the nail-bed discoloration is generally in the great toe and often bilateral in skiers who frequently lean forward. While more common with poorly fitting boots, skier's toe can also be seen in those whose boots fit well (272). However, the previous categorization can be arbitrary and virtually any toe or any combination of toes can be involved in any athletic activity (249).

Consequently, trauma to the nail bed and plate are the main etiologic factors in subungual hematoma (273). In general, the harder the surface, the greater the impact of the shoe upon the surface, and the more likely it is to develop subungual hematoma (274). Bleeding is caused by blunt trauma or repeated disturbance to the rich vascular nail bed. The collected blood, giving the nail its distinct dark red-to-black appearance, can cause an increase in pressure on the nerve endings and may therefore be intensely painful (273,275,276). Patients with onychogryphosis or other nail dystrophies are at greater risk for subungual hematomas (254).

The first indication of subungual hematoma, upon physical assessment, is the appearance of a dark red-to-black nail (267). If the hematoma is older or chronic, the color will generally be blue, purple, or black and will usually not be tender (267). However, it should be noted that subungual hematomas do not always result in nail discoloration (254).

The differential diagnosis for subungual hematoma includes melanoma, malignant tumors, melanocytic lesions, onychomycosis, subungual exostosis, and melanonychia striata (249,267). However, if the physician is unclear as to what the condition may be, a biopsy of the nail plate, nail bed and/or matrix may need to be performed as the possibility of a subungual melanoma must be considered (254,257,266,267,277). Nail melanomas are uncommon but do comprise 2% of all melanomas (263). The clinician should be especially suspicious for melanoma if there is leaching of pigment to the nail fold proximally to the proximal nail fold or laterally (Hutchinson's sign) or if there are a variety of hues overall (254).

The clinician should be aware that a significant percentage of patients with subungual melanoma describe a history of trauma. If there is no history of trauma, then the clinician should be especially suspicious of melanoma or melanocytic nevus (248,263). Physicians should record the percentage of the nail bed that is covered by the condition and any further trauma experienced by the affected digit (257). Radiographic imaging may be indicated to rule out fracture (257). To rule out onychomycosis, a simple KOH test and nail culture can be performed (see section in this chapter on onychomycosis) (264).

Treatment for subungual hematoma is typically unnecessary as these conditions generally heal naturally. This may take time as the nail will need to grow out moving at a rate that corresponds with the growth of the nail plate (248,270). However, if the patient is experiencing excruciating pain, then treatment is indicated to provide immediate relief, especially if the patient presents within 48 hours of the incident (267). Aseptic technique as well as universal precautions are recommended since the blood may spurt (257). However, if the affected digit is not sore, then it may be left alone; the subungual hematoma will eventually resolve due to growth of the nail plate (267,276).

The treatment option chosen will be dependent upon the extent of the trauma. Trephination is usually performed for hematomas affecting less than 50% of the nail. If painful, a digital nerve block may be necessary (273). If a digital block is necessary, we have described a technique which lessens pain with the use of an ice cube for 30 to 45 seconds before the needle is injected (278). Alternatively, we have also described the technique of vibration anesthesia using massagers to vibrate and distract the patient and fill the nerves with vibration so that less pain is felt (279). Our paper has the use of online videos describing the technique.

This procedure involves the use of a hot paperclip or an 18 gauge needle held with a hemostat or electric cauterizing lance, or a handheld cautery unit or a hand engine with a dental bur held perpendicularly above the center of the hematoma to make a puncture at the base of the nail using slow, careful, and steady pressure. This will relieve the pressure created by the increase of blood on the nail bed (257,275,276). The hole should be large enough for the blood to drain (276). This procedure should not be performed on patients wearing acrylic nails as they may be flammable (275). If the lesion is older than 48 hours, then nail avulsion may be indicated (267). Carbon dioxide laser may be used as well but requires specialized equipment (270). If the pain is manageable, conservative treatment including ice, analgesia, warm water soaks, and elevation may be used (257,277).

The subungual hematoma may also be relieved by drilling a needle and placing a capillary tube into the nail plate, which allows the blood to be extracted through capillary action (257). Moreover, new studies have shown the use of a 29-gauge, extrafine insulin syringe needle for the withdrawal of the hematoma to be effective (273). After the nail is trimmed and cleaned, the patient secures the nail. With care taken to avoid the nail bed, the physician places the needle under and parallel to the nail plate. The needle is then gently pushed back and forward creating a small hole; placing mild pressure on the nail will relieve the condition as blood will begin to drain (273). If the patient feels pain, the clinician may need to wait a few seconds before proceeding (273). If the blood persists, there may be a septum and evacuation of the other side may be necessary (273). Kaya et al. feel that the use of the extrafine 29-gauge insulin syringe is especially helpful for hematomas of the smaller nails (273). No matter how the drainage is performed, a sterile pressure dressing should be placed after the procedure in order to prevent further bleeding or infection (250,267).

The removal of the entire nail has been recommended if the hematoma affects more than 50% of the nail; the complete removal is mainly performed as a preventative measure to nail deformation and to preserve function (256,275,280). Although inconclusive, a retrospective review of papers involving the fingernail revealed that trephining is as likely as effective as complete removal of the nail, as long as there are no underlying injuries (256). This is true, in particular with regards to fingernail lesions, despite the level of severity of the hematoma (280).

If more than 25% of the nail is involved, sequelae may include onycholysis and shedding of the nail plate (54,253,267). Other possible complications include infection and temporary or permanent nail deformity.

Properly fitting shoes can prevent subungual hematomas (260,267). It is also recommended to cut nails straight across so as to prevent an unequal distribution of forces on the nail bed (248). Orthotic devices may be helpful in preventing the toes from being forced against the toe box (253). In addition, toe pads and side straps may help prevent anterior slipping of the foot in the shoe (271).

ONYCHOCRYPTOSIS, INGROWN TOENAIL

In onychocryptosis, also known as ingrown toenails, the large toenail acts as a foreign body when the spicule of the nail gets embedded in the nail fold, causing pain and inflammation. Tight, occlusive footwear compact the toes causing this condition. In addition, incorrect cutting of the nail and prior trauma may result in further nail embedment in the nail groove. This causes the body to develop a foreign body reaction, resulting in inflammation and pain (262,281). Ingrown toenails can affect athletes such as tennis players, basketball players, football players, runners, and dancers (54,282–284). Participants in the Special Olympics had double the rate of onychocryptosis compared to that of the general population although this was an observational survey without further laboratory or other evaluation (11).

Patients may have nails that experience overcurvature and are deep along the sulcus at the border (284). However, factors other than genes may play an important role, such as pressure on the affected toe(s). For example, in an obese person heavy weight is concentrated over a small area of the foot. Onychocryptosis is seen in men three times more frequently than in women (281). Older individuals are more susceptible to ingrown toenails because the nail tends to become more curved over time (283); however, the condition is observed in people of all ages (281).

An additional factor in onychocryptosis is caused by the irregular fit of the nail plate on its nail groove. This may be caused by trauma of the toe, cutting the nail too short, irregularly tight footwear and due to other forces on the affected toe. The nail will bury itself, causing inflammation, and occasionally bacteria or fungal infection. If not treated at this stage, the individual may experience further burial of the nail due to overgrowth of surrounding tissues (262).

Generally, onychocryptosis can be diagnosed clinically as patients generally present with pain in the lateral and distal nail fold to their internist or an ER, but also often to a podiatrist, dermatologist, or orthopedic surgeon. Upon clinical evaluation, the affected toe may appear inflamed with overgrowth of granulation tissue on the nail margin and in the surrounding region. Crusting and drainage may also be present. The patient usually experiences pain upon movement (262,281). Among the differential diagnosis are impetigo, lymphangitis, obesity, gout, osteomyelitis, paronychia, fracture, foreign body, bunion, pyogenic granuloma (Fig. 32.11), mucous cyst, subungual exostosis, candidiasis, periungual fibroma, cellulitis, *S. aureus* infection, and streptococcal infection (54,281).

Often no laboratory studies are required, but KOH prep, fungal, bacterial, and viral cultures may be indicated. Radiographic imaging may be necessary to rule out foreign body, fracture, subungual exostosis, or osteomyelitis (176).

If the condition is mild with only erythema and edema then initial treatment can be conservative, often a change in shoes to a more comfortable toe box or cutting the nail straight across is all that is necessary (262,281,285). Soaks and analgesics can be helpful. More advanced staged disease can be treated by stretching the soft tissue; the nail can then be trained by placing wool underneath, avoiding the nail from becoming embedded. Often, however, partial nail avulsion may be indicated, and occasionally full nail avulsion. This is accomplished using a digital nail block, though a metatarsal block may be preferable (286).

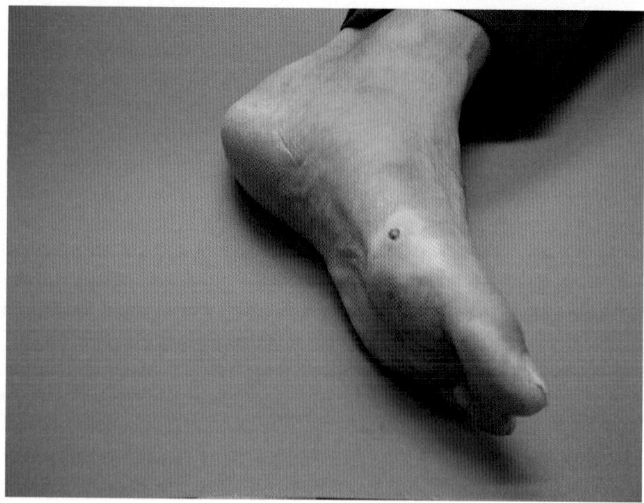

Figure 32.11. Pyogenic granuloma (the light area is vasoconstriction from injection of local anesthesia).

Then approximately a quarter to a third of the nail, including the affected area, can be removed. The clinician and patient may then decide to perform a matricectomy generally with 70% to 90% phenol. The decision to perform matricectomy can wait to see if the ingrown toenail is recurrent. The relief of pain after partial nail avulsion is rapid. Often a partial nail matricectomy is performed concomitantly. According to a Cochrane analysis, chemical matricectomy is preferred over surgical matricectomy, though the use of phenol can increase post-operative infection (287).

In order to prevent ingrown toenails, the use of wide, comfortable footwear should be implemented, along with toe caps, which serve by protecting the trauma-prone toe (54). Patients need to be instructed to cut the nail across and not toward the matrix.

PLANTAR HYPERHIDROSIS

Excessive sweating of the foot is known as plantar hyperhidrosis and can affect both men and women of all ages, but can be especially detrimental to athletic performance. Hyperhidrosis can be difficult to control. It is generally bilateral and symmetrical (Fig. 32.12), usually beginning in adolescence. It is believed that as much as 2.8% of the population may suffer from hyperhidrosis (288). This is consistent with studies done in Southeast Asia, which also show an incidence of about 3% (289). Besides the feet, the axillae, palms, and face are the most common sites of hyperhidrosis. Typically, about 44% of patients presenting with hyperhidrosis report it affecting their feet (290).

One study showed no significant difference in prevalence between men and women (289). However, a later study which surveyed two hyperhidrosis clinics, one in the US and one in Canada, did find a significant difference between males and

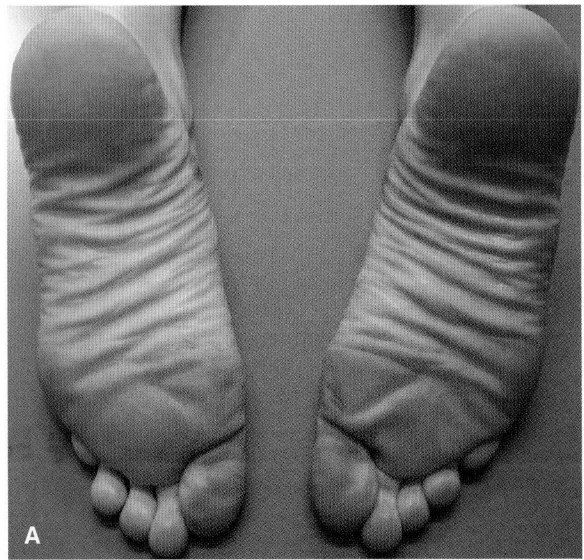

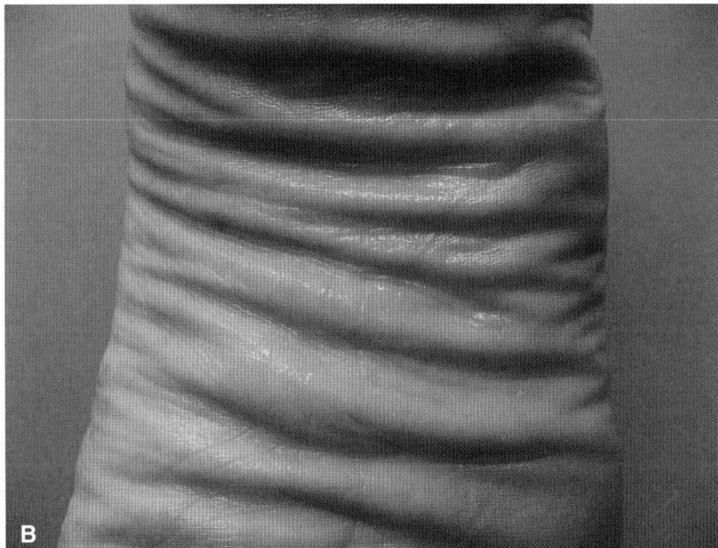

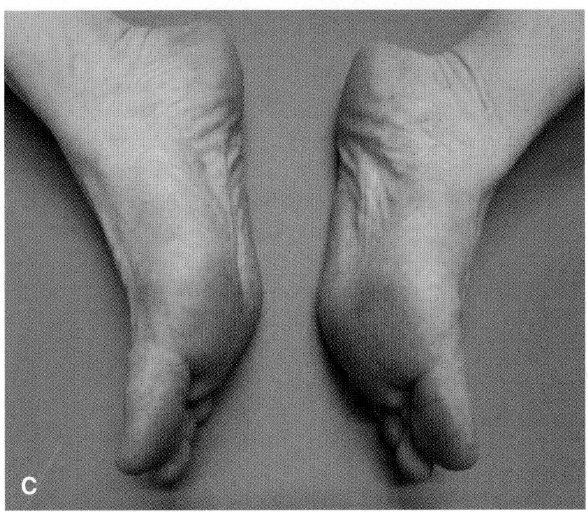

Figure 32.12. Hyperhidrosis. **A:** Hyperhidrosis before botulinum toxin type A treatment. Note the active sweating, even at rest. **B:** Close-up of hyperhidrosis with increased sweating before injection of botulinum toxin type A. **C:** Hyperhidrosis 2 weeks after injection of botulinum toxin type A. Note the dry surfaces of the feet.

females (291). Specifically, when both the Canadian and American patients were combined, 62.8% of the patients were female (292). The Canadian/American study also found that women at 46% were more likely than men at 25% to present with plantar hyperhidrosis (291).

Another difference between these two epidemiologic studies was the general age of onset. In the US study, the average age of onset was found to be 25 while the American/Canadian study found the average age to be closer to 14 years old (289,291). In addition, this study further differentiated the age of onset depending on the body part that was affected by hyperhidrosis (291). People with palmar or plantar hyperhidrosis were more likely to have onset of symptoms before puberty, while those with axillary hyperhidrosis were more likely to have onset post-puberty (291). Other associations found in the American/Canadian study were: 87.9% of patients were Caucasian, the mean age of the patients at both clinics was 25 years old, and 43.4% of patients were students (at any level) (291). Participants in the Special Olympics had a higher rate of plantar hyperhidrosis than that of the general population although this was an observational survey without further evaluation (11).

Hyperhidrosis is believed to also have a familial component. According to the American/Canadian survey, between 30% to 65% of patients have a positive family history (291). Hyperhidrosis is inherited via an autosomal dominant gene with variable levels of penetrance; if one parent has hyperhidrosis, the likelihood that a child will inherit it is about 25% (290).

Although the exact cause of hyperhidrosis is not known, it is believed that excessive sweating is not caused by a malfunction of the sweat glands, but perhaps an exaggerated response to emotional stimuli (291). Excessive sweating is triggered by stress or emotion, and does not occur during sleep or sedation (293).

There are two main causes of sweat: thermoregulation, which allows the body to dissipate heat, and emotional sweat (290). Whereas eccrine glands involved in thermoregulation are distributed throughout the body, but are most dense in the palms and soles (293), the sweat glands that may be related to emotion are limited to the face, axillae, palms, and soles (290). The symptoms of hyperhidrosis are probably due to a stimulus that is triggered in the anterior cingulated frontal cortex, while thermoregulation is regulated by the preoptic-anterior hypothalamus (290).

Plantar hyperhidrosis is often revealed by history, although many patients may never present with it because they may not be aware of available treatments. Physical examination will often reveal excessive sweating, but since hyperhidrosis can be episodic, the physical examination is often not confirmatory. Minor's starch-iodine test is often helpful in assessing the exact areas in which hyperhidrosis occurs, as sweating turns the areas dark purple (292).

Plantar hyperhidrosis can cause numerous secondary problems including bromhidrosis, pitted keratolysis, bacterial and fungal skin infections, and skin maceration (290,292,294). In addition, most patients have tried various over-the-counter methods of control, which have had little or no success (293,295). Functional impairment and disability from hyperhidrosis can be measured by the hyperhidrosis disease and severity scale or HDSS, as well as by the dermatology life quality index (DLQI) (296).

Treatment of hyperhidrosis is initiated by differentiating between primary and secondary hyperhidrosis (295). While primary hyperhidrosis is believed to be caused partly by an exaggerated emotional response, secondary hyperhidrosis is a result of various other conditions (295) that may cause excessive sweating such as fever and associated illnesses, endocrine and metabolic conditions, neurologic disorders, cardiovascular disorders, respiratory disorders, medication use, drug use, diabetes, menopause, and infection among various other etiologies (289).

When secondary hyperhidrosis is ruled out, then there are a number of different treatments for primary hyperhidrosis that can be successful.

The least invasive and typical first-step approach is the use of topical antisweating agents or antiperspirants. Historically, the most successful topical is 20% aluminum chloride hexahydrate in absolute anhydrous ethyl alcohol (drysol) (293). At this concentration, aluminum chloride is believed to block the sweat pores and cause the secretory cells to tatrophy (293). The most common method used is for the patient to apply the agent to the affected area at night and then wash it off the next morning with topical baking soda to minimize irritation (293). Compliance with regimens may become an issue because drysol can be excessively irritating (295). Another preparation that has been used is 55% aluminum chloride hexahydrate in 6% salicylic acid gel (295).

Systemic medications such as anticholinergics have been used with some success in the treatment of plantar hyperhidrosis but the doses used have associated toxicity; oral glycopyrrolate and sometimes clonidine can be useful periodically (293,297).

If topical medications are unsuccessful, iontophoresis, which is the use of electrical current via water or other solutions, can be tried. First used in 1952 and available to the public since 1984, iontophoresis is often very helpful and has few side effects (290,293). The mechanism behind the benefits of this treatment is not fully understood; however, various explanations exist (293). One theory is that the pulses may cause hyperkeratosis of the sweat pores, which prevents sweat from getting through to the surface (293). Others speculate that iontophoresis may work by disrupting the electrochemical gradient of sweat secretion and through a biofeedback mechanism (293). Although treatment plans vary, 30-minute sessions, once daily to several times weekly are often used (290). Traditionally, tap water has been used for iontophoresis; however, recently it has been shown that 0.05% glycopyrrolate solution is even more effective (290,298). Side effects from iontophoresis are minimal and mild and include slight pain, irritation, skin burns, and in some an aggravation of symptoms for a short period of time (45,293).

Botulinum toxin type A, better known as Botox®, and also termed onabotulinumtoxinA, is FDA approved for the treatment of axillary hyperhidrosis and is used off-label to treat plantar hyperhidrosis (299–301).

A competitive botulinum product, Dysport®, also termed abobotulinumtoxinA can be used as well and is also off-label for treating plantar hyperhidrosis. Botulinum toxin type A acts by blocking presynaptic acetylcholine at the neuromuscular junction (292). It is speculated that blocking the release prevents the nerves from being stimulated, thereby reducing sweating (292).

Botulinum toxin type A has been very successful in decreasing hyperhidrosis. For the most part, its greatest limitation is the patient's ability to handle the numerous injections needed (278). In the past, techniques including nerve blocks have been used but require additional expertise. In addition, it may be difficult for the patient to walk or drive home for a certain time after the procedure. Topical anesthetics have been used with little success. Needle-free devices, such as Dermojet, have been recommended as well (302).

Vibration therapy as first described by Smith, Comite et al. has been used in order to minimize the pain involved with botulinum toxin type A injections (279). The technique involves the use of one or two commercially available massagers, which are handled by the assistant; generally little training is needed for the assistant to be comfortable with the procedure. The massagers are applied a few seconds prior to the injections. Vibration acts to compete with nerves transmitting pain thereby lessening any possible discomfort. After the procedure is over, the massagers are no longer used and thus, as opposed to nerve blocks, do not have any short-term sequelae. For a demonstration of vibration anesthesia, please see the paper co-authored by this author. Demonstration videos are available online. This paper was the first dermatologic paper ever to show audiovisuals as part of a peer-reviewed paper (303).

While we still occasionally use vibration anesthesia, Smith, Comite, and Storwick later described the use of ice as another easier and successful alternative (278). The ice is placed on the area to be injected for anywhere from 3 to 10 seconds before the botulinum toxin is injected.

Recommended doses of onabotulinumtoxinA for plantar hyperhidrosis vary from 50 to 250 units per foot (295,299, 300,304). However as the dosage is increased, so does the theoretical risk for the formation of antibodies (305). Botulinum toxin type A injections may be effective for 3 months to about a year (293,300). Side effects are generally minor and may include bruising, hematomas, and transient weakness and the expense may be considerable (293). Anecdotally some patients report that treatment of palmar hyperhidrosis with botulinum toxin can aid their plantar hyperhidrosis but objective evidence is lacking (306).

Sympathectomy is the surgical technique used in the most severe cases of hyperhidrosis. As the most invasive treatment for this condition, it is usually preserved as a last resort because of possible complications (290). Performed since 1920, the procedure has a good success rate and is most often permanent (293). For plantar hyperhidrosis, lumbar sympathectomy is commonly avoided because of the possibility of permanent sexual dysfunction (293). However, newer techniques such as thoracic chain sympathectomy have had some success, in which there was some improvement for about 50% to 70% of patients (290). Although there are numerous possible complications, some extremely severe, the most common side effect is compensatory hyperhidrosis (290,293). This can be devastating and incurable as the patient may need to change clothes several times daily because of increased sweating. The most common areas for compensatory sweating are the trunk, buttocks, groin, and thighs (290). Sometimes this compensatory sweating can be controlled with the less invasive treatments including topical medications and botulinum toxin (293). Endoscopic thoracic sympathicolysis resulted in only 30% plantar anhidrosis in one study (307).

It should be noted that often multiple and varied treatments are necessary to have sufficient success as per the patient's expectations and as the initial treatment wears off. For example, some physicians recommend the use of topicals such as aluminum chloride in addition to botulinum toxin type A injections (295).

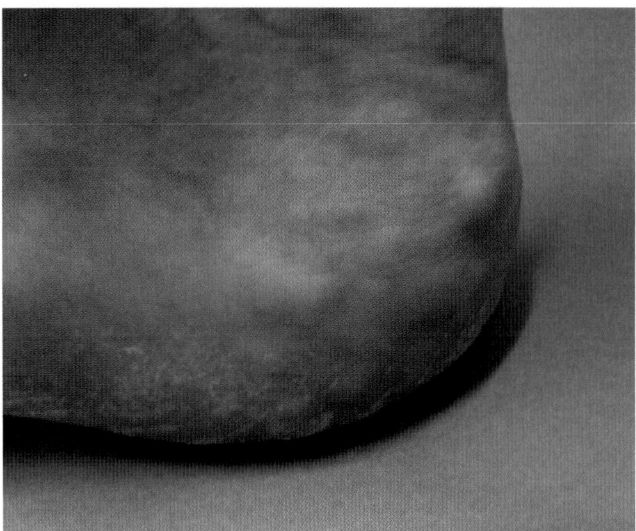

Figure 32.13. Piezogenic papules. These are better noted clinically when the patient bears weight or stands up.

SUBUNGUAL EXOSTOSIS

Subungual exostosis is a condition that sometimes can cause nail dystrophy and may need to be differentiated from a skin growth. Both ballet dancers who wear toe shoes, and cyclists who use toe clips seem to be at risk (308). The tumor may develop over the course of several months (54).

Although relatively rare, subungual exostosis mostly affects children and young adults (193). This condition most often affects the big toe approximately 80% of the time; however, the tumor has been found in other toes and fingers (54,309).

Subungual exostosis is a benign osteochondral tumor that grows from a distal phalanx (310). Although the exact cause is unknown, in many cases previous trauma may be involved. In other circumstances, chronic infection may play a role in triggering overgrowth (310). In addition, it is commonly thought that microtrauma may play a role; however, it is difficult to determine because usually the patient is unaware of the trauma (310).

Patients typically present with pain, nail dystrophy, and obvious radiographic features (311). Other common symptoms include expanding or ulcerating lesions on or near the nail bed (310). Subungual exostosis is usually diagnosed radiographically (311). Biopsy and histopathology are confirmatory. Recurrence occurs in 5% to 11% of cases (54).

The most effective form of treatment is surgical excision (310). The method is decided by the extent of damage to the nail bed.

PIEZOGENIC PEDAL PAPULES

Piezogenic pedal papules are skin-colored bumps caused by herniations of fat usually less than 1 cm in size around the heels (Fig. 32.13). These papules can affect athletes, most notably runners, triathletes, volleyball players, and basketball players (312). While the etiology is unknown, some believe the condition is linked to the inability of the heel fat to compartmentalize (313,314). The papules may be due to structural defects in the connective tissue and have been reported to be more common in patients with the Ehler–Danlos syndrome (315).

The prevalence of piezogenic pedal papules in athletes is unclear because out of the 466 cases reported in the literature, only 23 of those subjects were asked if they participated in sports (313). Of those 23 patients, 12 had piezogenic papules that were painful. However, the overall incidence of pain in piezogenic pedal papules was only about 7% (313). The pain may be due to ischemia caused by the associated nerves and vasculature accompanying the extrusion of fat (315–317). Though the papules are not commonly painful (313), discomfort from piezogenic pedal papules needs to be differentiated from plantar fasciitis (315) and other causes of musculoskeletal pain. One report describes the painful papules as being larger and histologically different: thickened dermis, loss of trabeculae of the subcutaneous tissue and loss of the normal compartments of the fat (317). One patient with foot pain needlessly had a triple arthrodesis before the correct diagnosis of piezogenic pedal papules was made (314).

If the diagnosis is unclear, one helpful diagnostic maneuver is to have the patient stand, as bearing weight can reveal the papules (313); when not weight-bearing, with heels off the ground, the papules may disappear (314). Biopsies are seldom required. The condition is benign and does not require treatment.

For those with painful piezogenic pedal papules, no one treatment has been proven effective. Among the treatments that have been reported with varying degrees of effectiveness are: surgery, minimizing standing and trauma, weight loss, cortisone injections (313), compression therapy (318), electro-acupuncture (316), heel cups (253,319) and deep punch biopsy (320). There is a case report of injections of bupivicaine and betamethasone curing painful piezogenic pedal papules in a male with Ehlers–Danlos syndrome type III (321).

REFERENCES

1. Derman W. Profile of Medical and Injury Consultations of Team South Africa During the XXVIIIth Olympiad, Athens 2004. *South African J Sports Med* 2008;20(3):72–76.
2. Cole GM. Plantar warts.http://www.emedicinehealth.com/plantar_warts/article_em.htm. Updated September 15, 2011. Accessed August 8, 2012

3. Esterowitz D, Greer KE, Cooper PH, et al. Plantar warts in the athlete. *Am J Emerg Med* 1995;13(4):441–443.
4. Lichon V, Khachemoune A. Plantar warts: A focus on treatment modalities. *Dermatol Nurs* 2007;19(4):372–375.
5. Skinner RB, Jr. Imiquimod. *Dermatol Clin* 2003;21(2):291–300.
6. Gentles JC, Evans EG. Foot infections in swimming baths. *Br Med J* 1973;3(5874): 260–262.
7. Conklin RJ. Common cutaneous disorders in athletes. *Sports Med* 1990;9(2):100–119.
8. Habif TP. Warts, Herpes Simplex, and other Viral Infections. *Clinical Dermatology*. 5th ed. Mosby; 2009.
9. Johnson LW. Communal showers and the risk of plantar warts. *J Fam Pract* 1995;40(2): 136–138.
10. Penso-Assathiany D, Flahault A, Roujeau JC. Warts, swimming pools and atopy: A case control study conducted in a private dermatology practice. *Ann Dermatol Venereol* 1999; 126(10):696–698.
11. Jenkins DW, Cooper K, O'Connor R, et al. Prevalence of podiatric conditions seen in special olympics athletes: Structural, biomechanical and dermatological findings. *Foot (Edinb)* 2011;21(1):15–25. doi: 10.1016/j.foot.2010.10.004.
12. Bae JM, Kang H, Kim HO, et al. Differential diagnosis of plantar wart from corn, callus and healed wart with the aid of dermoscopy. *Br J Dermatol* 2009;160(1):220–222. doi: 10.1111/j.1365-2133.2008.08937.x.
13. Young S, Cohen GE. Treatment of verruca plantaris with a combination of topical fluorouracil and salicylic acid. *J Am Podiatr Med Assoc* 2005;95(4):366–369.
14. Lever WF, Schaumburg-Lever G. *Histopathology of the Skin*. 6th ed. Philadelphia, PA: Lippincott; 1983:848.
15. Elder DE, Lever WF, Ovid Technologies I. Atlas and Synopsis of Lever's Histopathology of the Skin. 5th ed. 2007:478.
16. De Giorgi V, Massi D. Images in clinical medicine. Plantar melanoma–a false vegetant wart. *N Engl J Med* 2006;355(13):e13.
17. Omura EF, Rye B. Dermatologic disorders of the foot. *Clin Sports Med* 1994;13(4):825–841.
18. Lipke MM. An armamentarium of wart treatments. *Clin Med Res* 2006;4(4):273–293.
19. Gibbs S, Harvey I. Topical treatments for cutaneous warts. *Cochrane Database Syst Rev* 2006;(3):CD001781. doi: 10.1002/14651858.CD001781.pub2.
20. Johnson SM, Horn TD. Intralesional immunotherapy for warts using a combination of skin test antigens: A safe and effective therapy. *J Drugs Dermatol* 2004;3(3):263–265.
21. Litt JZ. Don't excise–exorcise. Treatment for subungual and periungual warts. *Cutis* 1978; 22(6):673–676.
22. de Haen M, Spigt MG, van Uden CJ, et al. Efficacy of duct tape vs placebo in the treatment of verruca vulgaris (warts) in primary school children. *Arch Pediatr Adolesc Med* 2006;160(11): 1121–1125.
23. Wenner R, Askari SK, Cham PM, et al. Duct tape for the treatment of common warts in adults: A double-blind randomized controlled trial. *Arch Dermatol* 2007;143(3):309–313.
24. Focht DR 3rd., Spicer C, Fairchok MP. The efficacy of duct tape vs cryotherapy in the treatment of verruca vulgaris (the common wart). *Arch Pediatr Adolesc Med* 2002;156(10):971–974.
25. Becerro de Bengoa Vallejo R, Losa Iglesias ME, Gomez-Martin B, et al. Application of cantharidin and podophyllotoxin for the treatment of plantar warts. *J Am Podiatr Med Assoc* 2008;98(6):445–450.
26. Ziolkowski P, Osiecka BJ, Siewinski M, et al. Pretreatment of plantar warts with azone enhances the effect of 5-aminolevulinic acid photodynamic therapy. *J Environ Pathol Toxicol Oncol* 2006;25(1-2):403–409.
27. Koenig RD, Horwitz LR. Verrucae plantaris–effective treatment with bleomycin: Review of the literature and case presentations. *J Foot Surg* 1982;21(2):108–110.
28. Shumack PH, Haddock MJ. Bleomycin: An effective treatment for warts. *Australas J Dermatol* 1979;20(1):41–42.
29. Hudson AL. Letter: Treatment of plantar warts with bleomycin. *Arch Dermatol* 1976; 112(8): 1179.
30. Bremner RM. Warts: Treatment with intralesional bleomycin. *Cutis* 1976;18(2):264–266.
31. Cordero AA, Guglielmi HA, Woscoff A. The common wart: Intralesional treatment with bleomycin sulfate. *Cutis* 1980;26(3):319–320, 322, 324.
32. Salk R, Douglas TS. Intralesional bleomycin sulfate injection for the treatment of verruca plantaris. *J Am Podiatr Med Assoc* 2006;96(3):220–225.
33. Saitta P, Krishnamurthy K, Brown LH. Bleomycin in dermatology: A review of intralesional applications. *Dermatol Surg* 2008;34(10):1299–1313.
34. Abess A, Keel DM, Graham BS. Flagellate hyperpigmentation following intralesional bleomycin treatment of verruca plantaris. *Arch Dermatol* 2003;139(3):337–339.
35. Bunney MH, Nolan MW, Buxton PK, et al. The treatment of resistant warts with intralesional bleomycin: A controlled clinical trial. *Br J Dermatol* 1984;111(2):197–207.
36. Czarnecki D. Bleomycin and periungual warts. *Med J Aust* 1984;141(1):40.
37. Miller RA. Nail dystrophy following intralesional injections of bleomycin for a periungual wart. *Arch Dermatol* 1984;120(7):963–964.
38. Urbina Gonzalez F, Cristobal Gil MC, Aguilar Martinez A, et al. Cutaneous toxicity of intralesional bleomycin administration in the treatment of periungual warts. *Arch Dermatol* 1986;122(9):974–975.
39. Iscimen A, Aydemir EH, Goksugur N, et al. Intralesional 5-fluorouracil, lidocaine and epinephrine mixture for the treatment of verrucae: A prospective placebo-controlled, single-blind randomized study. *J Eur Acad Dermatol Venereol* 2004;18(4):455–458.
40. Yazdanfar A, Farshchian M, Fereydoonnejad M, et al. Treatment of common warts with an intralesional mixture of 5-fluorouracil, lidocaine, and epinephrine: A prospective placebo-controlled, double-blind randomized trial. *Dermatol Surg* 2008;34(5):656–659.
41. Phillips RC, Ruhl TS, Pfenninger JL, et al. Treatment of warts with candida antigen injection. *Arch Dermatol* 2000;136(10):1274–1275.
42. Mitsuishi T, Sasagawa T, Kato T, et al. Combination of carbon dioxide laser therapy and artificial dermis application in plantar warts: Human papillomavirus DNA analysis after treatment. *Dermatol Surg* 2010;36(9):1401–1405. doi: 10.1111/j.1524-4725.2010.01648.x; 10.1111/j.1524-4725.2010.01648.x.
43. Maronn M, Salm C, Lyon V, et al. One-year experience with candida antigen immunotherapy for warts and molluscum. *Pediatr Dermatol* 2008;25(2):189–192.
44. Horn TD, Johnson SM, Helm RM, et al. Intralesional immunotherapy of warts with mumps, candida, and trichophyton skin test antigens: A single-blinded, randomized, and controlled trial. *Arch Dermatol* 2005;141(5):589–594.
45. Aksakal AA, Ozden MG, Atahan C, et al. Successful treatment of verruca plantaris with a single sublesional injection of interferon-alpha2a. *Clin Exp Dermatol* 2009;34(1):16–19.
46. Mullen BR, Guiliana JV, Nesheiwat F. Cimetidine as a first-line therapy for pedal verruca: Eight-year retrospective analysis. *J Am Podiatr Med Assoc* 2005;95(3):229–234.
47. Peter A, Gearhart MD. Staff Physician Department of Obstetrics and Gynecology, Pennsylvania Hospital. Human papillomavirus. http://emedicine.medscape.com/article/219110-overview. Updated 1997. Accessed January 1, 2009.
48. Huo W, Gao XH, Sun XP, et al. Local hyperthermia at 44 degrees C for the treatment of plantar warts: A randomized, patient-blinded, placebo-controlled trial. *J Infect Dis* 2010;201(8):1169–1172. doi: 10.1086/651506.
49. Shivakumar V, Okade R, Rajkumar V. Autoimplantation therapy for multiple warts. *Indian J Dermatol Venereol Leprol* 2009;75(6):593–595. doi: 10.4103/0378-6323.57721.
50. Apfelberg DB, Druker D, Maser MR, et al. Benefits of the CO2 laser for verruca resistant to other modalities of treatment. *J Dermatol Surg Oncol* 1989;15(4):371–375.
51. Robson KJ, Cunningham NM, Kruzan KL, et al. Pulsed-dye laser versus conventional therapy in the treatment of warts: A prospective randomized trial. *J Am Acad Dermatol* 2000;43 (2 Pt 1):275–280.
52. Schroeter CA, Pleunis J, van Nispen tot Pannerden C, et al. Photodynamic therapy: New treatment for therapy-resistant plantar warts. *Dermatol Surg* 2005;31(1):71–75.
53. Pecci M, Comeau D, Chawla V. Skin conditions in the athlete. *Am J Sports Med* 2009;37(2): 406–418.
54. Brian B. Adams. *Sports Dermatology*. Springer Science+Business Media, LLC Cincinnati OH; 2006:351.
55. Caputo R, De Boulle K, Del Rosso J, et al. Prevalence of superficial fungal infections among sports-active individuals: Results from the achilles survey, a review of the literature. *J Eur Acad Dermatol Venereol* 2001;15(4):312–316.
56. Auger P, Marquis G, Joly J, et al. Epidemiology of tinea pedis in marathon runners: Prevalence of occult athlete's foot. *Mycoses* 1993;36(1–2):35–41.
57. Lacroix C, Baspeyras M, de La Salmoniere P, et al. Tinea pedis in European marathon runners. *J Eur Acad Dermatol Venereol* 2002;16(2):139–142.
58. Field LA, Adams BB. Tinea pedis in athletes. *Int J Dermatol* 2008;47(5):485–492.
59. Mohrenschlager M, Seidl HP, Schnopp C, et al. Professional ice hockey players: A high-risk group for fungal infection of the foot? *Dermatology* 2001;203(3):271.
60. Purim KS, Bordignon GP, Queiroz-Telles F. Fungal infection of the feet in soccer players and non-athlete individuals. *Rev Iberoam Micol* 2005;22(1):34–38.
61. Pickup TL, Adams BB. Prevalence of tinea pedis in professional and college soccer players versus non-athletes. *Clin J Sport Med* 2007;17(1):52–54.
62. Attye A, Auger P, Joly J. Incidence of occult athlete's foot in swimmers. *Eur J Epidemiol* 1990;6(3):244–247.
63. Ajello L, Getz ME. Recovery of dermatophytes from shoes and shower stalls. *J Invest Dermatol* 1954;22(1):17–21; discussion, 21–24.
64. Kamihama T, Kimura T, Hosokawa JI, et al. Tinea pedis outbreak in swimming pools in japan. *Public Health* 1997;111(4):249–253.
65. English MP, Gibson MD. Studies in the epidemiology of tinea pedis. I. tinea pedis in school children. *Br Med J* 1959;1(5135):1442–1446.
66. Pleacher MD, Dexter WW. Cutaneous fungal and viral infections in athletes. *Clin Sports Med* 2007;26(3):397–411.
67. Adams BB. Skin infections in athletes. *Dermatol Nurs* 2008;20(1):39–44.
68. Levitt JO, Levitt BH, Akhavan A, et al. The sensitivity and specificity of potassium hydroxide smear and fungal culture relative to clinical assessment in the evaluation of tinea pedis: A pooled analysis. *Dermatol Res Pract* 2010;2010:764843. doi: 10.1155/2010/764843.
69. Leyden JJ, Kligman AM. Interdigital athlete's foot. the interaction of dermatophytes and resident bacteria. *Arch Dermatol* 1978;114(10):1466–1472.
70. Badillet G, Puissant A, Jourdan-Lemoine M, et al. The practice of judo and the risk of fungal contamination. *Ann Dermatol Venereol* 1982;109(8):661–664.
71. Bergstresser PR, Elewski B, Hanifin J, et al. Topical terbinafine and clotrimazole in interdigital tinea pedis: A multicenter comparison of cure and relapse rates with 1- and 4-week treatment regimens. *J Am Acad Dermatol* 1993;28(4):648–651.
72. Crawford F, Hollis S. Topical treatments for fungal infections of the skin and nails of the foot. *Cochrane Database Syst Rev* 2007;(3)(3):CD001434.
73. Evans EG, Dodman B, Williamson DM, et al. Comparison of terbinafine and clotrimazole in treating tinea pedis. *BMJ* 1993;307(6905):645–647.
74. Schopf R, Hettler O, Brautigam M, et al. Efficacy and tolerability of terbinafine 1% topical solution used for 1 week compared with 4 weeks clotrimazole 1% topical solution in the treatment of interdigital tinea pedis: A randomized, double-blind, multi-centre, 8-week clinical trial. *Mycoses* 1999;42(5–6):415–420.
75. Rotta I, Sanchez A, Goncalves PR, et al. Efficacy and safety of topical antifungals in the treatment of dermatomycosis: A systematic review. *Br J Dermatol* 2012;166(5):927–933. doi: 10.1111/j.1365-2133.2012.10815.x; 10.1111/j.1365-2133.2012.10815.x.
76. Romero-Cerecero O, Zamilpa A, Jimenez-Ferrer E, et al. Therapeutic effectiveness of ageratina pichinchensis on the treatment of chronic interdigital tinea pedis: A randomized, double-blind clinical trial. *J Altern Complement Med* 2012;18(6):607–611. doi: 10.1089/acm.2011.0319.

77. Bell-Syer SE, Hart R, Crawford F, et al. Oral treatments for fungal infections of the skin of the foot. *Cochrane Database Syst Rev* 2002;(2)(2):CD003584.
78. Levine N. Dermatologic aspects of sports medicine. *J Am Acad Dermatol* 1980;3(4):415–424.
79. Gupta AK, Ryder JE. How to improve cure rates for the management of onychomycosis. *Dermatol Clin* 2003;21(3):499–505, vii.
80. Daniel CR 3rd., Traditional management of onychomycosis. *J Am Acad Dermatol* 1996;35(3 Pt 2):S21–S25.
81. Karaca S, Kulac M, Cetinkaya Z, et al. Etiology of foot intertrigo in the district of afyonkarahisar, turkey: A bacteriologic and mycologic study. *J Am Podiatr Med Assoc* 2008;98(1):42–44.
82. Aste N, Atzori L, Zucca M, et al. Gram-negative bacterial toe web infection: A survey of 123 cases from the district of Cagliari, Italy. *J Am Acad Dermatol* 2001;45(4):537–541.
83. Schwartz RA. Hesselbirg JR. Gram-Negative Toe web Infection. <http://emedicine.medscape.com/article/1055306-print. Updated 2008>. Accessed February 4, 2012.
84. Fangman W, Burton C. Hyperkeratotic rim of gram-negative toe web infections. *Arch Dermatol* 2005;141(5):658.
85. Eaglstein NF, Marley WM, Marley NF, et al. Gram-negative bacterial toe web infection: Successful treatment with a new third generation cephalosporin. *J Am Acad Dermatol* 1983;8(2):225–228.
86. King DF, King LA. Importance of debridement in the treatment of gram-negative bacterial toe web infection. *J Am Acad Dermatol* 1986;14(2 Pt 1):278–279.
87. Fiorillo L, Zucker M, Sawyer D, et al. The pseudomonas hot-foot syndrome. *N Engl J Med* 2001;345(5):335–338.
88. Yu Y, Cheng AS, Wang L, et al. Hot tub folliculitis or hot hand-foot syndrome caused by pseudomonas aeruginosa. *J Am Acad Dermatol* 2007;57(4):596–600.
89. Michl RK, Rusche T, Grimm S, et al. Outbreak of hot-foot syndrome - caused by pseudomonas aeruginosa. *Klin Padiatr* 2012;224(4):252–255. doi: 10.1055/s-0031-1297949.
90. Rasmussen JE, Graves WH 3rd., Pseudomonas aeruginosa, hot tubs, and skin infections. *Am J Dis Child* 1982;136(6):553–554.
91. Kosatsky T, Kleeman J. Superficial and systemic illness related to a hot tub. *Am J Med* 1985;79(1):10–12.
92. Krivda S, Toner C. Pseudomonas Folliculitis. http://emedicine.medscape.com/article/1053170-medication. Updated 2006. Accessed February 5, 2009.
93. Centers for Disease Control and Prevention (CDC). Surveillance data from public spa inspections–United States, May-September 2002. *MMWR Morb Mortal Wkly Rep* 2004;53(25):553–555.
94. Vlahovic TC, Dunn SP, Kemp K. The use of a clindamycin 1%-benzoyl peroxide 5% topical gel in the treatment of pitted keratolysis: A novel therapy. *Adv Skin Wound Care* 2009;22(12):564–566. doi: 10.1097/01.ASW.0000363468.18117.fe.
95. Blaise G, Nikkels AF, Hermanns-Le T, et al. Corynebacterium-associated skin infections. *Int J Dermatol* 2008;47(9):884–890.
96. Stanton RL, Schwartz RA. Pitted keratolysis: A common foot problem. *Am Fam Physician* 1983;27(4):183–184.
97. Wohlrab J, Rohrbach D, Marsch WC. Keratolysis sulcata (pitted keratolysis): Clinical symptoms with different histological correlates. *Br J Dermatol* 2000;143(6):1348–1349.
98. Takama H, Tamada Y, Yano K, et al. Pitted keratolysis: Clinical manifestations in 53 cases. *Br J Dermatol* 1997;137(2):282–285.
99. Singh G, Naik CL. Pitted keratolysis. *Indian J Dermatol Venereol Leprol* 2005;71(3):213–215.
100. Longshaw CM, Wright JD, Farrell AM, et al. Kytococcus sedentarius, the organism associated with pitted keratolysis, produces two keratin-degrading enzymes. *J Appl Microbiol* 2002;93(5):810–816.
101. Lockwood LL, Gehrke S, Navarini AA. Dermoscopy of pitted keratolysis. *Case Rep Dermatol* 2010;2(2):146–148. doi: 10.1159/000319792.
102. Tamura BM, Cuce LC, Souza RL, et al. Plantar hyperhidrosis and pitted keratolysis treated with botulinum toxin injection. *Dermatol Surg* 2004;30(12 Pt 2):1510–1514.
103. Vazquez-Lopez F, Perez-Oliva N. Mupirocine ointment for symptomatic pitted keratolysis. *Infection* 1996;24(1):55.
104. Hochedez P, Caumes E. Hookworm-related cutaneous larva migrans. *J Travel Med* 2007;14(5):326–333.
105. Biolcati G, Alabiso A. Creeping eruption of larva migrans–a case report in a beach volley athlete. *Int J Sports Med* 1997;18(8):612–613.
106. Juzych LA. Cutaneous larva migrans clinical presentation. *Emedicinehealth* Available at http://emedicine.medscape.com/article/1108784-overview. Accessed August 15, 2012.
107. Jackson A, Heukelbach J, Calheiros CM, et al. A study in a community in brazil in which cutaneous larva migrans is endemic. *Clin Infect Dis* 2006;43(2):e13–e18. doi: 10.1086/ 505221.
108. Ang CC. Images in clinical medicine. cutaneous larva migrans. *N Engl J Med* 2010; 362(4):e10. doi: 10.1056/NEJMicm0808714.
109. Heukelbach J, Jackson A, Ariza L, et al. Prevalence and risk factors of hookworm-related cutaneous larva migrans in a rural community in brazil. *Ann Trop Med Parasitol* 2008; 102(1):53–61.
110. Purdy KS, Langley RG, Webb AN, et al. Cutaneous larva migrans. *Lancet* 2011;377 (9781):1948. doi: 10.1016/S0140-6736(10)61149-X.
111. Lydia A Juzych MD, Consulting Staff. Department of Dermatology, Henry Ford Health Sciences Center.Available at http://emedicine.medscape.com/article/1108784-overview. Updated 2008. Accessed January 1, 2009.
112. Yavuz M, Davis BL. Plantar shear stress distribution in athletic individuals with frictional foot blisters. *J Am Podiatr Med Assoc* 2010;100(2):116–120.
113. Reynolds KH, Halsmer SE. Injuries from ultimate frisbee. *WMJ* 2006;105(6):46–49.
114. Houston SD, Knox JM. Skin problems related to sports and recreational activities. *Cutis* 1977;19(4):487–491.
115. Mailler-Savage EA, Adams BB. Skin manifestations of running. *J Am Acad Dermatol* 2006;55(2):290–301. doi: 10.1016/j.jaad.2006.02.011.
116. Brennan FH Jr., Managing blisters in competitive athletes. *Curr Sports Med Rep* 2002; 1(6):319–322.
117. De Luca JF, Adams BB, Yosipovitch G. Skin manifestations of athletes competing in the summer olympics: What a sports medicine physician should know. *Sports Med* 2012;42(5):399–413. doi: 10.2165/11599050-000000000-00000; 10.2165/11599050-000000000-00000.
118. Knapik JJ, Reynolds K, Barson J. Influence of an antiperspirant on foot blister incidence during cross-country hiking. *J Am Acad Dermatol* 1998;39(2 Pt 1):202–206.
119. Knapik JJ, Reynolds K, Barson J. Risk factors for foot blisters during road marching: Tobacco use, ethnicity, foot type, previous illness, and other factors. *Mil Med* 1999; 164(2):92–97.
120. Gerhardt LC, Strassle V, Lenz A, et al. Influence of epidermal hydration on the friction of human skin against textiles. *J R Soc Interface* 2008;5(28):1317–1328.
121. Taylor CM, Riordan FA, Graham C. New football boots and toxic shock syndrome. *BMJ* 2006;332(7554):1376–1378. doi: 10.1136/bmj.332.7554.1376.
122. Spence WR, Shields MN. New insole for prevention of athletic blisters. *J Sports Med Phys Fitness* 1968;8(3):177–180.
123. Smith W, Walter J, Jr. Bailey M. Effects of insoles in coast guard basic training footwear. *J Am Podiatr Med Assoc* 1985;75(12):644–647.
124. Herring KM, Richie DH, Jr. Comparison of cotton and acrylic socks using a generic cushion sole design for runners. *J Am Podiatr Med Assoc* 1993;83(9):515–522.
125. Knapik JJ, Hamlet MP, Thompson KJ, et al. Influence of boot-sock systems on frequency and severity of foot blisters. *Mil Med* 1996;161(10):594–598.
126. Cohen PR, Eliezri YD, Silvers DN. Athlete's nodules. *J Am Acad Dermatol* 1991;24(2 Pt 1): 317–318.
127. Bender TW, 3rd. Cutaneous manifestations of disease in athletes. *Skinmed* 2003;2(1):34–40.
128. Dickens R, Adams BB, Mutasim DF. Sports-related pads. *Int J Dermatol* 2002;41(5):291–293.
129. Uchiyama M, Tsuboi R, Mitsuhashi Y. Athlete's nodule. *J Dermatol* 2009;36(11):608–611. doi: 10.1111/j.1346-8138.2009.00718.x.
130. Freeman DB. Corns and calluses resulting from mechanical hyperkeratosis. *Am Fam Physician* 2002;65(11):2277–2280.
131. Tlougan BE, Mancini AJ, Mandell JA, et al. Skin conditions in figure skaters, ice-hockey players and speed skaters: Part I - mechanical dermatoses. *Sports Med* 2011;41(9):709–719. doi: 10.2165/11590540-000000000-00000; 10.2165/11590540-000000000-00000.
132. Singh D, Bentley G, Trevino SG. Callosities, corns, and calluses. *BMJ* 1996;312(7043): 1403–1406.
133. Lipetz J, Kruse RJ. Injuries and special concerns of female figure skaters. *Clin Sports Med* 2000;19(2):369–380.
134. Kelechi TJ, Lukacs KS. Patient with dystrophic toenails, calluses, and heel fissures. *J Wound Ostomy Continence Nurs* 1997;24(4):237–242.
135. Silverberg N. Clavus. http://emedicine.medscape.com/article/1089594-overview. Updated 2007. Accessed February 5, 2009.
136. Strauss RM. Mountaineer's heel. *Br J Sports Med* 2004;38(3):344–345; discussion 345.
137. Fromer J. Talon Noir. *Arch Dermatol* 1971;104;452.
138. Verbov J. Calcaneal petechiae. *Arch Dermatol* 1973;107(6):918.
139. Basler RSW, Garcia MA. Acing Common Skin Problems in Tennis Players. *Phys Sportsmed* 1998;(12):37–44.
140. Mehregan AH. Black heel: A report of two cases. *Can Med Assoc J* 1966;95(11):584–585.
141. Metelitsa A, Barankin B, Lin AN. Diagnosis of sports-related dermatoses. *Int J Dermatol* 2004;43(2):113–119.
142. Crissey JT. Bedbugs: An old problem with a new dimension. *Int J Dermatol* 1981;20(6): 411–414.
143. Crissey JT, Peachey JC. Calcaneal petechiae. *Arch Dermatol* 1961;83:501.
144. Vakilzadeh F, Happle R. The tennis heel (black heel). *Z Hautkr* 1974;49(7):285–288.
145. Ayres S, Jr. Mihan R. Calcaneal petechiae. *Arch Dermatol* 1972;106(2):262.
146. Urbina F, Leon L, Sudy E. Black heel, talon noir or calcaneal petechiae? *Australas J Dermatol* 2008;49(3):148–151.
147. Levit F, Blankenship ML. Posttraumatic punctate hemorrhage of the skin: A better name than black heel. *Arch Dermatol* 1972;105(5):759.
148. Rufli T. Hyperkeratosis haemorrhagica. *Hautarzt* 1980;31(11):606–609.
149. Hafner J, Haenseler E, Ossent P, et al. Benzidine stain for the histochemical detection of hemoglobin in splinter hemorrhage (subungual hematoma) and black heel. *Am J Dermatopathol* 1995;17(4):362–367.
150. Garcia-Doval I, de la Torre C, Losada A, et al. Disseminated punctate intraepidermal haemorrhage: A widespread counterpart of black heel. *Acta Derm Venereol* 1999;79(5):403.
151. Zalaudek I, Argenziano G, Soyer HP, et al. Dermoscopy of subcorneal hematoma. *Dermatol Surg* 2004;30(9):1229–1232.
152. Izumi AK. Letter: Pigmented palmar petechiae (black palm). *Arch Dermatol* 1974;109(2): 261.
153. Smith M. Environmental and Sports-Related Skin Diseases. *Dermatol* 2003:2:1385–1400.
154. Moehrle M. Ultraviolet exposure in the ironman triathlon. *Med Sci Sports Exerc* 2001;33(8): 1385–1386.
155. Moehrle M, Heinrich L, Schmid A, et al. Extreme UV exposure of professional cyclists. *Dermatol* 2000;201(1):44–45.
156. Moehrle M. Outdoor sports and skin cancer. *Clin Dermatol* 2008;26(1):12–15.
157. Hamant ES, Adams BB. Sunscreen use among collegiate athletes. *J Am Acad Dermatol* 2005;53(2):237–241.
158. Jardine A, Bright M, Knight L, et al. Does physical activity increase the risk of unsafe sun exposure? *Health Promot J Austr* 2012;23(1):52–57.
159. Han A, Maibach HI. Management of acute sunburn. *Am J Clin Dermatol* 2004;5(1):39–47.
160. Wright MW, Wright ST, Wagner RF. Mechanisms of sunscreen failure. *J Am Acad Dermatol* 2001;44(5):781–784.
161. Bangha E, Elsner P, Kistler GS. Suppression of UV-induced erythema by topical treatment with melatonin (N-acetyl-5-methoxytryptamine). influence of the application time point. *Dermatology* 1997;195(3):248–252.
162. Ambros-Rudolph CM, Hofmann-Wellenhof R, Richtig E, et al. Malignant melanoma in marathon runners. *Arch Dermatol* 2006;142(11):1471–1474.

163. Almahameed A, Pinto DS. Pernio (chilblains). *Curr Treat Options Cardiovasc Med* 2008;10(2):128–135.
164. Goette DK. Chilblains (perniosis). *J Am Acad Dermatol* 1990;23(2 Pt 1):257–262.
165. Jacob JR, Weisman MH, Rosenblatt SI, et al. Chronic pernio. A historical perspective of cold-induced vascular disease. *Arch Intern Med* 1986;146(8):1589–1592.
166. Raza N, Sajid MD, Ejaz A. Chilblains at abbottabad, a moderately cold weather station. *J Ayub Med Coll Abbottabad* 2006;18(3):25–28.
167. Long CC, Holt PJ. Tobogganers thighs. *Clin Exp Dermatol* 1992;17(6):466–467.
168. Chan Y, Tang WY, Lam WY, et al. A cluster of chilblains in hong kong. *Hong Kong Med J* 2008;14(3):185–191.
169. Sallis R, Chassay CM. Recognizing and treating common cold-induced injury in outdoor sports. *Med Sci Sports Exerc* 1999;31(10):1367–1373.
170. Price RD, Murdoch DR. Perniosis (chilblains) of the thigh: Report of five cases, including four following river crossings. *High Alt Med Biol* 2001;2(4):535–538.
171. Goodfield M. Cold-induced skin disorders. *Pract* 1989;233(1480):1616, 1618–1620.
172. Fisher DA, Everett MA. Violaceous rash of dorsal fingers in a woman. diagnosis: Chilblain lupus erythematosus (perniosis). *Arch Dermatol* 1996;132(4):459, 462.
173. Cribier B, Djeridi N, Peltre B, et al. A histologic and immunohistochemical study of chilblains. *J Am Acad Dermatol* 2001;45(6):924–929.
174. Rustin MH, Newton JA, Smith NP, et al. The treatment of chilblains with nifedipine: The results of a pilot study, a double-blind placebo-controlled randomized study and a long-term open trial. *Br J Dermatol* 1989;120(2):267–275.
175. McMahon JA, Howe A. Cold weather issues in sideline and event management. *Curr Sports Med Rep* 2012;11(3):135–141. doi: 10.1249/JSR.0b013e3182578783.
176. Tlougan BE, Mancini AJ, Mandell JA, et al. Skin conditions in figure skaters, ice-hockey players and speed skaters: Part II - cold-induced, infectious and inflammatory dermatoses. *Sports Med* 2011;41(11):967–984. doi: 10.2165/11592190-000000000-00000; 10.2165/11592190-000000000-00000.
177. DeFranco MJ, Baker CL, 3rd. DaSilva JJ, et al. Environmental issues for team physicians. *Am J Sports Med* 2008;36(11):2226–2237.
178. Golant A, Nord RM, Paksima N, et al. Cold exposure injuries to the extremities. *J Am Acad Orthop Surg* 2008;16(12):704–715.
179. Castellani JW, Young AJ, Ducharme MB, et al. American college of sports medicine position stand: Prevention of cold injuries during exercise. *Med Sci Sports Exerc* 2006;38(11):2012–2029.
180. Golja P, Kacin A, Tipton MJ, et al. Hypoxia increases the cutaneous threshold for the sensation of cold. *Eur J Appl Physiol* 2004;92(1–2):62–68.
181. Cipollaro VA. Cryogenic injury due to local application of a reusable cold compress. *Cutis* 1992;50(2):111–112.
182. Washburn B. Frostbite: What it is–how to prevent it–emergency treatment. *N Engl J Med* 1962;266:974–989.
183. Seto CK, Way D, O'Connor N. Environmental illness in athletes. *Clin Sports Med* 2005;24(3):695–718, x.
184. Patel NN, Patel DN. Frostbite. *Am J Med* 2008;121(9):765–766.
185. Harirchi I, Arvin A, Vash JH, et al. Frostbite: Incidence and predisposing factors in mountaineers. *Br J Sports Med* 2005;39(12):898–901; discussion 901.
186. Morocco A. Sea urchin envenomation. *Clin Toxicol (Phila)* 2005;43(2):119–120.
187. Zoltan TB, Taylor KS, Achar SA. Health issues for surfers. *Am Fam Physician* 2005;71(12): 2313–2317.
188. Beeching NJ, Morgan HV, Lloyd AL. Sea-urchin granuloma of the toe. *Pract* 1982; 226(1371):1567–1571.
189. Auerbach PS. Envenomation by aquatic invertebrates. In: Auerbach PS, ed. *Medicine for the Outdoors: The Essential Guide to Emergency Medical Procedures and First Aid,* 5th ed. St. Louis, MO: Mosby; 2009.
190. Wu ML, Chou SL, Huang TY, et al. Sea-urchin envenomation. *Vet Hum Toxicol* 2003;45(6):307–309.
191. Liram N, Gomori M, Perouansky M. Sea urchin puncture resulting in PIP joint synovial arthritis: Case report and MRI study. *J Travel Med* 2000;7(1):43–45.
192. Perkins RA, Morgan SS. Poisoning, envenomation, and trauma from marine creatures. *Am Fam Physician* 2004;69(4):885–890.
193. O'Neal RL, Halstead BW, Howard LD, Jr. Injury to human tissues from sea urchin spines. *Calif Med* 1964;101:199–202.
194. Asada M, Komura J, Hosokawa H, et al. A case of delayed hypersensitivity reaction following a sea urchin sting. *Dermatologica* 1990;180(2):99–101.
195. Burke WA, Steinbaugh JR, O'Keefe EJ. Delayed hypersensitivity reaction following a sea urchin sting. *Int J Dermatol* 1986;25(10):649–650.
196. Baden HP, Burnett JW. Injuries from sea urchins. *South Med J* 1977;70(4):459–460.
197. Gungor S, Tarikci N, Gokdemir G. Removal of sea urchin spines using erbium-doped yttrium aluminum garnet ablation. *Dermatol Surg* 2012;38(3):508–510. doi: 10.1111/j.1524-4725.2011.02259.x; 10.1111/j.1524-4725.2011.02259.x.
198. Kucewicz A, Miller MA. Eosinophilic pneumonia associated with foot injury from a sea urchin. *Am J Emerg Med* 2007;25(7):862.e5–e6.
199. Guyot-Drouot MH, Rouneau D, Rolland JM, et al. Arthritis, tenosynovitis, fasciitis, and bursitis due to sea urchin spines. A series of 12 cases in reunion island. *Joint Bone Spine* 2000;67(2):94–100.
200. Naimer SA, Zvulunov A, Ben-Amitai D, et al. Plantar hidradenitis in children induced by exposure to wet footwear. *Pediatr Emerg Care* 2000;16(3):182–183.
201. Metzker A, Brodsky F. Traumatic plantar urticaria–an unrecognized entity? *J Am Acad Dermatol* 1988;18(1 Pt 1):144–146.
202. Bergfeld WF, Taylor JS. Trauma, sports, and the skin. *Am J Ind Med* 1985;8(4-5):403–413.
203. Prok Lori M, McGovern Thomas M. Poison ivy (toxicondendron) dermatitis. http://www.uptodate.com/contents/poison-ivy-toxicodendron-dermatitis Feb 15, 2012.
204. Goodall J. Oral corticosteroids for poison ivy dermatitis. *CMAJ* 2002;166(3):300–301.
205. Marks JG, Jr., Fowler JF, Jr., Sheretz EF, et al. Prevention of poison ivy and poison oak allergic contact dermatitis by quaternium-18 bentonite. *J Am Acad Dermatol* 1995;33(2 Pt 1): 212–216.
206. Crawford GH. http://emedicine.medscape.com/article/1090097-overview. Updated 2007. Accessed August 8, 2012.
207. Onder M, Atahan AC, Bassoy B. Foot dermatitis from the shoes. *Int J Dermatol* 2004; 43(8):565–567.
208. Kockentiet B, Adams BB. Contact dermatitis in athletes. *J Am Acad Dermatol* 2007; 56(6):1048–1055.
209. Carlsen KH, Kowalski ML. Asthma, allergy, the athlete and the olympics. *Allergy* 2008; 63(4):383–386. doi: 10.1111/j.1398-9995.2008.01630.x.
210. MacKnight JM, Mistry DJ. Allergic disorders in the athlete. *Clin Sports Med* 2005;24(3): 507–523, vii–viii.
211. Noakes TD. Running shoe anaphylaxis–a case report. *Br J Sports Med* 1983;17(3):213.
212. Fisher AA. Sports-related allergic dermatitis. *Cutis* 1992;50(2):95–97.
213. Foussereau J, Tomb R, Cavelier C. Allergic contact dermatitis from safety clothes and individual protective devices. *Dermatol Clin* 1990;8(1):127–132.
214. Heukelbach J, Feldmeier H. Epidemiological and clinical characteristics of hookworm-related cutaneous larva migrans. *Lancet Infect Dis* 2008;8(5):302–309.
215. Roberts JL, Hanifin JM. Athletic shoe dermatitis. contact allergy to ethyl butyl thiourea. *JAMA* 1979;241(3):275–276.
216. Jung JH, McLaughlin JL, Stannard J, et al. Isolation, via activity-directed fractionation, of mercaptobenzothiazole and dibenzothiazyl disulfide as 2 allergens responsible for tennis shoe dermatitis. *Contact Dermatitis* 1988;19(4):254–259.
217. Fisher AA. Sports-related cutaneous reactions: Part II. allergic contact dermatitis to sports equipment. *Cutis* 1999;63(4):202–204.
218. Ventura MT, Dagnello M, Matino MG, et al. Contact dermatitis in students practicing sports: Incidence of rubber sensitisation. *Br J Sports Med* 2001;35(2):100–102.
219. de Leeuw J, den Hollander P. A patient with a contact allergy to jogging cream. *Contact Dermatitis* 1987;17(4):260–261.
220. Kalavala M, Hughes TM, Goodwin RG, et al. Allergic contact dermatitis to peppermint foot spray. *Contact Dermatitis* 2007;57(1):57–58.
221. Romaguera C, Grimalt F, Vilaplana J. Shoe contact dermatitis. *Contact Dermatitis* 1988; 18(3):178.
222. Mandell JA, Tlougan BE, Cohen DE. Bunga pad-induced ankle dermatitis in a figure skater. *Dermatitis* 2011;22(1):58–59.
223. Ghaffari G, Craig T. The perceived obstacles in performing patch test to detect allergic contact dermatitis: A comparison between community allergists and directors of allergy training programs. *Ann Allergy Asthma Immunol* 2008;100(4):323–326.
224. Corazza M, Baldo F, Ricci M, et al. Efficacy of new barrier socks in the treatment of foot allergic contact dermatitis. *Acta Derm Venereol* 2011;91(1):68–69. doi: 10.2340/00015555-0932.
225. Meffert JM. Psoriasis. *emedicinehealth* Available at http://emedicine.medscape.com/article/1943419-overview. Accessed August 15, 2012.
226. Hofer A, Fink-Puches R, Kerl H, et al. Paired comparison of bathwater versus oral delivery of 8-methoxypsoralen in psoralen plus ultraviolet: A therapy for chronic palmoplantar psoriasis. *Photodermatol Photoimmunol Photomed* 2006;22(1):1–5.
227. Mehta BH, Amladi ST. Evaluation of topical 0.1% tazarotene cream in the treatment of palmoplantar psoriasis: An observer-blinded randomized controlled study. *Indian J Dermatol* 2011;56(1):40–43. doi: 10.4103/0019-5154.77550.
228. Lichon V, Khachemoune A. Lichen simplex chronicus. *Dermatol Nurs* 2007;19(3):276.
229. Lotti T, Buggiani G, Prignano F. Prurigo nodularis and lichen simplex chronicus. *Dermatol Ther* 2008;21(1):42–46.
230. Khaitan BK, Sood A, Singh MK. Lichen simplex chronicus with a cutaneous horn. *Acta Derm Venereol* 1999;79(3):243.
231. Gudnadottir G, Hilmarsdottir I, Sigurgeirsson B. Onychomycosis in icelandic swimmers. *Acta Derm Venereol* 1999;79(5):376–377.
232. Szepietowski JC, Reich A, Garlowska E, et al. Onychomycosis Epidemiology Study Group. Factors influencing coexistence of toenail onychomycosis with tinea pedis and other dermatomycoses: A survey of 2761 patients. *Arch Dermatol* 2006;142(10):1279–1284. doi: 10.1001/archderm.142.10.1279.
233. Haugh M, Helou S, Boissel JP, et al. Terbinafine in fungal infections of the nails: A meta-analysis of randomized clinical trials. *Br J Dermatol* 2002;147(1):118–121.
234. Sabadin CS, Benvegnu SA, da Fontoura MM, et al. Onychomycosis and tinea pedis in athletes from the state of rio grande do sul (brazil): A cross-sectional study. *Mycopathologia* 2011;171(3):183–189. doi: 10.1007/s11046-010-9360-z.
235. Kemna ME, Elewski BE. A U.S. epidemiologic survey of superficial fungal diseases. *J Am Acad Dermatol* 1996;35(4):539–542.
236. de Berker D. Clinical practice. fungal nail disease. *N Engl J Med* 2009;360(20):2108–2116. doi: 10.1056/NEJMcp0804878.
237. Blumberg M. http://emedicine.medscape.com/article/1105828-overview. Updated 2007. Accessed August 8, 2012.
238. Elewski BE. The effect of toenail onychomycosis on patient quality of life. *Int J Dermatol* 1997;36(10):754–756.
239. Dupuy A, Benchikhi H, Roujeau JC, et al. Risk factors for erysipelas of the leg (cellulitis): Case-control study. *BMJ* 1999;318(7198):1591–1594.
240. Hinojosa JR, Hitchcock K, Rodriguez JE. Clinical inquiries. which oral antifungal is best for toenail onychomycosis? *J Fam Pract* 2007;56(7):581–582.
241. Pavlovic MD, Bulajic N. Great toenail onychomycosis caused by syncephalastrum racemosum. *Dermatol Online J.* 2006;12(1):7.
242. Shemer A, Davidovici B, Grunwald MH, et al. Comparative study of nail sampling techniques in onychomycosis. *J Dermatol* 2009;36(7):410–414. doi: 10.1111/j.1346-8138.2009.00667.x.
243. Gupta AK, Ryder JE, Johnson AM. Cumulative meta-analysis of systemic antifungal agents for the treatment of onychomycosis. *Br J Dermatol* 2004;150(3):537–544.

244. O'Sullivan DP, Needham CA, Bangs A, et al. Postmarketing surveillance of oral terbinafine in the UK: Report of a large cohort study. *Br J Clin Pharmacol* 1996;42(5):559–565.
245. Chambers WM, Millar A, Jain S, et al. Terbinafine-induced hepatic dysfunction. *Eur J Gastroenterol Hepatol* 2001;13(9):1115–1118.
246. Sigurgeirsson B, Olafsson JH, Steinsson JB, et al. Long-term effectiveness of treatment with terbinafine vs itraconazole in onychomycosis: A 5-year blinded prospective follow-up study. *Arch Dermatol* 2002;138(3):353–357.
247. Piraccini BM, Sisti A, Tosti A. Long-term follow-up of toenail onychomycosis caused by dermatophytes after successful treatment with systemic antifungal agents. *J Am Acad Dermatol* 2010;62(3):411–414. doi: 10.1016/j.jaad.2009.04.062.
248. Mailler EA, Adams BB. The wear and tear of 26.2: Dermatological injuries reported on marathon day. *Br J Sports Med* 2004;38(4):498–501.
249. Scher RK. Occupational nail disorders. *Dermatol Clin* 1988;6(1):27–33.
250. Katchis, Stuart and Elliot Hershman. Broken nails to blistered heels. *Phys Sports Med* 1985; 3:415.
251. Adams BB. Sports dermatology. *Adolesc Med* 2001;12(2):vii, 305–322.
252. Rzonca EC, Lupo PJ. Pedal nail pathology: Biomechanical implications. *Clin Podiatr Med Surg* 1989;6(2):327–337.
253. Freiman A, Barankin B, Elpern DJ. Sports dermatology part 1: Common dermatoses. *CMAJ* 2004;171(8):851–853.
254. Helm TN, Bergfeld WF. Sports dermatology. *Clin Dermatol* 1998;16(1):159–165.
255. Chiarello S. Toe jam. *A.M.A. archives of dermatology* 1985;121:591.
256. Batrick N, Hashemi K, Freij R. Treatment of uncomplicated subungual haematoma. *Emerg Med J* 2003;20(1):65.
257. Gamston J. Subungual haematomas. *Emerg Nurse* 2006;14(7):26–34.
258. Witkowski JA, Parish LC. Athletic dermatology. *Int J Dermatol* 1978;17(9):714.
259. Powell FC. Sports dermatology. *J Eur Acad Dermatol Venereol* 1994;3:1.
260. Basler RS. Sports-related skin injuries. *Adv Dermatol* 1989;4:29–48; discussion 49.
261. Basler RS. Skin lesions related to sports activity. *Prim Care* 1983;10(3):479–494.
262. Mortimer PS, Dawber RP. Trauma to the nail unit including occupational sports injuries. *Dermatol Clin* 1985;3(3):415–420.
263. Tanzi EL, Scher R. Managing common nail disorders in active patients and athletes. *Phys Sports Med* 1999;27:35.
264. Gibbs RC. "Tennis toe". *Arch Dermatol* 1973;107(6):918.
265. Gibbs RC. Letter: Tennis toe. *JAMA* 1974;228(1):24.
266. Adams BB. Jogger's toenail. *J Am Acad Dermatol* 2003;48(5 Suppl):S58–S59.
267. Cohen PR, Schulze KE, Nelson BR. Subungual hematoma. *Dermatol Nurs* 2007;19(1):83–84.
268. Scher RK. Jogger's toe. *Int J Dermatol* 1978;17(9):719–720.
269. Bird N, Andreola V, Galli Lea. Medical care in the new york city marathon. *New York Running News.* 1980.
270. Helms A, Brodell RT. Surgical pearl: Prompt treatment of subungual hematoma by decompression. *J Am Acad Dermatol* 2000;42(3):508–509.
271. Pharis DB, Teller C, Wolf JE Jr., Cutaneous manifestations of sports participation. *J Am Acad Dermatol* 1997;36(3 Pt 1):448–459.
272. Englund SL, Adams BB. Winter sports dermatology: a review. *Cutis.* 2009;83(1):42–48.
273. Kaya TI, Tursen U, Baz K, et al. Extra-fine insulin syringe needle: An excellent instrument for the evacuation of subungual hematoma. *Dermatol Surg* 2003;29(11):1141–1143.
274. Kibler WB, Safran MR. Musculoskeletal injuries in the young tennis player. *Clin Sports Med* 2000;19(4):781–792.
275. Pirzada A, Waseem M. Subungual hematoma. *Pediatr Rev* 2004;25(10):369.
276. Oliver Mayorga BA. Hand, Subungal Hematoma Drainage. http://emedicine.medscape.com/article/82926-overview. Updated Dec. 13,2011. Accessed 2012.
277. Basler RS, Basler DL, Basler GC, et al. Cutaneous injuries in women athletes. *Dermatol Nurs* 1998;10(1):9–18; quiz 19–20.
278. Smith KC, Comite SL, Storwick GS. Ice minimizes discomfort associated with injection of botulinum toxin type A for the treatment of palmar and plantar hyperhidrosis. *Dermatol Surg* 2007;33(1 Spec No.):S88–S91.
279. Smith KC, Comite SL, Balasubramanian S, et al. Vibration anesthesia: A noninvasive method of reducing discomfort prior to dermatologic procedures. *Dermatol Online J* 2004;10(2):1.
280. Meek S, White M. Subungual haematomas: Is simple trephining enough? *J Accid Emerg Med* 1998;15(4):269–271.
281. Griffin LY. Common sports injuries of the foot and ankle seen in children and adolescents. *Orthop Clin North Am* 1994;25(1):83–93.
282. Gordon GM, Cuttic MM. Exercise and the aging foot. *South Med J* 1994;87(5):S36–S41.
283. Howse J. Disorders of the great toe in dancers. *Clin Sports Med* 1983;2(3):499–505.
284. Montgomery RM. Tennis and its skin problems. *Cutis* 1977;19(4):480–482.
285. Park DH, Singh D. The management of ingrowing toenails. *BMJ* 2012;344:e2089. doi: 10.1136/bmj.e2089.
286. Noel B. Anesthesia for ingrowing toenail surgery. *Dermatol Surg* 2010;36(8):1356–1357. doi: 10.1111/j.1524-4725.2010.01640.x.
287. Rounding C, Bloomfield S. Surgical treatments for ingrowing toenails. *Cochrane Database Syst Rev* 2005;(2)(2):CD001541. doi: 10.1002/14651858.CD001541.pub2.
288. Strutton DR, Kowalski JW, Glaser DA, et al. US prevalence of hyperhidrosis and impact on individuals with axillary hyperhidrosis: Results from a national survey. *J Am Acad Dermatol* 2004;51(2):241–248.
289. Eisenach JH, Atkinson JL, Fealey RD. Hyperhidrosis: Evolving therapies for a well-established phenomenon. *Mayo Clin Proc* 2005;80(5):657–666.
290. Vlahovic TC, Dunn SP, Blau JC, et al. Injectable botulinum toxin as a treatment for plantar hyperhidrosis: A case study. *J Am Podiatr Med Assoc* 2008;98(2):156–159.
291. Thomas I, Brown J, Vafaie J, et al. Palmoplantar hyperhidrosis: A therapeutic challenge. *Am Fam Physician* 2004;69(5):1117–1120.
292. Lear W, Kessler E, Solish N, et al. An epidemiological study of hyperhidrosis. *Dermatol Surg* 2007;33(1 Spec No.):S69–S75.
293. Benohanian A. Treatment of recalcitrant plantar hyperhidrosis with type-A botulinum toxin injections and aluminum chloride in salicylic acid gel. *Dermatol Online J* 2008;14(2):5.
294. Walling HW. Primary hyperhidrosis increases the risk of cutaneous infection: A case-control study of 387 patients. *J Am Acad Dermatol* 2009;61(2):242–246. doi: 10.1016/j.jaad.2009.02.038.
295. Stolman LP. Treatment of hyperhidrosis. *J Drugs Dermatol* 2003;2(5):521–527.
296. Doft MA, Hardy KL, Ascherman JA. Treatment of hyperhidrosis with botulinum toxin. *Aesthet Surg J* 2012;32(2):238–244. doi: 10.1177/1090820X11434506.
297. Walling HW, Swick BL. Treatment options for hyperhidrosis. *Am J Clin Dermatol* 2011;12(5): 285–295. doi: 10.2165/11587870-000000000-00000; 10.2165/11587870-000000000-00000.
298. Dolianitis C, Scarff CE, Kelly J, et al. Iontophoresis with glycopyrrolate for the treatment of palmoplantar hyperhidrosis. *Australas J Dermatol* 2004;45(4):208–212.
299. Vadoud-Seyedi J. Treatment of plantar hyperhidrosis with botulinum toxin type A. *Int J Dermatol* 2004;43(12):969–971.
300. Campanati A, Bernardini ML, Gesuita R, et al. Plantar focal idiopathic hyperhidrosis and botulinum toxin: A pilot study. *Eur J Dermatol* 2007;17(1):52–54.
301. Sevim S, Dogu O, Kaleagasi H. Botulinum toxin-A therapy for palmar and plantar hyperhidrosis. *Acta Neurol Belg* 2002;102(4):167–170.
302. Benohanian A. Palmar hyperhidrosis. needle-free anesthesia as an alternative to bier's block and peripheral nerve blockade for botulinum toxin therapy. *Dermatol Online J* 2006;12(6):26.
303. Huntley A, Comite SL, Smith KC. Audiovisual presentations in peer-reviewed medical literature. *Dermatol Online J* 2004;10(2):22.
304. Glaser DA, Hebert AA, Pariser DM, et al. Palmar and plantar hyperhidrosis: Best practice recommendations and special considerations. *Cutis* 2007;79(5 Suppl):18–28.
305. Wollina U, Konrad H. Managing adverse events associated with botulinum toxin type A: A focus on cosmetic procedures. *Am J Clin Dermatol* 2005;6(3):141–150.
306. Gregoriou S, Rigopoulos D, Makris M, et al. Effects of botulinum toxin-a therapy for palmar hyperhidrosis in plantar sweat production. *Dermatol Surg* 2010;36(4):496–498. doi: 10.1111/j.1524-4725.2010.01473.x.
307. Urena A, Ramos R, Masuet C, et al. An assessment of plantar hyperhidrosis after endoscopic thoracic sympathicolysis. *Eur J Cardiothorac Surg* 2009;36(2):360–363. doi: 10.1016/j.ejcts.2009.02.062.
308. Young RJ, 3rd., Wilde JL, Sartori CR, et al. Solitary nodule of the great toe. *Cutis* 2001; 68(1):57–58.
309. Ilyas W, Geskin L, Joseph AK, et al. Subungual exostosis of the third toe. *J Am Acad Dermatol* 2001;45(6 Suppl):S200–S201.
310. Suga H, Mukouda M. Subungual exostosis: A review of 16 cases focusing on postoperative deformity of the nail. *Ann Plast Surg* 2005;55(3):272–275.
311. Sanchez-Castellanos ME, Sandoval-Tress C, Ramirez-Barcena P. Subungual exostosis. *Arch Dermatol* 2007;143(9):1234.
312. Redbord KP, Adams BB. Piezogenic pedal papules in a marathon runner. *Clin J Sport Med* 2006;16(1):81–83.
313. Lin E, Ronen M, Stampler D, et al. Painful piezogenic heel papules. A case report. *J Bone Joint Surg Am* 1985;67(4):640–641.
314. Kahana M, Feinstein A, Tabachnic E, et al. Painful piezogenic pedal papules in patients with ehlers-danlos syndrome. *J Am Acad Dermatol* 1987;17(2 Pt 1):205–209.
315. Woodrow SL, Brereton-Smith G, Handfield-Jones S. Painful piezogenic pedal papules: Response to local electro-acupuncture. *Br J Dermatol* 1997;136(4):628–630.
316. Schlappner OL, Wood MG, Gerstein W, et al. Painful and nonpainful piezogenic pedal papules. *Arch Dermatol* 1972;106(5):729–733.
317. Shelley WB, Rawnsley HM. Painful feet due to herniation of fat. *JAMA* 1968;205(5): 308–309.
318. Boni R, Dummer R. Compression therapy in painful piezogenic pedal papules. *Arch Dermatol* 1996;132(2):127–128.
319. Levine N. Dermatologic aspects of sports medicine. *Dermatol Nurs* 1994;6(3):179–186; quiz 187–188.
320. Lebovits PE, Kouskoukis CE, Weidman AI. Piezogenic pedal papules. *Cutis* 1982;29(3): 276–277, 280.
321. Doukas DJ, Holmes J, Leonard JA. A nonsurgical approach to painful piezogenic pedal papules. *Cutis* 2004;73(5):339–340, 346.

Index

Note: Page numbers followed "f" denote figures; those followed by a "t" denote tables.

R

S